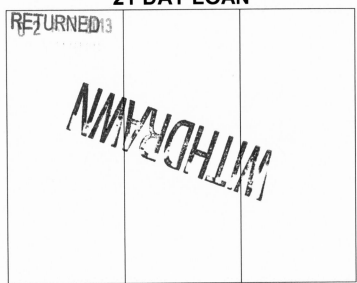

Intestinal Failure

Diagnosis, Management and Transplantation

Intestinal Failure

Diagnosis, Management and Transplantation

EDITED BY

Alan N. Langnas, DO

Chief, Section of Transplant Surgery
University of Nebraska Medical Center
Omaha, Nebraska, USA

Olivier Goulet, MD, PhD

Pediatric Gastroenterology-Hepatology and Nutrition
Reference Center for Rare Digestive Diseases
Integrated Program of Intestinal Failure, Home Parenteral Nutrition
and Intestinal Transplantation
University of Paris-Descartes
Necker Hospital
Paris, France

Eamonn M.M. Quigley, MD, FRCP, FACP, FACG, FRCPI

Alimentary Pharmabiotic Centre
Department of Medicine
National University of Ireland, Cork
Cork, Ireland

Kelly A. Tappenden, PhD, RD

Department of Food Science and Human Nutrition
University of Illinois at Urbana-Champaign
Urbana, Illinois, USA

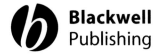

Blackwell
Publishing

© 2008 by Blackwell Publishing

Blackwell Publishing, Inc., 350 Main Street, Malden, Massachusetts 02148-5020, USA
Blackwell Publishing Ltd, 9600 Garsington Road, Oxford OX4 2DQ, UK
Blackwell Publishing Asia Pty Ltd, 550 Swanston Street, Carlton, Victoria 3053, Australia

First published 2008
1   2008

Library of Congress Cataloging-in-Publication Data

Intestinal failure : diagnosis, management and transplantation / edited by Alan
Langnas . . . [et al.].
   p.   ; cm.
   Includes bibliographical references and index.
   ISBN 978-1-4051-4637-1
   1. Intestines–Diseases. I. Langnas, Alan.
   [DNLM: 1. Intestines–physiopathology. 2. Intestinal Diseases–drug therapy.
   3. Intestinal Diseases–surgery. 4. Intestines–transplantation. WI 400 I6022 2008]
   RC860.I59 2006
   616.3′4–dc22
2007015740
ISBN: 978-1-4051-4637-1

A catalogue record for this title is available from the British Library

Set in 8.75/12pt Meridien by Aptara Inc., New Delhi, India
Printed and bound in Singapore by Fabulous Printers Pte Ltd

Commissioning Editor: Alison Brown
Editorial Assistant: Jennifer Seward
Development Editor: Elisabeth Dodds
Production Controller: Debbie Wyer

For further information on Blackwell Publishing, visit our website:
http://www.blackwellpublishing.com

The publisher's policy is to use permanent paper from mills that operate a sustainable forestry
policy, and which has been manufactured from pulp processed using acid-free and elementary
chlorine-free practices. Furthermore, the publisher ensures that the text paper and cover board
used have met acceptable environmental accreditation standards.

Contents

Contents

List of Contributors

Kareem M. Abu-Elmagd, MD, PhD, FACS
Professor of Surgery
Director, Intestinal Rehabilitation and Transplantation Center
University of Pittsburgh Medical Center
Pittsburgh, Pennsylvania, USA

Ahmed Abu-Shanab, MB BCh, MSc
(internal medicine)
Alimentary Pharmabiotic Centre
Department of Medicine
National University of Ireland, Cork
Cork, Ireland

Sue V. Beath, BSc, MRCP, FRCPCH
Consultant Paediatric Hepatologist
Birmingham Children's Hospital
West Midlands, UK

Enrico Benedetti, MD, FACS
Professor and Head, Department of Surgery
University of Illinois at Chicago
Chicago, Illinois, USA

Jean F. Botha, MBBCh, FCS(SA)
Assistant Professor
Department of Surgery
Section of Transplantation
University of Nebraska Medical Center
Omaha, Nebraska, USA

Alan L. Buchman, MD, MSPH
Professor of Medicine and Surgery
Feinberg School of Medicine
Division of Gastroenterology
Northwestern University
Chicago, Illinois, USA

Brenda Bursch, PhD
Professor of Psychiatry and Biobehavioral Sciences, and Pediatrics
David Geffen School of Medicine at UCLA
Los Angeles, California, USA

Virginie Colomb, MD, PhD
Pediatric Gastroenterology-Hepatology and Nutrition
Reference Center for Rare Digestive Diseases
Integrated Program for Intestinal Failure, Home Parenteral Nutrition
and Intestinal Transplantation
University of Paris-Descartes
Necker Hospital
Paris, France

Anthony J. Demetris, MD
Starzl Professor of Transplant Pathology
University of Pittsburgh Medical Center
Pittsburgh, Pennsylvania, USA

John K. DiBaise, MD
Associate Professor of Medicine
Mayo Clinic
Scottsdale, Arizona, USA

Carlo Di Lorenzo, MD
Professor of Clinical Pediatrics
Division of Pediatric Gastroenterology
The Ohio State University and Columbus Children's Hospital
Columbus, Ohio, USA

Christopher Duggan, MD, MPH
Associate Professor of Pediatrics, Harvard Medical School
Medical Director, Short Bowel Syndrome Program
Children's Hospital, Boston
Boston, Massachusetts, USA

Roger W. Evans, PhD
Consultant in Health Care
Rochester, Minnesota, USA

Douglas G. Farmer, MD
Associate Professor of Surgery
Director, Intestinal Transplant Program
Dumont-UCLA Transplant Center
Los Angeles, California, USA

Erin M. Fennelly, RD, CNSD
Georgetown University Transplant Institute
Washington, DC, USA

Yigael Finkel, MD, PhD
Associate Professor of Paediatrics
Department of Woman and Child Health
Karolinska Institutet
Stockholm, Sweden

Thomas Fishbein, MD
Professor of Surgery and Pediatrics
Director, Intestinal and Pediatric Liver Transplantation
Georgetown University Hospital
Washington, DC, USA

Alison Freifeld, MD
Director, Immunocompromised Host Infectious Diseases Program
Associate Professor
Department of Medicine
University of Nebraska Medical Center
Omaha, Nebraska, USA

Jonathan P. Fryer, MD
Associate Professor of Surgery
Director, Intestinal Transplantation
Feinberg School of Medicine
Northwestern University
Chicago, Illinois, USA

Simon M. Gabe, MSc, MD, FRCP
Consultant Gastroenterologist and Honorary Senior Lecturer
Lennard-Jones Intestinal Failure Unit
St Mark's Hospital
Harrow, UK

Raquel Garcia-Roca, MD
Department of Surgery
University of Minnesota
Minneapolis, Minnesota, USA

Jodi Gentleman, LCSW
Medical Social Worker
The Nebraska Medical Center
Omaha, Nebraska, USA

Olivier Goulet, MD, PhD
Pediatric Gastroenterology-Hepatology and Nutrition
Reference Center for Rare Digestive Diseases
Integrated Program for Intestinal Failure, Home Parenteral Nutrition
and Intestinal Transplantation
University of Paris-Descartes
Necker Hospital
Paris, France

David R. Grant, MD, FRCSC
Professor of Surgery
Surgical Director, Multi-Organ Transplantation
University Health Network
University of Toronto
Toronto, Ontario, Canada

Wendy J. Grant, MD
Assistant Professor of Surgery
Organ Transplantation Program
University of Nebraska Medical Center
Omaha, Nebraska, USA

Thomas G. Gross, MD, PhD
Gordon Teter Chair for Pediatric Cancer
Associate Professor, Department of Pediatrics, The Ohio
State University
Chief, Division of Hematology/Oncology/BMT, Columbus
Children's Hospital
Columbus, Ohio, USA

Rainer Gruessner, MD
Professor of Chairman
Department of Surgery
University of Arizona
Tucson, Arizona, USA

Gabriel J. Hauser, MD, MBA
Vice Chairman, Department of Pediatrics
Professor of Pediatrics, Physiology and Biophysics
Medical Director, Pediatric Inpatient Services
Chief, Pediatric Critical Care and Pulmonary Medicine
Georgetown University Children's Medical Center
Washington, DC, USA

Simon P. Horslen, MB ChB, FRCPCH
Professor of Pediatrics, University of Washington
Medical Director, Liver and Intestine Transplantation
Children's Hospital and Regional Medical Center
Seattle, Washington, USA

Paul E. Hyman, MD
Professor of Pediatric Gastroenterology and Behavioral Pediatrics
University of Kansas School of Medicine
Kansas City, Kansas, USA

Dominique M. Jan, MD
Professor of Clinical Surgery
Columbia University
College of Physicians and Surgeons
New York, New York, USA

Khursheed N. Jeejeebhoy, MBBS, PhD, FRCP, FRCPC
Professor Emeritus, Department of Medicine
University of Toronto
Toronto, Ontario, Canada

Francisca Joly, MD
Gastroenterology and Nutrition Support
Reference Centre for Rare Digestive Diseases
Integrated Program for Intestinal Failure, Home Parenteral Nutrition
and Intestinal Transplantation
Hôpital Beaujon
Clichy la Garenne, France

List of Contributors

Andre Kalil, MD
Department of Medicine
University of Nebraska Medical Center
Omaha, Nebraska, USA

Daniel S. Kamin, MD
Division of Gastroenterology and Nutrition
Children's Hospital, Boston
Boston, Massachusetts, USA

Stuart S. Kaufman, MD
Medical Director
Pediatric Liver and Intestinal Transplantation
Georgetown University Transplant Institute and
Children's National Medical Center
Washington, DC, USA

Sanja Kolaček, MD
Professor of Pediatrics
Head, Division of Pediatrics
Chief, Referral Center for Pediatric Gastroenterology and Nutrition
Children's Hospital Zagreb
Zagreb University Medical School
Zagreb, Croatia

Alan N. Langnas, DO
Chief, Section of Transplant Surgery
University of Nebraska Medical Center
Omaha, Nebraska, USA

Henri G. Leuvenink, PhD
Head of Surgical Research Laboratory
University Medical Center Groningen
University of Groningen
Groningen, The Netherlands

Marc S. Levin, MD
Associate Professor of Medicine
Division of Gastroenterology
Washington University School of Medicine; and
Staff Physician
St Louis VA Medical Center
St. Louis, Missouri, USA

Greger Lindberg, MD, PhD
Associate Professor
Department of Medicine
Division of Gastroenterology and Hepatology
Karolinska Institutet
Stockholm, Sweden

David A.J. Lloyd, MA, MRCP
Lennard-Jones Intestinal Failure Unit
St Mark's Hospital
Harrow, UK

Frances R. Malone, RN, ARNP, PhD
Division of Transplant Surgery
Children's Hospital and Regional Medical Center
Seattle, Washington, USA

Bernard Messing, MD, PhD
Gastroenterology and Nutrition Support
Reference Centre for Rare Digestive Diseases
Integrated Program for Intestinal Failure, Home Parenteral Nutrition
and Intestinal Transplantation
Hôpital Beaujon
Clichy la Garenne, France

Julije Meštrović, MD, PhD
Assistant Professor of Pediatrics
Head, Pediatric Intensive Care Unit
Spit University Hospital
Split, Croatia

Hayat Mousa, MD, FAAP
Medical Director, Center for Advanced Research in
Neuromuscular Gastrointestinal Disorders (C.A.R.I.N.G)
Associate Professor in Clinical Pediatrics, Division of
Gastroenterology
The Ohio State University College of Medicine and Public Health
Columbus, Ohio, USA

Kenneth A. Newell, MD, PhD
Professor of Surgery
Department of Surgery and the Emory Transplant Center
Emory University
Atlanta, Georgia, USA

Vincent B. Nieuwenhuijs, MD, PhD
Abdominal and Transplant Surgery
University Medical Center Groningen
Groningen, The Netherlands

Mihai Oltean, MD
Department of Surgery and Transplantation
Sahlgrenska University Hospital
Gothenburg, Sweden

Liam O'Mahony, BSc, PhD
Principal Investigator
Alimentary Pharmabiotic Centre
BioSciences Institute
University College Cork
Cork, Ireland

Fabrizio Panaro, MD
Division of Transplantation
University of Illinois at Chicago
Chicago, Illinois, USA

Leonard W. Penkoski, MSW, CSW
University of Nebraska Medical Center
Omaha, Nebraska, USA

Rutger J. Ploeg, MD, PhD
Professor of Surgery
Abdominal and Transplant Surgery
University Medical Center Groningen
Groningen, The Netherlands

Jeffrey S. Plotkin, MD
Associate Professor of Anesthesia and Surgery
Director, Transplant Anesthesia and Critical Care
Georgetown University Hospital
Washington, DC, USA

Rodrigo Quera, MD
Department of Internal Medicine
Gastroenterology
Hospital Clinico Universidad de Chile
Santiago de Chile, Chile

Eamonn M.M. Quigley, MD, FRCP,
FACP, FACG, FRCPI
Alimentary Pharmabiotic Centre
Department of Medicine
National University of Ireland, Cork
Cork, Ireland

Deborah C. Rubin, MD
Professor of Medicine Molecular Biology
   and Pharmacology
Washington University School of Medicine
St. Louis, Missouri, USA

Harry C. Sax, MD
Professor of Surgery
The Warren Alpert Medical School of
Brown University
Surgeon-in-Chief
The Miriam Hospital
Providence, Rhode Island, USA

Shimul A. Shah, MD
Assistant Professor of Surgery
Division of Organ Transplantation
University of Massachusetts Memorial Medical Center
University of Massachusetts Medical School
Worcester, Massachusetts, USA

James H. Sorrell, MD
Associate Professor
Department of Psychiatry
Nebraska Medical Center
Omaha, Nebraska, USA

Debra Sudan, MD
Professor of Surgery
Director, Intestinal Rehabilitation Program
University of Nebraska
Omaha, Nebraska, USA

Kelly A. Tappenden, PhD, RD
Department of Food Science and Human Nutrition
University of Illinois at Urbana-Champaign
Urbana, Illinois, USA

Giuliano Testa, MD, FACS
Associate Professor of Surgery
Director, Liver Transplantation and Hepatobiliary Surgery
University of Chicago Medical Center
Chicago, Illinois, USA

Jon S. Thompson, MD
Professor of Surgery
University of Nebraska Medical Center
Omaha, Nebraska, USA

Clarivet Torres, MD
Pediatric Gastroenterology – Hepatology
Liver-Intestinal Transplant
Georgetown University Hospital Children
National Medical Center
Medical Director, Intestinal Rehabilitation Program
Washington, DC, USA

Ramsey K. Umar, MD
Fellow, Divisions of Gastroenterology and Hepatology
Feinberg School of Medicine
Northwestern University
Chicago, Illinois, USA

Jon A. Vanderhoof, MD
Consultant, Division of Gastroenterology
Department of Medicine
Children's Hospital, Boston, Massachusetts, USA;
Lecturer of Pediatrics, Harvard Medical School
Boston, Massachusetts, USA; and
Vice-President, Global Medical Affairs
Mead Johnson Nutritionals
Evansville, Indiana, USA

List of Contributors

Jennifer N. Woodard
Division of Nutritional Sciences
University of Illinois at Urbana-Champaign
Urbana, Illinois, USA

Jeremy M. Woodward, MA,
PhD, FRCP
Consultant Gastroenterologist
Addenbrooke's Hospital
Cambridge, UK

Tong Wu, MD, PhD
Associate Professor of Pathology
Department of Pathology
Thomas E. Starzl Transplantation Institute
University of Pittsburgh Medical Center
Pittsburgh, Pennsylvania, USA

Rosemary J. Young, NP-C, MS, BSN
Boys Town National Research Hospital
Boys Town, Nebraska, USA

Foreword

What a privilege it is to have been a part of the greater medical community during the past fifty years; and to have had the opportunity to witness, and to have contributed in a small way to this special period of extraordinary and unprecedented discovery and advancement in virtually every aspect of basic and clinical research; and to experience the joy and satisfaction of the effective practical translation of the new knowledge and technology to the solution or amelioration of difficult and complex patient problems. Although remarkable progress has been made in the acquisition, assessment and useful application of a broad spectrum of medical knowledge, skill, experience, judgment and wisdom throughout the centuries of the past two millennia, advances in basic and clinical science, technology, health care delivery, public health, and preventive medicine during the past century have been especially unparalleled and enormous; and have greatly surpassed the total of all the knowledge in all of the disciplines related to medical and surgical endeavors throughout all previous recorded history. Each era has had its outstanding clinicians and investigators who have exhibited exceptional intellect, curiosity, courage, conscientiousness, competence, character, creativity, and vision in making significant, and often lasting, contributions to the optimal practice of the medicine and surgery of its time; and the twentieth century has produced many more such talented and productive clinically oriented scientists than any other equivalent period.

This unique volume, "Intestinal Failure; Diagnosis, Management and Transplantation," with its four able and distinguished editors who are all leading contributors to this relatively new field; and the impressive group of more than sixty-five internationally recognized additional authors who have joined them from nine countries, overtly manifests the magnitude and usefulness of the data, knowledge, and experience which have been amassed in this critically important area in a rather short time, largely as a result of multidisciplinary collaboration and cooperation. The comprehensive nature of this tome is suggested by its title and evident by its table of contents which logically and rationally groups its forty-two chapters into seven parts, covering virtually the full range of the field of intestinal failure from the relatively straightforward to the complex, and from the subtle to the sublime.

During the latter half of the past century, the basic laboratory development and successful clinical application of total parenteral nutrition has resulted in multiple significant changes in the modern practice of medicine, surgery and pediatrics, and many of their subspecialties. Arguably, none of the benefits of this technique have been more fundamental and lifesaving than the subsequent developments and advances in the understanding, operative procedures, and metabolic and nutritional management and support of patients with short bowel syndrome following massive intestinal resection. Moreover, primarily as a result of the remarkable salvage of most of these patients with this critically severe life-threatening situation, it was eventually recognized that a broader spectrum of disorders of alimentary tract function could be identified besides the "end game" short bowel syndrome; and that patients with these intestinal dysfunctions deserved our collective attention, investigation, and attempts to prevent, ameliorate or cure. Accordingly, the concept of intestinal failure inevitably and justifiably arose, and continues to evolve. Just as the most challenging individual pathophysiological (and frequently lethal) conditions involving the heart, lung, liver, and kidney often result in various degrees and types of failure of these organs and their associated systems, so to, it has become obvious that the relatively more extensive and expansive alimentary tract, together with its important appendages ranging from the salivary glands to the gallbladder, liver, and pancreas, can also exhibit various manifestations of failure. Intestinal failure has had both short and lengthy definitions and will likely undergo additional revisions as knowledge of this deceptively simple yet tremendously complex and adaptable organ system, and the various failures of its multiple components, accumulates from further study. Essentially, intestinal failure is a condition characterized by deficient, inadequate, ineffective, or non-existent performance of the appropriate and expected functions essential for the safe and optimal absorption of the fluids and nutrients required to maintain the normal physiologic activities of the body cell mass.

The current strategies of nutritional and metabolic support of the whole patient and of the primary organ systems, such as the cardiovascular, respiratory, renal, hepatic, intestinal, and central nervous system, must progress and advance to the cellular and subcellular levels if the ultimate goal of providing optimal nutritional, metabolic, immunologic, pharmacologic, and interventional support for all patients under all conditions at all times is to be realized. The intricate relationships among nutrient substrates, cellular biology, immunology, and the human genome are myriad, and their identification, classification, and beneficial application to the management of complex and/or critically ill patients will undoubtedly present new frontiers for basic and clinical investigation throughout the twenty-first century and beyond. This tome explores these promising possibilities and demonstrates clearly that knowledge of, and the judicious practice of, clinical nutrition, metabolism, immunology, cell biology, genetics, and organ transplantation require the most sophisticated integration of clinical skills and acumen with the basic science disciplines of biology, chemistry, physics, genomics, immunology, pharmacology, interventional therapeutics, and hybrids of these fundamental areas.

It has been a source of immense gratification for me to have lived through a most exciting era of basic discovery and efficacious clinical application of countless modalities and technological advances of nutritional and metabolic support to the rational management of a wide variety of nutritionally deficient and/or critically ill patients in virtually all medical and surgical disciplines. Measures for reducing the morbidity and mortality associated with all major pathophysiologic con-

ditions, and their management by improving the nutritional status of patients, have expanded vastly from the simple peripheral intravenous infusion of isotonic carbohydrate and electrolyte solutions to the complex and sophisticated parenteral and enteral provision of most or all of the nutrient requirements in myriad clinical situations during my professional lifetime of more than four decades. Today, clinical nutrition is advancing rapidly toward the provision of optimal nutrient substrates to individual cells or groups of cells, whether normal or compromised, and in reality represents the practice of clinical biochemistry. The continuing identification and classification of genetic control of all metabolic events in human beings is well on its way, and upon its completion, nutritional support will acquire an unprecedented degree of precision; and this molecular biologic revolution will transform the practice of medicine and surgery forever. A more recent genuine and heartfelt gratification for me has been the growth and development of invaluable and productive personal and professional relationships which have been spawned by the cooperation and collaboration among basic and clinical scientists throughout the world. This volume is exemplary evidence of some of the most objective and tangible success of such mutual endeavors and serves as an outstanding model for others.

Total parenteral nutrition, inaugurated successfully as a useful basic clinical nutritional technique more than forty years ago, has been instrumental directly in saving countless lives and has demonstrated emphatically the relevance of adequate nutritional support and nutrition status to achieving optimal clinical outcomes. These results have subsequently led to the monumental increase in the development and application of enteral feedings in patients with functioning gastrointestinal tracts, but whose oral intakes were inadequate to support normal bodily structure and functions. Furthermore, the consequent obvious need for specialized ambulatory and home parenteral and enteral nutritional support has fostered and advanced the unbridled development of home health care and home nutritional support. Initially, the primary goal of total parenteral nutrition was to meet the nutritional needs of malnourished patients who could not eat, would not eat, should not eat, or could not eat enough. Patients with short bowel syndrome, regardless of the etiology, were the prototype beneficiaries of the newly developed alternate feeding technique; and not only could they be fed adequately to survive their catastrophic condition, but they could "buy time" to allow and promote adaptation of the residual bowel to carry out normal or near normal absorptive functions. In patients who could not adapt sufficiently to reestablish adequate intestinal function, nutrient requirements unable to be met entirely by the intestinal tract could be supplemented intravenously as required. Some patients have been supported by parenteral nutrition at home for more than thirty years to date and have adapted quite well to the changes imposed on their lifestyles. On the other hand, some have had physical, psychological, emotional, and other problems including recurring sepsis, liver dysfunction, thrombosis and/or exhausted venous access, which have stimulated attempts either to undertake intensive intestinal rehabilitation measures to increase absorption using special regimens of enterocyte stimulation (growth factors) and enterocyte nutrients (glutamine) to promote optimal adaptation in order to wean patients from parenteral nutrition. Finally, when all reasonable conservative attempts to overcome or compensate for intestinal failure and its complications have proven inadequate, intestinal lengthening procedures and, ultimately, intestinal transplantation become the only viable therapeutic options at the present time. However, future innovative techniques, together with the natural maturation and modifications of medical technology and practices that are now occurring, and will continue to occur, are most exciting, promising, almost incomprehensible, and seemingly unlimited in dealing with this most challenging intestinal dilemma.

For the opportunity to contribute my thoughts through this foreword, I am grateful to the editors, who have already earned professional distinction as gifted, energetic and innovative investigators, teachers, practitioners, writers, advocates and leaders in all aspects of the vital field of nutritional support and management of intestinal failure. They have diligently and capably applied their innate and acquired qualities and talents throughout this comprehensive work product, together with their outstanding group of authors and co-authors, to provide a landmark reference book and practical manual, which will undoubtedly serve the needs of the entire range of individuals interested in providing safe, competent, integrated, and comprehensive management and support of patients with intestinal failure, from the novice students to the most experienced investigators and clinical practitioners. A unique aspect of this volume is that it concisely, and virtually completely, presents the up-to-date key information required for a thorough understanding of the full spectrum of intestinal failure from the basic fundamentals of nutritional biochemistry to the practical essentials in the successful management of the most critically ill and malnourished patients in a wide variety of conditions and situations. Thus, it can serve aptly and concurrently as a basic reference tome, as a convenient and practical handbook, and as a stimulus for anticipated innovative and ingenious future investigational endeavors.

Stanley J. Dudrick, MD, FACS
Chairman, Department of Surgery
Director, Program in Surgery
Saint Mary's Hospital/Yale University
School of Medicine
Professor of Surgery
Yale University School of Medicine

Preface

Intestinal failure is a rare, though devastating, condition that may threaten life, or seriously impair its quality, for those afflicted. These latter factors, together with the wide range of medical and surgical specialties that may become embroiled in the care of the intestinal failure patient, have led this topic to assume an importance in modern medicine that greatly exceeds that which its prevalence alone would demand. This has also been an area of tremendous clinical and research activity and much progress. Refinements in parenteral nutrition now permit long-term survival for many intestinal failure patients, while the advent of intestinal transplantation as a valid clinical option provides the hope of even greater independence. On embarking on the project we recognised a need to provide, in a single volume, an inclusive survey of the filed which encompassed advances in both basic science and clinical practice.

The goal of this volume, therefore, is to bring these developments together and in so doing to update the clinician, scientist and clinical investigator, alike, on the very latest information on the science and practice of intestinal failure and to present this in a manner that is accessible to all. We have endeavoured to provide the reader with a comprehensive survey of the pathogenesis, assessment and management of intestinal failure, in each instance providing the scientific background that underpins progress in each of these areas. Dilemmas in this area transcend science and medical practice and involve significant ethical, socio-economic and psychological issues; each is addressed to ensure a holistic approach to the topic.

We hope that this book will be your "go to" source on this topic and that it will also serve to advance understanding of the field, promote optimal patient care and stimulate further research.

Alan N. Langnas, DO
Olivier Goulet, MD, PhD
Eamonn M.M. Quigley, MD, FRCP, FACP,
FACG, FRCPI
Kelly A. Tappenden, PhD, RD

Abbreviations

2-MG	2-monoacylglycerol		**CSA**	cyclosporine
6-TG	6-thioguanine compounds		**CMV**	cytomegalovirus
ACR	acute cellular rejection		**CTL**	cytotoxic T lymphocytes
ACAT	acylcoenzyme A:cholesterol acyltransferase		**DD**	deceased donor
A.S.P.E.N.	American Society for Parenteral and Enteral Nutrition		**DC-SIGN**	Dendritic Cell Specific ICAM-3-Grabbing Non-integrin
ADCC	antibody-dependent cellular cytotoxicity		**DC**	dendritic cells
APC	antigen presenting cells		**DNA**	deoxyribonucleic acid
AIE	autoimmune enteropathy		**DG**	diacylglycerol
BPD	biliopancreatic diversion		**DRG**	diagnosis-related group
BINOCAR	British Isles Network of Congenital Anomaly Registers		**DPP IV**	dipeptidyl peptidase IV
			DGBP	distal gastric bypass
BAL	broncho-alveolar lavage		**DXA**	dual-energy X-ray absorptiometry
BB	brush border		**EBER**	EBV encoded RNA
CCR9	cadherin, chemokine receptor 9		**EBV-CTLs**	EBV-specific cytotoxic T-cells
CRDs	carbohydrate recognition domains		**EM**	electron microscopic
CARD	Caspase Activation and Recruit Domain		**ESLD**	end-stage liver disease
CMS	Center for Medicare and Medicaid Services		**ENS**	enteric nervous system
			EGF	epidermal growth factor
CMS	Centers for Medicare and Medicaid Services		**EBV**	Epstein-Barr Virus
			EGD	esophagogastroduodenoscopy
CVC	central venous catheter		**EVA**	ethyl vinyl acetate plastic
CVT	central venous thrombosis		**ESBLs**	extended-spectrum beta-lactamases
CCRs	chemokine receptors		**EJV**	external jugular vein
CHB	Children's Hospital Boston		**ECM**	extracellular matrix
COG	Children's Oncology Group		**FAE**	follicle associated epithelium
CIF	chronic intestinal failure		**FFA**	free fatty acids
CIP	chronic intestinal pseudo-obstruction		**FGID**	functional gastrointestinal disorders
CART	cocaine and amphetamine regulated transcript		**GBP**	gastric bypass
			GIST	gastrointestinal stromal tumors
CFUs	colony forming units		**GJ**	gastro-jejunal
CBC	complete blood counts		**GF**	germ-free
CEF	continuous enteral feeding		**GLP2**	glucagon-like peptide-2
CDAI	Crohn's Disease Activity Index		**Gln**	glutamine
cpm	cycles per minute		**GVHD**	graft-vs-host-disease
			GH	growth hormone
cAMP	cyclic adenosine monophosphate		**GALT**	gut-associated lymphoid tissue

HCRIS	Healthcare Cost Reporting Information System		**MMIHS**	megacystis microcolon intestinal hypoperistalsis syndrome
HO-1	hemoxygenase-1		**MLNs**	mesenteric lymph nodes
HSPG	heparan sulfate proteoglycan		**MVT**	mesenteric venous thrombosis
HTK	Histidine-Triptophane-Ketoglutarate		**MSSA**	methicillin-susceptible organisms
HD	Hodgkin's disease		**MTP**	microsomal triglyceride transfer protein
HPN	home parenteral nutrition		**MVA**	microvillous atrophy
hRFC	human reduced folate carrier		**MMC**	migrating motor complex
hTHTR-1	human thiamine transporter-1		**MNGIE**	mitochondrial neurogastrointestinal encephalomyopathy
HES	hydroxy-ethyl starch		**MAP**	mitogen activated protein
IC-DMP	ICCs of the deep muscular plexus		**mMVTx**	modified multivisceral transplantation
IRAKs	IL-1R associated kinases		**MALT**	mucosa-associated lymphoid tissue
IRAK-M	IL-1R-associated kinase M		**MAdCAM-1**	mucosal addressin cell adhesion molecule-1
IBAT	ileal bile acid transporter		**MODS**	multi-organ dysfunction syndrome
ICV	ileocecal valve		**MVT**	multivisceral transplant
IPEX	immune dysregulation, polyendocrino-pathy autoimmune enteropathy X-linked		**MVTx**	multivisceral transplantation
			MMF	mycophenolate mofetil
IgA	immunoglobulin A		**MyD88s**	MyD88 short
IMA	inferior mesenteric artery		**NHEs**	Na/Hexchangers
IVC	inferior vena cava		**NBS**	Narcotic Bowel Syndrome
IBD	inflammatory bowel disease		**NK**	natural killer
IGF-1	insulin-like growth factor 1		**NEC**	necrotizing enterocolitis
IGF-2	insulin-like growth factor 2		**NPC1L1**	Niemann-Pick C1-like 1 protein
IL-2	interleukin-2		**NPO**	nil per os
IJV	internal jugular vein		**NO**	nitric oxide
ICC	interstitial cells of Cajal		**NAFLD**	non-alcoholic fatty liver disease
IFALD	intestinal failure associated liver disease		**NHL**	non-Hodgkin lymphoma
IF	intestinal failure		**Nod**	nucleotide-binding oligomerization domain
ITR	Intestinal Transplant Registry		**NST**	nutrition support team
ITx	intestinal transplantation		**OASIS**	Oley A.S.P.E.N. Information System
IDI	intractable diarrhea of infancy		**PTH**	parathyroid hormone
IELs	intra-epithelial lymphocytes		**PN**	parenteral nutrition
IR	ischemia- and reperfusion		**PNAC**	parenteral nutrition associated cholestasis
I-ITx	isolated intestinal transplantation		**ppm**	parts per million
iLTx	isolated liver transplant		**PAMPs**	pathogen associated molecular patterns
JIB	jejunoileal bypass		**PRRs**	pattern recognition receptors
KGF	keratinocyte growth factor		**PELD**	pediatric end-stage liver disease
LMP	latent membrane protein		**PYY**	peptide YY
LPS	lipolysaccharidases		**PEG**	percutaneous endoscopic gastrostomy
L-ITx	liver intestinal transplantation		**PAS**	periodic acid Schiff
LD	living donor		**PIF**	permanent intestinal failure
LDITx	living donor segmental intestinal transplants		**PE**	physical exam
			PAF	platelet activating factor
LCTs	long chain triglycerides		**PEG**	polyethylene glycol
MEDPAR	Medicare Provider Review and Analysis			
MCTs	medium chain triglycerides			

PCR	polymerase chain reaction	**SMV**	superior mesenteric vein
PMNs	polymorphonuclear leukocytes	**SVC**	superior vena cava
PV	portal vein	**SOCS1**	suppressor of cytokine signaling 1
PTLD	post-transplant lymphoproliferative disease	**TCR**	T cell receptor
		TPMT	thiopurine methyltransferase
PDI	protracted diarrhea of infancy	**TRIF**	TIR-domain-containing adaptor protein inducing interferon
PE	pulmonary embolism		
QoL	quality of life	**TIRAP**	TIR-domain-containing adaptor protein
QALY	quality-adjusted life year	**TIR**	toll/interleukin-1 receptor
SSRIs	selective reuptake inhibitors	**TLRs**	toll-like receptors
STEP	serial transverse enteroplasty	**TPN**	total parenteral nutrition
SCID	severe combined immune deficiency	**TGF-α**	Transforming growth factor-α
SBS	short bowel syndrome	**TA**	transit-amplifying
SCFAs	short-chain fatty acids	**ITx**	transplantation of any intestine inclusive graft
SILT	simultaneous intestinal and liver transplant		
		TG	triacylglycerols
SIGIRR	single immunoglobulin IL-1R-related molecule	**TRAM**	TRIF-related adaptor molecule
		TRAIL	tumor necrosis factor related apoptosis inducing ligand
SIBO	small intestinal bacterial overgrowth		
SMVT	sodium-dependent multivitamin transporter	**TNF-α**	tumor necrosis-factor alpha
		UNOS	United Network for Organ Sharing
SVCT-1	sodium-dependent vitamin C transporter 1	**UW**	University of Wisconsin solution
		VRE	vancomycin-resistant enterococcus
subCVs	subclavian vein	**VIP**	vasoactive intestinal peptide
SMA	superior mesenteric artery	**VLDL**	very low density lipoproteins

1 Introduction

1 The History of Intestinal Failure and Transplantation

Alan N. Langnas

Major advances in modern medicine often have occurred in giant leaps rather than incrementally; progress in the management of intestinal failure has been no different. The ancient Greeks were the first to propose physiology to explain the workings of the human body. In the traditional Hellenic view, there were three dominant centers of the body: the liver, the heart, and the brain. The liver was thought to be the source of nourishment and growth [1]. This view went virtually unchallenged for 13 centuries. The demonstration of the circulation of blood by William Harvey brought an end to Galenic physiology and the beginnings of our ability to conceptualize a role for intravenous therapies. It was nearly 300 years later that the foundations for organ transplantation were laid down by a French surgeon working in the United States, Alexis Carrel. Dr Carrel effectively demonstrated the ability to anastamose blood vessels and attempt organ transplantation. These exciting discoveries of Sir William Harvey and Nobel Laureate Alexis Carrell provided the inspiration for numerous others and helped usher in the modern era of treatment for intestinal failure.

Early approaches to intestinal failure

Enteral nutritional support

Eating and the digestive process have intrigued mankind for thousands of years. In Hellenic times the

Intestinal Failure: Diagnosis, Management and Transplantation.
Edited by Alan N. Langnas, Olivier Goulet, Eamonn M.M. Quigley and Kelly A. Tappenden. © 2008 Blackwell Publishing. ISBN 978-1-4051-4637-1.

only enteral therapies available were alterations in diet or the use of enemas. Interestingly, and not dissimilarly to today, these ancient physicians used enemas in an attempt to improve overall health and treat a variety of other ailments [2,3]. The contents of these rectal infusions included eggs, brandy, wine, milk, and whey and wheat broths [3,4].

Enemas were the only practical method of infusion of nutrition until suitable tools to access the esophagus and stomach were devised. It was not until 1598 that the first description of a hollow tube attached to a bladder filled with food was used to feed directly into the esophagus [3,5]. Improvements on this included the development of a soft, flexible leather tube to provide access to the esophagus and stomach. This was the first time that the idea of an orogastric tube was proposed [3]. John Hunter was an early proponent of enteral feeding and suggested the use of a liquid composed of jellies, milk, water, wine, and eggs [3,6].

The development of parenteral support

The first giant step forward in the evolution of parenteral treatments for intestinal failure was the description of circulation by William (Figure 1.1). Harvey was born in England and studied at Cambridge. In 1600, he traveled to Padua to study anatomy and embryology under Fabricius. On returning to England, he swiftly established his reputation and by 1618 he was selected to be one of the royal physicians [1].

Harvey's challenge was to reconcile his observations from the numerous dissections he carried out with the Galenian description of circulation. Before Harvey's definitive work, the Greek explanation for blood flow stated that blood was created by the liver from chyle and was then drawn into the body by the heart

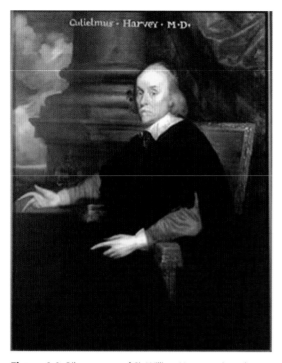

Figure 1.1 Oil on canvas of Sir William Harvey, artist unknown (1578 to 1657). (Source: http://www.rcplondon.ac.uk.)

forced from the heart in systole and that the amount of blood expelled in an hour by the heart far exceeded the blood volume of the animal. Harvey therefore proposed that the blood must flow in a circuit. His seminal experiment made use of a man's forearm and a tourniquet (Figure 1.2). A ligature was placed around the forearm and tightened to prevent any blood flow to the hand. The ligature was loosened slightly to allow for blood to flow into the hand but tight enough to prevent venous drainage. The hand became swollen and veins engorged. Although capillaries were yet to be discovered, Harvey suggested that a conduit must exist to get blood from the arteries to the veins and, thereby, complete the circuit [1,7].

Following the description of circulation the idea of intravenous infusions was not long in coming. The first reports of this included the intravenous injection of wine and ale in dogs which revealed effects similar to that seen with oral ingestion; later others successfully treated cholera patients with an intravenous infusion of an electrolyte solutions and milk [8,9,13]. The first attempts with fat infusions involved intravenous injections of olive oil in dogs. The dogs died rapidly [10]. By the 1800's physicians began administering fats subcutaneously. There were numerous reports by the end of the 19th century of subcutaneous injections of milk with egg yolk or cod liver oil [10]. Although this represented the first attempts at total parenteral nutrition, the injections were too painful to be practical [11]. It

in diastole. The new blood was then completely absorbed by the body. The cycle was then repeated with the liver creating new blood [1]. As described by Porter, Harvey's fundamental observation was that blood was

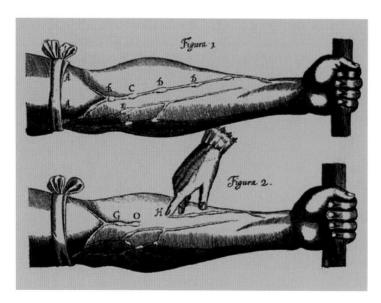

Figure 1.2 Illustration depicting one of Harvey's seminal experiments, which demonstrated that venous blood only travels toward the heart, from *Exercitatio Anatomica de Motu Cordus et Sanguinis in Animalibus*, 1628. (Source: http://www.life.uiuc.edu/ib/494/harvey.html.)

would be another 50 years before a commercial intravenous fat emulsion would be available in the United States.

By the late 1800s the first infusions of glucose and amino acid solutions in man were being reported [10,12,13]. While somewhat successful, the glucose infusions were associated with fever and chills. It was not known that the fevers were due to pyrogens or endotoxin in the solutions. By 1915 a dose response curve for the infusion of glucose was reported and in 1924 the use of continuous glucose infusions were being described [13,14]. The concept that proteins were broken down into amino acids was first described in the late 19th century and subsequently it was determined that polypeptides could be created from amino acids [15]. The first attempts at nonoral protein treatments included proctocylsis enemas and later two Danish scientists reported using intravenous protein infusions, comprised of hydrolyzed beef protein, into goats, and achieved a positive nitrogen balance [10,13,16]. The stage had now been set to usher in the modern era of the treatment of intestinal failure.

The development of modern parenteral nutrition

The development of any new field of study often requires the recognition of a specific medical problem, as well as cause-and-effect relationships. By the early 20th century improvements in anesthesia allowed surgeons to tackle more complex operations. As noted by Arvid Wretlind in a comprehensive review of this topic, postoperative complications compelled surgeons to examine a variety of factors including comorbidities such as the nutritional status of the patient. One of the first reports of a potential link between nutritional status and surgical outcomes was published in 1936 by Studley. He observed that patients with chronic peptic ulcer disease who had lost more than 20% of their weight before surgery died at a much greater rate when compared to patients who had lost less than 20% of their weight [17]. The origins of surgical nutrition became a strong impetus to take this bedside problem to the laboratory.

Another big step forward in the development of modern intravenous nutrition was made by Dr Robert Elman. Dr Elman was a surgeon practicing in St Louis whose specialty was the open treatment of burns.

Although before Dr Elman there had been reports of successful intravenous infusions of amino acids in goats, his seminal contribution was the demonstration that amino acids could be effectively and safely administered intravenously to humans [13,16,18]. The amino acid solutions were prepared as an enzymatic hydrolysate of casein and pancreas. This product was soon known as Amigen. As noted by Wretland, there were still concerns that intravenous amino acids would not be metabolized by the liver and could result in end-organ injuries, particularly to the brain [10]. Further experiments eventually demonstrated that the utilization of intravenous enzymatic casein hydrolysate was the same regardless of route of administration, whether intravenous or intraportal [19].

With the recognition that amino acid infusions were both relatively safe and effective, limits to its use were being noted. It was noted that the protein hydrolysates contained only 50% free amino acids, resulting in the delivery of only about 2 kcal/gram. This eventually led to the development of crystalline amino acids. Bansi was the first to introduce a crystalline L-amino acid solution in 1964 [20]. Numerous improvements took place, including the ability to manipulate the amino acid patterns in various products. Soon, limits to the effectiveness of parenteral nutrition were observed, including the development of essential fatty acid deficiencies. First, in order to provide adequate calories, the volume of administered fluids often exceeded 3 liters per day. This large amount of fluid was difficult for many patients to manage and diuretics were typically required. Second, attempts at administering high glucose concentration infusions (>10%) via peripheral veins resulted in thrombophlebitis. Central venous access was not yet routinely performed, and clinicians looked for other sources of parenteral calories. Intravenous alcohol was tried because of the relatively high caloric density (7 kcal/gm). While alcohol was a good source of energy, the side effects of the infusion prevented it from practical consideration. The next best candidate for increasing calories was the administration of fats. The infusion of fats also would prevent the development of fatty acid deficiencies and its clinical manifestations such as a skin rash.

Interest in developing a form of fat for intravenous infusion had been going on since the early 20th century. The first attempts at fat infusions in children occurred in the 1920s. The major limit to supplying this high caloric source was the need for an emulsifying agent. Cotton seed products became available in the 1950s, but side effects, including nausea, vomiting, fevers, rash, and liver dysfunction, limited its application [10]. The Food and Drug Administration (FDA) eventually stopped its use in 1964. In 1961, a Swedish scientist, Arvid Wretlind, found a relatively nontoxic formulation, soon to be known as Intralipid. The key to his success was combination of soy bean oil emulsified by egg yolk phospholipids in glycerol [10].

By 1968, all of the pieces were in place for Dr. Dudrick and coworkers at the University of Pennsylvania to demonstrate growth and development in beagle puppies with intravenous nutrition [21]. The beagle puppies were fed through an intravenous catheter placed in to the superior vena cava via the external jugular vein. Isocaloric oral calories were given to the littermate controls. The beagles that were fed entirely intravenously actually surpassed the controls in terms of weight gain and were equal in skeletal growth and activity level. This experimental work was the culmination of many years of clinical activity and leadership by Jonathan Rhoads in the Department of Surgery.

One major hurdle still persisted: safe access to the central venous circulation. Rhoads and colleagues at the University of Pennsylvania were using the "5 liter program" to provide adequate calories through a peripheral vein [22]. This approach required close monitoring of the patient and frequent use of diuretics. If patients could receive higher concentrations of glucose via a central vein, then these large volumes of fluid could be avoided. This group had begun placing catheters in the central venous system via the antecubital route in terminally ill cancer patients. At autopsy, numerous clots were noted along the catheter and a fear of pulmonary emboli limited its use [22]. In a first person account of these events Dudrick notes that a 1967 report of percutaneous infraclavicular venepuncture of the subclavian vein for the purpose of central venous pressure monitoring encouraged surgeons at the University of Pennsylvania to use this approach for the placement of a central venous catheter to administer parenteral nutrition [22,23]. It would now be possible and practical to provide long-term parenteral nutrition. Dudrick writes that in 1967, he was asked to consult on an unfortunate little girl born with intestinal atresia [22]. The child was destined to die by starvation. She weighed about 2 kg at the initiation of total parenteral nutrition. Over the ensuing 22 months of her life, she was able achieve growth, development, and a maximum weight of 8.3 kg [24]. The modern era of parenteral nutrition had begun.

The development of modern enteral nutrition

In parallel with the above described progress in parenteral nutrition came developments in enteral nutrition. As described in the comprehensive review by Chernoff, early attempts involved the placement of a weighted nasal-jejunal tube, but many physicians were not convinced that predigested protein hydroysates could be administered safely to humans. By the 1930s, it was accepted that these protein solutions could be fed to surgical patients [25]. Skim milk treated with acid, pepsin, and some vitamins was a common recipe [5]. Further advances led to the development of an infant formula that could be used for babies with allergies and other nonspecific gastrointestinal ailments. In 1943, Mulholland and coworkers demonstrated the benefits of enteral versus parenteral nutrition in the convalescing postoperative patient [3,26]. Soon thereafter, jejeunostomy feeding tubes were being placed at the time of surgery and the first enteral feeding pumps were in use.

Various enteral recipes were developed to create food that was well tolerated and provided the requisite balance of calories, nutrients, and vitamins. Many of these blenderized formulas were made in hospital kitchens [3]. One major advance came directly from the emerging programs at the National Aeronautics and Space Administration (NASA). Nutritionists were asked to develop a diet for astronauts with the central prerequisite being the production of a low fecal output. Elemental diets were a direct consequence of these efforts, although the astronauts were very critical regarding their taste [5,27]. Continued developments in enteral formulas over the past 20 years have resulted in the evolution of feeds for very specific clinical conditions, including renal, live, and pulmonary failure. Advances in enteral nutrition have been less dramatic than those seen with parenteral nutrition,

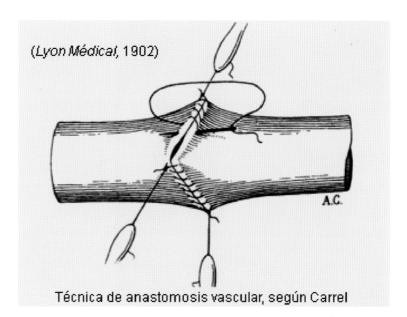

Figure 1.3 A drawing by Carrel, demonstrating a new technique for anastamosis blood vessel together.

but enteral nutrition remains cheaper, safer, and often more effective.

History of intestinal transplantation

The ancient beginnings of transplantation are represented in Greek mythology by the Chimera. Homer first describes the Chimera in the *Iliad* as a "thing of immortal make, not human, lion fronted and snake behind, goat in the middle" [28]. Today, the Chimera is used to describe objects that have the attributes of more than one source, often in the context of organ transplantation. The development of intestinal transplantation paralleled the development of other types of organ transplantation. The seemingly hopeless outcome of early attempts at intestinal transplantation needs to be seen in the context of an era where total parenteral nutrition had yet to be developed and all of these unfortunate patients were going to starve to death. The success that we see with intestinal transplantation today is based on progress in two interrelated areas, surgery and immunology.

The key to the development of solid organ transplantation was the ability to successfully and reliably restore blood flow to the transplanted organ by suturing donor and recipient blood vessels together. As noted by Sade in a paper describing Alexis Carrel, conventional surgical thinking in the late 1800's was that blood vessels could only be ligated not repaired [29]. A medical student at the University of Lyon, Alexis Carrel, challenged that surgical dogma; if other human tissue could be sewn back together why not blood vessels [29]? Carrel published his first articles on vacular anastamosis at that time [30,31] Figure 1.3. Disillusioned with his prospects in France, Carrel left Lyon in 1904 for the University of Chicago and, eventually, the Rockefeller Institute in New York where he continued his research. In the United States, he perfected the surgical technique by using finer sutures and developed the triangulation technique for anatamosing small blood vessels. His ability to anastamose blood vessels led him to attempt a variety of organ transplants in dogs, including that of the intestine [32]. By 1930 Carrel was developing a machine to preserve organs for transplantation and collaborated with the famous aviator Charles Lindberg. Working together for over 5 years they attempted to construct a device to perfuse and oxygenate organs [29,33]. Carrel was known as an innovative surgeon that placed a great deal of emphasis on intuition including the quote, "All great men are gifted with intuition. They know without reasoning of analysis what they need to know." Later in life he accepted a more controversial role in the French

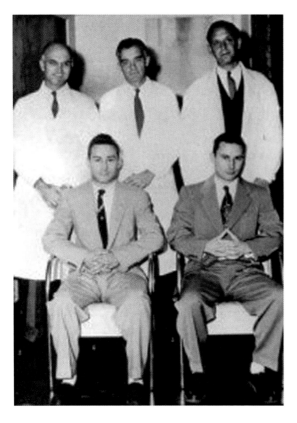

Figure 1.4 Photograph of the first successful kidney transplant team. Front row (left to right): Richard Herrick, kidney transplant recipient; Ronald Herrick, kidney donor. Back row (left to right): The Brigham transplant team: Dr Joseph E. Murray, surgeon for the recipient; Dr John P. Merrill, nephrologist and coleader of the team; and Dr J. Hartwell Harrison, urological surgeon for the donor. (Source: http://www.donatelife.org/transplant/murray.html.)

Vichy government after the Genman invasion of World War II. Carrel received the Nobel Prize for Physiology and Medicine in 1912 for his work in both vascular anastamosis and organ transplantation.

While Carrel seemingly overcame the technical limits of organ transplantation, the biology of organ transplantation was not known. At the beginning of World War II, many British pilots were being severely burned. The Brazilian-born British zoologist Peter Medawar was asked by the British government to determine why skin grafts taken from one individual would not graft permanently graft to another. Working with the plastic surgeon Thomas Gibson, they developed and studied a rabbit model of skin grafting. Their findings were the first to suggest that it was the immune system that was responsible for the destruction of the skin allograft [34]. Medawar received the Nobel Prize for Physiology and Medicine, in 1960, for this work. Finally, in 1954, Murray and coworkers, understanding the surgical and biologic basis of transplantation, became the

first to perform a successful kidney transplant between identical twins [35].

The technical foundations to intestinal transplantation can be linked to professors Lillehi and Starzl. At the University of Minnesota, Lillehei performed autotransplants and homotransplants of the intestine in dogs. These operations demonstrated many things including that the intestine could tolerate preservation outside the dog's body and would then function adequately following re-implantation [36,37]. Starzl later, reported the startling technical feat of transplanting what would be referred to today as a multivisceral transplant in dogs [36,38]. The early successes with kidney, liver, and heart transplants, combined with the fact that long-term parenteral nutrition would not be available until the mid-1970s, provided the impetus to surgeons to attempt the first human intestinal transplants. Over the next 25 years, numerous intestinal transplants were performed, but there were no survivors [36]. In 1987, using cyclosporine-based immunsesuppresssion, the Pittsburgh group transplanted a multivisceral graft consisting of a stomach, duodenum, pancreas, small bowel, colon, and liver into a 3-year-old girl [39]. The multivisceral allograft functioned for 6 months before the child died of lymphoma. The first long-term survivor of a small bowel transplant with enteral autonomy was reported in 1990 by Grant [40]. Finally, the introduction of the new antirejection agent tacrolimus in 1989 changed the transplant landscape, allowing for intestinal transplantation to evolve into a widely performed and successful transplant procedure.

References

1 Porter R. (1997) The greatest benefit to mankind: a medical history of humanity. About William Harvey. Available at: http://www.williamharvey.org/wm harvey.htm. [Accessed 15 May 2007]

2 McCamish MA, Bounous G, Geraghty ME. History of enteral feeding: past and present perspectives. In: Rombeau JL, Rolandelli RH, eds. Clinical Nutrition: Enteral and Tube Feeding. 3rd ed. Philadelphia: WB Saunders Co, 1997.

3 Harkness L. The history of enteral nutrition therapy: from raw eggs and nasal tubes to purified amino acids and early postoperative jejunal delivery. J Am Diet Assoc 2002;102:399–404.

4 Randall HT. The history of enteral nutrition. In: Rombeau JL, Caldwell M, eds. Clinical Nutrition, Vol. 1: Enteral Nutrition and Tube Feeding. Philadelphia: WB Saunders Co, 1983.

5 Chernoff R. History of tube feeding: an overview of tube feeding: from ancient times to the future. Nut Clin Pract 2006;21:408–410.

6 Keoshian LA, Nelsen TS. A new design for a feeding tube. Plast Reconstr Surg 1969;44:508–509.

7 Harvey W. Exercitatio Anatomica de Motu Cordis et Sanguinus in Animalbus. Francofurti: Guilielmi Fitzeri, 1628.

8 Latta T. Relative to the treatment of cholera by the copious injection of aqueous and saline fluids into the veins. Lancet 1831–1832;2:274–277.

9 Hodder EM. Transfusion of milk in cholera. Practitioner 1873;10:14–16.

10 Wretlind A. Recollections of pioneers in nutrition: landmarks in the development of parenteral nutrition. J Am Coll Nutr 1972;11:366–373.

11 Friedrich PL. Die künstliche subkutane Ernährung in der praktihschen Chirurgie. Arch Klin Chirurgie 1904-1912;73:507–516.

12 Biedl A, Kraus R. Ueber intravenöse traubenzucherinfusionen an menschen. Wien Klin Wochenschr 1896;9:55–58.

13 Woodyatt PD, Sansum WD, Wilder RM. Prolonged and accurately timed i.v. injections of sugar: a preliminary report. JAMA 1915;65:2067–2070.

14 Zimmerman B. Intravenous tubing for parenteral therapy. Science 1945;101:567–568.

15 Macht S. Three hundred years of parenteral nutrition: the history of intravenous nutritional therapy. Conn Med January 1980;44[1].

16 Henriques V, Andersen AC. Cited by Greenstein JP, Wintz M. Chemistry of the Amino Acids. Vol. 1. New York: John Wiley & Sons, 1961.

17 Studley HO. Percentage of weight loss: a basic indicator of surgical risk in patients with chronic peptic ulcer. JAMA 1936;106:458–460.

18 Elman R. Amino acid content of the blood following intravenous injection of hydrolyzed casein. Proc Soc Exp Biol Med 1937;37:437–440.

19 Lidstrom FI. The effect of intraportal administration of a dialyzed enzymatic casein hydrolysate (Aminosol) on the urinary excretion of amino acids and peptides: II, Amino acid concentration in the hepatic vein and a peripheral vein after intravenous infusions of Aminosol. Acta Chir Scand 1954;186(suppl):45–52.

20 Bansi HW, Jurgens P, Muller G, et al. Der stoffwechsel bei intravenoser applikation von nahrlosungen, insbesondere synthetisch zusammengestellter aminosaurelosungen. Klin Wochenschr 1964;42:332.

21 Dudrick SJ, Wilmore DW, Vars HM, Rhoads JE. Long-term total parenteral nutrition with growth, development, and positive nitrogen balance. Surgery 1968;64:134–142.

22 Dudrick SJ. History of vascular access. JPEN J Parenter Enteral Nutr 2006;30:S47–S56.

23 Mogil RA, DeLaurentis DA, Rosemond GP. The infraclavicular venipuncture. Arch Surg 1967;95:320–324.

24 Wilmore DW, Dudrick SJ. Growth and development of an infant receiving all nutrients exclusively by vein. JAMA 1968;203:860–864.

25 Stengel A, Ravdin IS. The maintenance of nutrition in surgical patients with a description of the orojejunal method of feeding. Surgery 1939;6:511–523.

26 Mulholland JH, Tui C, Wright AM, Vinci VJ. Nitrogen metabolism, caloric intake and weight loss in postoperative convalescence. Ann Surg 1943;117:512–534.

27 Winitz M, Graff J, Gallagher N, Narkin A, Seedman DA. Evaluation of chemical diets as nutrition for man-in-space. Nature 1965;205:741–742.

28 Chimera (mythology): wikipedia.org/wiki/Chimera_(mythology) [Accessed 15 May 2007]

29 Sade R. Transplantation at 100 years: Alexis Carrel, pioneer surgeon. Science Direct: *Ann Thorac Surg* 2005;80:2415–2418.

30 Carrel A. Anastomose bout a bout de la jugulaire et de la corotide primitive. *Lyon Med* 1902;99:114.

31 Carrel A. The operative technique for vascular anastamosis and transplantation of viscera. *Lyon Med* 1902;98:859.

32 Carrel A. The transplantation of organs a preliminary communication. *JAMA* 1905;45:1645–1646.

33 Carrel A, Lindbergh CA. Culture of whole organs. *Science* 1935;31:621.

34 Gibson T, Medawar PB. The behaviour of skin homografts in man. *J Anat* 1943;77:299–310.

35 Merrill JP, Murray JE, Harrison JH, Guild WR. Successful homotransplantation of the human kidney between identical twins. *JAMA* 1956;160:227–282.

36 Reyes J, Bueno J, Kocoshis S, et al. Current status of intestinal transplantation in children. *J Pediatr Surg* 1998;33:243–254.

37 Lillehei RC, Miller AV. The physiological response of small bowel of the dog to ischemia including prolonged in vitro preservation of the small bowel with successful replacement and survival. *Ann Surg* 1959;150:543–560.

38 Starzl TE, Kaupp HA Jr. Mass homotransplantation of abdominal organs in dogs. *Surg Forum* 1960;11:28–30.

39 Starzl TE, Rowe M, Todo S, et al. Transplantation of multiple abdominal viscera. *JAMA* 1989;261:1449–1457.

40 Grant D, Wall W, Mimeault R, et al. Successful small-bowel/liver transplantation. *Lancet* 1990;335:181–184.

2 Intestinal Physiology and Immunology

2 Intestinal Morphology, Intestinal Regeneration and the Promise of Tissue Engineering

David A.J. Lloyd and Simon M. Gabe

Key points

- Intestinal morphology reflects its role as an absorptive surface and a barrier against luminal contents.
- Small intestinal surface area is increased about 600-fold by a combination of micro- and macroscopic features.
- Both small and large intestinal mucosal surfaces are rapidly replaced as a result of the activity of stem cells found in the intestinal crypts.
- Understanding of stem cell dynamics and signaling has increased rapidly in recent years.
- Tissue engineering of intestinal mucosa has been performed in animal models and offers the possibility of a novel therapy for patients with short bowel syndrome.

Introduction

The morphology of the intestine reflects its two principle roles: the digestion and absorption of nutrients, and the maintenance of a barrier against the external environment. This chapter will briefly describe the basic macroscopic and microscopic structure of the small and large intestine and will review current understanding of the role of stem cells in intestinal regeneration. An improved knowledge of stem cell biology has led to the

Intestinal Failure: Diagnosis, Management and Transplantation.
Edited by Alan N. Langnas, Olivier Goulet, Eamonn M.M. Quigley and Kelly A. Tappenden. © 2008 Blackwell Publishing. ISBN 978-1-4051-4637-1.

production of tissue engineered intestine and progress in this exciting field will be explored.

Morphology of the intestine

Macroscopic structure

The gross anatomy of the small and large intestine is well characterized, well understood, and is the topic of numerous texts. As such, a detailed description is not warranted here. However, there are a number of points that are relevant in the context of intestinal failure, in particular the length of normal small intestine and the vascular supply of the small and large intestine.

The combined length of the jejunum and ileum ranges from 3 to $8^1/_2$ m [1]. The variability of small intestinal length between individuals is difficult to predict and therefore it is vitally important that the length of remaining intestine rather than the length of resected intestine is recorded at surgery. The absorptive area of the small intestine is increased about threefold by the presence of circular infoldings known as plicae circulares. These are most marked in the jejunum, becoming smaller and less frequent as the colon is approached. The length of the large intestine is less variable, being about 1–1.5 m long. It is separated from the small intestine by the ileocaecal valve; the importance of the presence or absence of the ileocaecal valve postoperatively will be discussed in further chapters.

Other than the upper half of the duodenum, which receives blood from the pancreaticoduodenal artery, a branch of the gastroduodenal artery, the small intestine receives its arterial blood supply from branches of the superior mesenteric artery. Blood supply to the

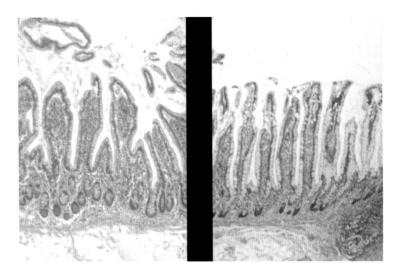

Figure 2.1 Cross-section through jejunum (left) and ileum (right) showing crypt-villus structure. (Images kindly supplied by P. Domizio.)

proximal large intestine, up to the distal third of the transverse colon, is also from branches of the superior mesenteric artery. However, the distal large intestine receives its blood supply via branches of the inferior mesenteric artery. Corresponding veins drain blood from both the small and large intestine into the portal circulation. It can be seen that the superior mesenteric artery and vein are of paramount importance to blood supply to and from the intestine and is the reason why infarction and thrombosis are so devastating.

Microscopic structure

Both the small and large intestine are composed of four distinct layers: the mucosa, the submucosa, the muscularis externa, and the serosa. The mucosa consists of a layer of columnar epithelium below which lies the lamina propria, a loose connective tissue layer containing blood vessels, lymphatics, and some lymphoid tissue. In the small intestine, the mucosa forms fingerlike projections known as villi. These are most pronounced in the ileum and serve to increase small intestinal surface area about tenfold. Each villus contains a dense capillary network, which lies just below the epithelium, and blind-ending lymphatic vessels, lacteals, which drain into lymphatics forming a plexus in the lamina propria. In between and in continuity with the villi are the intestinal crypts (Figure 2.1). These crypts contain intestinal epithelial stem cells which allow repopulation and repair of the small intestinal mucosa. Although the mucosa of the colon does not form villi, stem cells remain located in crypts.

Scattered throughout the lamina propria and submucosa of the small intestine, predominantly the ileum, are visible aggregates of lymphoid tissue known as Peyer's patches. The mucosa overlying the Peyer's patches is flattened and contains numerous antigen-sampling M cells. In the colon, the lamina propria contains larger numbers of smaller lymphoid nodules. The lamina propria is separated from the submucosa by a thin inner circular layer and an outer longitudinal layer of smooth muscle known as the muscularis mucosae. The submucosa contains a network of blood vessels and lymphatics as well as groups of neurons, which make up Meissner's plexus.

The muscularis externa, like the muscularis mucosae, consists of an inner circular layer and an outer longitudinal layer of smooth muscle. In the large intestine, the outer smooth muscle layer forms three bands known as teniae coli. Between the inner and outer smooth muscle layers are blood vessels and lymphatics, and neurons which make up Auerbach's plexus. The outer serosa is a thin layer of loose connective tissue containing vasculature and lymphatics, covered on the outer surface by mesothelium.

Mucosal cell types

There are five main epithelial cell lineages, all of which are derived from stem cells in the intestinal crypts. The most plentiful cells in the mucosal epithelium are columnar enterocytes, which make up the absorptive surface of the intestine. The apical surface of these cells consists of a layer of densely packed microvilli, visible with electron microscopy. Each enterocyte has about 3,000 microvilli on its apical surface and their presence increases small intestinal surface area about 20-fold. Intestinal enterocytes contain numerous transport proteins in their apical and basal membranes, which allow active and passive transport of nutrients from the gut. In addition, several digestive enzymes, such as disaccharidases, are bound to the enterocyte microvilli.

Located among the enterocytes are mucin-containing goblet cells. These cells produce mucus and other glycoproteins, which lubricate and protect the mucosal surface. Scattered enteroendocrine cells secrete peptide hormones, which exert endocrine and paracrine actions; the exact peptides secreted vary throughout the intestine. Paneth cells, unlike the other epithelial cell lines, are found at the crypt bases. They are characterised by granules containing lysozyme, tumour necrosis factor-α and defensins, and are believed to play an antibacterial role. Finally, M cells are believed to be involved in antigen sampling and transportation.

The lamina propria contains a wide range of cell types including smooth muscle cells, vascular endothelial cells and fibroblasts. Of particular interest are the intestinal subepithelial myofibroblasts. These cells are located in proximity to the mucosal epithelium and are believed to produce growth factors, including hepatocyte growth factor, which promote proliferation of the intestinal epithelial stem cells [2].

Regeneration of the intestinal mucosal epithelium

The intestinal mucosa has an impressive capacity for replication and regeneration both under normal physiological conditions and following injury. The entire small intestinal epithelium is replaced every 3–5 days. As mentioned previously, this regenerative capacity is dependent on the activity of intestinal epithelial stem cells found toward the base of the epithelial crypts.

Stem cell proliferation and epithelial cell differentiation

The majority of stem cell divisions are believed to result in a single daughter cell and a single stem cell, which

retains the original template DNA. These daughter cells then undergo further divisions to produce a population of transit-amplifying (TA) cells. These TA cells are rapidly proliferating and divide and further differentiate to produce the different epithelial cell lines. Stem cell daughter cells and TA cells retain their clonogenicity and are able to revert back to stem cells if the crypt is damaged and existing stem cells are lost. However, as the TA cells divide further, they lose their capacity for clonal expansion. Enterocytes, goblet cells, and enteroendocrine cells undergo further differentiation as they migrate upward toward the tip of the villus. They then are either shed into the intestinal lumen or undergo apoptosis. Each crypt contributes to the epithelium of a number of villi. Unlike the other cell lines, Paneth cells undergo differentiation as they migrate to the base of the crypts. The concept that a single intestinal stem cell can give rise to all intestinal epithelial cell lines is known as the Unitarian hypothesis and is supported by a significant body of evidence [3].

Although the hierarchical pattern of cell proliferation and differentiation from crypt to villus is firmly established, the exact number of the stems cells in each crypt is less clear. Historically, progress in this area has been hampered by a lack of reliable molecular stem cell markers, although the discovery of Musashi-1 and Hes1 as putative stem cell markers is encouraging [4]. It is believed that there are four to six stem cells in each crypt, which are located in a specific stem cell compartment also known as the "stem cell niche" (Figure 2.2). This niche comprises the intestinal epithelial stem cell, neighboring proliferating cells, and adjacent mesenchymal cells such as the pericryptal fibroblasts and intestinal subepithelial myofibroblasts [5]. These mesenchymal cells are believed to play an important role in the maintenance of the stem cell population and the control and regulation of proliferation via the secretion of various peptides including hepatocyte growth factor, keratinocyte growth factor, and tissue growth factor-β. There are complex signaling pathways between the different components of the stem cell niche, including the Wnt, hedgehog, and notch pathways. Our understanding of this signaling is increasing rapidly but is beyond the scope of this chapter and has been reviewed recently [3,6].

Although the majority of stem cell divisions result in one stem cell and one daughter cell as described

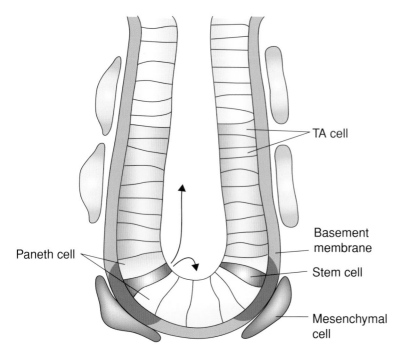

TA cell

Basement
membrane

Paneth cell

Stem cell

Mesenchymal
cell

Figure 2.2 Intestinal crypt. Stem cells (red) are found at the crypt bases. Stem cell progeny (yellow) known as transit amplifying (TA) cells migrate up the crypt undergoing further replication and differentiation. Basement membrane and mesenchymal cells (green) surround the stem cell niche. (Reprinted from Spradling et al. [5], with permission from Macmillan Publishers Ltd.)

earlier, division may be symmetrical, resulting in either two daughter cells or two stem cells. If the former occurs, then that stem cell will be lost from the crypt. This ultimately may lead to all cells in a crypt being descendants of a single stem cell. Conversely, if division results in two stem cells then the total number of stem cells in the crypt will increase. It has been proposed that increases in stem cell number may be triggers for crypt fission, a process vital to intestinal growth and repair after injury.

Stem cell plasticity

Stem cell plasticity refers to the ability of organ-specific stem cells from one tissue to produce cells of a different lineage and tissue. For example, adult bone marrow cells may be able to engraft into other tissues and differentiate into cell types specific to that organ, such as hepatocytes or skeletal myocytes. There is increasing evidence to support this hypothesis, especially from observations that Y-chromosome containing cells can be seen in the tissues of female recipients of bone marrow from male donors, although it has been argued that this may represent cell fusion rather than stem cell plasticity. In the small and large intestine, bone marrow

engraftment and differentiation into mesenchymal cells have been demonstrated in humans and mice [7]. The possibility that bone marrow derived cells could be used to populate and regenerate intestinal mucosa is clearly exciting and of particular relevance to the field of tissue engineering.

Tissue engineering of intestinal mucosa

Tissue engineering offers a novel approach to the treatment of short bowel syndrome. The basic concept is to seed intestinal tissue onto artificial, biodegradable scaffolds which will support the growth and development of organized intestinal "neomucosa." The use of autologous cells to create biocompatible tissue-engineered intestinal constructs has several benefits, including the stimulation of natural biological mechanisms for repair and remodeling, complete biocompatibility, the potential for further growth, and, of course, the avoidance of problems associated with transplantation. Potentially, the engineering of small intestine as a functional absorptive area could render patients with short bowel syndrome independent of parenteral nutrition.

Culturing intestinal epithelium

A necessary initial step in the creation of intestinal neomucosa has been the development of techniques to produce primary cultures of intestinal epithelium. In the early 1990s, Evans and colleagues described a method by which "organoid units" were derived from neonatal rat small intestine by partial digestion using a mixture of collagenase and dispase [8]. These organoid units are cellular aggregates consisting of polarised intestinal epithelium surrounding a core of mesenchymal cells. As digestion is incomplete, it is believed that the stem cell niche is maintained. Experiments have shown that the organoid units can be successfully cultured and maintained *in vitro* [8].

Generation of neomucosa

Tait and colleagues demonstrated that suspensions of organoid units transplanted into subcutaneous pockets in adult rodents could develop into small tubular structures, which consisted of a central lumen surrounded by a circumferential epithelial layer [9]. As early as 2 weeks after organoid unit transplantation, this epithelial layer had formed crypts and villi and was histologically similar to small intestinal mucosa. This neomucosa was shown to contain all epithelial cell lineages [9]. Although the majority of subsequent studies have used rodent tissue exclusively, it is noteworthy that Sattar and colleagues demonstrated that organoid units produced from human foetal small intestine could be successfully implanted subcutaneously into SCID mice to produce cysts of neomucosa similar to that described in rat models [10].

Growth of neomucosa on artificial scaffolds

A major challenge in the development of tissue engineered intestine is the production of a three-dimensional tubular structure with the correct orientation of mucosal, submucosal, and muscular layers. Artificial biodegradable scaffolds have been employed by several groups in an attempt to produce tubular structures lined with neomucosa [11,12] (see Figure 2.3). These scaffolds need to be flexible but also must maintain their structural integrity *in vivo*, and must be porous enough to allow cell migration and neovascularization to occur through the scaffold.

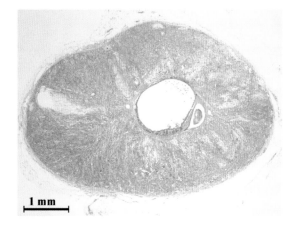

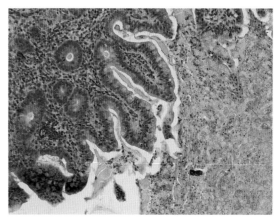

Figure 2.3 H&E staining of artificial scaffold 4 weeks after implantation of organoid units. There is evidence of mucosa and submucosa lining the entire circumference of the luminal surface of the scaffold. At high magnification, the appearance of the mucosa and submucosa lining the luminal surface of the scaffold is similar to that of normal small intestinal tissue. There is columnar epithelium containing mucin producing goblet cells, which has developed into crypts and villi. The submucosa contains macrophages, fibroblasts, and other inflammatory cells.

Vacanti and colleagues developed a model for the tissue engineering of intestinal neomucosa in which organoid units were seeded onto collagen coated polymer scaffolds, which were then implanted into the peritoneum of a rat model. By 2 weeks, the luminal surface of the tubular scaffold was covered with a layer of epithelium and between 2 and 6 weeks there was development of crypts and villi and evidence of epithelial maturation and cellular differentiation. Below the epithelium, smooth muscle-like cells and, possibly, early neural tissue were identified. Electrophysiological studies demonstrated the generation of transepithelial resistance, indicative of an active barrier, and evidence of active transport across the neomucosal membrane [13]. These scaffolds have been successfully reimplanted into native rat small intestine. When reassessed 5 months after reimplantation, the neomucosa had well-developed crypt-villus architecture similar to native small intestine; rates of proliferation and apoptosis were also similar [14]. Reimplanted neomucosa was significantly more developed than nonreimplanted tissue, suggesting a trophic effect of luminal bowel contents, and further studies have demonstrated that this can be amplified further by injection of GLP-2 [15]. This group has applied the same principles to other intestinal tissue and has produced tissue-engineered esophagus, stomach, and colon [16–18].

Functional capacity of neomucosa

Neomucosa produced by subcutaneous transplantation of organoid units has been shown to express brush border digestive enzymes [9, 19] and quantitative functional studies have demonstrated that the activity of these digestive enzymes was similar to that of age-matched control rat small intestine [19]. More recently, Grikscheit and colleagues implanted scaffolds containing tissue-engineered neomucosa into rats that had undergone 85% enterectomy and demonstrated that postoperative weight loss was reduced and subsequent weight gain enhanced [20]. Although this effect was attributed to the potential absorptive capacity of the implanted neointestine; it is possible that it may be, in part, mediated by the effects of the nonperistaltic neointestine on gut transit time.

Conclusions

Knowledge of intestinal regeneration and repair and, especially, of stem cell behaviour and function is increasing rapidly. This improved understanding has made it possible to produce experimental models of tissue-engineered intestine. Although the initial work is very encouraging, there are still significant limitations. One major problem is that the methodology employed is very inefficient with large quantities of neonatal tissue being required to produce a small

section of neointestine. Clearly, this significantly limits clinical application at present and future research will need to address the issues of yield and explore possible alternative sources of tissue with which to seed scaffolds. However, the concept of stem cell plasticity raises the possibility that one day bone marrow–derived stem cells might be used as substrates to produce significant quantities of artificially engineered intestine.

References

1 Nightingale J, Spiller R. *Normal Intestinal Anatomy and Physiology*. In: Nightingale J, ed. *Intestinal Failure*. London: Grenwich Medical Media, 2001:17–36.
2 Powell DW, Mifflin RC, Valentich JD, et al. Myofibroblasts. II. Intestinal subepithelial myofibroblasts. *Am J Physiol* 1999;277:C183–C201.
3 Leedham SJ, Brittan M, McDonald SA, Wright NA. Intestinal stem cells. *J Cell Mol Med* 2005;9:11–24.
4 Kayahara T, Sawada M, Takaishi S, et al. Candidate markers for stem and early progenitor cells, Musashi-1 and Hes1, are expressed in crypt base columnar cells of mouse small intestine. *FEBS Lett* 2003;535:131–135.
5 Spradling A, Drummond-Barbosa D, Kai T. Stem cells find their niche. *Nature* 2001;414:98–104.
6 Rizvi AZ, Hunter JG, Wong MH. Gut-derived stem cells. *Surgery* 2005;137:585–590.
7 Brittan M, Hunt T, Jeffery R, et al. Bone marrow derivation of pericryptal myofibroblasts in the mouse and human small intestine and colon. *Gut* 2002;50:752–757.
8 Evans GS, Flint N, Somers AS, Eyden B, Potten CS. The development of a method for the preparation of rat intestinal epithelial cell primary cultures. *J Cell Sci* 1992;101(Pt 1):219–231.
9 Tait IS, Flint N, Campbell FC, Evans GS. Generation of neomucosa in vivo by transplantation of dissociated rat postnatal small intestinal epithelium. *Differentiation* 1994;56:91–100.
10 Sattar A, Robson SC, Patel HR, Angus B, Campbell FC. Expression of growth regulatory genes in a SCID mouse-human model of intestinal epithelial regeneration. *J Pathol* 1999;187:229–236.
11 Choi RS, Vacanti JP. Preliminary studies of tissue-engineered intestine using isolated epithelial organoid units on tubular synthetic biodegradable scaffolds. *Transplant Proc* 1997;29:848–851.
12 Lloyd DA, Ansari TI, Gundabolu P, et al. A pilot study investigating a novel subcutaneously implanted pre-cellularised scaffold for tissue engineering of intestinal mucosa. *Eur Cell Mater* 2006;11:27–33.

13 Choi RS, Riegler M, Pothoulakis C, et al. Studies of brush border enzymes, basement membrane components, and electrophysiology of tissue-engineered neointestine. *J Pediatr Surg* 1998;33:991–996.

14 Tavakkolizadeh A, Berger UV, Stephen AE, et al. Tissue-engineered neomucosa: morphology, enterocyte dynamics, and SGLT1 expression topography. *Transplantation* 2003;75:181–185.

15 Ramsanahie A, Duxbury MS, Grikscheit TC, et al. Effect of GLP-2 on mucosal morphology and SGLT1 expression in tissue-engineered neointestine. *Am J Physiol Gastrointest Liver Physiol* 2003;285:G1345–G1352.

16 Grikscheit T, Ochoa ER, Srinivasan A, et al. Tissue-engineered esophagus: experimental substitution by onlay patch or interposition. *J Thorac Cardiovasc Surg* 2003;126:537–544.

17 Maemura T, Ogawa K, Shin M, et al. Assessment of tissue-engineered stomach derived from isolated epithelium organoid units. *Transplant Proc* 2004;36:1595–1599.

18 Grikscheit TC, Ogilvie JB, Ochoa ER, et al. Tissue-engineered colon exhibits function in vivo. *Surgery* 2002;132:200–204.

19 Tait IS, Penny JI, Campbell FC. Does neomucosa induced by small bowel stem cell transplantation have adequate function? *Am J Surg* 1995;169:120–125.

20 Grikscheit TC, Siddique A, Ochoa ER, et al. Tissue-engineered small intestine improves recovery after massive small bowel resection. *Ann Surg* 2004;240:748–754.

3 Basic Physiology of Motility, Absorption and Secretion

Greger Lindberg

Key points

- Intestinal motor activity can adapt to the type of food that has been ingested and this probably facilitates digestion and absorption of nutrients.

- The absorption of glucose and galactose into enterocytes is mainly by a sodium-dependent co-transporter called SGLT-1, whereas facilitated transport with the carrier GLUT-2 is used for the transport of sugars out of enterocytes.

- Virtually all dipeptides and tripeptides use the same proton-dependent peptide co-transporter PEPT1 for entry into enterocytes. This transporter is also important for the absorption of certain antibiotics and antiviral agents.

- Colipase is secreted from the pancreas as procolipase. The pentapeptide enterostatin that is cleaved off to form active colipase, has been suggested to be a specific satiety signal for the ingestion of fat.

- Chloride secretion in the small bowel is in part regulated by activity in the enteric nervous system.

The small intestine is the most indispensable part of the gastrointestinal tract. This is where foods are digested, dispersed, and absorbed as nutrients from the gut lumen into the bloodstream. The structural and functional properties of the gastrointestinal tract specifically serve the purposes of food digestion and absorption. Many different systems participate in the actions that together make it possible for us to uti-lize meat and vegetables as the main sources of protein, and starch, sugars and fat as sources of energy. The three functions of the small bowel that work in concert to achieve this are motility, secretion, and absorption.

Motility

The motor activity of the small intestine is largely governed by the enteric nervous system (ENS), which is part of the autonomic nervous system. The nerve cells of the ENS are grouped into two anatomically distinct plexuses, the myenteric plexus, which is located between the outer longitudinal muscle layer and the inner circular muscle layer, and the submucosal plexus. The ENS communicates with sympathetic ganglia (celiac and superior mesenteric ganglions) and the vagus nerve, and via these also with the spinal cord and the brain. In addition to parasympathetic and sympathetic input, the ENS receives input from sensory nerves in the mucosa and the bowel wall as well as paracrine and endocrine signals and input from mast cells of the immune system. The ENS forms a complex network of circuits between sensory neurons, interneurons and motor neurons with extensive convergence and divergence of connections (Figure 3.1). Within this system, a large number of chemicals serve as transmitters of signals. Acetylcholine and norepinephrine are the main transmitters of parasympathetic and sympathetic input, respectively. Acetylcholine, serotonin, vasoactive intestinal peptide (VIP), nitric oxide (NO), and somatostatin are used by interneurons. Acetylcholine and tachykinins are found in nerves that are excitatory to the muscle

Intestinal Failure: Diagnosis, Management and Transplantation. Edited by Alan N. Langnas, Olivier Goulet, Eamonn M.M. Quigley and Kelly A. Tappenden. © 2008 Blackwell Publishing. ISBN 978-1-4051-4637-1.

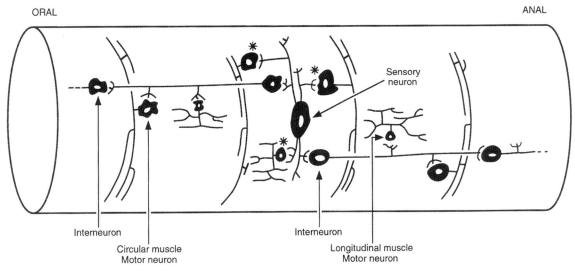

ORAL · ANAL

Sensory neuron

Interneuron

Circular muscle
Motor neuron

Interneuron

Longitudinal muscle
Motor neuron

Figure 3.1 Schematic representation of the neuronal circuits responsible for motility reflexes in the small intestine of the guinea pig. Sensory neurons provide synaptic inputs to motor neurons (monosynaptic reflexes are shown by asterisks) and to interneurons (di- and multisynaptic reflexes). Interneurons connect with other interneurons in chains and also innervate motor neurons. Each part of the intestine contains multiple overlapping circuits of this type, with extensive convergence and divergence of connections. (Modified from Furness et al. [1], with permission from Blackwell Publishing.)

and VIP and NO in inhibitory nerves. The same nerve can also contain more than one transmitter.

Another important component in the regulation of small bowel motor activity is the network of interstitial cells of Cajal (ICC). ICCs are specialized cells of mesenchymal origin that generate and propagate electrical slow waves. The ability to generate slow waves is unique to the ICC and makes them the pacemaker cells of the gut. ICCs are electrically coupled to smooth muscle cells via gap junctions. When the slow wave reaches the muscle cell, depolarization and activation of voltage-dependent Ca^{2+}-channels occurs (Figure 3.2). This may, or may not, lead to the generation of spikelike action potentials and muscle contraction. The response of smooth muscle cells to slow wave depolarization is believed to be a function of neural, hormonal, and paracrine regulation of ion channel expression and availability [3]. However, not all ICCs have the same mission in gut motility. Whereas ICCs located around the myenteric plexus (IC-MY) are thought to be responsible for generating and propagating slow waves, other types of ICC are situated at the interface between varicose nerve fibers and smooth muscle cells and they receive, transduce, and conduct neural signals to the smooth muscle cells. In the small bowel, the latter type is represented by the ICCs of the deep muscular plexus (IC-DMP).

Motor activity in the fed state

The slow wave rhythm in the proximal part of the small bowel is 11–12 cycles per minute (cpm) but the rhythm decreases along the gut and, in the terminal ileum, is about 8 cpm. Slow waves determine when a contraction can occur. Thus, in the duodenum, contractions can occur no more often than once every 5 seconds. When the musculature contracts the lumen is partially or totally occluded and the local intraluminal pressure increases. Most contractions in the small bowel are local events and involve only 1–4 cm of bowel at a time. Their effect on luminal contents depends on the state of the musculature above and below the contraction. If a contraction is not coordinated with muscle activity above and below the site of contraction, the content will be displaced in both oral and aboral direction. Such action will serve the purpose of mixing the content and exposing it to the epithelium. Contractions that are coordinated with adjacent sites will lead to propulsion of content. This is usually in the aboral direction,

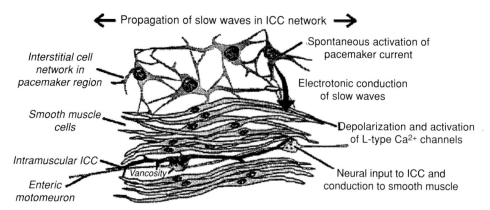

Figure 3.2 Model for the generation and modulation of electrical activity in gastrointestinal smooth muscle by interstitial cells of Cajal (ICC). Interstitial cell networks in pacemaker regions express the ionic mechanisms necessary to generate slow waves. These events can actively propagate through the ICC network via gap junctions connecting ICCs. Slow waves electrotonically conduct into smooth muscle cells, which are also electrically coupled to ICCs but appear to lack the mechanism for regenerating slow waves. Slow waves depolarize the smooth muscle cells, and activate voltage-dependent (L-type) Ca^{2+} channels. If threshold depolarization is achieved, Ca^{2+} action potentials are elicited. If threshold is not achieved, the activation of inward current in smooth muscle cells is manifest as an increase in the plateau phase of slow waves. (Modified from Horowitz et al. [2], with permission from Annual Reviews.)

but retropulsion also can occur over shorter or longer distances. In the fed state, the motor activity of the small bowel exhibits a mixture of contractile patterns that probably reflect the composition of ingested food (Figure 3.3). In dogs, ingestion of a nondigestible cellulose gel was associated with intense motor activity in the jejunum [4]. When fat was added to the meal a pattern of discrete clustered contractions was seen, whereas the addition of glucose led to an almost complete inhibition of motor activity. Neural, paracrine and endocrine regulation of fed motor activity is not well understood. Some of the regulation may well reside in the ENS but a normal response to food also requires extrinsic nerves. This can be deduced from the failure of the extrinisically denervated intestine to respond adequately to food stimulation in dogs [5] and the findings of abnormal intestinal fed motor activity after small bowel transplantation [6]. No systematic study of the effects of different nutrients on small bowel motor activity has been done in humans.

Motor activity in the fasting state

In the fasting state, there is a cyclic pattern with migrating activity complexes recurring irregularly at an interval that averages 80 minutes but that can range from 18 to 145 minutes [7]. The activity complex constitutes the third phase (phase III) of the migrating motor complex (MMC) (Figure 3.4). The activity complex consists of a 30–50 cm–long segment within which propagated contractions move in the aboral direction. The propagation velocity of individual contractions is the same as the propagation velocity of slow waves (about 120 cm/min), whereas the whole complex moves much slower (1–12 cm/min in the proximal jejunum). Phase III of the MMC is coordinated with intestinal secretion and secretion of bile and bicarbonate. It is believed to serve a housekeeping function, cleansing the intestinal lumen from debris, bacteria and cells shed from the mucosa. The control of the MMC resides within the ENS since it is preserved in the extrinsically denervated gut, but extrinsic neural activity can modify MMC characteristics such as cycle length.

Digestion and absorption

Digestion is the chemical breakdown of ingested foods by enzymes secreted by glandular cells in the mouth, chief cells in the stomach, acinar cells in the pancreas,

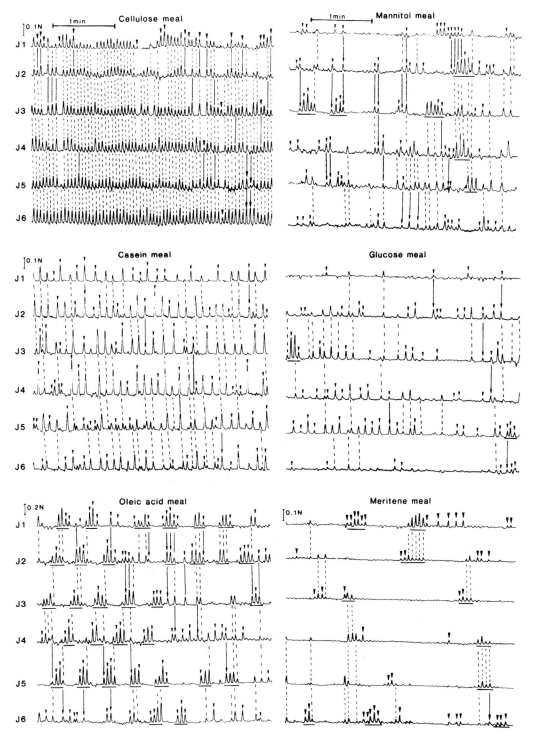

Figure 3.3 Jejunal motor patterns in dogs after different meals. Dashed lines indicate propagative contractions that led to contraction waves spreading over various distances; solid lines indicate simultaneously occurring contractions at adjacent recording sites that interrupt the propagation of contraction waves; triangles indicate stationary contractions occurring at one recording site only; clusters of contractions are underlined. All nutrients added to the control cellulose meal decreased the number of contraction waves and increased the incidence of stationary contractions. Clusters of contractions were most obvious after the oleic acid meal. (Reproduced from Schemann et al. [4], with permission from the American Gastroenterological Association.)

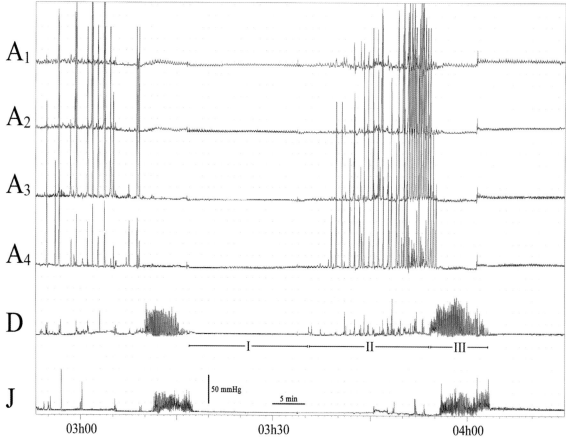

Figure 3.4 Normal fasting motor activity, as depicted by antro-duodeno-jejunal manometry in a healthy volunteer. Intraluminal pressures were monitored using a six-channel catheter with four sensors located 3 cm apart in the pyloric region, one sensor in the distal duodenum, and one sensor in the jejunum. This is part of a nocturnal recording that shows two migrating activity complexes and one complete MMC with phases I, II, and III.

and brush border enzymes from mucosal cells of the small intestine (Figure 3.5). Some of the digestive processes start already in the mouth where salivary amylase and, to some extent, lingual lipase are mixed with food during chewing. In the stomach, pepsin and gastric lipase, which are both active in the acidic environment of the stomach, contribute to the digestive process during mixing and grinding of food. The main part of digestion occurs, however, in the small intestine, and the exocrine pancreas is the most important source of enzymes used in the luminal digestion of food. Enzymes in the brush border of enterocytes carry out the final steps of digestion in the so-called membrane phase of digestion.

Carbohydrates

The average daily intake of carbohydrates is about 300 grams and this corresponds to about half of the caloric intake per day. About 50% of ingested carbohydrates are starch and 30% are sucrose. Other carbohydrates that we ingest more or less daily include lactose, maltose, glucose, fructose, and nondigestible carbohydrates such as cellulose and hemicellulose. Starch consists of two types of polymers, amylose, and amylopectin. Amylose is a straight-chain polymer of glucose linked by α-1,4-bonds. Glucose molecules also build up amylopectin but in addition to α-1,4-bonds amylopectin has α-1,6-bonds at every 20–30 glucose molecules. Amylopectin is quantitatively the largest

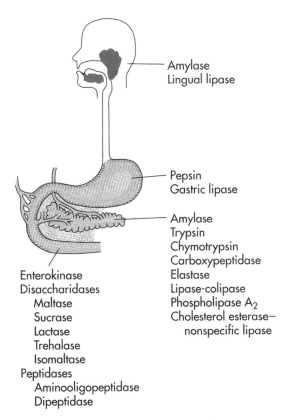

Amylase
Lingual lipase

Pepsin
Gastric lipase

Amylase
Trypsin
Chymotrypsin
Carboxypeptidase
Elastase
Lipase-colipase
Phospholipase A$_2$
Cholesterol esterase—
   nonspecific lipase

Enterokinase
Disaccharidases
   Maltase
   Sucrase
   Lactase
   Trehalase
   Isomaltase
Peptidases
   Aminooligopeptidase
   Dipeptidase

Figure 3.5 Sources of the principal luminal and membrane-bound digestive enzymes. (Reproduced from Johnson [8], with permission from Elsevier.)

carbohydrate in our food. Some of the digestion of starch takes place in the mouth with hydrolysis of α-1,4-bonds by salivary amylase, but most of the digestion occurs in the small intestine where digestion by pancreatic amylase produces maltose, maltotriose, and α-dextrins. The final steps of starch digestion are carried out by brush border carbohydrases, such as glycoamylase, sucrase, and isomaltase (Figure 3.6). The end product of starch digestion is glucose. Glycogen is a polysaccharide similar to amylopectin but with many more α-1,6-bonds. Humans, as well as animals, produce glycogen in order to store glucose in the liver and in muscle cells. Ingested glycogen from food mainly comes from liver and, to a lesser extent, meat. Glycogen follows the same digestive route as amylopectin. The main source of animal-derived sugar in the Western diet is lactose in milk. Lactose, sucrose, and trehalose are disaccharides that are digested only by brush border enzymes. The digestion of lactose by lactase yields glucose and galactose. Sucrose is split into fructose and glucose by sucrase, and trehalose into glucose by trehalase.

The absorption of glucose and galactose into enterocytes is mainly by the Na$^+$-dependent glucose-galactose co-transporter (SGLT-1) carrier (Figure 3.7). SGLT-1 is driven by an ATP-dependent Na$^+$ pump that maintains a sodium gradient that drags sodium, together with glucose or galactose, in the SGLT-1 carrier from the lumen into the cell. Fructose is transported into enterocytes using a different method called facilitated diffusion and this involves the carrier GLUT-5. Contrary to SGLT-1, GLUT-5 does not require energy and it cannot be energized to increase the rate of absorption. Glucose, galactose, and fructose leave the enterocyte via facilitated transport using the GLUT-2 carrier in the basolateral membrane. The reserve capacity of the small intestine to absorb monosaccharides and to transport them to the blood is about twice the average daily load of carbohydrates [10]. There is pronounced adaptation to diet, but the regulation of carbohydrate uptake is incompletely understood. The immediate regulation of carbohydrate digestion and absorption is governed by chemoreceptors and osmoreceptors in the jejunum, which can influence the emptying rate of the stomach.

Proteins

Protein consumption accounts for only 12%–15% of the daily energy intake. The main reason for protein intake is, however, not energy needs but the need for amino acids as building bricks for the synthesis of all of the proteins on which human life has been founded. The liver can synthesize several amino acids but eight amino acids are essential to humans, that is, they cannot be synthesized. These include tryptophan, lysine, methionine, phenylalanine, threonine, valine, leucine, and isoleucine. Two others, histidine and arginine, are essential for children.

The digestion and absorption of proteins are more complicated than those for carbohydrates. The average daily intake of protein in the Western world lies between 70 and 100 g. In addition, endogenous protein from secretions along the gastrointestinal tract adds another 50–60 g protein per day to the digestive system. Proteins are digested to short peptides and single amino acids. Digestion begins in the stomach, where pepsin

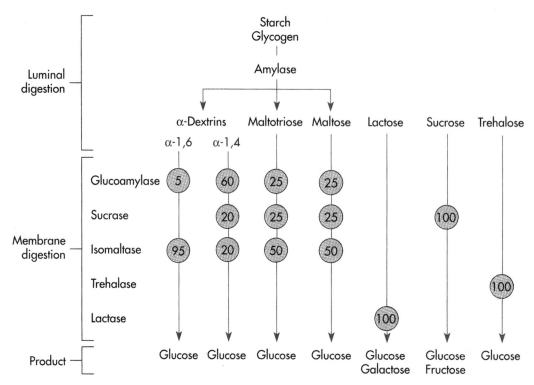

Figure 3.6 Summary of carbohydrate digestion. Circled numbers denote the approximate percentage of substrate hydrolyzed by a particular brush border enzyme. The same carrier (SGLT-1) actively transports glucose and galactose into enterocytes, while fructose is absorbed by facilitated diffusion using GLUT-5. (Reproduced from Johnson [8], with permission from Elsevier.)

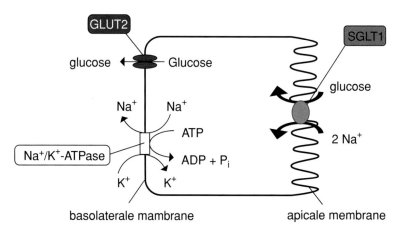

Figure 3.7 Transport of glucose in the intestinal epithelium. Absorption of glucose into enterocytes is catalyzed by the Na^+ dependent SGLT-1 co-transporter, located at the apical membrane. Glucose leaves the cell via a facilitated transport mechanism that utilizes SGLUT-5 at the basolateral membrane. The SGLT-1 trans- port system in energized by ATP that drives the Na^+/K^+-ATPase at the basolateral membrane. (Reproduced from Scheepers et al. [9], with permission from the American Society for Parenteral and Enteral Nutrition (A.S.P.E.N.).)

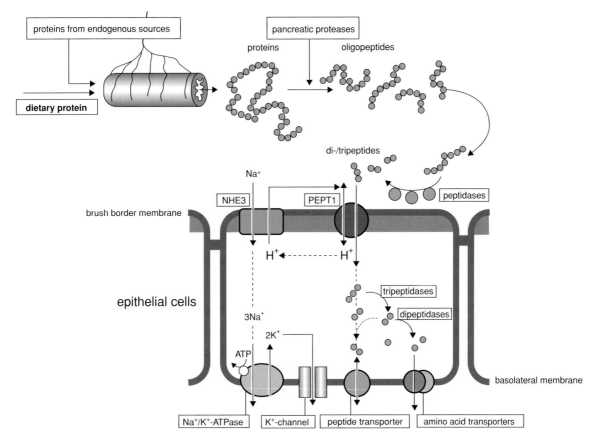

Figure 3.8 Integrated model depicting the generation of di- and tripeptides from the hydrolysis of luminal proteins and the pathways involved in the cellular uptake of peptides and mediated by PEPT1 in the apical membrane of intestinal epithelial cells. Following apical influx, di- and tripeptides are sequentially hydrolyzed by multiple cytosolic hydrolases. This is followed by the basolat-eral efflux of the amino acids via different amino acid-transporting systems. Peptides not undergoing hydrolysis can exit the cell by a basolateral peptide-transporting system, not yet identified on a molecular basis. (Reproduced from Daniel et al. [11], with permission from Annual Reviews.)

is activated in the acidic environment from pepsinogen secreted by the chief cells of the stomach. Secretion of pepsinogen takes place in response to food intake. Pepsin is an endopeptidase that hydrolyzes interior peptide bonds of proteins and polypeptides and pepsin has specificity for peptide bonds involving aromatic L-amino acids.

Pancreatic proteases carry out most of the luminal digestion of proteins. The secretion of pancreatic proteases is stimulated by cholecystokinin and secretin, which are released from mucosal I cells and S cells on the arrival of chyme into the intestine. Trypsin, chymotrypsin, and elastase are endopeptidases that cleave interior peptide bonds, whereas carboxypeptidase A

and B are exopeptidases that hydrolyze external peptide bonds. All pancreatic proteases are secreted as inactive precursors. Trypsinogen is the inactive precursor for trypsin. Enterokinase in the brush border of duodenal enterocytes activates some of the trypsinogen by cleaving off a hexapeptide. Active trypsin then activates the bulk of trypsinogen and also the precursors for the other pancreatic proteases, chymotrypsinogen, proelastase, procarboxypeptidase A, and procarboxypeptidase B. The luminal digestion of protein yields peptides and free amino acids (Figure 3.8). About 40% of protein is digested to free amino acids. Brush border peptidases continue the digestion of peptides longer than three amino acids, but dipeptides, tripeptides, and free amino acids are absorbed into the enterocytes. There are many different carriers for free amino acids, some of which are Na^+-dependent, others not, whereas dipeptides and tripeptides are transported using a single transporter, the H^+-dependent peptide co-transporter PEPT1 [11]. Although there are several thousand different peptides with two to three aminoacids, PEPT1 is capable of transporting the majority of them. The PEPT1 transporter has specificity for substrates with oppositely charged head groups separated by a carbon backbone with a distance of 5.5–6.3 Å [12]. PEPT1 utilizes water to shield off electric charges of amino acid side chains. Another important feature of this transporter is that it can transport a large number of peptidomimetic substances including aminocephalosporins, aminopenicillins, certain angiotensin-converting enzyme inhibitors, and amino acid-conjugated nucleoside-based antiviral agents.

Dipeptides are usually absorbed faster than a corresponding mixture of the same amino acids in free form. This, and the fact that peptide solutions have a lower osmolarity than the corresponding mixture of free amino acids, provides the rationale for using protein hydrolysates with short peptides rather than free amino acids in solutions for enteral nutrition [13].

Cytoplasmic peptidases in the enterocytes further hydrolyze dipeptides and tripeptides to free amino acids but some oligopeptides are transported out of the enterocytes into the blood using yet unknown transport mechanisms. Free amino acids leave the enterocyte via several different transporters at the basolateral membrane. Again, some of the transporters are Na^+-dependent, whereas others are not.

Lipids

Dietary lipids include several complex organic compounds such as phospholipids, sterols, hydrocarbons, and waxes but the dominant lipids in the human diet are triacylglycerols (TG), also known as triglycerides. Other important lipids are the fat-soluble vitamins (A, D, E, and K). Between 20% and 40% of the daily caloric intake come from lipids, although a general recommendation is that fat consumption should not exceed 30% of the total caloric intake. Lipids are insoluble in water, and this property makes the digestion and absorption of lipids very different from the digestion of carbohydrates and peptides. In order for lipids to be absorbed into enterocytes, they need to be partitioned into water-soluble micelles. Micelles are small (30–100 Å) particles formed by bile salts, phospholipids, and cholesterol in bile and products from enzymatic digestion of lipids. Micelles are rounded structures in which the outer surface is rendered hydrophilic by the polar sides of bile salts and phospholipids whereas the inner core is hydrophobic and can assimilate nonpolar lipids.

The digestion of lipids begins in the stomach. Lingual lipase from the salivary glands and gastric lipase are both acidic lipases with activity optima in the acidic environment of the stomach. In humans, the amount of lingual lipase is small and gastric lipase is the predominant acidic lipase. The two enzymes hydrolyze TG with a preference for medium-chained TG to diacylglycerol (DG) and free fatty acids (FFA). The acidic lipases do not hydrolyze either phospholipids or cholesterol esters. Another important part of lipid digestion is the emulsification of fat that is geberated by the grinding and mixing of food in the antrum. The emulsification of fat into small (diameter 0.5–1 μm) lipid droplets significantly increases the area of the oil-water interface and this is necessary for the action of pancreatic lipase in the upper small bowel.

Pancreatic lipase is secreted from the pancreas in its active form. Bile acids can inactivate pancreatic lipase by displacing it at the oil-water interface. This is prevented by colipase, a polypeptide that is secreted as procolipase together with pancreatic lipase and activated by trypsin. Colipase has the ability to take the place of bile acids at the oil-water interface. Lipase will bind to a specific site on colipase, once the colipase has attached to a fat droplet [14]. Colipase can also bind to micelles and this makes it possible for products of digestion by pancreatic lipase to enter directly into micelles. Pancreatic lipase hydrolyzes the outer, 1 and 3 ester linkages of TG to form 2-monoacylglycerol (2-MG) and FFA. 2-MG is the predominant form of MG that is absorbed by the small intestine.

The pentapeptide that is cleaved off from procolipase is called enterostatin and this peptide has been suggested to be a specific satiety signal for the ingestion of fat [15]. In rats, enterostatin has been shown to inhibit the intake of fat. It also has been shown that the secretion of procolipase increases in response to increases in both carbohydrates and proteins in food, and without a corresponding increase in the secretion of pancreatic lipase. Thus, it is possible that enterostatin can act as a general modulator of food intake. The action of enterostatin appears to depend on an intact afferent vagal function.

Pancreatic cholesterol esterase is a nonspecific esterase that hydrolyzes cholesterol esters, as well as esters of vitamins A, D, and E, phospholipids and all three ester linkages of acylglycerols. Cholesterol esterase is identical to the carboxyl ester hydrolase, which is found in human milk. Cholesterol esterase activity is enhanced by the presence of bile salts. A unique property of cholesterol esterase is its ability to form polymers. The formation of polymers protects the enzyme from proteolytic inactivation. Cholesterol esterase is secreted from the pancreas mainly as dimers and tetramers.

Phospholipids are digested in the small bowel only. Phosphatidylcholine is the dominating phospholipid in bile, where it takes part in the formation of mixed micelles. Phosphatidylcholine and dietary phospholipids are hydrolyzed by pancreatic phospholipase A_2, which is secreted from the pancreas as a precursor and activated by trypsin digestion. The activation of phospholipase A_2 requires calcium and its enzymatic action depends upon the presence of bile acids. Phospholipase A_2 has a preference for the hydrolysis of phospholipids at the 2-position, thus producing lysophospholipids and FFA.

Dietary cholesterol mainly comes as free sterol and only 10–15% as cholesteryl esters, which need to undergo enzymatic hydrolysis by cholesterol esterase before free cholesterol can be absorbed. The same enzyme also hydrolyzes plant sterol esters, which make up only a small portion of the dietary lipids.

The uptake of the products of lipid digestion into enterocytes is incompletely understood. Incorporation into micelles is crucial for the presentation of lipids to the brush border membrane. A water layer, often referred to as the unstirred water layer, covers the luminal side of the brush border. Solute molecules in the lumen gain access to the brush border membrane by diffusion across the unstirred water layer but the water layer prevents molecules that are insoluble in water from reaching the brush border. FFA and MG have little solubility in water and hence very few molecules will reach the brush border membrane. Solubilization in micelles increases the aqueous concentration of FFA and MG 100–1,000 times [16]. Transport of FFA and MG over the brush border membrane is mainly thought to occur by diffusion but there is also evidence that FFA can be absorbed by a carrier-mediated process [17,18].

Cholesterol uptake has similarly been hypothesized to be mainly by passive diffusion but again evidence exists that at least part of the sterol uptake may be protein mediated. The Niemann-Pick C1-like 1 protein (NPC1L1) has been put forward as a putative intestinal sterol influx transporter [19]. Cholesterol uptake is also regulated by active efflux of cholesterol and other sterols from enterocytes into the lumen. Two efflux proteins have been identified, both in the adenosine triphosphate-binding cassette, ABCG5 and ABCG8 [20].

Cholesterol and fatty acids absorbed by enterocytes are assembled in the endoplasmic reticulum into large intestinal lipoproteins called chylomicrons. Triacylglycerols are resynthesized via the monoglyceride acylation pathway and to some extent via the phosphatidic acid pathway. Cholesterol is esterified with FFA to cholesterylesters by acylcoenzyme A:cholesterol acyltransferase (ACAT). Newly synthesized TG and cholesterylesters are transferred to apolipoprotein B48 via the microsomal triglyceride transfer protein (MTP) to form an early, immature version of the chylomicron. These are transported in pre-chylomicron transport vesicles to the Golgi apparatus [21], where the chylomicrons are matured with additional TG, phospholipids, apoproteins, fat-soluble vitamins (A, D, E, and K) and glycosylation of the protein component. The chylomicrons are then transported to the basolateral membrane where they exocytose into the interstitial space and traverse the basement membrane to reach the lacteals.

Very low density lipoproteins (VLDL) are also produced by the enterocytes and, during fasting, these are the only lipoproteins produced by the small intestine. After a meal, the production of chylomicrons is increased in response to the amount of lipids being absorbed. It is unclear if production of VLDL is similarly increased. VLDLs are similar to chylomicrons but are smaller in size. Whether or not VLDL and chylomicrons are produced along the same production line has not been clarified. After exocytosis at the basolateral membrane VLDL, in a maner similar to chylomicrons, migrate to the lacteals, but some of them may also enter the blood stream. Although the majority of ingested lipids leave the enterocytes as chylomicrons or VLDL, some lipids, like short- and medium-chain fatty acids, may leave the mucosal cells in their free forms and enter the blood without being reesterified.

Bile acid reabsorption

The enterohepatic circulation of bile acids ensures that about 95% of the bile acids that are secreted into the gut lumen are reabsorbed in the small intestine. Bile acids are synthesized in the liver from cholesterol. Most of the bile acids are conjugated to taurine or glycine before being secreted into the bile. Reabsorption of bile acids is both by passive and active transport mechanisms. More hydrophobic bile acids, such as those with fewer hydroxyl groups and those that have become deconjugated, are absorbed passively throughout the small intestine. The hydrophilic bile acids are absorbed in the ileum by a specific sodium-coupled transporter protein, the ileal bile acid transporter (IBAT). The bile acids leave the ileal enterocytes by an anionic exchange process mediated by a transporter located in the basolateral membrane. The absorption of bile acids is specific to the distal ileum and functional or structural loss of this part of the small bowel may lead to malabsorption of bile acids.

Water and electrolytes

Large quantities of water are necessary for digestion and absorption. The small intestine receives between 7 and 10 liters of water per day. About 2 liters are ingested in food or drinks, saliva adds another liter of water, gastric juice 2 liters, pancreatic juice 2 liters, bile 1 liter, and intestinal secretion 1 liter. Most of the water is absorbed in the small intestine and only about 600 ml enters the colon. The absorption of water is, in general, the result of passive movement across the epithelial membrane in response to osmotic and hydrostatic pressures. In the absence of food, the osmotic pressure in the intestinal lumen mainly comes from the presence of ions. When food products enter the duodenum, there is rapid osmotic equilibration with the osmotic pressure of plasma. Water is absorbed from hypotonic solutions and is secreted into the lumen in response to hypertonic solutions. Water movement for the purpose of osmotic equilibration is mainly via the intercellular spaces with their relatively permeable junctions.

In the duodenum, the concentrations of Na^+ and K^+ are about the same as in plasma (140 mmol/1 and 4 mmol/1, respectively). The major anion is Cl^-. Sodium concentrations decrease along the small intestine and in the ileum $[Na^+]$ is about 125 mmol/1. The concentration of K^+ increases to about 9 mmol/1 in the ileum. Important anions in the ileum are Cl^- and HCO_3^-. Na^+ is transported from the lumen into enterocytes using four different mechanisms: the previously mentioned co-transport of Na^+ with nutrients, such as glucose/galactose or amino acids, the counter-transport of Na^+ for H^+, the co-transport of Na^+ with Cl^-, and to a small extent the movement of Na^+ by diffusion through water-filled channels. In the duodenum and jejunum, the first two mechanisms dominate, whereas in the ileum co-transport with Cl^- is the main mechanism for Na^+-absorption. Despite a large influx of Na^+ into enterocytes, the intracellular levels of Na^+ are kept low. The low levels of intracellular Na^+ are maintained by an efficient ion-pump at the basolateral membrane, the Na^+, K^+-activated ATPase. This enzyme-carrier molecule pumps 3 Na^+-ions out of the cell for every 2 K^+ ions pumped in, thus also maintaining a potential difference across the basolateral membrane known as the electrogenic potential.

The absorption of Cl^- is mainly by co-transport with Na^+ but in the distal ileum there is also countertransport of Cl^- into the enterocytes in exchange for metabolically produced HCO_3^-. Crypt cells have channels for Cl^- secretion in their apical membranes. These channels are activated by cyclic adenosine monophosphate (cAMP) and Ca^{++}. Activation occurs physiologically after a meal possibly as part of neural activity [22]. This mechanism is probably also responsible for the secretion of Cl^- that occurs in association with phase-III of the MMC. Other processes can activate secretion of Cl^-, and these include the actions of gastrointestinal hormones such as VIP, neurotransmitters, and paracrine secretions such as prostaglandins. The secretion of water and Cl^- is probably an important defense mechanism that enables the gut to flush out intestinal contents. The activation of the Cl^- channels in crypt cells also seems to be a target for bacterial toxins, such as cholera toxin, which can activate this process. Increased secretion from the small intestine may lead to loss of water and electrolytes, if secretion exceeds the absorptive capacity of the colon. Under normal conditions, the colon absorbs about 500 ml of water per day, but it is able to absorb up to 4–6 liters of water. In absence of the colon, even minor increases of intestinal secretion may lead to substantial losses of fluids and electrolytes.

Vitamins

Vitamins are organic compounds that we cannot synthesize; yet they are vital to our metabolic function. We must, therefore, rely on external sources for these compounds. One such source is our diet but bacteria in our large bowel also produce a number of the vitamins. Bacterial production and uptake by the colonic mucosa has been shown for vitamin K, thiamine (vitamin B_1), riboflavin (vitamin B_2), folate, pantothenic acid, and biotin (vitamin H). One vitamin, niacin (vitamin B_3) can actually be synthesized from the amino acid tryptophan. All other vitamins need to be digested and absorbed from the food. Absorption of vitamins is mainly by specific transport systems. The fat-soluble vitamins (A, D, E, and K) require solubilization in bile salt micelles before reaching the brush border membrane. Vitamin A is absorbed as β-carotene but the transporter for its uptake is not known. Vitamins E and D are believed to be absorbed passively through micellar absorption, whereas vitamin K utilizes a specific transporter. Specific transporters also have been identified for thiamine (human thiamine transporter-1, hTHTR-1), biotin and pantothenic acid (sodium-dependent multivitamin transporter, SMVT), ascorbic acid (sodium-dependent vitamin C transporter 1, SVCT-1), folate (human reduced folate carrier, hRFC), and cobalamin (vitamin B_{12}). The latter is transported to the ileum by haptocorrin, then binds to intrinsic factor (IF) and the IF-B_{12} complex is endocytosed once it has bound to the membrane receptor, cubulin. In addition, a sodium-independent carrier has been suggested for facilitated transport of riboflavin (vitamin B_2). Carriers for niacin (vitamin B_3) and pyridoxine (vitamin B_6) have not, as yet, been identified.

References

1 Furness JB, Bornstein JC, Pompolo S, et al. The circuitry of the enteric nervous system. *Neurogastroenterol Motil* 1994;6:241–253.

2 Horowitz B, Ward SM, Sanders KM. Cellular and molecular basis for electrical rhythmicity in gastrointestinal muscles. *Annu Rev Physiol* 1999;61:19–43.

3 Sanders KM, Koh SD, Ward SM. Interstitial cells of cajal as pacemakers in the gastrointestinal tract. *Annu Rev Physiol* 2006;68:307–343.

4 Schemann M, Ehrlein HJ. Postprandial patterns of canine jejunal motility and transit of luminal content. *Gastroenterology* 1986;90:991–1000.

5 Quigley EM, Spanta AD, Rose SG, Lof J, Thompson JS. Long-term effects of jejunoileal autotransplantation on myoelectrical activity in canine small intestine. *Dig Dis Sci* 1990;35:1505–1517.

6 Mousa H, Bueno J, Griffiths J, et al. Intestinal motility after small bowel transplantation. *Transplant Proc* 1998;30:2535–2536.

7 Scott SM, Knowles CH, Wang D, et al. The nocturnal jejunal migrating motor complex: defining normal ranges by study of 51 healthy adult volunteers and meta-analysis. *Neurogastroenterol Motil* 2006;18:927–935.

8 Johnson LR. Digestion and absorption. In: Johnson LR, Gerwin TA, eds. *Gastrointestinal Physiology*. 6th ed. St. Louis, Missouri: Mosby, Inc., 2001;119–141.

9 Scheepers A, Joost HG, Schurmann A. The glucose transporter families SGLT and GLUT: molecular basis of normal and aberrant function. *JPEN J Parenter Enteral Nutr* 2004;28:364–371.

10 Ferraris RP, Diamond J. Regulation of intestinal sugar transport. *Physiol Rev* 1997;77:257–302.

11 Daniel H. Molecular and integrative physiology of intestinal peptide transport. *Annu Rev Physiol* 2004;66:361–384.

12 Doring F, Will J, Amasheh S, et al. Minimal molecular determinants of substrates for recognition by the intestinal peptide transporter. *J Biol Chem* 1998;273:23211–23218.

13 Steinhardt HJ, Wolf A, Jakober B, et al. Nitrogen absorption in pancreatectomized patients: protein versus protein hydrolysate as substrate. *J Lab Clin Med* 1989;113:162–167.

14 Erlanson-Albertsson C. Pancreatic colipase. Structural and physiological aspects. *Biochim Biophys Acta* 1992;1125:1–7.

15 Berger K, Winzell MS, Mei J, Erlanson-Albertsson C. Enterostatin and its target mechanisms during regulation of fat intake. *Physiol Behav* 2004;83:623–630.

16 Phan CT, Tso P. Intestinal lipid absorption and transport. *Front Biosci* 2001;6:D299–319.

17 Chow SL, Hollander D. A dual, concentration-dependent absorption mechanism of linoleic acid by rat jejunum in vitro. *J Lipid Res* 1979;20:349–356.

18 Stremmel W. Uptake of fatty acids by jejunal mucosal cells is mediated by a fatty acid binding membrane protein. *J Clin Invest* 1988;82:2001–2010.

19 Altmann SW, Davis HR, Jr., Zhu LJ, et al. Niemann-Pick C1 Like 1 protein is critical for intestinal cholesterol absorption. *Science* 2004;303:1201–1204.

20 Duan LP, Wang HH, Wang DQ. Cholesterol absorption is mainly regulated by the jejunal and ileal ATP-binding cassette sterol efflux transporters Abcg5 and Abcg8 in mice. *J Lipid Res* 2004;45:1312–1323.

21 Kumar NS, Mansbach CM, 2nd. Prechylomicron transport vesicle: isolation and partial characterization. *Am J Physiol*. 1999;276(2 Pt 1):G378–86.

22 Cooke HJ. "Enteric tears": chloride secretion and its neural regulation. *News Physiol Sci* 1998;13:269–274.

4 Immunology of the Small Intestine

Liam O'Mahony

Key points

- The mucosal immune system must tolerate harmless antigens and protect against pathogens.

- Antigens and microbes are continually sampled via specialized lymphoid follicles (e.g. Peyer's patches) for immunological processing.

- Dendritic cell—T cell interactions are critical for the induction and maintenance of antigen tolerance.

- Pattern recognition receptors, such as TLRs, discriminate between different microbial species within the gut and receptor signaling shapes both the innate and adaptive immune response.

- Environment factors, such as the commensal flora, promote and condition mucosal immunity.

Introduction

The gastrointestinal tract is home to the largest accumulation of leukocytes in the body, where they are constantly being exposed to a wide array of foreign antigens. Complex signaling networks between multiple cell types ensure that the appropriate balance is maintained between immune protection from infection and tolerance of harmless antigens, such as the resident bacterial flora. Disturbance of this balance results in inappropriate immune activation, as observed in patients with Inflammatory Bowel Disease.

The small intestine is highly adapted to facilitate immunological sampling of intestinal contents. Specialized epithelial cells, M cells, actively transport

Intestinal Failure: Diagnosis, Management and Transplantation.
Edited by Alan N. Langnas, Olivier Goulet, Eamonn M.M. Quigley and Kelly A. Tappenden. © 2008 Blackwell Publishing.
ISBN 978-1-4051-4637-1.

antigen to underlying lymphoid follicles for immunological processing, whereas dendritic cells extend dendrites between epithelial cells in order to sample adherent bacterial species. This chapter will focus on the mechanisms by which the intestinal immune system samples luminal antigen and the controlling features that determine immunological tolerance. This phenomenon is still poorly described in the noninflamed human small intestine and a significant portion of our understanding of small intestinal immunology described here is derived from animal models and resected diseased tissue.

Cellular organization of the mucosal immune system

The gut mucosal immune system is constantly stimulated by luminal contents and bacteria, keeping it in a state of controlled "physiological" inflammation. Whereas its primary function is to protect the epithelial surfaces and the underlying tissues from potentially harmful environmental agents and microorganisms, the mucosal immune system must also tolerate nonharmful antigens and commensal microorganisms. The ability to tolerate a wide range of exogenous antigens is a unique feature of the mucosal system that is not seen with the systemic immune system [1]. Immunological tolerance is defined as specific immunological nonreactivity to a specific antigen resulting from a previous exposure to the same antigen. This process is accomplished by specific cell types within the intestine (e.g. regulatory T cells) and will be discussed in more detail later in this chapter.

The mucosal immune system is organised into organised and diffuse gut associated lymphoid tissues (GALT). The organized GALT includes Peyer's patches,

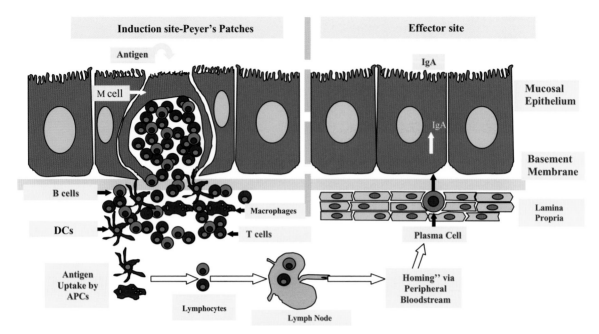

Figure 4.1 Antigen is actively sampled by M cells overlying Peyer's patches. Antigen presenting cells within the Peyer's patch prime T and B lymphocytes, which migrate to draining lymph nodes. Effector cells, such as plasma cells, return to intestinal sites to exert their protective functions.

mesenteric lymph nodes, and solitary lymphoid follicles in the gut wall where antigen uptake, processing, and presentation are facilitated (Figure 4.1). In contrast, diffuse GALT is a nonorganized system whereby individual cells, such as intra-epithelial lymphocytes (IELs), are dispersed throughout nonlymphoid tissue. Finally, epithelial cells themselves provide a barrier to antigen translocation and actively participate as sensors of luminal contents via the expression of toll-like receptors (TLRs).

Organized GALT

Peyer's patches are aggregates of lymphoid tissue found predominantly in the terminal ileum and can contain multiple lymphoid follicles. An average adult has approximately 200 Peyer's patches. The Peyer's patch has the classical anatomical appearance of a secondary lymphoid organ, with defined T and B cell regions (Figure 4.2). The Peyer's patch can be divided into five distinct compartments.

a Follicle associated epithelium (FAE). The FAE that overlies the Peyer's patch contains enterocytes and M cells, so-called because of the microfold or membra-

nous structure of their apical surface. These specialized cells lack certain brush border enzymes and readily transport luminal substances across the epithelial barrier to underlying lymphoid cells. Goblet cells are noticeably absent from the FAE, thereby, ensuring that mucus does not hamper the attachment of luminal antigens to the surface of M cells. M cells take up antigen by endocytosis and transport is via a transcellular rather than a paracellular route [2].

b Subepithelial dome. The dome is located above the follicle and consists of lymphocytes and dendritic cells.

c Lymphoid follicle. These are located below the muscularis mucosae and consist of germinal centres containing proliferating B cells, follicular dendritic cells, and macrophages.

d Corona. The corona surrounds the follicle and consists of lymphocytes expressing IgM and IgD on their cell surface.

e Interfollicular region. This area is characterized by the presence of high endothelial venules surrounded by lymphocytes, primarily T cells.

Antigens transported across M cells are sampled by the dendritic cells residing beneath the subepithelial dome region underlying the FAE. Dendritic cell

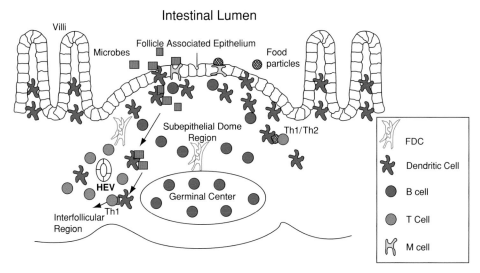

Figure 4.2 The anatomical appearance of the Peyer's patch resembles that of a classical secondary lymphoid follicle.

sampling of antigen in the Peyer's patch is believed to be a critical step in the induction of adaptive immunity [3]. Three different dendritic cell populations have been identified within the mouse Peyer's patch. CD11b+ dendritic cells are present within the subepithelial dome region and primarily secrete IL-10 on *in vitro* stimulation [4]. CD8$\alpha\alpha$+ dendritic cells reside within the T cell-rich interfollicular region, whereas double negative dendritic cells (CD11b and CD8$\alpha\alpha$ negative) are found throughout the Peyer's patch. CD8$\alpha\alpha$+ dendritic cells and double negative dendritic cells share functional characteristics, as both secrete IL-12 and induce predominantly Th1 responses. Recruitment of dendritic cells to the Peyer's patch is accomplished by secretion of the chemokines CCL19 and CCL21, which trigger the dendritic cell-expressed chemokine receptor CCR7. Only CD11b+ dendritic cells express CCR6, which ensures their migration to the CCR6 ligand, CCL20, which is secreted by the FAE [5]. The precise mechanism(s) by which dendritic cells coordinate the initiation of polarized immune responses to defined oral antigens *in vivo* is still unclear and warrants further investigation.

Antigens sampled within the Peyer's patch are transported via antigen presenting cells to the mesenteric lymph nodes (MLNs). Within the MLNs, interactions between dendritic cells, T cells and B cells occur resulting in the induction of protective mucosal immunity or tolerance. Dendritic cells containing live commensal micro-organisms have been detected within MLNs and these dendritic cells are restricted to the mucosal immune compartment by the barrier function of the MLNs [6]. This allows a mucosal immune response to occur without inducing unnecessary systemic immunity to these organisms. Provided MLNs are intact, the result of repeated intestinal commensal priming is to induce IgA selectively and locally, thereby, forming one of the layers of the mucosal barrier that limits bacterial penetration.

Diffuse GALT

The diffuse GALT is comprised of IELs and lamina propria mononuclear cells. IELs are a specialized subset of T cells, which are predominantly CD8+ and a significant percentage express the $\gamma\delta$ T cell receptor. $\gamma\delta$ T cells have a restricted T cell receptor (TCR) repertoire, compared to conventional $\alpha\beta$ T cells, which may be driven, in part, by the cytokine IL-15 [7]. As their name suggests, these cells are found between epithelial cells and are dispersed along the entire length of the intestinal tract. Their exact role in intestinal immunity is unclear but studies suggest that, because of their interaction with intestinal epithelial cells, they contribute to the generation of the suppressor T cells necessary for the maintenance of gut homeostasis as well as promoting gut healing following injury [8]. Inappropriate IEL activity can result in pathology, such as that observed in celiac disease [9]. In this instance, gluten exposure results in increased levels of IL-15, which up-regulates NKG2D receptor expression on IELs and MICA (MHC class I related A protein) expression on enterocytes. The interaction between these receptors results in enterocyte death and immune pathology.

In addition to IELs, dendritic cells are found to associate with epithelial cells [10]. Dendritic cells open the tight junctions between epithelial cells, send dendrites outside the epithelium, and directly sample bacteria. Because of their ability to express tight-junction proteins such as occludin, claudin 1, and zonula occludens 1, dendritic cell sampling ensures that the integrity of the epithelial barrier is preserved. This provides for an additional antigen sampling system to directly assess the bacterial species adherent to the epithelial cells.

Within the lamina propria, a complex mixture of lymphoid cells is present including macrophages, dendritic cells, mast cells, neutrophils, eosinophils, T cells, and B cells. These are primarily effector cells that have been activated within lymphoid follicles and have been recruited to the mucosa via the circulatory system. Terminally differentiated B cells produce vast amounts of the immunoglobulin IgA, which is transported via epithelial cells into the lumen. Secretory IgA (sIgA) is the most important immunoglobulin in the intestine and is a major contributor to the generation of mucosal adaptive immunity to luminal micro-organisms. Approximately 3 g of sIgA are delivered into the human intestinal lumen each day [11]. It is believed that sIgA inhibits interactions between bacteria and epithelial cells by binding potential pathogens and preventing them from attaching to the underlying epithelial layer [12]. IgA antibodies cannot bind complement and therefore do not have the ability to elicit an inflammatory response. In addition, sIgA facilitates the removal of antigen from the host by trapping it within the mucus layer. The immune response to both commensal and pathogenic organisms results in sIgA production but only the response to pathogens activates pro-inflammatory lymphocytes.

Epithelial cells

Although epithelial cells mediate nutrient absorption for the host, these cells also provide essential immunological functions. The tight intercellular junctions between epithelial cells ensure the exclusion of pro-inflammatory substances and microbes from subepithelial tissues. In addition, epithelial cells express a number of receptors (discussed in more detail later in this chapter), which result in the induction of chemokine production when activated by their appropriate ligand. For example, when bacterial flagellin binds TLR5, this interaction results in the secretion of IL8 and CCL20, ensuring rapid recruitment of mononuclear cells to the site of infection. Epithelial cells are thought to actively promote an anti-inflammatory state within the mucosa. Epithelial cell-conditioned dendritic cells release interleukins 10 and 6, but not interleukin 12, and they promote the polarization of T cells toward a T helper type 2 response, even after exposure to a T helper type 1-inducing pathogen [13]. Paneth cells are specialized epithelial cells that reside at the base of the small intestinal crypts of Lieberkuhn. Paneth cells release an array of antimicrobial molecules including α-defensins. α-defensins are cationic antimicrobial peptides containing three disulphide bonds, which disrupt the membrane integrity of target microbes. Paneth cell-derived antimicrobial molecules protect host cells from ingested pathogens by limiting the numbers of microbes colonizing the crypts and lumen. Interestingly, decreased levels of Paneth cell-derived α-defensins have been observed in patients with Crohn's disease affecting the ileum but not in Crohn's patients with disease limited to the colon [14], implicating impaired α-defensin production as a susceptibility factor for ileal Crohn's disease.

The molecular basis underpinning antigen recognition

In addition to the well-described antigen presentation system of the adaptive immune system, which results in the clonal expansion of antigen specific lymphocytes, the initial phase of the host response to antigens involves pattern recognition receptors (PRRs) that recognize evolutionary conserved microbial structures. Stimulation of different PRRs induces distinct patterns of gene expression, which not only leads to the activation of innate immunity but also instructs the development of antigen-specific acquired immunity. A number of PRRs are expressed by epithelial cells but they are more broadly expressed by macrophages and dendritic cells. There are a number of receptor types.

Table 4.1 Ligands recognized by each of the toll-like receptors.

	Activating Ligand
TLR-1	Tri-acyl bacterial lipoprotein
TLR-2	Peptidoglycan, Lipoteichoic acid
TLR-3	Double-stranded RNA
TLR-4	Lipopolysaccharide
TLR-5	Flagellin
TLR-6	Di-acyl bacterial lipoprotein
TLR-7	Single strand RNA
TLR-8	Single strand RNA
TLR-9	Unmethylated CpG DNA
TLR-10	Unknown
TLR-11	Uropathogenic bacteria

Toll-like receptors (TLRs) are phylogenetically conserved receptors that recognize pathogen associated molecular patterns (PAMPs). At least 11 members of the TLR family are known and they recognize a number of different components of bacteria and viruses (Table 4.1). Dendritic cells express TLRs and TLR signaling triggers dendritic cell maturation, which leads to the up-regulation of MHC and co-stimulatory molecules and the expression of pro-inflammatory cytokines. It is through this maturation process that dendritic cells acquire their unique ability to prime naïve T cells. Different types of dendritic cells (i.e. myeloid and plasmacytoid) express distinct arrays of TLRs, supporting the concept that they have developed through distinct evolutionary pathways to recognize different microbial antigens [15]. Intestinal epithelial cells express a number of TLRs including TLR4, TLR5, and TLR9. TLR4 recognises lipopolysaccharide (LPS—a component of the outer membrane of gram-negative bacteria), bacterial CPG DNA is the ligand for TLR9, whereas TLR5 binds flagellin. TLRs also play an important role in maintaining epithelial integrity, thus contributing to the mutualistic relationship that exists between the commensal flora and the gut epithelium. For example, epithelial cell recognition of TLR2 or TLR9 ligands strengthens gut barrier function. In addition, colonic epithelial cells in mice deficient in MyD88 (TLR intracellular adaptor protein) fail to express the cytoprotective proteins hsp25 and hsp72. As a result, these mice are highly susceptible to a chemically induced inflammatory bowel disease.

The intracellular signaling pathways activated by TLR ligands are still under investigation but the current published data can be summarized as follows (Figure 4.3). All TLRs have an extracellular region, which contains leucine-rich repeat motifs, and a cytoplasmic tail, which has a Toll/interleukin-1(IL-1) receptor (TIR) domain. TLR-signaling pathways originate from the TIR domain, as a result of its recruitment of TIR-domain-containing adaptors—such as MyD88 (myeloid differentiation primary-response protein 88), TIRAP (TIR-domain-containing adaptor protein), TRIF (TIR-domain-containing adaptor protein inducing interferon), and TRAM (TRIF-related adaptor molecule). Recruitment of these adaptors to the TIR domains initiates a signaling cascade through IL-1R associated kinases (IRAKs) and the adaptor TRAF-6, which, in turn, activate protein kinase cascades culminating in the activation of NF-κB and the mitogen activated protein (MAP) kinases p38, INK, and ERK1/2. Signaling through each TLR requires MyD88 for the production of inflammatory cytokines. However, a MyD88-independent pathway exists, and following signaling through TLR3 or TLR4, it leads to the production of type I interferons. TRIF is essential for the MyD88-independent pathway of TLR3 and TLR4 signaling, as well as for the TLR4-mediated production of inflammatory cytokines. TRAM is involved specifically in the TLR4-mediated, MyD88-independent pathway, whereas TIRAP mediates the TLR2- and TLR4-mediated, MyD88-dependent pathway. The TLR-signaling pathways are negatively regulated by TLR-inducible molecules—such as IRAK-M (IL-1-receptor (IL-1R)-associated kinase M), SOCS1 (suppressor of cytokine signaling 1), MyD88s (MyD88 short), SIGIRR (single immunoglobulin IL-1R-related molecule), and ST2 [16]. These negative regulators operate via multiple mechanisms. MyD88s prevents IRAK-4 recruitment, whereas IRAK-M also interferes with IRAK function by preventing IRAK dissociation from the signalling complex. ST2 negatively regulates NF-κB activation through TLR2, TLR4, and TLR9, but not TLR3 by sequestration of the downstream adaptor molecules MyD88 and Mal. SIGIRR also seems to operate via sequestration of signaling molecules, thus preventing further signal propagation. These mechanisms of down-regulating TLR activation are important for the appropriate activation of the host response to bacteria, thus avoiding excessive damage to the host.

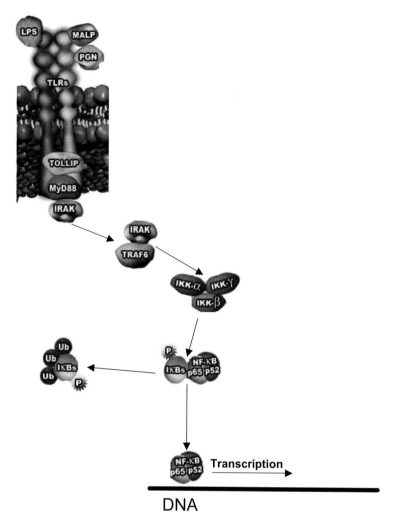

Figure 4.3 TLR signaling activates NF-κB via multiple intracellular events. Recruitment of the adaptors MyD88, IRAK, and TRAF-6 results in IKK kinase activation. The IKK complex phosphorylates the NF-κB inhibitor IκB resulting in its removal from NF-κB and is targeted for proteosomal degradation. The free NF-κB translocates into the nucleus and initiates transcription of target genes.

Their role in maintaining mucosal tolerance has yet to be elucidated.

The second class of PRRs are the nucleotide-binding oligomerization domain (Nod) molecules, Nod 1 and Nod 2 (also referred to as Caspase Activation and Recruit Domain (CARD) 4 and CARD 15). These are found in the cytosol of epithelial and immune cells. Nod1/CARD4 recognises a muropeptide motif mainly derived from gram-negative bacterial peptidoglycan, whereas Nod2/CARD15 detects a muramyl dipeptide that is common to a wide variety of bacteria. The identification of Nod2 as a susceptibility gene for Crohn's disease highlights the potential role of pattern-recognition

receptors and their ligands in diseases such as IBD [17].

Antigen presenting cells, such as dendritic cells, express C-type lectin receptors (CLRs), which bind carbohydrate structures that are present on a variety of pathogens and host cells. Based on their molecular structures, they include two types of receptors: type I C-type lectin (a type I transmembrane protein with several carbohydrate recognition domains [CRDs]) and type II C-type lectin (a type II transmembrane protein with a single CRD). Both types are considered to function mainly as pattern recognition receptors for antigen capture and, additionally, play a role in

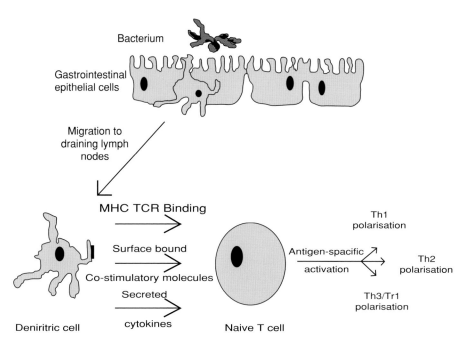

Bacterium

Gastrointestinal
epithelial cells

Migration to
draining lymph
nodes

MHC TCR Binding

Surface bound

Co-stimulatory molecules

Secreted

Deniritric cell   cytokines   Naive T cell

Antigen-spacific
activation

Th1
polarisation

Th2
polarisation

Th3/Tr1
polarisation

Figure 4.4 Dendritic within the gut directly sample luminal contents and present the antigen to T cells (MHC-TCR interactions). In addition, dendritic cells provide further information to the T cell concerning the nature of the antigen being presented via surface bound receptor-ligand interactions and the secretion of cytokines. Responding T cells are thereby instructed to differentiate into Th1, Th2, or Th3/Tr1 cells.

interactions between dendritic cells and other cells. Typically, immune activation does not ensue on antigen binding to CLRs; rather, these receptors induce immune tolerance by default, and require simultaneous signaling through TLRs. Although multiple CLRs can be expressed by dendritic cells, the best described is the type II receptor Dendritic Cell Specific ICAM-3-Grabbing Non-integrin (DC-SIGN or CD209). DC-SIGN recognizes viruses such as HIV-1 and Ebola, but also recognizes bacteria such as *Mycobacterium tuberculosis* and *Lactobacillus casei* [18].

Cellular basis of immunological tolerance

The effector mechanisms that have evolved to protect the host from invading pathogens could, if unregulated, also result in a potentially lethal immune response. Therefore, powerful controlling mechanisms must be in place to protect from inappropriate immune activation.

Antigen presenting cells are important for inducing immune responses and for the maintenance of tolerance (Figure 4.4). Dendritic cells that express antigen, but do not express adequate levels of co-stimulatory molecules, induce T cell anergy. However, experimental evidence suggests that this type of antigen presentation alone does not result in long-term functional unresponsiveness. In addition, dendritic cells can express ligands, which preferentially engage inhibitory receptors on T cells. PD-1 and CTLA-4 are two such receptors that may promote T cell tolerance [19]. The mechanism by which triggering of these receptors results in T cell tolerance is unknown but is related in part to the level of stimulatory ligand expression by dendritic cells and the production of cytokines such as IL-2 and IL-10. Interestingly, engagement of the dendritic cell receptor DC-SIGN by *Lactobacillus casei*, a commensal bacterium, results in a dendritic cell phenotype that promotes T regulatory cells, thus implicating this signaling system as a potent mechanism for the induction of tolerance to the commensal flora.

The ability of CD25$^+$ regulatory T cells (Treg) cells to inhibit immune pathology has been well documented in animal models. Naturally occurring Tregs are found in peripheral lymphoid organs and constitute 5–15% of peripheral CD4$^+$ T cells in the naïve mouse and 1–2% of circulating CD4+ T cells in humans. They constitutively express the α chain of the interleukin-2 (IL-2) receptor, otherwise known as CD25, and are thought to arise directly from the thymus because thymectomized mice develop multi-organ autoimmune disease 3 days after birth. In addition to expressing CD25, Treg cells also express the $\alpha\beta$ T cell receptor. The transcription factor Foxp3 is a unique feature of CD4+CD25+ Tregs, which distinguishes them from CD4+CD25− T cells. Foxp3 is required for Treg cell development and function while its expression in nonregulatory cells is sufficient to drive a suppressor phenotype [20]. Another distinguishing feature of CD25$^+$ Treg cells is their inability to produce the T cell growth factor IL-2. Indeed, Treg cells will inhibit IL-2 production by non-Treg responder T lymphocytes *in vitro* effectively halting T cell proliferation and clonal expansion. Typically, CD4$^+$CD25$^+$ T cells are in an activated state (CD45RA$^-$RO$^+$) and are continuously interacting with their environment.

In addition to naturally occurring CD4$^+$CD25$^+$ Treg cells, inducible regulatory T cells such as $T_{Reg}1$ (T_R1) or T helper type 3 (T_H3) cells have been described. T_R1 cells primarily secrete IL-10 with low amounts of IL-4 and TGF-β and have been shown to suppress macrophage production of pro-inflammatory cytokines as well as preventing the development of Th1 effector cells [21]. Co-transfer of murine T_R1 clones prevented the development of colitis in susceptible murine models. Antigen-induced activation of the T_R1 cells *in vivo* was required for this immunosuppression, as colitis was only inhibited in recipients receiving ovalbumin in their drinking water. T helper type 3 cells also arise after oral administration of antigen and can prevent development of immune pathology in animal models by producing high amounts of TGF-β and low amounts of IL-10, IL-4, and IFN-γ. Thus, regulatory T cells, not only arise in the thymus in response to self-antigen but also can be generated in the mucosal immune system, ensuring tolerance to harmless antigens.

Both cell contact–dependent and –independent mechanisms have been described for the immune suppressive activity of CD25+ Tregs. CTLA-4 cell surface expression counteracts the stimulating effects of CD28 ligation thus preventing T cell proliferation and cytokine production. Indeed, tolerance cannot be induced in CTLA-4 deficient mice [22]. CD25$^+$ Treg interaction with dendritic cells promotes the production of indolemine 2,3 dioxygenase which prevents effector T cells from responding to antigen [23]. The production of immunosuppressive cytokines plays a key role in mediating CD25$^+$ Treg suppression *in vivo* as pretreatment with anti-IL-10R or anti-TGF-β antibodies prevented their ability to inhibit colitis in a susceptible animal model [24]. There is convincing evidence that IL-10 and TGF-β are growth factors for Treg cells. Treg cells can be cloned *in vitro* by inclusion of IL-10 in the culture medium. Using a mechanism dependent on IL-10 and TGF-β, these clones were able to suppress antigen-specific activation of T cells *in vitro*, as well as being able to prevent development of colitis in mice lacking their own regulatory T cells. The majority of studies examining regulatory T cell activity have used animal models and whether any dysfunction in human regulatory T cells is associated with a breakdown in immunological tolerance in humans is unclear. Nevertheless, the development of strategies to enhance T regulatory cell activity and numbers for treatment of mucosal inflammatory activity are warranted.

Immune function in intestinal failure

Although it is clear from this discussion that the intestinal immune system has powerful controlling mechanisms in place that protect against damaging inflammatory responses, immune mediated disorders do occur in susceptible individuals. Crohn's disease and ulcerative colitis, collectively referred to as inflammatory bowel disease (IBD), are chronic aggressive disorders, with distinct features. Ulcerative colitis is characterized by inflammation with superficial ulcerations limited to the mucosa of the colon. Inflammation usually starts in the rectum and continuously spreads throughout the large intestine. Crohn's disease, however, is characterized by a discontinuous pattern, potentially affecting the entire gastrointestinal tract. In contrast to ulcerative colitis, inflammation in Crohn's disease patients is transmural with large ulcerations and occasionally granulomas are observed. Genetic factors, immune system responsiveness and environmental factors (such as the composition and metabolic activity of the gut flora) are all believed to play a role in the progression of these inflammatory states. Specific polymorphisms in the NOD2 gene are associated with susceptibility to Crohn's disease [25]. Although the exact role of this mutation in Crohn's disease remains unclear, NOD2 mutations may lead to an ineffective immune response to bacterial components and ineffective clearance of intracellular bacteria in human intestinal epithelia resulting in mucosal inflammation [26]. Experimental animal models of both Crohn's-like and colitis-like disease have revealed some of the mediators responsible for intestinal inflammation. IL-10 knock out mice spontaneously develop colitis, as do mice deficient in regulatory CD4/CD25 positive T cells [27]. Colonization with an enteric flora is required for full expression of disease. Indeed, the gastrointestinal flora is a common factor driving the inflammatory process, irrespective of the underlying genetic predisposition and immunological effector mechanism. The enteric flora may drive intestinal inflammation in susceptible individuals via disruption of the mucosal barrier (allowing increased uptake of luminal antigens), mimicry of self-antigens and activation of the mucosal immune system via modulation of transcription factors such as NF-κB. The linkage between the presence of bacteria and mucosal inflammation is supported by the observation that interruption of the faecal stream has been associated with clinical improvement. Crohn's disease lesions can be induced by direct instillation of faecal contents into apparently unaffected loops of bowel in susceptible individuals [28]. Thus, inflammatory bowel disease can be viewed as the consequence of loss of immunological tolerance to components of the gastrointestinal flora, which is reflected in patient serology and cellular immune reactivity to enteric flora antigens [29].

Enhanced mucosal permeability is thought to play a pivotal role in the maintenance of a chronic inflammatory state such as that seen in patients with IBD and graft versus host disease. Barrier function is mediated, in part, by the presence of the epithelial cell plasma membrane, whereas the paracellular space is sealed by the tight junction. Certain tight junction proteins such as claudins and occludin have been identified, whereas the identity and role of many others remain enigmatic. The tight junction complex is intimately interconnected with cytoskeletal elements which stabilize the tight junction and may be critical for its regulation. Tight junction permeability is plastic and is responsive to physiological, infectious and immunological signals [30]. For example, the physiological response to glucose includes a drop in paracellular permeability as a result of actomyosin contraction. Certain bacteria (e.g. enteropathogenic E Coli, EPEC) hijack this response by directly inducing myosin light chain phosphorylation, resulting in diminished barrier function. In addition, pro-inflammatory cytokines such as TNF-α and IFN-γ influence myosin phosphorylation leading to barrier dysfunction. Thus, one can visualize a model for colitis involving reduced barrier function, which allows bacteria access to the lamina propria, resulting in immune activation and involving pro-inflammatory cytokines, which further confounds tight junction integrity thereby locking the intestinal system into an inflammatory cycle of intestinal leakiness and immune activation. Usually, anti-inflammatory mediators such as IL-10 and TGF-β limit this cascade but, in genetically susceptible individuals, intestinal leakiness may result in colitis. In the case of graft versus host disease, the gastrointestinal tract is not only a target organ but is also a critical amplifier of systemic symptoms primarily because of the loss of barrier function [31]. Chemotherapy and radiotherapy damage the gastrointestinal epithelium allowing endotoxin penetration and activation of host macrophages resulting in pro-inflammatory cytokine secretion. Cytokine secretion by activated host cells further impairs barrier function while also promoting donor Th1 T cell cytotoxicity mediated via Fas and perforin pathways.

The intestine remains the most difficult organ to transplant due primarily to the unique immunological challenges that the intestinal environment encounters. The lymphoid content of the intestine is significant (i.e. mesenteric lymph nodes, GALT and mucosal lymphocytes) and is directly responsible for graft versus host disease [32]. However, although depletion of lymphoid tissue from the graft reduces the risk of graft versus host disease, this is not accompanied by a reduced risk of organ rejection. This is, in part, a result of the presence of endotoxin, which crosses the impaired mucosal barrier and drives the inflammatory response, as outlined above. In addition, the epithelial cells themselves may function as antigen presenting cells in such an environment resulting in immune activation. It is essential to promote the development of regulatory or tolerogenic lymphocytes in order to preserve intestinal integrity. However, the signals required are only beginning to be elucidated. Interestingly, high dose immunosuppression can be counterproductive and new lower dose immunosuppressive protocols have had some success suggesting that a certain level of immunological signaling within the gut facilitates tolerance [33].

Influence of the bacterial flora on intestinal immune activity

The single most important environmental factor that impacts on intestinal immune signaling is the presence of micro-organisms. Although most studies have focused on the gut's immune response to pathogens, exposure to pathogens is, in reality, a rare occurrence in the gut in contrast to its lifelong coexistence with vast numbers of nonpathogenic micro-organisms. Studies in germ-free (GF) mice have revealed dramatic alterations in the anatomy and function of both the mucosal and systemic immune compartments [34]. GF mice have hypoplastic Peyer's patches that contain few germinal centres, as well as greatly reduced numbers of IgA-producing plasma cells and lamina propria CD4+ T cells. The lymph nodes and spleen are poorly organized and the mice are hypogammaglobulinaemic. Acquisition of a bacterial flora results in the normalization of these abnormalities. Thus, the commensal bacteria drive and condition the mucosal immune system.

This observation has led investigators to further examine the therapeutic potential of specific bacterial species in driving regulatory immune responses within the mucosa. Murine studies have demonstrated that the deliberate administration of commensal, or probiotic, bacteria to susceptible colitis models results in reduced inflammatory activity associated with reduced pro-inflammatory cytokine production and a maintenance of regulatory cytokine production [35]. This suggests that certain bacterial strains can drive immunoregulatory responses via direct interaction with the mucosal immune system. In humans, dendritic cells isolated from mesenteric lymph nodes preferentially secrete the regulatory cytokines IL-10 and TGF-β when co-incubated with commensal bacterial, although the same dendritic cells preferentially secrete pro-inflammatory cytokines, but not regulatory

cytokines, when exposed to the pathogenic organism *Salmonella typhimurium* [36]. This suggests that intestinal dendritic cells exposed to commensal organisms *in vivo* may drive development of regulatory T cell activity resulting in improved immunological tolerance.

Clinical studies in humans assessing the impact of probiotic consumption on the symptoms of IBD are conflicting and are often confounded by small numbers [37]. However, the best evidence for probiotic efficacy in patients with IBD has been seen with a cocktail of eight different strains, which effectively maintains remission in patients with pouchitis. Probiotic treatments also have been examined for the treatment of IBS. Although the majority of bacterial strains examined have no demonstrable efficacy, consumption of one commensal bacterium *Bifidobacterium infantis* 35624 resulted in significant improvement of symptoms [38]. Interestingly, an imbalance in cytokine signaling networks observed in IBS patients was normalised by *Bifidobacterium infantis* 35624 consumption, suggesting an association between probiotic-induced immunoregulation and clinical efficacy.

These studies and others promote the further investigation of commensal micro-organisms for the treatment of mucosal disease, in particular, where a breakdown in tolerance is suspected. However, the mechanism of action of probiotics is uncertain and is likely to depend on the individual strain itself and the clinical condition for which it is used.

Conclusions

Immunity is traditionally defined as host resistance against disease caused by reinfection with the same agent. However, the small intestine is exposed to a wide variety of antigens that do not cause disease. Therefore, when considering immunity within the small intestine, it is important to understand the type of immune response required for this unique environment. The development of mucosal tolerance during evolution ensures that certain protective responses can be generated (e.g. sIgA) and damaging pro-inflammatory responses simultaneously avoided. Although the cellular and molecular basis for this phenomena are still poorly understood, the deliberate induction of antigen tolerance within the intestine may be of therapeutic benefit to patients suffering from gastrointestinal and autoimmune disorders.

References

1 Brandtzaeg P, Pabst R. Let's go mucosal: communication on slippery ground. *Trends Immunol* 2004;25:570–577.

2 Gebert A, Rothkotter HJ, Pabst R. M cells in Peyer's patches of the intestine. *Int Rev Cytol* 1996;167:91–159.

3 Brandtzaeg P, Baekkevold ES, Farstad IN, et al. Regional specialization in the mucosal immune system: what happens in the micro-compartments? *Immunol Today* 1999;20:141–151.

4 Iwasaki A, Kelsall BL. Unique functions of CD11b+, CD8 alpha+, and double-negative Peyer's patch dendritic cells. *J Immunol* 2001;166:4884–4890.

5 Iwasaki A, Kelsall BL. Localisation of distinct Peyer's patch dendritic cell subsets and their recruitment by chemokines macrophage inflammatory protein (MIP)-3alpha, MIP-3beta, and secondary lymphoid organ chemokine. *J Exp Med* 2000;191:1381–1394.

6 Macpherson AJ, Uhr T. Induction of protective IgA by intestinal dendritic cells carrying commensal bacteria. *Science* 2004;303:1662–1665.

7 Zhao H, Nguyen H, Kang J. Interleukin 15 controls the generation of the restricted T cell receptor repertoire of gamma delta intestinal intraepithelial lymphocytes. *Nat Immunol* 2005;6:1263–1271.

8 Hayday A, Theodoridis E, Ramsburg E, Shires J. Intraepithelial lymphocytes: exploring the Third Way in immunology. *Nat Immunol* 2001;2:997–1003.

9 Koning F. Celiac disease: caught between a rock and a hard place. *Gastroenterology* 2005;129:1294–1301.

10 Rescigno M, Urbano M, Valzasina B, et al. Dendritic cells express tight junction proteins and penetrate gut epithelial monolayers to sample bacteria. *Nat Immunol* 2001;2:361–367.

11 Conley ME, Delacroix DL. Intravascular and mucosal immunoglobulin A two separate but related systems of immune defense? *Ann Intern Med* 1987;106:892–899.

12 Macpherson AJ, Hunziker L, McCoy K, Lamarre A. IgA responses in the intestinal mucosa against pathogenic and non-pathogenic microorganisms. *Microbes Infect* 2001;3:1021–1035.

13 Rimoldi M, Chieppa M, Salucci V, et al. Intestinal immune homeostasis is regulated by the crosstalk between epithelial cells and dendritic cells. *Nat Immunol* 2005;6:507–514.

14 Wehkamp J, Harder J, Weichenthal M, et al. NOD2 (CARD15) mutations in Crohn's disease are associated with diminished mucosal alpha-defensin expression. *Gut* 2004;53:1658–1664.

15 Kadowaki N, Ho S, Antonenko S, et al. Subsets of human dendritic cell precursors express different toll-like receptors and respond to different microbial antigens. *J Exp Med* 2001;194:863–869.

16 Liew FY, Xu D, Brint EK, O'Neill LA. Negative regulation of toll-like receptor-mediated immune responses. *Nat Rev Immunol* 2005;5:446–458.

17 Inohara N, Ogura Y, Fontalba A, et al. Host recognition of bacterial muramyl dipeptide mediated through NOD2: implications for Crohn's disease. *J Biol Chem* 2003;275:5509–5512.

18 Koppel EA, van Gisbergen K, Geijtenbeek TBH, van Kooyk Y. Distinct functions of DC-SIGN and its homologues L-SIGN (DC-SIGNR) and mSIGNR1 in pathogen recognition and immune regulation. *Cell Microbiol* 2005;7:157–165.

19 Probst HC, McCoy K, Okazaki T, Honjo T, van den Broek M. Resting dendritic cells induce peripheral CD8+ T cell tolerance through PD-1 and CTLA-4. *Nat Immuol* 2005;6:280–286.

20 Fontenot JD, Gavin MA, Rudensky AY. Foxp3 programs the development and function of CD4+CD25+ regulatory T cells. *Nat Immunol* 2003;4:330–336.

21 Thorstenson KM, Khoruts A. Generation of anergic and potentially immunoregulatory CD25+CD4 T cells in vivo after induction of peripheral tolerance with intravenous or oral antigen. *J Immunol* 2001;167:188–195.

22 Greenwald RJ, Boussiotis VA, Lorsbach RB, Abbas AK, Sharpe AH. CTLA-4 regulates induction of anergy in vivo. *Immunity* 2001;14:145–155.

23 Mellor AL, Chandler P, Baban B, et al. Specific subsets of murine dendritic cells acquire potent T cell regulatory functions following CTLA4-mediated induction of indoleamine 2,3 dioxygenase. *Int Immunol* 2004;23:1391–1401.

24 Powrie F, Carlino J, Leach MW, Mauze S, Coffman RL. A critical role for transforming growth factor-beta but not interleukin 4 in the suppression of T helper type 1-mediated colitis by CD45RB(low) CD4+ T cells. *J Exp Med* 1996;183:2669–2674.

25 Hugot JP, Chamaillard M, Zouali H, et al. Association of NOD2 leucine-rich variants with susceptibility to Crohn's disease. *Nature* 2001;411:599–603.

26 Hisamatsu T, Suzuki M, Reinecker HC, et al. CARD15/NOD2 Functions as an antibacterial factor in human intestinal epithelial cells. *Gastroenterology* 2003;124:993–1000.

27 Wirtz S, Neyrath MF. Animal models of intestinal inflammation: new insights into the molecular

pathogenesis and immunotherapy of inflammatory bowel disease. *Int J Colorectal Dis* 2000;15:144–160.

28 D'Haens GR, Geboes K, Peeters M, et al. Early lesions of recurrent Crohn's disease caused by infusion of intestinal contents in excluded ileum. *Gastroenterology* 1998;114:262–267.

29 Duchmann R, Kaiser I, Mayet W, et al. Tolerance exists towards resident intestinal flora but is broken in active inflammatory bowel disease (IBD). *Clin Exp Immunol* 1995;102:448–455.

30 Clayburgh DR, Shen L, Turner JR. A porous defense: the leaky epithelial barrier in intestinal disease. *Lab Invest* 2004;84:282–291.

31 Iwasaki T. Recent advances in the treatment of Graft-Versus-Host Disease. *Clin Med Res* 2004;2:243–252.

32 Pirenne J, Kawai M. Tolerogenic protocols for intestinal transplantation. *Transplant Immunol* 2004;13:131–137.

33 Pirenne J, Koshiba T, Geboes K. Complete freedom from rejection after intestinal transplantation using a new tolerogenic protocol combined with low immunosuppression. *Transplantation* 2002;73:966–968.

34 Macpherson AJ, Harris N. Interactions between commensal intestinal bacteria and the immune system. *Nat Rev Immunol* 2004;4:478–485.

35 McCarthy J, O'Mahony L, O'Callaghan L, et al. Double blind, placebo controlled trial of two probiotic strains in interleukin 10 knockout mice and mechanistic link with cytokine balance. *Gut* 2003;52:975–980.

36 O'Mahony L, O'Callaghan L, McCarthy J, et al. Differential cytokine response from dendritic cells to commensal and pathogenic bacteria in different lymphoid compartments in humans. *Am J Physiol Gastrointest Liver Physiol* 2006;290:839–845.

37 Shanahan F. Probiotics in inflammatory bowel disease—therapeutic rationale and role. *Adv Drug Deliv Rev* 2004;56:809–818.

38 O'Mahony L, McCarthy J, Kelly P, et al. Lactobacillus and bifidobacterium in irritable bowel syndrome: symptom responses and relationship to cytokine profiles. *Gastroenterology* 2005;128:541–551.

5 Intestinal Adaptation

The Biology of the Intestinal Response to Resection and Disease

Marc S. Levin and Deborah C. Rubin

Key points

- The intestinal adaptive response to resection is complex and has been characterized by studies of its structural, functional, cellular and molecular components.

- Parameters of adaptation include intestinal mass, length and thickness, and morphometric measures including villus length, crypt depth and mucosal surface area.

- Alterations in multiple intestinal cell kinetic parameters, including rates of crypt cell proliferation, enterocyte migration and apoptosis, result in the adaptive phenotype.

- Future studies that focus on the molecular and cellular basis of the adaptive response are critical for defining targeted therapies that will enhance structural and functional small bowel surface area following its loss as a result of resection or disease.

Introduction

The small intestine contains a perpetually proliferating and differentiating epithelium that endows it with the ability to regenerate and adapt to the loss of functional surface area. This adaptive response is characterized by crypt cell hyperplasia, villus lengthening, and increased absorptive function. Based on studies in a variety of animal models, it is evident that the underlying mechanisms responsible for the adaptive response share some

Intestinal Failure: Diagnosis, Management and Transplantation.
Edited by Alan N. Langnas, Olivier Goulet, Eamonn M.M. Quigley and Kelly A. Tappenden. © 2008 Blackwell Publishing. ISBN 978-1-4051-4637-1.

common features with those underlying a variety of physiologic and pathophysiological states. Examples include the rapid augmentation of intestinal absorptive capacity that occurs in response to refeeding after starvation, hibernation, or total parenteral nutrition.

There is evidence supporting an adaptive response in humans, however, controlled quantitative and mechanistic analyses are not practical. Therefore, adaptation has been best characterized in rodent, rabbit, pig, and canine resection models. For these experiments, intestinal surface area is reduced by partial resection or bypass and the remnant remaining in continuity is studied at intervals post-op. Using these models, direct comparisons between resected and sham resected animals are feasible. Parameters of adaptation that are commonly used in experimental studies include intestinal mass, length and thickness; morphometric measures, including villus length, crypt depth, and mucosal surface area; and measures reflecting rates of crypt cell proliferation, enterocyte migration, and apoptosis. Although the mechanistic basis of the adaptive response has only been partially elucidated, it is clear that changes in rates of crypt cell proliferation, programmed cell death, and enterocyte migration are important contributors. In addition, there is evidence that individual enterocytes exhibit a more differentiated phenotype resulting in enhanced absorptive capacity per cell (e.g., [1]).

The adaptive response is biphasic in rodent intestinal resection models

There are two phases of the adaptive response [2,3] in rodent intestinal resection models. The early phase

(16 h to 48 h after resection) is characterized by rapid cellular proliferation producing villus lengthening. Some authors have observed an increase in microvillus surface area whereas others have reported decreased microvillar surface area. Increased expression of enterocyte-specific genes such as cellular retinol binding protein II and apolipoprotein A IV also occurs [1]. Significant increases in the overall number and percentage of both Paneth and goblet cells within the intestinal epithelium occur by 12 h [4]. By 48 h, the transport of nutrients such as glucose and glutamine are increased (e.g., [5]). The late phase (at 1–2 weeks, maximum by 4–6 weeks) is characterized by increased functional capacity, increased villus lengthening, and crypt deepening resulting from accelerated cellular proliferation and increased enterocyte migration rates.

Functional response—absorption of fluids, electrolytes and nutrients

Although different species can tolerate different degrees of resection, the ability to survive free of parenteral nutritional support following intestinal resection depends on the magnitude of residual functional intestinal capacity, compensatory mechanisms, and the adaptive restitution. Evidence for functional adaptation in humans includes the observation that parenteral fluid and electrolyte requirements decline with time and many patients are able to be weaned off parenteral nutrition. In addition, when directly studied, intestinal absorption of water and sodium were enhanced in patients after massive small bowel resections when compared to control subjects, (e.g., [6]). Glucose, galactose, and amino acid absorption also improved significantly after resection [7] and calcium absorption continued to increase for more than 2 years after a major bowel resection [8]. Additional support for the presence of an adaptive response in the human intestine is provided by the morphologic and functional changes that occur following segmental small bowel transplants [9,10].

Functional adaptation has been demonstrated and subjected to further study in animal models. These studies suggest that changes in the expression of apical membrane Na/H exchangers (NHEs) NHE2 and NHE3 [11], Na+/glucose cotransporters, such as the apical Na-dependent transporter SGLT1 [12] and the basolat-

eral glucose transporter GLUT2 (unpublished observation Levin MS), all contribute to the enhanced fluid and electrolyte absorption.

Diamond and colleagues have shown, in the rat model, that functional adaptation (at least in terms of glucose transport) is incomplete and is largely the result of increased intestinal surface area resulting from cellular hyperplasia [13]. Nevertheless, the hypothesis that adaptation is the result of simple hyperplasia with elongated villi populated by relatively immature enterocytes has been challenged by studies examining the activities of brush border enzymes and the expression of enterocyte specific genes involved in nutrient trafficking. These studies clearly indicate that there is an enterocyte specific response, which contributes to the absorption of some nutrients [1,14,15]. For example, after jejunal resection ileal enterocytes acquired α-glucosidase activities that were fourfold higher than control cells [14]. Similarly, the expression of many enterocyte-specific genes (e.g. liver fatty acid binding protein, intestinal fatty acid binding protein, apolipoprotein-AIV, ileal lipid binding protein) were all increased in the remnant ileum following submassive small bowel resection [1,15].

An additional important compensatory mechanism is the contribution of the cecal flora which helps to maintain energy balance by salvaging carbohydrates and producing short chain fatty acids. Increased fermentation and increases in cecal mass observed in experimental models of short bowel syndrome suggest that fermentation plays an increased role in energy balance after resection [13].

Mechanisms of adaptation: regulation of crypt cell proliferation and programmed cell death are important mechanisms for intestinal homeostasis and adaptation

Crypt cell proliferation
The gut epithelium is continually renewed by balanced cell proliferation, migration, differentiation, and death. Crypt cell proliferation is markedly increased after partial resection of the proximal small intestine. In rodent resection models, evidence of stimulated proliferation is apparent as early as 12–16 hours postoperatively, (e.g. the proportion of proliferating cells, based on BrdU-labeling increased from 15% to 30% [16]).

Although the extrinsic signals inducing the early increase in proliferation are not well defined, a clear role for intracellular polyamines has been established. Decreasing polyamine synthesis reduces crypt proliferation [17] whereas increasing polyamine levels by stimulating ornithine decarboxylase or inhibiting diamine oxidase activity [18] enhances adaptation. Based on studies in p21 null mice, the mitogenic response to intestinal resection was shown to also require the cyclin-dependent kinase inhibitor p21 (WAF1/CIP1). Furthermore, in vitro studies indicate that the epidermal growth factor receptor mediated induction of enterocyte proliferation is likely mediated by a mitogen-activated protein kinase-dependent increase in p21 [19]. In the p21 null mice, adaptation-induced stimulation of apoptosis still occurred, thus suggesting that proliferation and apoptosis are differentially regulated in the adapting intestine [20,21]. Proadaptive factors such as retinoic acid stimulate proliferation and inhibit apoptosis [16,22–24], whereas others primarily modulate one or the other of these processes. The intestinotrophic effects of glucagon-like peptide-2 (GLP2) in the intact small bowel occur by stimulation of proliferation and inhibition of apoptosis, whereas, the proadaptive effects of GLP2 after partial small bowel resection appear to be primarily due to stimulation of proliferation.

Apoptosis

In most resection models of intestinal adaptation, crypt cell apoptosis is increased in the adapting remnant intestine. Apoptosis occurring in the crypts presumably functions to remove damaged stem cells and regulate cell numbers. As cells migrate toward the villus tip, cell position and interactions with the extracellular environment influence the initiation of apoptosis and/or anoikis (i.e. cell death initiated after loss of contact with the extracellular matrix [ECM] or changes in the interaction with the ECM) [25]. However, as a result of methodological differences, there is conflicting data regarding the incidence of villus apoptosis and anoikis in the adapting gut.

Studies in wild type and genetically engineered mice showed that the increase in crypt apoptosis occurs in conjunction with a shift toward greater expression of pro-apoptotic (relative to pro-survival) members of the Bcl-2 gene family [26,27] and is independent of p53 [28]. Reversal of this shift by overexpressing intestinal

Bcl-2 in transgenic mice resulted an enhanced adaptive response [29]. Experiments in Bax null mice indicate that apoptosis is mediated by Bax [27,30] and this probably occurs via the extrinsic cell death pathway [27], although the specific ligand and cell membrane receptors that trigger this response have not been identified.

Experiments in knockout mice suggest that signaling is not mediated by the tumor necrosis factor receptor-1 or the FAS death receptors [31], therefore, the role of the tumor necrosis factor related apoptosis inducing ligand (TRAIL) receptor is being investigated. The observed enhanced adaptive response in Bcl2 overexpressing transgenic mice and in Bax null mice mice has fueled interest in defining the mechanistic basis of adaptation-induced apoptosis since inhibiting apoptosis may provide a clinically useful means to promote adaptation in patients with short bowel syndrome [27,29]. In addition, the augmented adaptive response in Bax null mice mice occurred without increased crypt cell proliferation, suggesting that adaptation induced Bax-dependent apoptosis may be the primary factor limiting the magnitude of the adaptive response in the mouse model [27].

Stem cell response to intestinal resection

It is well established that following resection, villus epithelial hyperplasia occurs, villi are longer, and there are increased numbers of all four differentiated cell types. However, novel observations in mice suggest that the initial response of the stem cell to resection is to rapidly increase the numbers of secretory cells [4], specifically goblet and Paneth cells; this increase is sustained as long as 1–4 weeks after resection. Trans-differentiation of enterocytes to goblet cells was also suggested to occur in the first 12 hours following resection. These data provide evidence that the secretory cell population of the small bowel may play an important role in initiating the adaptive response. The increase in goblet cell density post-resection may be mediated, at least in part, by epidermal growth factor (EGF) because this response is blocked in *waved* mice, which have a spontaneous mutation in the EGF receptor tyrosine kinase resulting in a nonfunctional receptor, and in mice that have been treated with an EGF inhibitor [32]. Further studies to elucidate the stem cell response to small bowel resection may provide the basis for future, novel therapies.

Increased enterocyte migration and changes in the ECM contribute to the adaptive response

The intestinal epithelium is continuously renewed as proliferating daughter cells differentiate into one of the four principal intestinal epithelial cell types during a complex, bidirectional migration process. Enterocytic, goblet, and enteroendocrine cells migrate from the crypts onto the villi and Paneth cells migrate to the base of the crypts. The factors that regulate these precise migration patterns in the normal gut epithelium are still being elucidated, as are the changes that occur following small bowel resection. In rodent models, epithelial cell migration rate is increased following intestinal resection, and remains elevated for months after surgery [2,3]. In the normal intestine, members of the ephrinB1 and ephrinB2/B3 receptor family are important in determining the localization and migration patterns of Paneth cells; mice in which the ephrin B3 receptor gene is deleted exhibit profound abnormalities in Paneth cell localization [33]. In addition, Fox11 deficient mice also showed marked alterations in Paneth cell position, likely as a result of changes in EphB/Ephrin B regulation. A gut-specific and inducible deletion of the Apc gene resulted in a marked decrease in epithelial cell migration associated with loss of differentiation of enterocytes, goblet, and enteroendocrine cells, and an increase in Paneth cells and markers of Paneth cell differentiation [34].

Epithelial-matrix interactions are of critical importance in regulating migration of epithelial cells from the crypt to the villus tip. In the normal intestine, this process appears to be regulated by components of the basic membrane and extracellular matrix, including collagen IV, e-cadherins, laminin, and integrins [22,35,39]. Evidence supporting a role for collagen IV and laminin in mediating epithelial cell migration after resection comes from studies in vitamin A deficient rats [22]. In this model, epithelial cell migration was decreased in remnant ileum, associated with decreased crypt cell proliferation and increased apoptosis. Analysis of matrix components revealed decreases in collagen IV and laminin but not fibronectin expression.

The inhibition of hedgehog (Hh) signaling also affects epithelial cell migration following resection. Hedgehog proteins (including Indian Hh and Desert Hh) are produced by the small bowel (Sonic Hh is predominantly produced in the stomach), and act on adjacent stromal cells that express Patched or Patched 2 receptors for Hh signaling. Systemic administration of antibodies that block hedgehog signaling in the gut resulted in increased migration and apoptosis [36] in mice following 50% small intestinal resection. This was associated with increased expression of integrin-$\beta 1$ but no change in collagen IV or e-cadherin. Others have shown that Hh signaling affects morphogenetic cell movements in embryonic life [40]. These results suggest a novel role for Hh signaling in the gut, and also indicate the potential importance of epithelial-mesenchymal cross-talk in regulating migration.

Enteroendocrine cells also may signal to the epithelium to regulate cell migration [41]. Peptide YY and neuropeptide Y have been shown to increase expression of markers of enterocyte differentiation and to decrease CD63, a tetraspanin involved in cell adhesion. Treatment of epithelial cells with these peptides resulted in increased cell migration in concert with increased expression of matrix metalloproteinase 3.

Humoral mediators

Luminal nutrients and enteric secretions are clearly required for a full adaptive response. In addition to luminal factors, there is ample evidence that humoral factors are important mediators of adaptation. For example, studies in parabiotic rats [42] and pigs [43] demonstrated that partial small intestinal resection in one member of the pair stimulated intestinal growth in the unoperated member. Compared to controls undergoing transection or laparotomy, serum obtained from rodents or dogs after small bowel resection has been shown to stimulate proliferation of intestinal cell lines. Studies in rodent models have identified a variety of factors with proadaptive properties, that is, stimulation of crypt cell proliferation, enterocyte migration, or enterocyte differentiation, or inhibition of apoptosis in the intestinal remnant following partial enterectomy. For some of these there is also support for an endogenous role in adaptation. Experimental data supporting a direct role in adaptation is strongest for glucagon-like peptide 2 (GLP-2), growth hormone (See Chapter 25) and EGF.

Glucagon-like peptide 2

GLP-2 has been shown to have specific trophic effects in the normal intestine and the remnant following partial resection. GLP-2 is an intestine-specific 33 AA peptide product of post-translational processing of proglucagon, which is produced by intestinal enteroendocrine cells. Endogenous GLP-2 is rapidly cleaved by brush border dipeptidyl peptidase IV (DPP IV); therefore, studies addressing the therapeutic potential of GLP-2 have utilized DPP IV resistant analogs (e.g. substitution of glycine for alanine at position two) or have been done in conjunction with a DPP IV inhibitor or in DPP-IV deficient transgenic mice. The observation that DPP IV mRNA levels are reduced in the remnant adapting intestine are consistent with a role for endogenous GLP-2 in adaptation [44]. The physiologic effects of GLP-2 are mediated by a specific receptor that is a member of the class II glucagon-secretin G protein-coupled receptor superfamily. The receptor is not expressed in enterocytes and intestinal expression appears to be limited to subsets of enteric neurons and enteroendocrine cells [45,46]. Therefore, the intestinal effects of GLP-2 on mucosal growth and adaptation are thought to be indirect.

Data supporting a role for GLP-2 in small bowel adaptation include studies in rats demonstrating increased absorptive capacity [47], villus height [48] and mucosal antioxidant capacity following partial resection and administration of GLP-2 analogs (reviewed in [49]). In humans, administration of GLP-2 has been associated with increased nutrient absorption, villus height, crypt depth, and mitotic index leading to increased intestinal weight and decreased fecal output [50].

Growth hormone (GH)\Insulin-like Growth Factors 1 and 2 (IGF-1, IGF-2)

Human growth hormone has been approved for use in the treatment of patients with short bowel syndrome (see Chapter 25). In rodent models, the trophic effects of GH are primarily mediated through IGF-1 signaling, although the trophic effects of combined GH and IGF-1 are greater than either alone (reviewed in [51]). IGF-1, secreted by the liver and by intestinal lamina propria mesenchymal cells, binds to IGF-1 receptors leading to stimulation of crypt cell proliferation and inhibi-

tion of apoptosis. The availability of IGF-1 is modulated by interactions with IGF binding proteins. In rodents, systemic administration of IGF-1 or analogs with enhanced bioavailability due to reduced affinities for IGF binding proteins stimulated small bowel growth after partial small bowel resection [52,54]. However, levels of IGF-1 in serum and intestinal tissues do not increase postresection. Thus, the observed reduction in the expression of IGF binding protein-3 has been invoked as a mechanism for the putative proadaptive effects of endogenous IGF-1 in resection models of adaptation [55].

Epidermal growth factor

EGF binds to receptors found on the brush border and basolateral cell membrane of cells distributed throughout the digestive tract. Sources of luminal EGF include salivary and Brunner's gland secretions, breast milk and pancreaticobiliary secretions. Epidermal growth factor and related peptides (e.g. transforming growth factor-α and amphiregulin) that bind to the EGF receptor (EGFR) stimulate intestinal growth and promote injury repair by increasing crypt cell proliferation and inhibiting apoptosis. Studies in resection models suggest that EGFR signaling contributes to the adaptive response (reviewed in [56]). For example, adaptation is increased by intestinal overexpression of an EGF transgene or by administration of exogenous EGF, whereas adaptation is reduced by sialectomy, or by mutation of the EGFR as occurs in waved-2 mice or by oral administration of a selective EGFR inhibitor. The trophic effects of EGFR signaling are mediated by increases in proliferation and inhibition of apoptosis that result in increased intestinal length and mucosal thickness with longer villi and deeper crypts. Based on the observation that EGF administration can also enhance nutrient absorption in animal resection models, a pilot study was conducted in infants with chronic short bowel syndrome. Administration of oral EGF enhanced carbohydrate absorption and tolerance of enteral feeds in all five study patients [57].

Other factors with limited data suggestive of proadaptive properties in animal models include the following:

Neurotensin

Neurotensin is an intestinal peptide that is most abundant in the ileum and is secreted by enteroendocrine cells in response to fat and other nutrients. In rats, neurotensin can reverse intestinal hypoplasia induced by an elemental diet and, in the small bowel resection model, neurotensin can stimulate adaptation [58,59].

Hepatocyte growth factor

Hepatocyte growth factor, a heterodimeric protein, which binds to the c-met tyrosine kinase that is expressed in many tissues, including the small intestine, has been shown to stimulate intestinal proliferation and absorption. In rats, luminal or systemic perfusion of hepatocyte growth factor after partial small bowel resection increased absorption of galactose and glycine and augmented mucosal mass [60].

Leptin

Leptin is a 16-kD protein that acts through the leptin receptor to control body weight by regulating food intake and energy expenditure. Leptin has been studied in rodent resection models of adaptation because it is trophic to the intact small bowel. These studies have shown that parenteral leptin enhanced the adaptive response by stimulating crypt cell proliferation and carbohydrate absorption [61,62]. Concordant with a pro-adaptive role, the intestinal proliferative response to resection was impaired in leptin deficient mice [63].

Keratinocyte growth factor (KGF)

Keratinocyte growth factor, a member of the fibroblast growth factor (fibroblast growth factor 7) is a potent mitogen for epithelial cells. In the gut, it is produced by intraepithelial lymphocytes and stromal fibroblasts. Modified KGF has been approved for clinical use to prevent and treat chemotherapy-induced mucositis. KGF has been studied in rat models of short bowel syndrome. In some of these, KGF stimulated small intestinal and colonic crypt cell proliferation, in addition to increasing intestinal and colonic goblet cell number and the expression of the cytoprotective trefoil peptide TFF3 [47,64]. KGF administration also increased transport of electrolytes, glucose, and amino acids in the remnant small intestine [65].

Nutrient mediators

It is well established in animal models that the adaptive response is optimal when nutrients are provided enterally (reviewed in [66]; see Chapter 24). Concordant with the induction of intestinal atrophy that occurs in the normal intestine when nutrition is provided exclusively via parenteral routes, the adaptive response is diminished by exclusive parenteral feeding. The pro-adaptive benefits of luminal nutrients are likely related to stimulation of pancreatic and biliary secretions that are enterotrophic, direct nutrient effects, stimulation of secretion of humoral mediators, increased intestinal blood flow, and bacterial metabolism of unabsorbed nutrients (e.g. production of short chain fatty acids from undigested carbohydrates). In addition, oral feedings may enhance the release of salivary epidermal growth factor. Animal studies have identified several putative pro-adaptive nutrients. The relative trophic effects of some of these nutrients can be summarized as follows. Complex diets are superior to elemental diets for promoting adaptation. In order of descending potency, free fatty acids, long chain triglycerides, medium chain triglycerides, carbohydrates, and proteins can stimulate aspects of the adaptive response. In addition, in several studies, nutrients, including short chain fatty acids, arginine, and retinoic acid were also pro-adaptive, at least when administered parenterally. The use of luminal factors and intestinotrophic nutrients, including glutamine and short chain fatty acids, are discussed in detail in Chapter 24.

Role of enteric nervous system and submucosa

The role of the enteric nervous system in the adaptive response is still being clarified. A classic study described jejunectomized pigs that underwent vagal deafferentation and had a diminished adaptive response with an absence of compensatory hypertrophy, despite unaltered food intake, compared to pigs that underwent resection but whose vagi remained intact [43]. The role of the vagus in food intake and obesity is being extensively investigated, but its role in the adaptive response remains unclear. Newer data implicate the cocaine and amphetamine regulated transcript (CART) as having a role in neuronal adaptation following resection or bypass. CART was first isolated from rat brain as a transcript induced by cocaine or amphetamine administration. It is also expressed in the peripheral nervous system and, specifically, in myenteric neurons of the small and large intestine [67]. In a model of ileal atrophy induced by bypassing the gut, CART mRNA-expressing neurons increased in number [67,68]. These data and other studies suggest that CART may function as a neuroprotective agent, to preserve and maintain enteric neurons. Following massive small bowel resection in the dog, concentrations of vasoactive intestinal peptide (VIP) were reduced by 50% in the mucosa and muscle layers [69]. Similarly, VIP immunoreactive nerve fibers were markedly decreased following gut resection in piglets [70]. Interestingly, VIP and neuropeptide Y expressing nerves also decreased in number in bypassed intestine, but nitric oxide synthase expressing neurons increased in an atrophy model [71]. The role of GLP-2 in gut adaptation is discussed elsewhere, but it is interesting to note that the GLP-2 receptor is expressed on enteric nerves [45,72] as well as enteroendocrine cells [46] and myofibroblasts [73]; thus, GLP-2's effects on crypt cell proliferation may well be mediated indirectly through the enteric nervous system.

Conclusions

The intestinal adaptive response to resection is complex and has been characterized in studies of its structural, functional, cellular, and molecular components. Our understanding of the molecular basis of this response has advanced greatly in the past several years, but the underlying pathways, cell-specific responses and potential regulators still remain to be elucidated. Although there are clearly differences between adaptation in animal models and humans, future studies that address these mechanisms will undoubtedly facilitate the design of targeted therapies to enhance the adaptive response and increase functional small bowel surface area in patients with short bowel syndrome.

References

1 Rubin DC, Swietlicki EA, Wang JL, Dodson BD, Levin MS. Enterocytic gene expression in intestinal adaptation: evidence for a specific cellular response. *Am J Physiol* 1996;270:G143–G152.

2 Dowling RH. Cellular and molecular basis of intestinal and pancreatic adaptation. [Review]. *Scandinavian J Gastroenterol—Suppl* 1992;193:64–67.

3 Bristol JB, Williamson RC. Nutrition, operations, and intestinal adaptation. [Review]. *JPEN: J Parenter Enteral Nutr* 1988;12:299–309.

4 Helmrath MA, Fong JJ, Dekaney CM, Henning SJ. Rapid expansion of intestinal secretory lineages following a massive small bowel resection in mice. *Am J Physiol Gastrointest Liver Physiol* 2006.

5 Welters CF, Dejong CH, Deutz NE, Heineman E. Intestinal function and metabolism in the early adaptive phase after massive small bowel resection in the rat. *J Pediatr Surg* 2001;36:1746–51.

6 Weinstein LD, Shoemaker CP, Hersh T, Wright HK. Enhanced intestinal absorption after small bowel resection in man. *Arch Surg* 1969;99:560–562.

7 Althausen TL, Doig RK, Uyeyama K, Weiden S. Digestion and absorption after massive resection of the small intestine. II. Recovery of the absorptive function as shown by intestinal absorption tests in two patients and a consideration of compensatory mechanisms. *Gastroenterology* 1950;16:126–139.

8 Gouttebel MC, Saint Aubert B, Colette C, et al. Intestinal adaptation in patients with short bowel syndrome. Measurement by calcium absorption. *Dig Dis Sci* 1989;34:709–715.

9 Benedetti E, Baum C, Cicalese L, et al. Progressive functional adaptation of segmental bowel graft from living related donor. *Transplantation* 2001;71:569–571.

10 Jao W, Sileri P, Holaysan J, et al. Morphologic adaptation following segmental living related intestinal transplantation. *Transplant Proc* 2002;34:924.

11 Musch MW, Bookstein C, Rocha F, et al. Region-specific adaptation of apical Na/H exchangers after extensive proximal small bowel resection 10.1152/ ajpgi.00528.2001. *Am J Physiol Gastrointest Liver Physiol* 2002;283:G975–985.

12 Hines OJ, Bilchik AJ, Zinner MJ, et al. Adaptation of the Na+/glucose cotransporter following intestinal resection. *J Surg Res* 1994;57:22–27.

13 O'Connor TP, Lam MM, Diamond J. Magnitude of functional adaptation after intestinal resection. *Am J Physiol Regul Integr Comp Physiol* 1999;276:R1265–1275.

14 Chaves M, Smith MW, Williamson RC. Increased activity of digestive enzymes in ileal enterocytes adapting to proximal small bowel resection. *Gut* 1987;28:981–987.

15 Dodson BD, Wang JL, Swietlicki EA, Rubin DC, Levin MS. Analysis of cloned cDNAs differentially expressed in adapting remnant small intestine after partial resection. *Am J Physiol* 1996;271(2 Pt 1):G347–G356.

16 Wang JL, Swartz-Basile DA, Rubin DC, Levin MS. Retinoic acid stimulates early cellular proliferation in

the adapting remnant rat small intestine after resection. *J Nutr* 1997;127.

17 Luk GD, Baylin SB. Inhibition of intestinal epithelial DNA synthesis and adaptive hyperplasia after jejunectomy in the rat by suppression of polyamine biosynthesis. *J Clin Invest* 1984;74:698–704.

18 Erdman SH, Park JH, Thompson JS, et al. Suppression of diamine oxidase activity enhances postresection ileal proliferation in the rat. *Gastroenterology* 1989;96:1533–1538.

19 Sheng G, Bernabe KQ, Guo J, Warner BW. Epidermal growth factor receptor-mediated proliferation of enterocytes requires p21waf1/cip1 expression. *Gastroenterology* 2006;131:153–164.

20 Stern LE, Falcone RA, Kemp CJ, et al. p21 (WAF1/CIP1) is required for the mitogenic response to intestinal resection. *J Surg Res* 2000;90:45–50.

21 Stehr W, Bernal NP, Erwin CR, Bernabe KQ, Guo J, Warner BW. Roles for p21waf1/cip1 and p27kip1 during the adaptation response to massive intestinal resection 10.1152/ajpgi.00235.2005. *Am J Physiol Gastrointest Liver Physiol* 2006;290:G933–941.

22 Swartz-Basile DA, Wang L, Tang Y, et al. Vitamin A deficiency inhibits intestinal adaptation by modulating apoptosis, proliferation, and enterocyte migration. *Am J Physiol Gastrointest Liver Physiol* 2003;285:G424–G432.

23 Swartz-Basile DA, Rubin DC, Levin MS. Vitamin A status modulates intestinal adaptation after partial small bowel resection. *JPEN J Parenter Enteral Nutr* 2000;24:81–88.

24 Wang L, Tang Y, Rubin DC, Levin MS. Chronically administered retinoic acid has trophic effects in the rat small intestine and promotes adaptation in a resection model of short bowel syndrome 10.1152/ajpgi.00567.2006. *Am J Physiol Gastrointest Liver Physiol* 2007;292:G1559–G1569.

25 Hall PA, Coates PJ, Ansari B, Hopwood D. Regulation of cell number in the mammalian gastrointestinal tract: the importance of apoptosis. *J Cell Sci* 1994;107(Pt 12):3569–3577.

26 Helmrath MA, Shin CE, Erwin CR, Warner BW. The EGF backslash EGF-receptor axis modulates enterocyte apoptosis during intestinal adaptation. *J Surg Res* 1998;77:17–22.

27 Tang Y, Swartz-Basile DA, Swietlicki EA, et al. Bax is required for resection-induced changes in apoptosis, proliferation, and members of the extrinsic cell death pathways. *Gastroenterology* 2004;126:220–230.

28 Shin CE, Falcone RA, Kemp CJ, et al. Intestinal adaptation and enterocyte apoptosis following small bowel resection is p53 independent. *Am J Physiol Gastrointest Liver Physiol* 1999;277:G717–G724.

29 Welters CFM, Piersma FE, Hockenbery DM, Heineman E. The role of apoptosis during intestinal adaptation after small bowel resection. *J Pediatr Surg* 2000;35:20–24.

30 Stern LE, Huang F, Kemp CJ, et al. Bax is required for increased enterocyte apoptosis after massive small bowel resection. *Surgery* 2000;128:165–170.

31 Knott AW, O'Brien DP, Juno RJ, et al. Enterocyte apoptosis after enterectomy in mice is activated independent of the extrinsic death receptor pathway. *Am J Physiol Gastrointest Liver Physiol* 2003;285:G404–G413.

32 Jarboe MD, Juno RJ, Stehr W, et al. Epidermal growth factor receptor signaling regulates goblet cell production after small bowel resection. *J Pediatr Surg* 2005;40:92–7.

33 Batlle E, Henderson JT, Beghtel H, et al. Beta-catenin and TCF mediate cell positioning in the intestinal epithelium by controlling the expression of EphB/ephrinB. *Cell* 2002;111:251–263.

34 Andreu P, Colnot S, Godard C, et al. Crypt-restricted proliferation and commitment to the Paneth cell lineage following Apc loss in the mouse intestine. *Development* 2005;132:1443–1451.

35 Sanders MA, Basson MD. Collagen IV-dependent ERK activation in human Caco-2 intestinal epithelial cells requires focal adhesion kinase. *J Biol Chem* 2000;275:38040–38047.

36 Tang Y, Swietlicki EA, Jiang S, et al. Increased apoptosis and accelerated epithelial migration following inhibition of hedgehog signaling in adaptive small bowel postresection. *Am J Physiol Gastrointest Liver Physiol* 2006;290:G1280–G1288.

37 Qureshi FG, Leaphart C, Cetin S, et al. Increased expression and function of integrins in enterocytes by endotoxin impairs epithelial restitution. *Gastroenterology* 2005;128:1012–1022.

38 Hermiston ML, Gordon JI. In vivo analysis of cadherin function in the mouse intestinal epithelium: essential roles in adhesion, maintenance of differentiation, and regulation of programmed cell death. *J Cell Biol* 1995;129:489–506.

39 Hermiston ML, Wong MH, Gordon JI. Forced expression of E-cadherin in the mouse intestinal epithelium slows cell migration and provides evidence for nonautonomous regulation of cell fate in a self-renewing system. *Genes Dev* 1996;10:985–996.

40 Charron F, Stein E, Jeong J, et al. The morphogen sonic hedgehog is an axonal chemoattractant that collaborates with netrin-1 in midline axon guidance. *Cell* 2003;113:11–23.

41 Lee M, Hadi M, Hallden G, Aponte GW. Peptide YY and neuropeptide Y induce villin expression, reduce adhesion, and enhance migration in small

intestinal cells through the regulation of CD63, matrix metalloproteinase-3, and Cdc42 activity. *J Biol Chem* 2005;280:125–36.

42 Williamson RC, Buchholtz TW, Malt RA. Humoral stimulation of cell proliferation in small bowel after transection and resection in rats. *Gastroenterology* 1978;75:249–254.

43 Laplace JP. Compensatory hypertrophy of the residual small intestine after partial enterectomy. A neurohumoral feedback? *Ann Rech Vet* 1980;11:165–77.

44 Dunphy JL, Justice FA, Taylor RG, Fuller PJ. mRNA levels of dipeptidyl peptidase IV decrease during intestinal adaptation. *J Surg Res* 1999;87:130–3.

45 Bjerknes M, Cheng H. Modulation of specific intestinal epithelial progenitors by enteric neurons. *Proc Natl Acad Sci U S A* 2001;98:12497–502.

46 Yusta B, Huang L, Munroe D, et al. Enteroendocrine localization of GLP-2 receptor expression in humans and rodents. *Gastroenterology* 2000;119:744–55.

47 Washizawa N, Gu LH, Gu L, et al. Comparative effects of glucagon-like peptide-2 (GLP-2), growth hormone (GH), and keratinocyte growth factor (KGF) on markers of gut adaptation after massive small bowel resection in rats. *JPEN J Parenter Enteral Nutr* 2004;28:399–409.

48 Scott RB, Kirk D, MacNaughton WK, Meddings JB. GLP-2 augments the adaptive response to massive intestinal resection in rat. *Am J Physiol Gastrointest Liver Physiol* 1998;275:G911–921.

49 Martin GR, Beck PL, Sigalet DL. Gut hormones, and short bowel syndrome: The enigmatic role of glucagon-like peptide-2 in the regulation of intestinal adaptation. *World J Gastroenterol* 2006;12:4117–4129.

50 Estall JL, Drucker DJ. Glucagon-like peptide-2. *Ann Rev Nutr* 2006;26:391–411.

51 Lund PK. Molecular basis of intestinal adaptation: the role of the insulin-like growth factor system. *Ann N Y Acad Sci* 1998;859:18–36.

52 Ney DM. Effects of insulin-like growth factor-I and growth hormone in models of parenteral nutrition. *JPEN J Parenter Enteral Nutr* 1999;23(6 Suppl):S184–9.

53 Vanderhoof JA, McCusker RH, Clark R, et al. Truncated and native insulinlike growth factor I enhance mucosal adaptation after jejunoileal resection. *Gastroenterology* 1992;102:1949–1956.

54 Lemmey AB, Martin AA, Read LC, et al. IGF-I and the truncated analogue des-(1–3)IGF-I enhance growth in rats after gut resection. *Am J Physiol* 1991;260 (2 Pt 1):E213–E219.

55 Albiston AL, Taylor RG, Herington AC, et al. Divergent ileal IGF-I and IGFBP-3 gene expression after small

bowel resection: a novel mechanism to amplify IGF action? *Mol Cell Endocrinol* 1992;83:R17–R20.

56 Warner BW, Erwin CR. Critical roles for EGF receptor signaling during resection-induced intestinal adaptation. *J Pediatr Gastroenterol Nutr* 2006;43(Suppl 1):S68–S73.

57 Sigalet DL, Martin GR, Butzner JD, et al. A pilot study of the use of epidermal growth factor in pediatric short bowel syndrome. *J Pediatr Surg* 2005;40:763–768.

58 Evers BM, Izukura M, Townsend CM, Jr., et al. Neurotensin prevents intestinal mucosal hypoplasia in rats fed an elemental diet. *Dig Dis Sci* 1992;37:426–431.

59 de Miguel E, Gomez de Segura IA, Bonet H, et al. Trophic effects of neurotensin in massive bowel resection in the rat. *Dig Dis Sci* 1994;39:59–64.

60 Kato Y, Yu D, Schwartz MZ. Enhancement of intestinal adaptation by hepatocyte growth factor. *Journal of Pediatric Surgery Papers Presented at the 28th Annual Meeting of the* 1998;33:235–239.

61 Pearson PY, O'Connor DM, Schwartz MZ. Novel effect of leptin on small intestine adaptation. *J Surg Res* 2001;97:192–5.

62 Sukhotnik I, Vadasz Z, Coran AG, et al. Effect of leptin on intestinal re-growth following massive small bowel resection in rat. *Pediatr Surg Int* 2006;22:9–15.

63 Kiely JM, Noh J-H, Pitt HA, Swartz-Basile DA. Impaired intestinal cell proliferation and cell death in leptin-deficient obese mice. *JPEN J Parenter Enteral Nutr* 2005;29:30–35.

64 Johnson WF, DiPalma CR, Ziegler TR, et al. Keratinocyte growth factor enhances early gut adaptation in a rat model of short bowel syndrome. *Vet Surg* 2000;29:17–27.

65 Yang H, Wildhaber BE, Teitelbaum DH. 2003 Harry M. Vars Research Award. Keratinocyte growth factor improves epithelial function after massive small bowel resection. *JPEN J Parenter Enteral Nutr* 2003;27:198–206; discussion 206–207.

66 Tappenden KA. Mechanisms of enteral nutrient-enhanced intestinal adaptation. *Gastroenterology* 2006; 130(2 Suppl 1):S93–S99.

67 Ekblad E, Kuhar M, Wierup N, Sundler F. Cocaine- and amphetamine-regulated transcript: distribution and function in rat gastrointestinal tract. *Neurogastroenterol Motil* 2003;15:545–557.

68 Ekblad E. CART in the enteric nervous system. *Peptides* 2006;27:2024–30.

69 Adrian TE, Thompson JS, Quigley EM. Time course of adaptive regulatory peptide changes following massive small bowel resection in the dog. *Dig Dis Sci* 1996;41:1194–1203.

70 Vento P, Kiviluoto T, Pakarinen M, et al. Nerve terminals containing neuropeptides decrease in number after massive proximal small bowel resection in the piglet. *Dig Dis Sci* 1998;43:1102–1110.

71 Ekelund KM, Ekblad E. Structural, neuronal, and functional adaptive changes in atrophic rat ileum. *Gut* 1999;45:236–245.

72 Guan X, Karpen HE, Stephens J, et al. GLP-2 receptor localizes to enteric neurons and endocrine cells expressing vasoactive peptides and mediates increased blood flow. *Gastroenterology* 2006;130:150–164.

73 Orskov C, Hartmann B, Poulsen SS, et al. GLP-2 stimulates colonic growth via KGF, released by subepithelial myofibroblasts with GLP-2 receptors. *Regul Pept* 2005;124:105–112.

3 Intestinal Failure: Definition and Pathophysiology

.

6 Intestinal Failure: Definitions and Classifications

Dominique M. Jan

Key points

- There are numerous definitions of intestinal failure; some are anatomic while others are functional.
- Various classifications of intestinal failure also have been proposed.
- Prognosis often can be predicted by the location and length of remnant bowel in patients with short bowel syndrome.
- Intestinal rehabilitation should be considered in patients capable of absorbing oral nutrients.
- Transplantation remains reserved for patients with irreversible IF associated with life threatening complications.

Intestinal failure (IF) is a clinical condition of temporary or permanent intestinal malabsorption. As there is a relatively safe artificial support system in the form of parenteral nutrition (PN), IF must be differentiated from other examples of vital organ failure. Mortality and morbidity rates for most patients on PN are low and have continued to decrease with advances in supportive techniques and their application. Ongoing research continues to explore therapeutic interventions to optimize adaptation and promote the absorptive function of the intestine.

Implicit in the concept of intestinal failure is a prolonged and potentially long-term requirement for PN, as long as it persists. Irreversible IF requires long-term and indefinite PN. When complications secondary to IF

Intestinal Failure: Diagnosis, Management and Transplantation.
Edited by Alan N. Langnas, Olivier Goulet, Eamonn M.M. Quigley and Kelly A. Tappenden. © 2008 Blackwell Publishing.
ISBN 978-1-4051-4637-1.

occur, the issue of intestinal transplantation (ITx) will be raised. The prognosis of IF is related to the cause, the age-adjusted length of the intestinal remnant, the anatomical location of the resected intestine and the occurrence of complications. The aim of this review is to discuss:

Definitions of IF
Causes of IF
Classifications of IF

Introduction

Until the late 1960s, malnutrition secondary to intestinal malabsorption was an irreversible and fatal condition. All attempts of intestinal transplantation failed. Whereas Lillehei et al. [1] reported the first case of bowel transplantation in humans in October 1967, up to 1970 all patients who received an intestinal graft died of technical complications, sepsis, or rejection. Over the same period of time, total parenteral nutrition was developed successfully by Dudrick, Wilmore, and their colleagues [2]. In their initial report, they documented 30 subjects receiving total parenteral nutrition who were able to achieve positive nitrogen balance, maintain weight, heal wounds, and close fistulae.

After these initial successes of PN, the new technique was introduced into the clinical mainstream, and indications for its use have expanded tremendously. Thereafter, numerous nontransplant strategies that may allow patients to discontinue or curtail the use of total parenteral nutrition have been used in the treatment of patients with short-bowel syndrome. The creation of reversed intestinal segments was popular in the 1960s, the aim of this operation was to produce a sort of functional partial small bowel obstruction that would slow intestinal transit time, thereby, encouraging greater nutrient absorption and decreasing diarrhea and nutrient loss. The results were mixed to questionable.

Cyclosporine revived interest in small-intestinal transplantation; however, clinical results were disappointing because most grafts were lost to rejection. The most significant contribution to progress in intestinal transplantation was the introduction of tacrolimus, in 1990, by Starzl and his colleagues [3].

Definition of IF

Most commonly intestinal failure is defined as the critical reduction of functional gut mass below the minimal amount necessary for adequate digestion and absorption to satisfy body nutrient and fluid requirements. This is often combined with an estimate of small intestinal length. However, the definition of IF can be a matter of debate. Thus, newer definitions of IF now include the measurement of fecal energy loss, rather than residual bowel length, for patients with short bowel syndrome (SBS) [4].

In addition to anatomic and nutritional criteria for defining IF, a biological marker of gut functional mass has been recently proposed [5]. Citrulline is a nonessential amino acid that is mostly produced by enterocytes and not incorporated into peptides or proteins. A postabsorptive plasma level of citrulline, lower than 20 µmol/L (half the normal value in controls) and detected beyond the 2-year period of adaptation after the reestablishment of bowel continuity after extensive small-bowel resection is significantly associated with permanent intestinal failure. This biochemical marker cannot be used in the presence of renal insufficiency. It is correlated to remnant small-bowel length and absorptive capacity; it is more predictive of permanent intestinal failure (negative and positive predictive values of 86% and 95%, respectively) than remnant length of small bowel alone [6]. In fact, citrulline seems to reflect the absorptive function of the remaining short gut. It is interesting to note that in children with SBS, a similar citrulline threshold (19 µmol/L) was recently found to be similarly predictive for both length of remnant small bowel and likelihood of tolerance of enteral nutrition among a group of patients being weaned off HPN [7]. Combining the length of the remnant bowel

with the citrulline level offers the advantage of better defining appropriate HPN candidates for either complementary (pharmacologic trophic gut factors or reconstructive surgery) or alternative treatments for permanent intestinal failure.

A more simple but practical approach would be to define the degree of IF according to the amount of PN required for maintenance of nutritional status in adults and of growth in children [10]. This definition provides a parameter that is independent of the length or function of the remnant gut. This is also a good way to track progress with any intervention. For example, a patient treated with a novel agent can to be stated to have reduced PN requirements from 5 to 3 days per week. This would also take into account the issue of hyperphagia that occurs in some patients without discernable evidence of absorption of nutrients. This definition would facilitate both comparisons between programs and multicenter trials.

The causes of intestinal failure

Causes of IF in children
The natural history of IF is variable and is largely influenced by the underlying disorder. In children, the etiology of intestinal failure is dominated by congenital disorders or severe and permanent diseases of early onset which necessitate protracted or indefinite support with PN.

Short Bowel Syndrome (SBS) was one of the first recognized causes of IF [11]. However, with the increasing and successful use of long-term PN during the last decades, several other causes of IF have emerged such as severe extensive motility disorders, including extended Hirschsprung's disease, chronic intestinal pseudo-obstruction, and, more recently, congenital diseases of enterocyte development.

Definition of SBS
SBS is characterized by a state of malabsorption after extensive loss or resection of the small bowel. It is an anatomical and functional definition. The length of resection results in insufficient nutritive supply requiring artificial nutrition. Long-term PN allows infants and children with SBS to grow normally during the long period required for adaptation of the remnant small intestine. In addition to the requirement

for PN, the child with SBS-related IF may benefit from other established medical and surgical interventions intended to improve function of the remnant small intestine.

SBS is the most frequent cause of protracted IF in children [12,13]. The major consequence of resection of the small bowel is malabsorption. This is primarily because of the reduction of the absorptive surface area. SBS may be secondary to congenital anomalies of the digestive tract. Accordingly, therefore, most patients with SBS present at or near birth. Atresia may occur anywhere in the small intestine. SBS is more common with multiple intestinal atresias and the "apple peel" deformity caused by interruption of the superior mesenteric artery, in which there is a proximal jejunal atresia and the distal bowel becomes coiled around a long marginal artery. Gastroschisis can lead to SBS as the result of prenatal bowel ischemia, or postnatal necrotizing enterocolitis. Overall, approximately 5% of gastroschisis patients develop short bowel syndrome secondary to extensive intestinal resection [14]. Hirschsprung's disease, involving the small bowel as well as the entire colon, could be an eventual cause of SBS. When the aganglionosis extends to involve more than 50 cm of the ileum demonstrated SBS is likely [15,16]. In patients born with a normal gastrointestinal tract, the most frequent indication for extensive resection is necrotizing enterocolitis (NEC), especially in premature infants. NEC results from ischemic injury to the small bowel, which most often has to be resected [17]. Typically, an extensive resection of the ileum and proximal colon proves necessary and the function of the remnant small intestine is often compromised.

Midgut volvulus from malrotation causes ischemia and necrosis with subsequent extensive resection. Volvulus also may occur in children in relation to benign tumors, such as lymphangioma, mesenteric cysts, and, in older children, desmoid tumors. The functional consequences of SBS depend on the length and site of the resected small intestine, on the one hand, and the cause of resection as well as the age of the patient at the onset of SBS, on the other. All theses factors influence the capacity of the remnant gut to function and the potential for adaptation.

The small bowel length doubles during the last trimester of gestation, suggesting that a short bowel remnant does not have the same prognosis in a preterm infant as in a full-term baby [18]. Despite this potential for growth and other factors determining the outcome, it is classical to consider different groups of patients after small bowel resection, according to the length of the small intestine measured along the antimesenteric border. A short resection leaves more than 50% of the native small intestine, a large resection leaves between 20 to 50% of the native small bowel, and an extensive resection leaves less than 20% of the small bowel or less than 40 cm without the ileocecal valve (ICV), [11]. Large and massive resections are more likely to lead to temporary or permanent IF.

Prognosis depends not only on the overall length resected but also the portion of small bowel resected [19]. Jejunal resection is better tolerated for a variety of reasons. The most important may be that the jejunum has a limited capacity to adapt relative to the ileum. Possibly of equal importance, the ileum is the site of synthesis for gastrointestinal hormones such as enteroglucagon. This helps explain why jejunal resection is better tolerated that ileal resection [20].

Outcome of children with SBS

The medical management of patients with SBS aims to promote gut adaptation and to recover intestinal function sufficient to achieve intestinal autonomy (PN weaning). Nutritional support provides an optimal nutritional status allowing normal growth and development, whereas, for infants or children, oral feeding skills have to be acquired or maintained. PN is the cornerstone of management, but as much nutrition as possible should be provided to the patient via the intestine in order to improve the physiological processes of SB adaptation and villous hyperplasia. Early use of the gastrointestinal tract, especially by oral feeding (to enhance gastrointestinal secretions, stimulate salivary production of epidermal growth factor and promote gallbladder motility), is recommended.

Until 30 years ago, the prognosis after extensive bowel resection was poor, especially in the neonatal period. The onset of parenteral and enteral feeding in daily practice has transformed the outcome during the past 3 decades [8,19,21]. More than 90% of infants and children now survive after extensive small bowel resection in the neonatal period. The duration of PN dependency varies according to the intestinal length and the presence of the ileocecal valve. By multivariate analysis, PN duration is significantly influenced by the length of residual short bowel and the absence of ICV [21]. After PN weaning, patients grow up normally with a normal puberty and final height as expected from genetic target height. Thus, with favorable anatomic prognostic factors and a short duration of initial PN, normal long-term growth may be predicted. However, long-term nutritional status and bone mineralization have to be monitored carefully. Conversely, poor anatomic factors and protracted initial PN require careful monitoring of growth and may, sometimes, require nutritional support to be restarted. Patients permanently dependent on PN need other, innovative, therapeutic approaches.

Factors such as functional (absorption and motility) capacity of the remnant small intestine and small bowel bacterial overgrowth (SBBO) emerge as being critical in predicting outcome. A small number of patients will acquire intestinal autonomy only very slowly, if at all, because of major degrees of bowel dilation and the presence of dysmotility. In such patients, different surgical approaches have been proposed for increasing nutrient and fluid absorption. Surgical procedures aimed at slowing intestinal transit (intestinal valves, reversed intestinal segments) have been attempted and have been extensively reviewed, whereas clinical results are conflicting. Longitudinal intestinal lengthening and tailoring (LILT) was first proposed for selected patients with dilated bowel segments, in 1980 [22,23]. LILT has the theoretical advantage of not only tapering the dilated segment, but also of using the divided intestine to increase total small bowel length. This procedure allows improvement in more than 50%. Since 2003, an alternative to the LILT have been proposed, a Serial Transverse EnteroPlasty (STEP) to lengthen the bowel [24]. The only definitive contraindications to these reconstructive procedures are patients with severe liver disease or cirrhosis.

However, this procedure may be achieved successfully after isolated liver transplantation for liver disease secondary to intestinal failure and SBS [22]. SBBO is a frequent complication that causes mucosal inflammation, which may exacerbate further nutrient malabsorption [20]. SBBO increases the risk of intestinal bacterial translocation, and exacerbates hepatotoxicity related to PN. SBBO is likely to occur in the case of ICV resection, poor motility in a dilated small bowel segment, or when a tight anastomosis is present. Therapy

is difficult, the use of antibiotics is a matter of debate and should be used very cautiously according to their effects. First, the use of a broad-spectrum antimicrobial therapy must be limited in view of the high risk of emergence of multiresistant strains of bacteria and the deleterious impact on colonic physiology of disturbing the bacterial flora. The use of probiotics might be helpful but is not yet validated in SBS pediatric patients and should be used very cautiously regarding the addition of exogenous flora to an already overgrown small bowel bacterial flora [19]. Whenever possible, performing an intestinal tapering procedure or resecting a tight anastomosis may be mandatory to obtain the disappearance of bacterial overgrowth.

Other causes of IF

Intestinal neuromuscular motility disorders

Total colonic aganglionosis with jejuno-ileal involvement is a rare form of Hirschsprung disease (HD). HD affects 1 in 5000 newborns and is defined as an absence of ganglion cells in a variable length of distal bowel. The receptor tyrosine kinase gene RET is the most common gene in which a mutation may be found. In 80% of infants, the aganglionosis is confined to the rectum and sigmoid, but it may extend to encompass the entire colon (total colonic aganglionosis) or very rarely (1% of HD) affect the entire intestine. When the normal ganglionic small bowel is shorter than 50 cm, the probability for permanent PN dependency is high. There is no surgical procedure to improve the intestinal absorption. Thus, total colonic aganglionosis with jejuno-ileal involvement is equivalent to SBS without colon [15,16].

Chronic intestinal pseudo-obstruction syndrome (CIPOS) is a very heterogeneous condition in terms of clinical presentation, histopathological features, severity of motility disorders, and outcome [25]. Patients with the most severe form of CIPOS, myopathic or neuropathic with or without urinary tract involvement, are very uncomfortable because of the association of enterostoma, gastrostomy tube, central line, and sometimes vesicostomy. Intestinal transplantation becomes a logical option but may prove challenging in view of the usual history of multiple prior surgical procedures and the frequent presence of associated disorders such as uropathy or peripheral neuropathy. Congenital diseases of enterocyte development such as microvillus atrophy (MVA) and intestinal epithelial dysplasia (IED) or "tufting enteropathy" cause IF [21,26]. There is strong evidence that both disorders are inherited in an autosomic recessive manner. Onset of either disorder is within the first few days or weeks of life in the form of severe watery diarrhea. Most patients suffering from a constitutive disorder of intestinal epithelial cells remain permanently dependent on PN and are logical candidates for intestinal transplantation.

Causes of intestinal failure in adults

Short Bowel Syndrome represents nearly 80% of long-term HPN adult patients [13,27]. In adults the minimal lengths of a normal small bowel are 100 cm with no colon in continuity, 60 cm with some remaining colon, and 35 cm with the full colon (and the ileocecal valve). Short Bowel Syndrome in the adult population may be secondary to: ischemia (21%), Crohn's disease (16%), desmoid tumor, Gardner's syndrome and familial polyposis (24%), trauma (12%), volvulus (9%), and a miscellaneous group of rare causes (e.g. radiation enteritis, postbariatric surgery) (20%) [28]. Patients with Crohn's disease represent a very distinctive group of patients with intestinal failure [29,30]. Intestinal failure in Crohn's disease may occur secondary to extensive primary disease or to multiple resections. The latter occur mainly in the context of unplanned resections for intrabdominal sepsis. In considering such patients for intestinal transplantation the risk of recurrent disease must be considered. Short Bowel Syndrome post mesenteric venous thrombosis can be associated with hypercoagulable states related to inherited thrombotic disorders, such as Factor V Leiden mutation, deficiencies of anticoagulant proteins (protein S, protein C, and antithrombin III) [31,32].

Classification (linked to the management of IF)

The initial definition of intestinal failure was "a reduction in functioning gut mass below the minimal amount necessary for adequate digestion and absorption of nutrients." Two principles apply to obtain the minimum required level of PN dependence in a patient: to avoid exclusive or total intravenous feeding as

much as possible and to implement enteral feeding as much as possible.

Patient management

The goals of the management of intestinal failure are multiple: to cure the IF and achieve a full recovery by weaning PN, to procure a safe artificial support to minimize the complications and, in the case of definite IF, to offer the patient the best quality of life with, or without, intestinal transplantation. So the objectives of a center for intestinal rehabilitation is to define the candidacy for rehabilitation or temporary IF, the candidacy for long-term and definite PN or irreversible IF and candidacy for transplantation or irreversible IF with complications [33] (Figure 6.1).

Rehabilitation is considered for any patient who demonstrates ar a tolerance for oral feeding. Children who have tolerated continuous tube feeding and who have more than 20 cm of jejunoileum when the ileocecal valve is in situ, or more that 40 cm without the ICV should be considered for rehabilitation. In adults, the likelihood of weaning from HPN can be variously predicted, according to the length of remaining, depending on the three main anatomic types of SBS: end-jejunostomy (no colon in continuity), jejunocolonic (some part of the colon is in continuity), and jejuno-ileal (the full colon is in continuity): for these three scenarios, the minimal lengths of a normal small bowel are 100 cm, 60 cm, and 35 cm, respectively [34]. The probability of weaning patients off PN becomes less than 10% if weaning is not obtained during the first 4 years of PN in children and 2 years in adults. Management of HPN must be an integrated part of the management of the disease that has led to intestinal failure. We have new tools that permit better delineation, among short bowel patients, of transient from permanent (i.e. irreversible intestinal failure). The prognosis is better in HPN patients having a short but functioning gut rather than in patients with a longer but nonfunctioning gut [35].

Patients with no chance of intestinal rehabilitation are candidates for long-term PN. It is important to set up a minimum level of PN dependence during HPN management. PN dependence can be viewed as the minimal input of water, minerals, protein, and energy

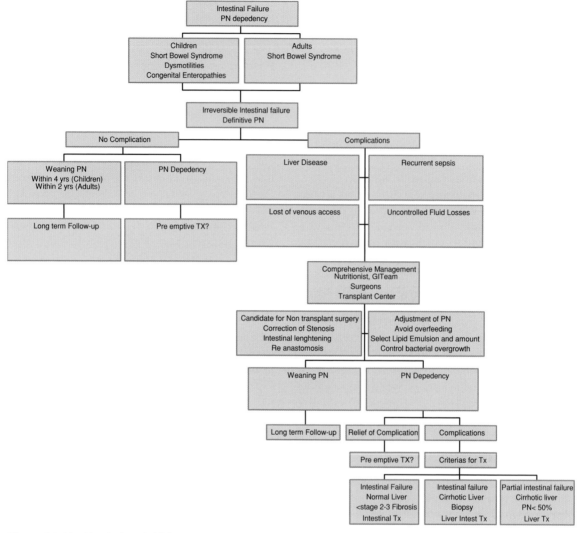

Figure 6.1 Algorithm for intestinal failure management.

for patient's equilibrium. Insufficient oral intake or oral failure, not directly dependent on the intestinal condition, is another caveat that compromises oral autonomy and also may induce a higher-than-needed PN delivery. Management should focus on the avoidance of complications, in particular liver disease and sepsis. Intestinal failure–associated liver disease develops in 40% to 60% of infants who require long-term total parenteral nutrition (TPN) for intestinal failure and 15% to 40% of adults on home parenteral nutrition [36,37]. Progression to biliary cirrhosis and the development of portal hypertension and liver failure occurs in a minor-

ity but is more common in infants and neonates than in adults. Sepsis remains the main cause of death in this group. This point raises the question of preemptive transplantation.

The remaining group contains those patients who should be enrolled in a transplant program. In the United States, Medicare pays for intestinal transplantation in patients who failed PN, including those with liver failure, thrombosis of at least two or more major vessels channels and frequent line infections (more than two sepsis a year). This definition is probably much too restrictive and we should consider for

Table 6.1 Patient population with intestinal failure. (Reproduced from Pironi et al. [27], with permission from Blackwell Publishing.)

	Adults (N = 688)	Pediatrics (N = 166)
Gender (No.)		
Male/female	293/395	87/79
Age (yr)	52.9 ± 15.2 (18.5–88.0)	6.1 ± 5.1 (0.2–18.0)
Cause of intestinal failure (No. (%))		
Short bowel syndrome	514 (74.7)	87 (52.4)
Motility disorder	124 (18.0)	38 (22.9)
Extensive Enteropathy	35 (5.1)	41 (24.7)
Primary disease in the pediatric population		
Congenital short bowel		42 (25.3)
Congenital mucosal disease		29 (17.5)
Chronic intestinal pseudo-obstruction		29 (17.4)
Volvulus		13 (16.5)
Necrotizing enterocolitis		13 (7.8)
Hirschsprung's disease		9 (5.4)
Crohn's disease		6 (3.6)
Primary disease in the adult population		
Mesenteric ischemia	**185 (26.9)**	
Crohn's disease	**159 (23.1)**	
Radiation enteritis	**73 (10.6)**	
Chronic intestinal pseudo-obstruction	**72 (10.5)**	
Surgical complications	55 (8.0)	
Familial polyposis	21 (3.0)	
Cancer	17 (2.5)	

intestinal transplantation, patients with intestinal failure and high morbidity or "low acceptance of PN." This should include patients with "nonreconstructible gastrointestinal tract," and those with difficult electrolyte management. The European Survey [27] reported that about 15% of adult and 35% of pediatric patients currently on PN for IF were candidates for transplantation, but only a few (about 15% of both adult and pediatric candidates) were considered to need ITx immediately (Table 6.1).

This may point out uncertainties about timing for patient referral and the need for guidelines on this key point. Late referral for ITx may be associated with higher mortality rates, because of the difficulty in matching up donor organs, especially in children. Data from the International Transplant Registry show lower survival rates in patients who required hospital-ization immediately before transplantation because of a poor clinical status [28]. At present, candidacy for ITx because of intestinal failure with high morbidity may be taken into account only when a careful revision of the treatment protocol has failed to improve the patient outcome. Patients unwilling to continue PN and asking for a preemptive intestinal transplantation should be aware that no study has yet clearly demonstrated a difference in quality of life between stable patients on long-term PN and transplanted patients [27].

Conclusions

Intestinal failure is less frequent than liver, heart, or renal failure but it remains a life-threatening clinical situation. Parenteral nutrition is the first line treatment in irreversible IF. A comprehensive management directed in an intestinal rehabilitation center demonstrated the safety of the long-term PN, increases the chance to be off PN and if the IF is irreversible to improve the survival after intestinal transplantation [38].

References

1 Lillehei RC, Idezuki Y, Feemster JA, et al. Transplantation of stomach, intestine, and pancreas: experimental and clinical observations. *Surgery* 1967;62:721–741.

2 Dudrick SJ, Wilmore DW, Vars HM, et al. Can intravenous feeding as the sole means of nutrition support growth in the child and restore weight loss in an adult? An affirmative answer. *Ann Surg* 1969;169:974–984.

3 Lee KK, Stangl MJ, Todo S, et al. Successful orthotopic small bowel transplantation with short-term FK 506 immunosuppressive therapy. *Transplant Proc* 1990;22:78–79.

4 Nordgaard I, Hansen BS, Mortensen PB. Importance of colonic support for energy absorption as small-bowel failure proceeds. *Am J Clin Nutr* 1996;64:222–231.

5 Crenn P, Coudray-Lucas C, Thuillier F, et al. Postabsorptive plasma citrulline concentration is a marker of absorptive enterocyte mass and intestinal failure in humans. *Gastroenterology* 2000;119:1496–1505.

6 Crenn P, Vahedi K, Lavergne-Slove A, et al. Plasma citrulline: a marker of enterocyte mass in villous atrophy-associated small bowel disease. *Gastroenterology* 2003;124:1210–1219.

7 Rhoads JM, Plunkett E, Galanko J, et al. Serum citrulline levels correlate with enteral tolerance and bowel length in infants with short bowel syndrome. *J Pediatr* 2005;146:542–547.

8 Goulet O, Ruemmele F. Causes and management of intestinal failure in children. *Gastroenterology* 2006;130(Suppl 1):S16–S28.

9 Pappas PA, Tzakis AG, Saudubray JM, et al. Trends in serum citrulline and acute rejection among recipients of small bowel transplants. *Transplant Proc* 2004;36:345–347.

10 Howard L, Ament M, Fleming CR, et al. Current use and clinical outcome of home parenteral and enteral nutrition therapies in the United States. *Gastroenterology* 1995;109:355–365.

11 Goulet O, Baglin-Gobet S, Talbotec C, et al. Outcome and long-term growth after extensive small bowel resection in the neonatal period: a survey of 87 children. *Eur J Pediatr Surg* 2005;15:95–101.

12 Goulet OJ, Revillon Y, Jan D, et al. Neonatal short bowel syndrome. *J Pediatr* 1991;119:18–23.

13 Bakonyi Neto A, Takegawa B, Ortolan E, et al. Demographic of short gut syndrome: increasing demand is not followed by referral of potential candidates for small bowel transplantation. *Transplant Proc* 2004;36:259–260.

14 Driver CP, Bruce J, Bianchi A, et al. The contemporary outcome of gastroschisis. *J Pediatr Surg* 2000;35:1719–1723.

15 Yann R, Yves A, Dominique J, et al. Improved quality of life by combined transplantation in Hirschsprung's disease with a very long aganglionic segment. *J Pediatr Surg* 2003;38:422–424; discussion 422–424.

16 Bond GJ, Reyes JD. Intestinal transplantation for total/near-total aganglionosis and intestinal pseudo-obstruction. *Semin Pediatr Surg* 2004;13:286–292.

17 Vennarecci G, Kato T, Misiakos EP, et al. Intestinal transplantation for short gut syndrome attributable to necrotizing enterocolitis. *Pediatrics* 2000;105: E25.

18 Touloukian RJ, Smith GJ. Normal intestinal length in preterm infants. *J Pediatr Surg* 1983;18:720–723.

19 DiBaise JK, Young RJ, Vanderhoof JA. Intestinal rehabilitation and the short bowel syndrome: part 1. *Am J Gastroenterol* 2004;99:1386–1395.

20 DiBaise JK, Young RJ, Vanderhoof JA. Intestinal rehabilitation and the short bowel syndrome: part 2. *Am J Gastroenterol* 2004;99:1823–1832.

21 Goulet O, Sauvat F, Jan D. Surgery for pediatric patients with chronic intestinal pseudo-obstruction syndrome. *J Pediatr Gastroenterol Nutr* 2005;41(Suppl 1):S66–S68.

22 Bianchi A. From the cradle to enteral autonomy: the role of autologous gastrointestinal reconstruction. *Gastroenterology* 2006;130(Suppl 1):S138–S146.

23 Bianchi A. Autologous gastrointestinal reconstruction for short bowel syndrome. *Br J Hosp Med (Lond)* 2007;68: 24–27.

24 Kim HB, Fauza D, Garza J, et al. Serial transverse enteroplasty (STEP): a novel bowel lengthening procedure. *J Pediatr Surg* 2003;38:425–429.

25 Faure C, Goulet O, Ategbo S, et al. Chronic intestinal pseudoobstruction syndrome: clinical analysis, outcome, and prognosis in 105 children. French-Speaking Group of Pediatric Gastroenterology. *Dig Dis Sci* 1999;44:953–959.

26 Herzog D, Atkison P, Grant D, et al. Combined bowel-liver transplantation in an infant with microvillous inclusion disease. *J Pediatr Gastroenterol Nutr* 1996;22:405–408.

27 Pironi L, Hébuterne X, Van Gossum A, et al. Candidates for intestinal transplantation: a multicenter survey in

Europe. *Am J Gastroenterol* 2006;101:1633–1643; quiz 1679.

28 Grant D, Abu-Elmagd K, Reyes J, et al. 2003 report of the intestine transplant registry: a new era has dawned. *Ann Surg* 2005;241: 607–613.

29 Thompson JS, Iyer KR, DiBaise JK, et al. Short bowel syndrome and Crohn's disease. *J Gastrointest Surg* 2003;7:1069–1072.

30 Kaila B, Grant D, Pettigrew N, et al. Crohn's disease recurrence in a small bowel transplant. *Am J Gastroenterol* 2004;99:158–162.

31 Rhee RY, Gloviczki P. Mesenteric venous thrombosis. *Surg Clin North Am* 1997;77:327–338.

32 Grant D, Wall W, Mimeault R, et al. Successful small-bowel/liver transplantation. *Lancet* 1990;335: 181–184.

33 Fishbein TM, Schiano T, LeLeiko N, et al. An integrated approach to intestinal failure: results of a new program with total parenteral nutrition, bowel rehabil-itation, and transplantation. *J Gastrointest Surg* 2002;6: 554–562.

34 Messing B, Crenn P, Beau P, et al. Long-term survival and parenteral nutrition dependence in adult patients with the short bowel syndrome. *Gastroenterology* 1999;117:1043–1050.

35 Messing B, Joly F. Guidelines for management of home parenteral support in adult chronic intestinal failure patients. *Gastroenterology* 2006;130(Suppl 1):S43–S51.

36 Kelly DA. Intestinal failure-associated liver disease: what do we know today? *Gastroenterology* 2006;130(Suppl 1):S70–S77.

37 Gupte GL, Beath SV, Kelly DA, et al. Current issues in the management of intestinal failure. *Arch Dis Child* 2006;91:259–264.

38 Fryer J, Pellar S, Ormond D, et al. Mortality in candidates waiting for combined liver-intestine transplants exceeds that for other candidates waiting for liver transplants. *Liver Transpl* 2003;9:748–753.

7 Causes of Intestinal Failure in the Newborn

Yigael Finkel

Key points

- Appropriate surgical management of congenital and neonatal intestinal catastrophes will allow most neonates and infants to survive.

- The long-term medical management should include therapies adapted to each stage of intestinal failure based on a multidisciplinary approach in centers involving pediatric surgery, pediatric gastroenterology, parenteral nutrition expertise and home-parenteral nutrition program.

- Growth may be achieved on long-term parenteral nutrition.

- Appropriate medical management should especially aim to prevent PN related complications such as vascular thrombosis and catheter related sepsis as well as IF related end stage liver disease (see Chapter 21).

- Long term PN and home PN are the cornerstone of management (see Chapter 14) together with appropriate feeding favoring early oral feeding (see Chapter 17).

- Non transplant surgery may be indicated in selected patients fulfilling the criteria with appropriate timing (see Chapter 26)

- Isolated liver Tx for SBS, however successful in many cases, should be avoided with careful measures to prevent liver disease (see Chapter 30)

Intestinal Failure: Diagnosis, Management and Transplantation.
Edited by Alan N. Langnas, Olivier Goulet, Eamonn M.M. Quigley and Kelly A. Tappenden. © 2008 Blackwell Publishing. ISBN 978-1-4051-4637-1.

Congenital or acquired disorders of the gastrointestinal tract of the newborn infant may cause intestinal failure requiring long-term parenteral nutrition. On the basis of pathogenesis, the causes of intestinal failure in this age-group can be classified as:

1 Anatomic reduction of the gut.
2 Neuromuscular disease involving the GI tract.
3 Congenital diseases of the intestinal epithelium.

In Table 7.1, the four most common conditions that cause intestinal failure in infants are presented (Table 7.1).

Congenital malformations

Gastroschisis

Gastroschisis is an abdominal wall defect characterized by an intact umbilical cord, evisceration of bowel through a defect in the abdominal wall, generally to the right of the cord, and with no membrane covering (Figure 7.1). Gastroschisis was described as early as 1733 by Calder. It was not until 1952, however, that it was distinguished from the other major abdominal wall defect, omphalocele [5].

Incidence

Recent European epidemiological studies of gastroschisis show a real increase in prevalence of gastroschisis since 1980, probably a result of unknown environmental factors [6], and a regional variation within United Kingdom ranging from 1.8 to 3.2 per 10,000 registered births [7]. Recent data from the British Isles Network of Congenital Anomaly Registers (BINOCAR) show that the prevalence of gastroschisis is even higher at 4.0 per 10,000 total births for the period 2002 to 2004. There has been a significant increase over the past 10 years

Table 7.1 Etiology of short bowel syndrome in children.

	USA (1)	CANADA (2)	France (3)	International (4)
• Atresia	30%	30%	39%	23%
• Volvulus	10%	10%	24%	24%
• Gastroschisis	17%	12.5%	14%	14%
• NEC	43%	35%	14%	27%

(Reproduced from Groulet and Sauvat. *Curr Opin Clin Nutr Metab Care* 2006;304–13, with permission from Lippincott Williams and Wilkins.)

from 2.5 to 4.4 per 10,000 total births over the period 1994 to 2003. Around 40% of babies with gastroschisis are born to mothers under the age of 20 years compared with only 9% of overall births.

Pathogenesis and etiology

In 1963, Duhamel [8] suggested that an early teratogenic event might prevent differentiation of the embryonic mesenchyme, thereby, reducing the mesenchymal support leading to a disruption of the abdominal wall. Recent theories have focused on dysplastic abdominal wall formation, perhaps related to a vascular abnormality resulting in a thinned area of abdominal wall) which

ruptures because of intraabdominal pressure [9]. Arguments for genetic factors for gastroschisis are supported by familiar incidence [10]. An association between maternal medication during pregnancy and an increased risk of gastroschisis has been reported [11].

Clinical management

Prenatal diagnosis of abdominal wall defects is routine. This allows one to choose delivery time and place and facilitates the preparation of the surgical team. The outcome for infants with gastroschisis seems not to be

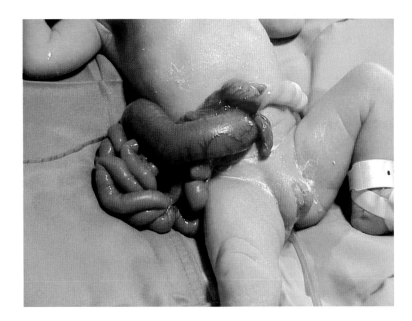

Figure 7.1 Gastroschisis. (Courtesy Dr Henrik Ehrén.)

influenced by mode of delivery, according to one meta-analysis [12]. However, most clinicians agree on the need for caesarean section in cases where the liver is extracorporeal.

Repair technique

The reduction of the abdominal contents should be performed within hours after delivery to avoid fluid losses and compromise to intestinal circulation with care to avoid marked increase of abdominal pressure during reduction of the herniated viscera into the abdomen. There is no evidence either supporting, or refuting, the use of ward reduction of gastroschisis rather than performing this procedure under anaesthesia in an operating room [13]. If reduction is not possible, a prosthetic silo created from silastic or Teflon is recommended.

Problems leading to IF

Survival for gastroschisis is over 85% [14]. However, feeding intolerance is highly prevalent in infants with gastroschisis caused by one or a combination of factors, such as bowel hypomotility, intestinal atresia, perforation, the presence of necrotic bowel segments, and the development of ovules. Intestinal atresia occurs in approximately 10 to 20% of infants with gastroschisis, and contributes to feeding delays and long-term parenteral nutrition.

Malrotation and midgut volvulus

Malrotation leading to volvulus should be regarded as a surgical time bomb with early clincial signs indistinguishable from less serious disorders of intestinal obstruction in infants. It is one of the four most common conditions that lead up to intestinal failure in infants.

Incidence

The incidence of malrotation in children 1–18 years of age is 5.3 per million population [15]. Population-based figures for prematures and infants are unavailable.

Embryology

At the fifth gestational week the fetal small intestine forms a loop which extrudes into the umbilical cord. The fetal gut subsequently undergoes enlargement, elongation and return of the hernial contents. The final placement of the intestine into the abdominal cavity is achieved by rotation and fixation of the fetal gut. Three steps in rotation have been identified although they are not fully proven and were lately contested [16].

   The general belief is that separate clinical entities may arise from impairment in each of the stages respectively. Although strict evidence is lacking the theory of stages in gut-rotation allows a comprehensible explanation of the various clinical presentations of malrotation. Failure of rotation in the first abdominal wall closure stage is seen in infants with omphalocele. Abnormity rotation of the second stage results may cause nonrotation of the gut, which is rare. The third and fourth parts of the duodenum are vertically placed along the right side of the superior mesenteric artery, the small bowel is on the right side and the colon to the left of the midline. In reversed rotation the duodenum is placed across anterior of with the cecum and the colon are placed behind the superior mesenteric vessels. Malrotation occurs when the rotation is not completed and typically the cecum does not reach the right ileal fossa and is found suphepatically or in a central position in the abdomen. The fixation of the gut may be aberrant and bands may form between the duodenum and the right colon. In cases of anomalous third stage the fixation of the midgut and cecum may be deficient.

Clinical management

Midgut volvulus in the newborn may develop as a result of anomalous rotation but also may occur without malrotation, more often so in premature infants with lax tissue [17]. Intrauterine midgut volvulus is thought to be the cause of intestinal atresia typ III b (see later). The symptoms of midgut volvulus are indistinguishable from other disorders with intestinal obstruction; vomiting, often bile-stained and abdominal

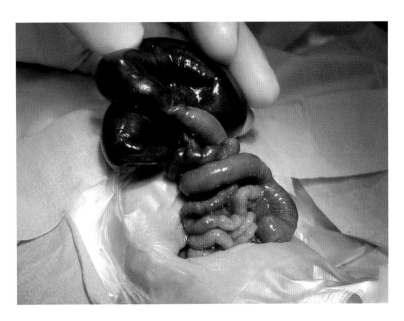

Figure 7.2 Volvulus. (Courtesy Dr Henrik Ehrén.)

distension in infants. Abdominal pain accompanied by bilious vomits are more common symptoms of malrotation in children >1 year of age. Barium enema and upper gastrointestinal series, Doppler flow of the superior mesenteric vessels, and laparoscopy are used to confirm the diagnosis.

The surgical management of midgut volvulus comprises expedience, detorsion of the volvulus, restoration of circulation, separation of adhesions between bowel loops, and attempts to preserve bowel length. A conservative resection of only obviously necrotic tissue is recommended and bowel with questionable viability should be left in situ for a second look 24–36 hours later (18) (Figure 7.2).

Intestinal atresia

The intestinal atresias are categorised according to their localisation. Duodenal lesions are classified by the method of Gray and Skandalakis. A type I defect represents a mucosal web with normal muscular wall (most common); type II, a short fibrous cord connecting the 2 atretic ends of the duodenum; and type III (least common), in which there is complete separation of the atretic ends. According to the classification of jejunoileal atresias by Martin and Zerella [19] and by

Grosfeld et al. [20], a type I defect represents a mucosal defect with an intact mesentery, a type II defect consists of a fibrous cord connecting the atretic bowel ends, a type IIIa lesion denotes an atretic segment with a V-shaped mesenteric gap defect, whereas a type IIIb defect defines the apple peel deformity, in which there is a proximal jejunal atresia and the distal bowel is supplied by a single retrograde blood vessel. In a type IV defect, multiple instances of atresias ("string of sausage" effect) are present. Atresia affecting the colon is, in most cases, a type IIIa defect, according to this classification [21] (Figure 7.3).

Etiology

There are two major theories regarding the etiology of intestinal atresia. Tandler presented, in 1900, his theory of a lack of revacuolization of the solid cord stage of intestinal development and Louw and Barnard [23] suggested that a late intrauterine mesenteric vascular accident is the cause of most jejunoileal and colonic atresias. Interestingly, the hypothesis on lack of revacuolization as the probable cause for most cases of duodenal still persists in many review articles. Jejunoileal atresias probably occur as a result of intestinal volvulus, intussusception, internal hernia, or strangulation

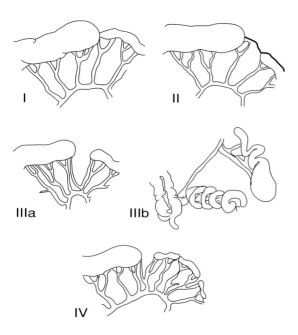

I
II
IIIa
IIIb
IV

Figure 7.3 Classification of jejunoileal atresia describes the pathology as type I (mucosal web), type II (fibrous cord), type IIIa (mesenteric gap defect), type IIIb ("apple peel"), or type IV (multiple atresias). (Reproduced from Welch et al. [22], with permission from Elsevier.)

in a tight gastroschisis or omphalocele defect. Familial instances of jejunoileal and colonic atresias also have been observed, suggesting that genetic factors may play a part in these cases.

Duodenal atresia is associated with prematurity, congenital anomalies including pancreatic anomalies; intestinal malrotation; esophageal atresia; Meckel's diverticulum; variants of imperforate anus; congenital heart disease; central nervous system lesions; renal anomalies; and, rarely, biliary tract anomalies. Down syndrome occurs in 25–30% of patients.

Prenatal diagnosis

The number of cases of intestinal atresia that are identified prenatally has increased as a result of the routine use of ultrasonographic monitoring of fetal development. Prenatal ultrasonography may identify the presence of maternal polyhydramnios and distension of the stomach and duodenum with swallowed amniotic fluid. These observations are often associated with a high risk of duodenal atresia. A notable number of jejunoileal and colonic atresias, however, remain undetected by prenatal ultrasonography.

Presentation

Typically, there are signs of bowel obstruction including bilious vomiting, abdominal distension, and failure to pass meconium in instances of lower obstruction. Most infants with duodenal obstruction do not have significant abdominal distension.

Clinical management

Preoperatively, management includes an orogastric sump tube to decompress the stomach, intravenous fluid resuscitation, and evaluation for associated cardiac or renal malformations. The operative management of intestinal atresia is individualized. Although the operative mortality has been reduced considerably over the last decades, infants with gastroschisis associated with atresia still have a prolonged length of hospital stay and higher morbidity and mortality. Multiple atresias or postoperative complications may lead to long-term TPN, while delayed or absence of bowel adaptation results in intestinal failure.

Intestinal atresia associated with immune-deficiency

Intestinal atresia has been reported to be associated with immunodeficiency. The first report involved three siblings with multiple-level intestinal atresias. One sib had severe combined immunodeficiency syndrome and clinical histories of the other two sibs strongly suggested a congenital immunodeficiency syndrome [24]. One report on three siblings each in two nonrelated families pointed to an association with Fanconi's anemia in three of seven pregnancies (two boys, one girl) suggesting an autosomal recessive mode of transmission. In a second family, identical multiple atresias occurred in two female siblings born 18 months apart and a third child with a duodenal stenosis. Overwhelming sepsis and a T cell dysfunction was seen in the postoperative period, which had partially corrected by follow-up at 5 months. This rare syndrome appears to have an autosomal recessive mode of transmission [25]. In one case-report of an infant with multiple segmental areas of atresia of the small and large bowel, with histologic features characteristic of the hereditary form of the disease posttransfusion graft-versus-host disease developed first, and then immunodeficiency was found [26]. In case of multiple intestinal atresias attention should be given to possible associated immune disorder and irradiation of blood products is recommended pending evaluation of immune system status. Donor immune reconstitution was reported in a child with multiple intestinal atresia and SCID who underwent liver and small-bowel transplantation. The child did not experience intestinal graft rejection but only a mild GVHD and it was postulated that this child engrafted a donor-derived immune system [27].

Necrotizing enterocolitis

Necrotizing enterocolitis (NEC) is an inflammatory bowel necrosis and a major cause of morbidity and mortality for preterm infants. Ninety percent of NEC occurs in premature infants and the incidence of NEC is inversely correlated with gestational age and birth weight.

Epidemiology

A large epidemiological study from the United States revealed an incidence of NEC of 2.8% [28]. Although the odds of death or major morbidity for very low birth weight (VLBW) infants who are born at non-subspecialty perinatal centers is twice that of infants who are born at subspecialty centers (despite controlling for demographic) this is not the case for the outcome of NEC [29]. Most studies report that the overall incidence of NEC in premature infants has remained unchanged over the last decades. However, one recent study in Australia observed a significant reduction in 24–28 weeks gestational age infants over the time period 1986–1999 [30].

Etiology and pathology

NEC does not occur in utero and 90% of the cases occur after infants have been fed. This points to the likelihood that the ingested feeds and the gut functions influenced by feeding per se may initiate the events that lead to NEC and the factors involved can be summarized as follows:

1 immature intestinal host defenses and blood flow regulation
2 bacterial colonization
3 inflammatory responses.

The host defenses of the gastrointestinal tract comprise physical barriers, that is, mucous membranes, intestinal epithelia, tight junctions, and mucin. Increased bacterial adherence to the mucosal membrane can be caused by decreased peristaltic activity caused by immaturity and by the presence of more adhesion sites caused by a different pattern of carbohydrate residues on the cell surfaces in the immature intestine [31].

Mucosal injury and immune stimulation by bacteria or bacterial products may lead to an inflammatory cascade that results in the ischemic necrosis, acute and chronic inflammation, bacterial overgrowth, and tissue repair seen in histopathological specimens of NEC. Several inflammatory mediators have been implicated in the pathogenesis of NEC: Platelet activating factor (PAF), toll-like receptors [32,33] excessive cytokine and nitric oxide (NO) production, disordered

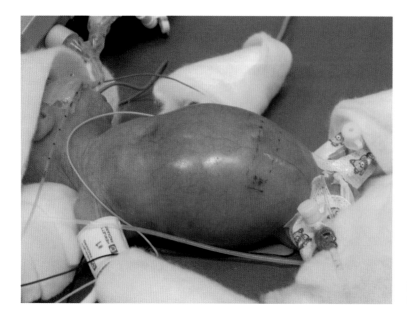

Figure 7.4 Distended abdomen with NEC. (Courtesy Dr Henrik Ehrén.)

enterocyte signaling and dysfunction of the intestinal barrier have all been implicated as playing a role in the genesis of NEC. The inflammatory process, in NEC, primarily affects the terminal ileum and proximal colon but also can be widespread throughout the large and small intestine.

Feeding strategies involving comparisons of either rapid or slow increases in daily feed volumes to prevent NEC, have shown conflicting results [34,35]. A meta-analysis of transpyloric versus intragastric feeding did not reveal any difference in NEC between the two feeding methods [36]. Several studies have shown that infants who are fed human milk are less likely to develop NEC compared to formula-fed infants.

Clinical features

NEC presents with variable symptoms, including abdominal distension, feeding intolerance, gastric aspirates and bilious vomiting (Figure 7.4). Local tenderness or an abdominal mass may be defined on clinical examination and progression to pneumoperitoneum and sepsis with respiratory failure, shock and death may follow. The progression of this disease has been staged by Bell staging system [37] (Table 7.2). Laboratory studies may reveal leukocytosis, thrombocytope-

nia, electrolyte imbalance and acidosis, and coagulopathy. The typical radiological features of NEC are listed in the staging system of Bell. Thrombocytopenia is commonly observed in infants with severe NEC. A rapid fall in platelet count has a high specificity and positive predictive value for intestinal gangrene in NEC. Mortality in NEC can be 20–50% and as high as 60% in those infants who require surgery. NEC is associated with long-term morbidity and prolonged parenteral nutrition, multiple surgical procedures, and intestinal failure.

Treatment

Therapy of NEC includes stopping feeds, nasogastric decompression, fluid and electrolyte resuscitation, broad-spectrum antibiotics and, in selected cases, respiratory support. Severity, whether mild or critical, determines the duration of medical therapy. Parenteral antibiotics and nutrition and nil by mouth are usually prescribed for 7–14 days.

The indications for surgery are:

1 presence of pneumoperitoneum, indicating perforation of the intestine

2 clinical deterioration despite maximal medical treatment

Table 7.2 Bell staging system.

Stage	Systemic signs	Intestinal signs	Rediologic signs
Stage 1: Suspected NEC	Temperature instabililty, apnea, bradycardia, lethargy	Abdominal distension, gastric residue, vomiting, hematochezia	Normal or mild ileus
Stage 2: Definite NEC	Same as 1	Same as 1 plus abdominal tenderness	Prenumatoisis intestinalis or portal air
Stage 3: Advanced NEC	Shock, DIC, metabolic acidosis, thrombocytopenia, neutropenia	Peritonitis	Pneumoperitoneum

(Reproduced from Bell et al. [37], with permission from Lippincott Williams and Wilkins.)

3 abdominal mass with persistent intestinal obstruction or sepsis

4 development of intestinal stricture.

A laparoscopy may be useful to verify the need of surgical treatment and can be performed even in small infants by trained paediatric surgeons [38]. There is controversy regarding the preferred method of surgical management of NEC. The options are primary peritoneal drainage or laparotomy. At laparotomy, resection of affected bowel with formation of high enterostomy or primary anastomosis of remaining gut, are well accepted techniques. In infants suffering NEC, which involves extensive inflammation of both the large and the small intestine, a proximal, diverting jejonostomy or the "clip and drop" technique have been advocated [39]. These infants will develop intestinal failure needing long-term parenteral nutrition.

Is it possible to lower the risk of NEC with probiotics?

Recently, the first controlled studies of probiotics in VLBW children was published. The first study [40] involved 367 VLBW (<1500 g) infants who were all enterally fed and survived beyond the 7th day after birth. All infants received human breast milk, which was supplemented in the treated group (n = 180) with *Lactobacillus acidophilus* and *Bifidobacterium infantis* twice daily until discharge. The incidence of NEC or death was significantly lower in the probiotic-supplemented

group compared to placebo controls (5% vs. 12.8%) in these high-risk premature infants. In addition, no case of severe NEC was observed in the supplemented group compared to 3% in the control group. The second study [41] was performed in 145 premature infants assigned to a control group or treatment group, which were supplemented by a mixture of *Bifidobacterium infantis, Streptococcus thermophilus,* and *Bifidobacterium bifidum.* The NEC incidence was reduced to 4% in probiotic-supplemented infants compared to 16.4% (p = 0.03) in the nonsupplemented control group. In addition, NEC was less severe in the probiotic-supplemented group. The underlying molecular mechanisms of this NEC-prevention by probiotic supplementation remain unclear. With regard to safety concerns in the use of viable bacterial organisms in immunodeficient or compromised patients, such as premature infants, the studies of Lin et al. and Bin-Nun et al. did not reveal any complications, such as increased risk of septicaemia or others, related to the use of probiotics.

Total or near-total intestinal aganglionosis

Hirschsprung's disease (HD) is a congenital disorder characterised an interruption of the craniocaudal migration of neuroblasts and an absence of ganglionic innervation of the affected bowel causing intestinal obstruction. In 75–80% of the cases, the aganglionosis is confined to the rectum and sigmoid colon. Manifestation of the disease has been linked to mutations in genes that encode the crucial signals for the development of the enteric nervous system-the RET and EDNRB signaling pathways. The Phox2b gene is involved in neurogenesis and regulates Ret expression in mice, in which disruption of the Phox2b results in a de Vries PA. HD-like phenotype. Total or near-total aganglionosis (TAG or NTAG) is a rare form of HD, affecting less than 1% of children with HD. Recently, the concomitant existence of total bowel aganglionosis and congenital central hypoventilation syndrome in a neonate with Phox2b gene mutation was described [42].

Clinical management

Abdominal distension and bilious vomiting within the first week of life are the main clinical features of this condition. The extent of the aganglionotic segment of the small intestine and the appropriate placing of an ostomy should be guided by perioperative histopathologcial examinations of biopsies. In infants left with less than 50 cm of small intestine one can presume a definite and irreversible diagnosis of intestinal failure requiring long-term parenteral nutrition. In contrast to conditions of anatomical short bowel, there is no possibility for the remnant bowel to undergo adaptation and growth allowing for intestinal independency myotomy-myectomy, first described by Ziegler [43], and later by Shimotake et al. and Saxton et al. [44,45], has been suggested to improve the situation with respect to enteral nutrition in these patients. However, it has been reported that complications are the rule rather than the exception after this procedure.

Although several surgical techniques have been proposed for the use of the remnant aganglionic small-bowel in TAG, at present there is no evidence to recommend any. It is, rather, recommended to avoid recurrent surgery for lengthening, tapering, STEP, or longitudinal myotomy. All surgical procedures that could lead to a reduction of the abdominal cavity size will thereby impair the probable intestinal transplantation procedure. Over the last few years, the use of parenteral nutrition and new surgical techniques, including small-bowel transplantation, have slightly improved the prognosis of this condition previously

regarded as fatal. Aganglionosis has been estimated to account for approximately 8% of patients with a primary indication for pediatric intestinal transplantation [46]. A general view is therefore that early referral to an expert unit to review the indications for small bowel transplantation is essential for the child with TAG [47].

References

1 Andorsky DJ, Lund DP, Lillehei CW, et al. Nutritional and other postoperative management of neonates with short bowel syndrome correlates with clinical outcomes. *J Pediatr* 2001;139:27–33.

2 Wales PW, de Silva N, Kim JH, et al. Neonatal short bowel syndrome: a cohort study. *J Pediatr Surg* 2005;40:755–762.

3 Goulet O, Baglin-Gobet S, Talbotec C, et al. Outcome and long-term growth after extensive small bowel resection in the neonatal period: a survey of 87 children. *Eur J Pediatr Surg* 2005;15:95–101.

4 Koffeman GI, van Gemert WG, George EK, Veenendaal RA. Classification, epidemiology and aetiology. *Best Pract Res Clin Gastroenterol* 2003;17:879–893.

5 Moore TC, Stokes GE. Gastroschisis, report of two cases treated by a modification of the Gross operation for omphalocele. *Surgery* 1952;33:112–120.

6 Dolk H. EUROCAT: 25 years of European surveillance of congenital anomalies. *Arch Dis Child Fetal Neonatal Ed* 2005;90:F355–F358.

7 Rankin J, Pattenden, S Abramsky L, et al. Prevalence of congenital anomalies in five British regions, 1991–99. *Arch Dis Child Fetal Neonatal Ed* 2005;90:F374–F379.

8 Duhamel B. Embryology of exomphalos and allied malformations. *Arch Dis Child 1963*;38:142–147.

9 De Vries PA. The pathogenesis of gastroschisis and omphalocele. *J Pediatr Surg* 1980;15:245–251.

10 Torfs CP, Velie EM, Oechsli FW, et al. A population-based study of gastroschisis: demographic, pregnancy and lifestyle risk factors. *Teratology* 1994;50:44–53.

11 Werler MM, Sheehan JE, Mitchell AA. Maternal medication use and risks of gastroschisis and small intestinal atresia. *Am J Epidemiol* 2002;155:26–31.

12 Segel SY, Marder SJ, Parry S, et al. Fetal abdominal wall defects and mode of delivery: a systematic review. *Obstet Gynecol* 2001;98:867–873.

13 Davies MW, Kimble RM, Woodgate PG. Ward reduction without general anaesthesia versus reduction and repair under general anaesthesia for gastroschisis in

newborn infants. The Cochran Database of systematic review 2002;Issue 3.

14 Snyder CL. Outcome analysis for gastroschisis. *J Pediatr Surg* 1999;34:1253–1256.

15 Malek, M, Burd, R. Surgical treatment of malrotation after infancy: a population-based study. *J Pediatr Surg* 2005;40:285–289.

16 Kluth D, Kaestner M, Tibboel D, Lambrecht W. Rotation of the gut: fact or fantasy? *J Pediatr Surg* 1995;30:448–453.

17 Usmani SS, Kenigsberg K. Intrauterine volvulus without malrotation. *J Pediatr Surg* 1991;26:1409–1410.

18 Ford EG, Senac MO Jr, Srikanth MS, Weitzman JJ. Malrotation of the intestine in children. *Ann Surg* 1992; 215:172–178.

19 Martin LW, Zerella JT. Jejunoileal atresia: a proposed classification. *J Pediatr Surg* 1976;11:399–403.

20 Grosfeld JL, Ballantine TVN, Shoemaker R. Operative management of intestinal atresia and stenosis based on pathologic findings. *J Pediatr Surg* 1979;14:368–375.

21 Gray SW, Skandalakis JE. *Embryology for Surgeons.* Philadelphia, Pa: WB Saunders Co, 1972;147–148.

22 Welch KW, Randolph JG, Ravitch MM, O'Neill JA Jr, Rowe MI, eds. *Pediatric Surgery* 4th ed, St Louis, Mo: Mosby-Year Book Inc, 1996.

23 Louw JH. Resection and end-to-end anastomosis in the management of atresia and stenosis of the small bowel. *Surgery* 1967;62:940–950.

24 Moreno LA, Gottrand F, Turck D, et al. Severe combined immunodeficiency syndrome associated with autosomal recessive familial multiple gastrointestinal atresias: study of a family. *Am J Med Genet* 1990;37:143–146.

25 Moore SW, de Jongh G, Bouic P, et al. Immune deficiency in familial duodenal atresia. *J Pediatr Surg* 1996;31:1733–1735.

26 Walker MW, Lovell MA, Kelly TE, et al. Multiple areas of intestinal atresia associated with immunodeficiency and posttransfusion graft-versus-host disease. *J Pediatr* 1993;123:93–95.

27 Gilroy RK, Coccia PF, Talmadge JE, Hatcher LI, Pirrucello SJ, Shaw BW Jr, Rubocki RJ, Sudan DL, Langnas AN, Horslen SP. Donor immune reconstitution after liver-small bowel transplantation for multiple intestinal atresia with immunodeficiency. *Blood* 2004;103:1171–1174.

28 Guthrie SO, Gordon PV, Thomas V, et al. Necrotising enterocolitis among neonates in the United States. *J Perinatol* 2003;23:278–285.

29 Warner B, Musial J, Chevier T, Donovan T. The effect of birth hospital types on the outcome of very low birth weight infants. *Pediatrics* 2004;113:35–41.

30 Luig M, Lui K, NICUS group Epidemiology of necrotising enetrocolitis—Changing trends in extremely premarure infants over 14 years. *J Paediatr Child Health* 2005;41:169–173.

31 Dai, D, Nanthkumar, NN, Newburg, DS, Walker, WA. Role of oligosaccharides and glycoconjugates in Intestinal Host Defense *J Pediatr Gastr Nutr* 2000;30(Suppl 2):S23–S33.

32 Ewer AK, Al-Salu W, Marshall JM, et al. The role of platelet acticating factor in a neonatal piglet model of necrotising enterocolitis. *Gut* 2004;53:207–213.

33 Caplan MS, Simon D, Jilling T. The role of PAF, TLR and the inflammatory response in neonatal necrotizing enterocolitis. *Semin Pedatr Surg* 2005;14:145–151.

34 Berseth CL Bisquera JA, Paje VU. Prolonging small feeding volumes early in life decreases the incidence of necrotiing enterocolitis in VLBW infants. *Pediatrics* 2003;111:529–534.

35 Salhorra A, Ramji S. Slow versus fast enteral feed advancement in VLBW infants. *Indian Pediatr* 2004;41:435–441.

36 McGuire P. Systematic review of transpyloric versus gastric tube feeding for preterm infants. *Arch Dis Child Fetal Neonatal* 2004;89:F289–F292.

37 Bell MJ, Ternberg JL, Feigin RD, et al. Neonatal necrotizing enterocolitis. *Ann Surg* 1978;187:1–7.

38 Pierro A. The surgical management of necrotising enterocolitis. *Early Human Development* 2005;81:79–85.

39 Vaughan WG, Grosfeld JL, West K, et al. Avoidance of stomas and delayed anastomosis for bowel necrosis the "clip and drop-back" technique. *J Pediatr Surg* 1996;31: 542–545.

40 Lin HC, Su BH, Chen AC, et al. Oral probiotics reduce the incidence and severity of necrotizing enterocolitis in very low birth weight infants. *Pediatrics* 2005;115:1–4.

41 Bin-Nun A, Bromiker R, Wilschanski M, et al. Oral probiotics prevent necrotizing enterocolitis in very low birth weight neonates. *J Pediatr* 2005;147:192–196.

42 Ou-Yang MC, Yang SN, Hsu YM, et al. Concomitant existence of total bowel aganglionosis and congenital central hypoventilation syndrome in a neonate with PHOX2B gene mutation. *J Pediatr Surg* 2007;42: 9–11.

43 Ziegler MM, Royal RE, Brandt J, et al. Extended myectomy-myotomy. A therapeutic alternative for total intestinal aganglionosis. *Ann Surg* 1993;218:504–509.

44 Shimotake T, Go S, Tomiyama H, et al. Proximal jejunostomy with or without myectomy-myotomy

modification in five infants with total intestinal agan-glionosis: An experience with surgical treatments in a single institution. *J Pediatr Surg* 2002;37:835–839.

45 Saxton ML, Ein SH, Hoehner J, Kim PC. Near-total in-testinal aganglionosis: long-term follow-up of a morbid condition. *J Pediatr Surg* 2000;35:669–672.

46 Grant D, Abu-Elmagd K, Reyes J, et al.; on behalf of the Intestine Transplant Registry. 2003 report of the intes-tine transplant registry: a new era has dawned. *Ann Surg* 2005;241:607–613.

47 Sharif K, Beath SV, Kelly DA, et al. New perspective for the management of near-total or total intestinal agan-glionosis. *J Pediatr Surg* 2003;38:25–28.

8 Congenital Enteropathies Causing Permanent Intestinal Failure

Olivier Goulet

Key points

- Congenital enteropathies are increasingly recognized as an important cause of intestinal failure in infancy and early childhood.

- It is important, clinically, to differentiate between protracted diarrhea of infancy (PDI), on the one hand, and intractable diarrhea (IDI) of infancy, on the other; the former ultimately resolves, the latter does not.

- The classification of IDI is based on clinical presentation and histological criteria. The main causes are: microvillous inclusion disease or microvillous atrophy, tufting enteropathy or intestinal epithelial dysplasia, syndromatic or phenotypic diarrhea, and autoimmune enteropathy.

- Progress has been made in understanding the genetic and molecular basis of these disorders.

- Management involves nutritional support and, for autoimmune enteropathies, intensive immunosuppression and even bone marrow transplantation. Congenital disease of epithelium development such as microvillous inclusion disease or tufting enteropathy require intestinal transplantation.

Among the causes of permanent intestinal failure (PIF), congenital enteropathies involving the development of the intestinal mucosa have an ever-increasing prominence [1]. The syndrome of intractable diarrhea of

Intestinal Failure: Diagnosis, Management and Transplantation.
Edited by Alan N. Langnas, Olivier Goulet, Eamonn M.M. Quigley and Kelly A. Tappenden. © 2008 Blackwell Publishing. ISBN 978-1-4051-4637-1.

infancy (IDI) was first described by Avery et al. in 1968 based on the following features: diarrhea occurring in a newborn younger than 3 months of age, lasting more than 2 weeks with three or more negative stool cultures for bacterial pathogens [2]. Most cases were managed in hospital using intravenous fluids; diarrhea, however, was persistent and intractable with a high mortality rate from infection or malnutrition [3]. The definition, presentation, and outcome of this syndrome have changed considerably over during the last three decades as a result of major improvements in nutritional management and a better understanding of the pathology of the small bowel mucosa. An early onset of severe diarrhea of infancy has been recently reported [4,5], and the term "severe diarrhea requiring parenteral nutrition" was proposed [4,5]. Diarrhea sometimes persists for years despite prolonged bowel rest and various therapeutic trials. In most cases, such as constitutive enterocyte disorders or autoimmune enteropathy, the situation rapidly becomes life-threatening and these patients depend, for their survival, on long-term parenteral nutrition (PN). Table 8.1 shows the diagnostic heterogenity of 65 cases with severe diarrhea requiring PN for more than one month, as recently analyzed in a French multicenter study [6]. Two major subtypes can be differentiated: patients with "protracted diarrhea of infancy" (PDI), which can be expected to resolve despite its initial severity. PDI can result from a sensitisation to a common food protein (e.g. cow's milk), or it can be secondary to a severe infection of the digestive tract (postenteritis syndrome) [7]. The second group is characterized by an "intractable diarrhea of infancy" (IDI) with onset within the first 2 years of life. It is important to distinguish between IDI and PDI because children with PDI always recover, sometimes only after several

Table 8.1 Causes and outcomes of protracted and intractable diarrhea of infancy.

Cause	Patients (n)	Deceased (n)
Protracted diarrhea	**39**	**1**
Multiple food intolerance	15	0
Infectious enteritis	14	0
Colitis (including 2 CMV)	6	1
CDG syndrome	1	0
Ganglioneuroblastoma	1	0
Unknown	2	0
Intractable diarrhea	**21**	**3**
Abnormalities of the enterocyte	6	1
– intestinal epithelial dysplasia	3	0
– microvillous atrophy	5	3
Autoimmune enteropathy	3	0
Phenotypic diarrhea	4	0
Undefined		

weeks or months of parenteral or enteral nutrition. In contrast, patients with IDI will remain dependent on parenteral nutrition or—in the case of autoimmune enteropathy—lifelong massive immunosuppression or bone marrow transplantation [8].

Current classification of intractable diarrhea of infancy

An attempt to classify IDI with villous atrophy a on the basis of immunohistological criteria and emphasizing the role of activated T cells in the intestinal mucosa, has been proposed [9]. A multicenter survey from ESPGHAN collected cases of IDI and villous atrophy according to precisely defined light microscopic characteristics and resulted in the delineation of several types of IDI [10]. The first is characterized by a mononuclear cell infiltration of the lamina propria and is considered to be associated with activated T cells. The second histological pattern features the early onset of severe diarrhea, villous atrophy without mononuclear cell infiltration of the lamina propria and specific histological abnormalities involving the epithelium. To date, several types of primary epithelial abnormalities inducing IDI have been identified. The first described was microvillous atrophy (MVA) or microvillous inclusion disease and, more recently, tufting enteropathy or intestinal epithelial dysplasia [11]. Some patients are small for gestational age and present with phenotypic abnormalities corresponding to the previously described syndromatic diarrhea [12].

Microvillous atrophy

In 1978, Davidson et al. reported five infants with severe, persistent diarrhea beginning in the newborn period, in whom light microscopy revealed crypt hypoplastic villous atrophy [13]. Electron microscopic (EM) examination of small intestinal biopsies from three of the patients showed severe brush-border (BB) abnormalities and increased liposome-like bodies, and in one, intracytoplasmic cysts made up of the brush border. Further children were reported with these characteristic cytoplasmic inclusions of the BB membrane [6,14]. From these clinical and histological descriptions, MVA has been established as a distinct disease within the syndrome of IDI, based on the characteristic morphological features. MVA, in its typical form, is a congenital disorder of intestinal epithelial cells presenting as intractable neonatal diarrhea [14].

Clinical features

In general, infants develop severe watery diarrhea within the first days after birth. Stool volumes may be as high that 250–300 ml/kg body weight per day, with electrolyte concentrations similar to those seen in small intestinal fluid. This disorder is particularly life-threatening because massive diarrhea leads to rapid dehydration and electrolyte imbalance with subsequent metabolic decompensation within a few hours. Severe watery diarrhea persists despite bowel rest. The differential diagnosis may include congenital chloride diarrhea or sodium malabsorption diarrhea, which can be easily distinguished from MVA by assessments of blood and stool electrolytes [15–17]. In contrast, the clinical presentation of MVA may, sometimes, be very atypical as a pseudo-obstruction-type syndrome featuring distended loops of small bowel and colon filled with fluid. Usually, the onset of diarrhea in MVA is within the first few days (early-onset or congenital form). However,

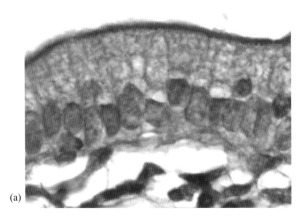

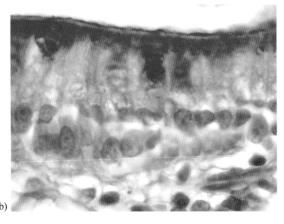

Figure 8.1 Periodic acid-schiff (PAS) staining. (a) Normal mucosa, normal PAS, brush border staining. (b) Abnormal accumulation of PAS, positive material in the apical cytoplasme of epithelial cells in microvillous inclusion disease.

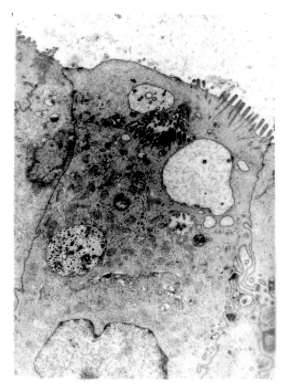

Figure 8.2 Microvillous inclusion disease. Electron microscopy of jejunal biopsy specimen. The brush border is almost absent. The cytoplasm contains a microvillous inclusion.

in few patients the onset of diarrhea is delayed (first month) and less severe (late-onset form).

Histopathological analysis

The diagnosis may be easily performed on the basis of light microscopic examination of duodenal or jejunal biopsy specimens. On haematoxylin-eosin staining, the mucosa appears flattened with hypoplastic villous atrophy. Highly characteristic for this disorder is the accumulation of periodic acid Schiff (PAS)–positive secretory granules within the apical cytoplasm of enterocytes [17–19] (Figure 8.1). At the ultrastructural level, microvilli are found to be rare or absent on

intestinal epithelial cells and inclusions of microvilli in the cytoplasm of enterocytes are seen; the latter defines this entity [20]. A valuable new tool for the light microscopic diagnosis of MVA was recently proposed [21,22]. CD-10 is a membrane-associated neutral peptidase, shown to have a linear brush-border staining pattern in the normal small intestine. In contrast to this surface staining pattern seen in different populations (normal intestine, celiac disease, autoimmune enteropathy, allergy), all MVA cases revealed prominent intracytoplasmic CD-10 immunoreactivity in surface enterocytes [21]. Similar results were obtained with PAS, polyclonal carcinoembryonic antigen, and alkaline phosphatase, three stains known to show cytoplasmic staining of surface enterocytes in MVA [23]. On electron microscopy, surface epithelial cells show absent or grossly abnormal microvilli, as well as numerous vesicular bodies of various size, and the characteristic microvilous inclusions (Figure 8.2). Crypt cells are almost normal morphogically, but do not contain increased numbers of apical vesicles and vesicular bodies. Microvillous inclusions, as well as increased secretory granules, are also present in the large bowel, an area more easily accessible for biopsy, especially in early infancy.

Pathophysiology and mode of transmission

A defect in the membrane trafficking of immature and/or differentiating enterocytes has been proposed as a basic etiopathogenic mechanism in MVA [20,23]. This membrane defect results in complete intestinal failure. It has been speculated that the disease is associated with a disorder of the cytoskeleton of enterocytes, which produces an abnormal assembly of microvilli. Intestinal microvillous dystrophy was reported as being a hypothetical variant of MVA [24]. The underlying pathogenesis of MVA is still unclear. When analyzing the turnover of sucrase-isomaltase, as a representative brush border protein, there is clear evidence that the direct and indirect constitutive pathways are intact in MVA [20]. These observations are compatible with the hypothesis that there is a block in the exocytosis of an unidentified brush border-related material, as exhibited by the accumulation of PAS-positive secretory granules, a result of a deficient molecular myosin-actin based transport system [19]. Secretory granule accumulation is the first abnormality detected in the epithelial cell life cycle, and the formation of microvillous inclusions appears subsequently in older cells [14,19]. Indeed, in both congenital and late onset microvillous atrophy, microvilli appear near normal in regions where secretory granules first accumulate, and microvilli reappear on surface epithelial cells in atypical microvillous atrophy, despite their severe reduction in the crypt epithelium [14] This indicates that a defect in microvillous biosynthesis is not the basis of the disease. Therefore, a defect in endocytosis is rather unlikely. More recently, by investigating the secretory granules, Phillips et al. suggested that MVA involves a defect in exocytosis of the glycocalyx that might impair normal cell functions [23]. Indeed, in MVA, there is an accumulation within the epithelium of a neutral glycosubstance that contained acetylated sialic acid. Blood group antigens are detected on the brush bor-

der, in mucus, and within goblet cells in normal mucosa, whereas in MVA they are additionally expressed within the apical cytoplasm of epithelial cells mirroring the PAS abnormality. Immunoelectron microscopy localized expression to secretory granules. It is speculated that the abnormal staining pattern reflects the accumulation of glycocalyx-related material. Whether the consequences of this abnormality are sufficient to explain the severity of the clinical picture in microvillous atrophy awaits further investigation.

Considering the number of cases with affected siblings and the frequency of consanguinity among patients in families of affected infants, this disease appears to be transmitted as an autosomal recessive trait [25–27]. No candidate gene has, to date, been identified. MVA has been reported in a girl with autosomal dominant hypochondroplasia [26]. The gene defect of this disease was recently localized on chromosome region 4p16.3, which might help in elucidating the genetic basis of MVA.

Long-term outcome
MVA is a congenital constitutive intestinal epithelial cell disorder leading, in its typical early-onset form, to PIF. The largest multicenter survey of 23 MVA patients [14] revealed an extremely reduced life expectancy with a 1-year survival rate of less than 25%. Most children died of septic complications, liver failure, or metabolic decompensation. A few cases of MVA, especially those with the late-onset form, may survive with limited stool output and may require only partial PN. Treatment with corticosteroïds, colostrum, or epidermal growth factor have not been successful, but octreotide has been used with partial success in one patient [14]. In contrast to the dismal outcomes reported before the 1980s, PN now allows most infants and children with MVA to survive. However, complications related to inadequate PN do limit long-term survival. In addition, and in the absence of any associated renal disease, some of these infants and children used to develop chronic fluid and electrolyte imbalance and acidosis with consequent growth impairment. Others, because of repeated episodes of dehydration in the absence of supplemental calcium and phosphate intake, developed nephrocalcinosis. Finally, even with adequate long-term PN and normal growth, most children continue to manifest high and disabling levels of stool output that require daily fluid and electrolyte

replacement and result in a high risk for severe dehydration. Thus, intestinal transplantation became the only definitive treatment for this rare intestinal disease.

Several cases of successful transplantation for MVA have been reported [28–32]. Transplantation involved isolated intestine [28,31] or combined with the liver [29,30]. In reports of these cases, there has been an open discussion on whether or not the colon should be transplanted together with the small bowel. We recently reported on patients with early-onset congenital MVA [32]. Two patients died before they could be put on the waiting list for SbTx, one patient is still awaiting SbTx. We performed cadaveric intestinal transplantation (ITx) on 7 patients aged between 3 and 11 years using tacrolimus, steroids, and IL-2 blockers. Three isolated ITx were performed and four combined liver and intestinal transplants. The right colon was included in five of these grafts (two isolated ITx). Six patients (86%) have survived with a median follow-up of 3 years (range 1–8 years).

MVA has clearly become a logical indication for ITx. Management involves nutritional support and the prevention of water-electrolytes imbalance. Because of high daily fluid losses, these patients are very difficult to manage safely on cyclical parenteral nutrition. Repeated water and electrolyte imbalance may impair renal function and cause tubular injury and nephrocalcinosis. Most patients receive continuous parenteral nutrition with subsequent poor quality of life and increased risk of PN-related metabolic complications as a result of the need for continuous infusion of PN. Thus, the appropriate strategy requires early referral for transplantation of a patient in good nutritional status. In our experience, the youngest patient with MVA was successfully transplanted at 11 months of age and is doing very well 2 years later. ITx alone, or in combination with liver transplantation, should be offered to children with MVA as an initial option rather than subjecting them to permanent PN dependency or death [32,33].

Intestinal epithelial dysplasia (IED) or tufting enteropathy

Three cases of severe diarrhea neonatal with abnormal epithelial morphology, were reported by Reifen et al as 'tufting enteropathy" [34]. We identified nine cases

of severe neonatal diarrhea, which were clearly different from MVA [11]. Further studies in these patients allowed us to define that IED is a constitutive epithelial disorder involving both the small intestine and the colon [35]. In our experience, IED seems to be especially common among patients of Arabic origin, from the Middle East or North Africa. A particular characteristic of this disease is its clinical and histological heterogenicity and its association with malformations or other epithelial diseases.

Clinical features

Typically, these patients present during the first weeks of life with severe diarrhea. Most have consanguineous parents or an affected sibling and some died during the first months of life with severe diarrhea of unknown origin [36]. Usually, diarrhea persists despite of bowel rest but is, typically, less severe than that which occurs in MVA. Attempts at continuous enteral feeding (CEF), with a protein hydrolysate or aminoacids, worsen the diarrhea; newborns rapidly fail to thrive and develop severe protein-energy malnutrition. Given the early onset of diarrhea, MVA may be suspected clinically in these children; however, morphological analysis of small and large bowel biopsies readily allows differentiation between these entities.

Histological presentation

Villous atrophy is present but is variable in severity. In the most typical form, abnormalities are localized mainly in the epithelium and include a disorganisation of surface enterocytes with focal crowding, resembling tufts (Figure 8.3). These characteristic "tufts" of extruding epithelium, first described by Reifen et al. [34], are seen toward the villous tip and may affect up to 70% of all villi. The tufting process is not limited to the small intestine but also involves the colonic mucosa [11]. This appearance also can be observed in the crypt epithelium and, in addition, crypts often have an abnormal appearance with dilatation and such features as pseudocysts and abnormal regeneration with branching [11]. A study of basement membrane components demonstrated an abnormal deposition of laminin and heparan sulfate proteoglycan (HSPG) at that level compared to biopsy specimens from patients with coeliac disease or autoimmune enteropathy [11]. Relative to

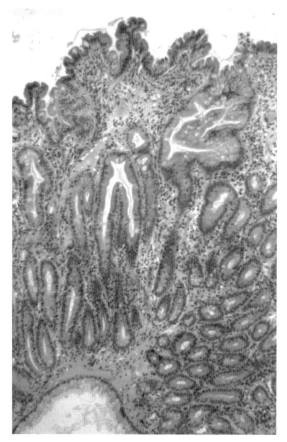

Figure 8.3 Intestinal epithelial dysplasia. Partial villous atrophy with crypt hyperplasia or pseudocystic crypt appearance, branching pictures, and disorganization of surface epithelium.

controls, there was a faint and irregular deposition of laminin at the epithelial-lamina propria interface, whereas HSPG were large and lamellar suggestive of an abnormal development of the basement membrane as the origin of the epithelial abnormalities. By contrast, we observed, by immunohistochemistry, an increased expression of desmoglein in IED, and ultrastructural changes in desmosomes, which were increased in length and number [35] (Figure 8.4).

IED is most often suspected after ruling out MVA and the final diagnosis is made rather late by performing repeated intestinal biopsies which demonstrate a transition from a relatively normal appearance in early life (featuring only nonspecific villous atrophy with or without monocellular cell infiltration of the lamina propria) to the later appearance of the characteristic

tufts. In addition, it is unusual and technically difficult to show any specific abnormalities in the basement membrane components, integrins or desmosomes in the mucosa, in the absence of tufts. Another difficulty is related to the infiltration of the lamina propria by T cells supporting the hypothesis of an immune-related enteropathy, as previously described, especially when tufts are missing. One could speculate that defective cell adhesion increases intestinal permeability with a subsequent inflammatory reaction. In a mouse model of dysfunctional E-cadherin, this primary disorder of epithelial permeability or integrity was responsible for secondary T cell mediated mucosal damage [37]. Murch et al. described this type of lesion in infants with epithelial dysplasia [38].

Associated disorders

Several cases of IED have been reported as being associated with phenotypic abnormalities; for example, Dubowitz syndrome or malformative syndrome [39,40]. An association between congenital IDI and choanal atresia was recently reported in four children [39]. We have observed a number of associated malformations, including rectal or esophageal atresia and have, recently, reported a nonspecific punctiform keratitis associated with conjonctival dysplasia, involving about 60% of patients [36]. This associated keratitis is very intriguing because it is also an epithelial disease that might help to elucidate the molecular basis of the intestinal epithelial disease. The fact that some children have no ophtalmological symptoms confirms the heterogeneity of the disease.

Interestingly, Lachaux et al. have recently reported a case of a newborn presenting with pyloric atresia and intractable diarrhea [41]. Light microscopic examination showed extensive desquamation extending from the gastric fundus to the rectum with only a few epithelial cells remaining at the base of the crypts. Electron microscopy of the gut revealed normal desmosomes but a cleavage located between the lamina propria and the basal pole of the enterocytes. This newly disease is thought to be related to a congenital deficiency of $\alpha_6\beta_4$ integrin. This integrin is known to be defective in epidermolysis bullosa, in which gross epidermal shedding occurs, although the cutaneous expression of $\alpha_6\beta_4$ integrin appeared to be normal in this case of IDI. This is consistent with a mutation within an intestinal isoform of the $\alpha_6\beta_4$ integrin, or a deficiency of

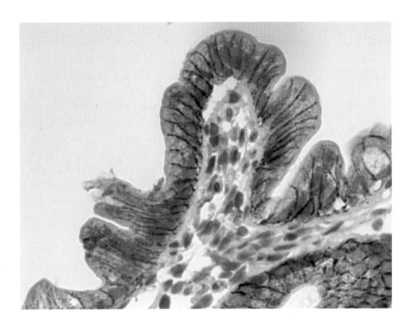

Figure 8.4 Intestinal epithelial dysplasia. Increased expression of desmoglein staining of the tight junction in a patient with intestinal epithelial dysplasia.

a related and immuno-histochemically cross-reactive intestinal integrin [42,43]. Rather like epidermolysis bullosa, which shares several similarities at the ultrastructural and possibly molecular level, there are likely to be several distinct mutations that may result in this phenotype.

Pathophysiology and mode of transmission

When compared to biopsy specimens from patients with coeliac disease or autoimmune enteropathy, IED was shown to be associated with an abnormal appearance of the basement membrane [11]. Basement membrane molecules are involved in epithelial-mesenchymal cell interactions, which are fundamental to intestinal development and differentiation [44–47]. Alterations suggestive of abnormal cell-cell and cell-matrix interactions were seen in patients with IED, without any evidence of abnormalities in epithelial cell polarization and proliferation [35]. Alterations included an abnormal distribution of the adhesion molecule $\alpha_2\beta_1$ integrin along the crypt-villous axis. The integrin $\alpha_2\beta_1$ is involved in the interaction of epithelial cells with various basement membrane components, such as laminin and collagen. To date, the pathophysiological mechanisms resulting in an increased immunohistochemical expression of desmoglein and the ultrastructural changes seen in desmosomes remain

unclear [35]. A mouse in which the gene encoding the transcription factor Elf3 is disrupted develops morphologic features resembling epithelial dysplasia in infants [48]. In this mouse model, there is abnormal morphogenesis of villi, whereas progenitor crypt cells appear normal. The enterocytes in Elf3-deficient mice produce low levels of the type 2 receptor for transforming growth factor-beta, which induces the differentiation of immature intestinal epithelia. It remains to be determined, in the human infant, whether the the observed modifications of epithelial morphology are primary or secondary. Both clinical studies the findings in experimental animal models should provide clues to the pathogenesis of these epithelial abnormalities and to the severity of this neonatal diarrhea syndrome. Tufts correspond to nonapoptotic epithelial cells at the villous tips that are no longer in contact with the basement membrane. It can be speculated that a defect of normal enterocyte apoptosis at the end of their lifespan, or an alteration in cell-cell contact dynamics, is responsible for this effect. Whether or not the tufts are the primary abnormality in this disorder or represent a secondary phenomenon remains to be determined.

A genetic basis for this disorder is suspected based on the the clear association with parental consanguinity or disease in siblings. These features suggest an autosomal recessive transmission. The gene involved in this congenital inherited autosomal recessive disease has not, as yet, been identified.

Outcome

This neonatal diarrhea, which resists all treatments requires permanent PN. However, it seems that some infants have a rather milder phenotype than others [49]. Because of the preservation of some degree of intestinal function and a more limited volume of stool output, some patients need only partial long-term PN with infusions three to four times per week. However, careful monitoring should be performed to avoid progressive growth retardation or liver disease. In most patients, the severity of intestinal malabsorption and diarrhea make them totally dependent on daily long-term PN with subsequent risk of complications. For some patients with severe persistent diarrhea, the risk of water and electrolyte imbalance, although lower than in MVA, still demands adapted PN and an appropriate long-term strategy. Thus, IED becomes another indication for intestinal transplantation [50–53].

Other congenital enteropathies

Phenotypic diarrhea

The so-called phenotypic diarrhea, that is, an IDI syndrome associated with phenotypic abnormalities and immune deficiency is a rare and recently reported disease [12]. The patients present with diarrhea starting within the first 6 months of life (<1 month in most cases) and have several features in common. They are small for gestional age and have an abnormal phenotype [12]. All have facial dysmorphism with prominent forehead, broad nose, and hypertelorism. They have a distinct abnormality of hair, *tricorrhexis nodosa*, in which the hair is woolly, difficult to manage, easily pulled out and poorly pigmented even in children of Middle Eastern origin. Among the congenital forms of hair dysplasia, *tricorrhexis nodosa* is very common and can be present in several pathologic conditions [54–57]. In addition, the previously reported patients had defective antibody responses, despite normal serum immunoglobulin levels, and defective antigen-specific skin tests, despite positive proliferative responses in vitro [12]. Small bowel biopsy specimen from patients with syndromatic diarrhea show moderate or severe villous atrophy with an inconsistent degree of

mononuclear cell infiltration of the lamina propria and an absence of epithelial abnormalities. Histologically, there are no specific abnormalities. The prognosis of this type of intractable diarrhea of infancy is poor because most patients have died between the ages of 2 and 5 years, some in relation to the early onset of liver disease [12]. The cause of this diarrhea is unknown and relationships between low birth weight, dysmorphism, severe diarrhea, trichorrhexis, and immune deficiency are unclear. The coexistence of morphological, trichological and immunological abnormalities with an early-onset intractable diarrhea syndrome whose severity is disproportionate to the degree of mucosal architectural abnormality (consistent with a primary enterocyte abnormality) present suggests either a mutation within several genes, inherited together by linkage disequilibrium, or, more probably, an interference with a higher level of control, such as a patterning gene. The characteristic hair abnormalities may allow a more focused search for candidate mutations, as relatively few genes have been implicated in hair development [58–60].

In our experience, surviving patients have not, as yet, been transplanted as their PN dependency has been variable on long-term follow-up; their growth and neurological development, however, have been impaired.

Autoimmune enteropathy

"Autoimmune enteropathy" (AIE) is a new, well-recognized, and distinct entity, which features a severe enteropathy [61,62]. The identification of a disease that features mutations in the *FOXP3* gene as its basic defect and that presents as AIE points to a defect in regulatory T cell homeostasis [63]. *FOXP3* is primarily expressed by CD4+CD25+regulatory T cells and is a potent transcriptional suppressor and key modulator of T cell functions. A nonfunctional *FOXP3* leads to a tremendous hyperactivation of T cells, resulting in autoimmune aggression, such as seen in patients with immune dysregulation, polyendocrinopathy autoimmune enteropathy X-linked (IPEX) syndrome, a subgroup of AIE [62–64]. Based on the presence of such profound immune dysregulation new treatment strategies emerged for AIE. The use of T cell immunosuppressive drugs, such as tacrolimus combined to steroids, seem to be beneficial in some patients; however, long-term remission was not always possible [64]. Bone marrow transplantation might be the treatment of choice in those patients who do not respond to immunosuppression [8]. However, initial, encouraging results remain to be confirmed as, to date, long-term outcomes have not been reported. A new mutation within an upstream noncoding region of FOXP3 results in a variant of IPEX syndrome in which autoimmune and severe immunoallergic symptoms are associated [66].

Autoimmune enteropathy is not an indication for intestinal transplantation because most patients currently respond to immunosuppressive treatment combined with parenteral or enteral feeding. Patients not responding to this management should receive bone marrow transplantation.

The foregoing list of congenital enteropathies is not exhaustive because other forms with abnormal small bowel mucosa have been described, including mitochondrial DNA rearrangements [67], congenital enterocyte heparan sulphate deficiency [68], phosphomannose isomerase deficiency [69], and carbohydrate-deficient glycoproteins syndrome with a presentation that features both hepatic and intestinal manifestations [70], or severe intractable diarrhea as the recently described congenital malabsorptive diarrhea due to a mutation in the neurogenin-3 gene [71]. Most of these diseases do not involve the digestive tract alone and cause intestinal failure of variable intensity. They are not currently recognized as indication of intestinal transplantation.

Conclusion

Congenital enteropathies are increasingly recognized as important cause of intestinal failure in infancy and early childhood. Indications for intestinal transplantation involve only microvillous atrophy or tufting enteropathy, whereas phenotypic diarrhea and autoimmune enteropathy are not considered as indications.

Pretransplant management involves nutritional support and prevention of IF-related liver disease as well as renal injury related to water electrolyte imbalance.

References

1 Goulet O, Ruemmele F. Causes and management of intestinal failure in children. *Gastroenterology* 2006; 130:S16–28.

2 Avery GB, Villacivencio O, Lilly JR, Randolph JG. Intractable diarrhea in early infancy. *Pediatrics* 1968; 41:712–722.

3 Ricour C, Navarro J, Frederich A, et al. La diarrhée grave rebelle du nourrisson (à propos de 84 observations). *Arch Fr Pediat* 1977;34:44–59.

4 Guarino A, Spagnulo MI, Russo S, et al. Etiology and risk factors of severe and protracted diarrhea. *J Pediatr Gastroenterol Nutr* 1995;20:173–178.

5 Catassi C, Fabiani E, Spagnuolo MI, et al. Severe and protracted diarrhea: results of the 3-year SIGEP multicenter survey. *J Pediatr Gastroenterol Nutr* 1999;29:63–68.

6 Goulet O, Besnard M, Girardet JP, Lachaux A, Sarles J and the French Speaking Group of Hepatology, Gastroenterology and Nutrition. *Clin Nutr* 1998;17:9 (A).

7 Vernacchio L, Vezina RM, Mitchell AA, et al. Characteristics of persistent diarrhea in a community-based cohort of young US children. *J Pediatr Gastroenterol Nutr* 2006;43:52–58.

8 Baud O, Goulet O, Canioni D, et al. Treatment of the immune dysregulation, polyendocrinopathy, enteropathy, and X-linked syndrome (IPEX) by allogeneic bone marrow transplantation. *N Engl J Med* 2001;38:1758–1762.

9 Cuenod B, Brousse N, Goulet O, et al. Classification of intractable diarrhea in infancy using clinical and immunohistological criteria. *Gastroenterology* 1990; 99:1037–1043.

10 Goulet O, Brousse N, Canioni D, et al. Syndrome of intractable diarrhea with persistent villous atrophy in early childhood: A clinicopatological survey of 47 cases. *J Pediatr Gastroenterol Nutr* 1998;26:151–161.

11 Goulet O, Kedinger M, Brousse N, et al. Intractable diarrhea of infancy: a new entity with epithelial and basement membrane abnormalities. *J Pediatr* 1995;127:212–219.

12 Giraut D, Goulet O, Ledeist F, et al. Intractable diarrhea syndrome associated with phenotypic abnormalities and immune deficiency. *J Pediatr* 1994;125:36–42.

13 Davidson GP, Cuiz E, Hamilton JR, Gall DG. Familial enteropathy: a syndrome of protracted diarrhea from birth, failure to thrive, and hypoplastic villous atrophy. *Gastroenterology* 1978;75:783–790.

14 Phillips AD, Schmitz J. Familial microvillous atrophy: A clinicopathological survey of 23 cases. *J Pediatr Gastroenterol Nutr* 1992;14:380–396.

15 Hihnala S, Hoglund P, Lammi L, et al. Long-term clinical outcome in patients with congenital chloride diarrhea. *J Pediatr Gastroenterol Nutr* 2006;42:369–375.

16 Muller T, Wijmenga C, Phillips AD, et al. Congenital sodium diarrhea is an autosomal recessive disorder of

sodium/proton exchange but unrelated to known candidate genes. *Gastroenterology* 2000;119:1506–1513.

17 Ruemmele FM, Schmitz J, Goulet O. Microvillous inclusion disease (microvillous atrophy). *Orphanet J Rare Dis* 2006;1:22.

18 Bell SW, Kerner JA Jr, Sibley RK. Microvillous inclusion disease. The importance of electron microscopy for diagnosis. *Am J Surg Pathol* 1991;15:1157–1164.

19 Phillips AD, Szfranski M, Man L-Y, Wall W. Periodic acid Schiff staining abnormality in microvillous atrophy: photometric and ultrastructural studies. *J Pediatr Gastroenterol Nutr* 2000;30:34–42.

20 Phillips A, Fransen J, Hauri HP, Sterchi E. The constitutive exocytotic pathway in microvillous atrophy. *J Pediatr Gastroenterol Nutr* 1993;17:239–246.

21 Groisman GM, Amar M, Livne E. CD10: A Valuable Tool for the Light Microscopic Diagnosis of Microvillous Inclusion Disease (Familial Microvillous Atrophy). *Am J Surg Pathol* 2002;26:902–907.

22 Youssef N, Ruemmele F, Goulet O, Patey N. CD-10 expresion in microvillous inclusion disease. CD10 expression in a case of microvillous inclusion disease. *Ann Pathol.* 2004;24:624–627.

23 Phillips AD, Brown A, Hicks S, et al. Acetylated sialic acid residues and blood group antigens localise within the epithelium in microvillous atrophy indicating internal accumulation of the glycocalyx. *Gut* 2004;25:1764–1771.

24 Raafat F, Green NJ, Nathavitharana KA, Booth IW. Intestinal microvillous dystrophy: a variant of microvillous inclusion disease or a new entity? *Hum Pathol* 1994;53:1243–1248.

25 Nathavitharana KA, Green NJ, Raafat F, Booth IW. Siblings with microvillous inclusion disease. *Arch Dis Child* 1994;71:71–73.

26 Heinz-Erian P, Schmidt H, Le Merrer M, et al. Congenital microvillous atrophy in a girl with autosomal dominant hypochondroplasia. *J Pediatr Gastroenterol Nutr* 1999;28: 28203–28205.

27 Michail S, Collins JF, Xu H, et al. Abnormal expression of brush-border membrane transporters in the duodenal mucosa of two patients with microvillous inclusion disease. *J Pediatr Gastroenterol Nutr* 1998;27: 536–542.

28 Oliva MM, Perman JA, Saavedra JM, et al. Successful intestinal transplantation for microvillous inclusion disease. *Gastroenterology* 1994;106:771–774.

29 Herzog D, Atkinson P, Grant D, et al. Combined bowel-liver transplantation in an infant with microvillous inclusion disease. *J Pediatr Gastroenterol Nutr* 1996;22:405–408.

30 Randak C, Langnas AN, Kaufman SS, et al. Pretransplant management and small bowel-liver transplantation in an infant with microvillous inclusion disease. *J Pediatr Gastroenterol Nutr* 1998;27:333–337.

31 Bunn SK, Beath SV, Mckeirnan PJ, et al. Treatment of Microvillous Inclusion Disease by Intestinal Transplantation. *J Pediatr Gastroenterol Nutr Pediatr* 2000;31:176–180.

32 Ruemmele FM, Brousse N, Goulet O. Autoimmune enteropathy—molecular concepts. *Curr Opin Gastroenterol* 2004;20:587–591.

33 Croft NM, Howatson AG, Ling SC, et al. Microvillous inclusion disease: an evolving condition. *J Pediatr Gastroenterol Nutr* 2000;31:185–189.

34 Reifen RM, Cutz E, Griffiths AM, Ngan BY, Sherman PM. Tufting enteropathy a newly recognized clinicopathological entity associated with refractory diarrhea in infants. *J Pediatr Gastroenterol Nutr* 1994;18:379–385.

35 Patey N, Scoazec JY, Cuenod-Jabri B, et al. Distribution of cell adhesion molecules in infants with intestinal epithelial dysplasia (tufting enteropathy). *Gastroenterology* 1997;113:833–843.

36 Goulet O, Salomon J, Ruemmele F, et al. Intestinal epithelial dysplasia (tufting enteropathy). *Orphanet J Rare Dis* 2007;20.

37 Hermiston ML, Gordon JI. Inflammatory bowel disease and adenomas in mice expressing a dominant negative N-cadherin. *Science* 1995;270:1203–1207.

38 Murch S, Graham A, Vermault A, et al. Functionnaly significant secondary inflammation occurs in a primary epithelial enteropathy. *Pediatr Gastroenterol Nutr* 1997;24: 467.

39 Krantz M, Jansson U, Rectors S, et al. Hereditary intractable diarrhea with choanal atresia. A new familial syndrome. *J Pediatr Gastroenterol Nutr* 1997;24:470.

40 Abely M, Fromont Hankard G, et al. Intractable infant diarrhea with epithelial dysplasia associated with polymalformative syndrome. *J Pediatr Gastroenterol Nutr* 1998;29:348–352.

41 Lachaux A, Bouvier R, Loras I, et al. Isolated deficient alpha6beta4 integrin expression in the gut associated with intractable diarrhea. *J Pediatr Gastroenterol Nutr* 1999;24:395–401.

42 Beaulieu JF. Differential expression of the VLA family of integrins along the crypt-villous axis in the human small intestine. *J Cell Sci* 1992;102:427–436.

43 Simon-Assmann P, Duclos B, Orian-Rousseau V, et al. Differential expression of laminin isoforms and alpha 6-beta 4 integrin subunits in the developing human and mouse intestine. *Dev Dyn* 1994;201:71–85.

44 Simon-Assmann P, Bouziges F, Vigny M, Kedinger M. Origin and deposition of basement membrane. Heparan

Sulfate Proteoglycan in the developing intestine. *J Cell Biol* 1989;109:1837–1848.

45 Simo P, Simon-Assmann P, Bouziges F, et al. Changes in the expression of laminin during intestinal development. *Development* 1991;112:477–487.

46 Simo P, Bouziges F, Lissitzky JC, et al. Dual and asynchronous deposition of laminin chains at the epithelial mesenchymal interface in the gut. *Gastroenterology* 1992;102:1835–1845.

47 Simon-Assmann P, Kedinger M. Heterotypic cellular cooperation in gut morphogenesis and differentiation. *Cell Biol* 1993;4:221–230.

48 Ng Ayn, Waring P, Ristevski S, et al. Inactivation of the transcription factor Elf3 in mice results in dysmorphogenesis and altered differentiation of intestinal epithelium. *Gastroeneterology* 2002;122:1455–1466.

49 Cameron DJS, Barnes GL. Successful Pregnancy Outcome in Tufting Enteropathy. *J Pediatr Gastroenterol Nutr* 2003;36:158.

50 Lacaille F, Cuenod B, Colomb V, et al. Successful Combined liver and small bowel transplantation in a child with epithelial dysplasia. *J Pediatr Gastroenterol Nutr* 1998;2:230–233.

51 Goulet O. Intestinal transplantation. *Curr Opin Clin Nutr Metab Care* 1999;2:315–321.

52 Goulet O, Salomon J, Ruemmele F, et al. Intestinal epithelial dysplasia (Tufting enteropathy). *Orphanet J Rare Dis* 2007;20.

53 Paramesh AS, Fishbein T, Tschernia A, et al. Isolated Small Bowel Transplantation for Tufting Enteropathy. *J Pediatr Gastroenterol Nutr* 2003;36:138–140.

54 Itin PH, Pittelkow MR. Trichothiodystrophy: review of sulfur-deficient brittle hair syndromes and association with the ectodermal dysplasia. *J Am Acad Dermatol* 1990;22:705–717.

55 Happle R, Traupe H, Gröbe H, Bonsmann G. The tay syndrome (congenital ichthyosis with trichothiodystrophy). *Eur J Pediatr* 1984;141:147–152.

56 Stefanini M, Vermeulen W, Weeda G, et al. A new nucleotide-excision-repair gene associated with the disorder trichothiodystrophy. *Am J Hum Genet* 1993;53:817–821.

57 Mariani E, Facchini A, Honorati MC, et al. Immune defects in families and patients with xeroderma pigmentosum and trichothiodystrophy. *Clin Exp Immunol* 1992;88:376–382.

58 Verloes A, Lombet J, Lambert Y, et al. Tricho-hepato-enteric syndrome: further delineation of a distinct syndrome with neonatal hemochromatosis phenotype, intractable diarrhea, and hair anomalies. *Am J Med Gen* 1997;68:391–395.

59 De Vries E, Visser DM, Van Dongen JJM, et al. Oligoclonal gammopathy in "phenotypic diarrhea." *J Pediatr Gastroenterol Nutr* 2000;30:349–350.

60 Fabre A, Andre N, Breton A, et al. Intractable diarrhea with "phenotypic anomalies" and tricho-hepato-enteric syndrome: two names for the same disorder. *Am J Med Genet A* 2007;584–588.

61 Ruemmele FM, Brousse N, Goulet O. Autoimmune enteropathy. Edited by: Walker A, Goulet O, Kleinman R, Shneider P, Sherman P, Sanderson I. Pediatric Gastroitestinal Disease. Hamilton, Ontario, Canada: Bc Decker, 2004;959–965.

62 Wildin RS, Ramsdell F, Peake J, et al. X-linked neonatal diabetes mellitus, enteropathy and endocrinopathy syndrome is the human equivalent of mouse scurfy. *Nat Genet* 2001;27:18–20.

63 Wildin RS, Smyk-Pearson S, Filipovich AH. Clinical and molecular features of the immunodysregulation, polyendocrinopathy, enteropathy, and X-linked (IPEX) syndrome. *J Med Genet* 2002;39:537–545.

64 Kobayashi I, Shiari R, Yamada M et al. Novel mutations of *FOXP3* in two Japanese patients with immune dysregulation, polyendocrinopathy, enteropathy, and X-linked syndrome (IPEX). *J Med Genet* 2001;38:874–876.

65 Gambineri E, Torgerson Tr, Ochs HD. Immune dysregulation, polyendocrinopathy, enteropathy, and X-linked inheritance (IPEX), a syndrome of systemic autoimmunity caused by mutations of *FOXP3*, a critical regulator of T-cell homeostasis. *Curr Opin Rheumatol* 2003;15:430–435.

66 Torgerson TR, Linane A, Moes N, et al. Severe food allergy as a variant of IPEX syndrome caused by a deletion in a noncoding region of the FOXP3 gene. *Gastroenterology* 2007;1705–1717.

67 Cormier-Daire V, Bonnefont JP, Rustin P, et al. Mitochondrial DNA rearrangements with onset as chronic diarrhea with villous atrophy. *J Pediatr* 1994;124:63–70.

68 Murch S, Winyard PJD, Koletzko S, et al. Congenital enterocyte heparan sulphate deficiency with massive albumin loss, secretory diarrhea and malnutrition. *Lancet* 1996;347:1299–1301.

69 Jaeken J, Matthij G, Saudubray JM, et al. Phosphomannose isomerase deficiency: a carbohydrate-deficient glycoproteins syndrome with hepatic-intestinal presentation. *Am J Hum Genet* 1998;62:1535–1539.

70 Oren A, Houwen RH. Phosphomannoseisomerase deficiency as the cause of protein-losing enteropathy and congenital liver fibrosis. *J Pediatr Gastroenterol Nutr* 1999;29:231–232.

71 Wang J, Cortina G, Wu SV, et al. Mutant neurogenin-3 in congenital malabsorptive diarrhea. *N Engl J Med* 2006;270–280.

9 Causes of Intestinal Failure in the Adult

Harry C. Sax

Key points

- There are multiple etiologies leading to the requirement for bowel resection.
- The development of intestinal failure is dependent on both length and quality of the remaining bowel.
- Extra intestinal manifestations of the primary disease process can affect long term prognosis and alter surgical and medical options.
- Surgical interventions, when indicated, should anticipate and address the potential for additional procedures in the future.
- Although small bowel transplantation remains the ultimate salvage for intestinal failure, residual bowel function can be optimized.

Introduction

The "short bowel syndrome" is a misnomer. Although many patients who have intractable diarrhea, malabsorption, and electrolyte abnormalities do have inadequate absorptive length, many others suffer because of poor physiologic function. This chapter will outline common, non-IBD, etiologies of intestinal failure, discuss basic diagnostic and therapeutic interventions, and touch on strategies that can be employed intraoperatively to optimize function. Other chapters in this text provide more detail of the treatment decisions

Intestinal Failure: Diagnosis, Management and Transplantation.
Edited by Alan N. Langnas, Olivier Goulet, Eamonn M.M. Quigley and Kelly A. Tappenden. © 2008 Blackwell Publishing.
ISBN 978-1-4051-4637-1.

involved in the care of the patient with IBD or morbid obesity.

What leads to massive resection?

The need for massive bowel resection may arise from a large number of disorders, which can be conveniently grouped into the following broad categories: ischemia, infiltrative processes, malignancy, and trauma, including ionizing radiation.

Ischemia occurs when perfusion is no longer adequate to overcome capillary pressure in the wall of the bowel. This can be caused by inadequate inflow, increased wall tension due to intestinal obstruction, or impediments to venous outflow. The celiac axis supplies the stomach, duodenum, and foregut to the proximal jejunum; the superior mesenteric artery (SMA) perfuses the remainder of the small bowel and the colon to the splenic flexure, and the inferior mesenteric artery (IMA) the remainder of the colon. The most devastating embolic event is to the SMA, seen in patients with atrial fibrillation or severe atherosclerotic peripheral vascular disease [1]. Patients present with sudden onset of severe abdominal pain, yet often have a very benign abdominal examination. Diagnosis is often based on history, although CT scanning with intravenous contrast may show variable perfusion of the bowel, associated with mucosal edema. In a patient with a high index of suspicion, some clinicians move directly to angiography, in hopes of initiating directed thrombolytic therapy. Surgical intervention is aimed at restoring flow through embolectomy or bypass, and performing minimal resection of clearly nonviable bowel, often with a "second look" procedure within 48 hours.

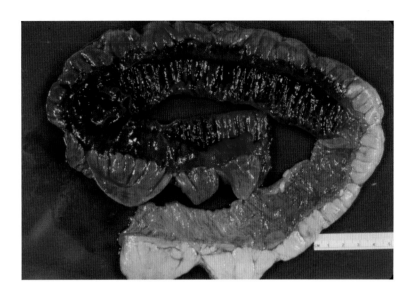

Figure 9.1 Segmental bowel resection due to internal hernia. Note the sharply defined demarcation of viability.

Closed loop obstructions and incarcerated hernias also cause ischemia and can progress to gangrene. Although inflow and outflow are reduced, the main culprit is progressive distension of the bowel, increasing wall tension and decreasing perfusion. Included in this category are internal hernias, where a loop of bowel slips beneath an adhesive band or through a naturally occurring foramen. In many cases, this can also lead to a volvulus, as the partial fixation allows the bowel to twist upon itself (Figure 9.1). An increasing number of patients who have undergone Roux en Y Gastric bypass are at risk for internal hernia as new potential spaces are created when the Roux limb is brought into an ante-colic, ante-gastric position [2,3]. These patients are especially difficult to diagnose, as many have preexisting nausea and vomiting. Further, if the pancreaticobiliary limb is entrapped, a closed loop obstruct can occur, with massive dilation of the distal stomach and duodenum, oftentimes associated with pancreatitis. There is no role for angiography in this situation, as prompt surgical intervention is indicated.

Mesenteric venous thrombosis (MVT) is a difficult diagnosis, as the onset tends to be more gradual than in the case of an embolus. MVT is associated with some psychotropic medications and digitalis toxicity, but is also seen in patients who are institutionalized, and may have become progressively dehydrated and immobile.

Previously healthy individuals with hypercoagulable states, such as Protein S or C deficiency, may present with MVT as the first manifestation of the disease [4]. It is difficult to declot mesenteric veins surgically, and therapy is initially aimed at systemic anticoagulation or thrombolytic therapy, followed by segmental resection.

The infiltrative processes include desmoid and carcinoid tumors and amyloidosis. Desmoids, which are associated with Gardner's syndrome, are ubiquitous in location and create multiple areas of dense fibrosis and desmoplastic reaction. Spontaneous enterocutaneous fistulae can appear. Gardner's patients often have undergone total proctocolectomy to treat the primary disease and prevent progression to cancer. This creates great risks for further malabsorption after small bowel resection. In addition, abdominal wall desmoids are often treated with radiation, leading to underlying enteritis in the remaining bowel. Many of these patients come to transplant, often as a staged enterectomy [5]. Carcinoid tumors, although often isolated, can occur throughout the bowel. They elicit significant desmoplastic reaction in the mesentery, which often requires much wider bowel resection than would be necessary for the tumor alone. In situations in which metastatic disease to the liver has already occurred, diarrhea is a prominent component, and more limited resection, coupled with adjuvant therapy, is warranted and discussed later in this chapter. Amyloidosis, a systemic disease involving multiple systems, infiltrates the bowel wall, causing motility disorders. The underlying cardiac and hepatic dysfunction may, however, be the more life threatening issues. Adenocarcinoma of the small bowel and isolated small bowel lymphoma are rare and seldom require massive resection. The small bowel is more likely to be secondarily involved by direct extension from gynecologic tumors or colon cancer. Retroperitoneal sarcomas often surround mesenteric vasculature and, if complete resection is attempted, the small bowel may be sacrificed, unless vascular continuity can be restored. Gastrointestinal stromal tumors (GIST) arise in the wall of the bowel, but often infiltrate the mesentery and can be multiple in nature. Limited primary resection is indicated in cases of obstruction or necrosis. The availability of highly effective signal transduction inhibitors, such as Gleevac, can induce shrinkage of c Kit positive GIST tumors, and limit the extent of resection [6].

External trauma to the bowel from blunt or penetrating injury is an increasingly common indication for bowel resection. Blunt trauma is predominantly decellerative as a result of the widespread use of seat and shoulder belts. Although these prevent fatal head and neck injury, much of the kinetic energy is transferred to the small bowel mesentery when forward acceleration of the viscera abruptly ceases, leading to avulsion of the blood supply. Penetrating trauma can involve direct vascular injury but is more likely to cause direct multiple perforations. In situations in which individual debridement and closure of multiple enterotomies in close proximity is untenable, segmental resection may be necessary. Bowel segments deemed marginal, in terms of viability, following a blast injury can be stapled off and no primary anastomosis performed; a second look celiotomy is then performed when the patient is more stable. The vast majority of small bowel trauma is iatrogenic, occurring during abdominal exploration for other conditions. Dense intra-abdominal adhesions requiring lysis can lead to long segments of deserosalized or perforated bowel. In general, primary repair should be attempted, unless this leads to narrowing. Given the high morbidity of an enterocutaneous fistula, it may be appropriate to sacrifice marginal bowel to allow an anastomosis to be performed in healthy tissue. Although the time interval from insult to injury is typically prolonged, an increasing number of patients are developing bowel dysfunction from radiation therapy given in the past for treatment of malignancies of the pelvis or for lymphoma. Radiation enteritis follows a continuum from an acute, inflammatory, hyperemic phase through relative quiescence to a progressive fibrosis and obstruction associated with obliterative vasculitis. Although the classic appearance of pale, somewhat fibrotic bowel suggests affected areas there is a field effect such that normal appearing bowel, which would remain after resection, is incapable of undergoing adaptation, and may itself progress to fibrosis. There are scattered reports of the use of stricturoplasty, as opposed to resection, in this situation [7].

Although this chapter does not focus on specific surgical techniques, certain intraoperative maneuvers can aid in the patient's long-term care. Patients with short gut who will require long-term TPN invariably develop cholelithiasis and may present with a laboratory picture of cholestasis. Prophylactic cholecystectomy should be performed and a baseline liver biopsy obtained. Enteral access in the form of gastrostomy will allow supplemental tube feedings. The colon provides additional absorptive capacity of both fluids and nutrients; thus, intestinal continuity should be maintained if at all possible. It is also reasonable to create an end sigmoid colostomy, which allows easier care of high volume outputs. Patients with intractable diarrhea will often limit oral intake, even if it is tenable, to reduce the discomfort of perineal excoriation. In those patients in whom a long defunctionalized segment is anticipated, placement of a jejunostomy allows refeeding of proximal ostomy output and may reduce the amount of parenteral support needed. Finally, as these patients often require multiple celiotomies, placement of an adhesion barrier, such as Seprafilm, can increase the ease of any subsequent intervention.

When is all not enough?

Intestinal failure can occur in patients who have undergone no resection but have significant intrinsic disease. Primary etiologies include motility disorders, such as pseudoobstruction, malabsorptive disorders like celiac

Table 9.1 Etiologies of intestinal failure.

Iatrogenic	Ischemic	Infiltrative	Obstructive	Functional
Blunt trauma	Arterial embolism	Desmoid tumors	Adhesive	Pseudoobstruction
Penetrating trauma	Venous Occlusion	Carcinoid	Internal hernia	IBD
Operative misadventure	Low flow/Shock	Amyloidosis	Radiation enteritis	Bacterial overgrowth
		Malignancy		

sprue, infection, and secretory diseases as seen in carcinoid or AIDS associated colitis.

The classic motility disorder is Hirschprung's disease, seen in newborns. In this situation, a lack of myenteric ganglia prevents normal defecation (see Chapter 12, "Motility Disorders," for further details). Adult motility disorders are far more heterogeneous, are not uniformly associated with nerve loss, and are discussed elsewhere in this text.

Malabsorption, in spite of normal bowel length, occurs with intrinsic mucosal diseases such as Crohn's disease, and in those situations where significant small intestinal bacterial overgrowth is present, as may occur with partial obstruction or defunctionalized bowel loops. Malabsorption from bacterial overgrowth, is an important complication of many disorders that produce intestinal failure, and can be diagnosed by breath testing, jejunal sampling and assessing the response to empiric antibiotic therapy.

Although not true intestinal failure, significant malabsorption is a hallmark of infestation by tapeworms or other parasites. A strong suspicion of relevant exposure as well as analysis of stool aids in the diagnosis.

The carcinoid syndrome occurs when tumors have direct access to the systemic circulation, such as occurs with metastatic hepatic disease or when the primary is located in the rectum or bronchus. In addition to diarrhea, the patient manifests classic flushing of the face and extremities. Diagnosis is made by elevation of urinary 5-HIAA and localization with octreotide nuclear scanning, computerized tomography, or contrast studies. Treatment is aimed at resection of the primary, or palliation with a short- or long-acting somatostatin analogue.

With improvements in retroviral therapy, long-term survival from HIV is now common. Nonetheless, in advanced disease, a protein-losing enteropathy can develop and lead to wasting and secondary colonic infections, especially with *cryptosporidium*, are common. Patients can also develop Kaposi's sarcoma of the small bowel, which tends to multifocal or lymphomas. The use of TPN was once avoided, for fear of increased line infection rates. More recent reports suggest that long-term TPN can be provided to HIV patients safely, if meticulous line care is accomplished [8].

Summary

Intestinal failure can occur due to massive resection of healthy bowel, a lesser resection of inherently diseased bowel, or even in patients with full length bowel in continuity. A careful diagnostic evaluation, including review of the operative reports and pathology, allows the development of a well thought–out plan to optimize function.

References

1 Greenwald DA, Brandt LJ, Reinus JF. Ischemic bowel disease in the elderly. *Gastroenterol Clin North Am* 2001;6: 445–473.

2 Iannelli A, Facchiano E, Gugenheim J. Internal hernia after laparoscopic Roux-en-Y gastric bypass for morbid obesity. *Obes Surg* 2006;16:1265–1271.

3 Capella RF, Iannace VA, Capella JF. Bowel obstruction after open and laparoscopic gastric bypass surgery for morbid obesity. *J Am Coll Surg* 2006;203:328–335.

4 Aaolu N, Mustafa NA, Turkyilmaz S. Prothrombotic disorders in patients with mesenteric vein thrombosis. *J Invest Surg* 2003;16:299–304.

5 Fishbein T, Schiano T, Jaffe D. et al. Isolated intestinal transplantation in adults with nonreconstructible GI tracts. *Transplant Proc* 2000;32:1231–1232.

6 Schnadig ID, Blanke CD. Gastrointestinal stromal tumors: imatinib and beyond. *Curr Treat Options Oncol* 2006;7:427–437.

7 Dietz DW, Remzi FH, Fazio VW. Strictureplasty for obstructing small-bowel lesions in diffuse radiation enteritis—successful outcome in five patients. *Dis Colon Rectum* 2001;44:1772–1777.

8 Skiest DJ, Grant P, Keiser P. Nontunneled central venous catheters in patients with AIDS are associated with a low infection rate. *J Acquir Immune Defic Syndr Retrovirol* 1998;17:220–226.

10 Intestinal Failure Related to Bariatric Surgery

Jon S. Thompson

Key points

- Morbidly obese patients may undergo bariatric surgery to induce malabsorption.
- Procedures performed include jejunoileal bypass, biliopancreatic diversion, and distal gastric bypass.
- Malabsorptive bariatric procedures can lead to intestinal failure.
- Patients undergoing bariatric procedures are at risk for short bowel syndrome due to postoperative complications.
- Although some problems (incisional hernia, adhesive obstruction) are related to any abdominal procedure, bariatric operations have specific complications (internal hernia, mesenteric ischemia, bypassed segment) to be considered.
- Surgical reconstruction of the bariatric procedure is often necessary to correct intestinal failure.

Introduction

Paradoxically, morbidly obese patients undergoing bariatric procedures are at risk for developing intestinal failure. This can occur in patients undergoing malabsorptive procedures which bypass significant portions of the intestine. Historically, these patients underwent intestinal bypass. More recently, biliopancreatic diversion and revisional procedures after gastric bypass put patients at risk for intestinal failure

Intestinal Failure: Diagnosis, Management and Transplantation.
Edited by Alan N. Langnas, Olivier Goulet, Eamonn M.M. Quigley and Kelly A. Tappenden. © 2008 Blackwell Publishing.
ISBN 978-1-4051-4637-1.

(Table 10.1). There have now been several reports of short bowel syndrome (SBS) as a postoperative complication of bariatric procedures. Although gastrointestinal reconstruction is a treatment option in many patients with malabsorptive procedures, others, including the SBS patients, require prolonged nutritional support and some eventually require transplantation.

Intestinal failure related to malabsorptive procedures

Intestinal bypass

Jejunoileal bypass (JIB) was widely performed for morbidly obese patients for approximately one decade 30 years ago [1–3]. Several techniques were employed but generally involved connecting approximately 30–35 cm of proximal jejunum to 10–20 cm of the terminal ileum in an end-to-end or end-to-side fashion (Figure 10.1). The resultant malabsorption causes weight loss but at the expense of a variety of complications. Early complications include fluid and electrolyte disturbances, with hypokalemia, hypocalcemia, and hypomagnesemia. These improve with time, as does diarrhea. However, steatorrhea persists and vitamin supplementation is required. One-fourth of patients develop protein malnutrition which requires therapy. Bone disease, oxalate nephropathy, and urinary stones are other complications, occurring in one-third of patients.

The bypassed intestinal segment itself maybe the source of several problems. Dermatis and migratory polyarthralgias occur in 10–15% of patients related to stasis and bacterial overgrowth and enteritis in the bypassed intestine. The blind loop syndrome occurs with gas-bloat, cramps, and worsening of diarrhea. Perhaps

Table 10.1 Bariatric procedures and the gastrointestinal tract.

	Jejunoileal bypass	Biliopancreatic diversion	Roux-en-Y gastric bypass	Distal gastric bypass
Stomach	intact	200–250 cc s/p sleeve or distal resection	30 cc pouch s/p bypass or resection	30 cc pouch s/p bypass or resection
Duodenum	in continuity	bypassed	bypassed	bypassed
Small Intestine	30–35 cm proximal jejunum plus 10–20 cm ileum: long bypassed segment	250 cm alimentary limb: common channel 50–100 cm	up to 150 cm Roux limb: common channel >250 cm	greater than 150 cm Roux limb; common channel 50–100 cm
Colon	intact	intact	intact	intact

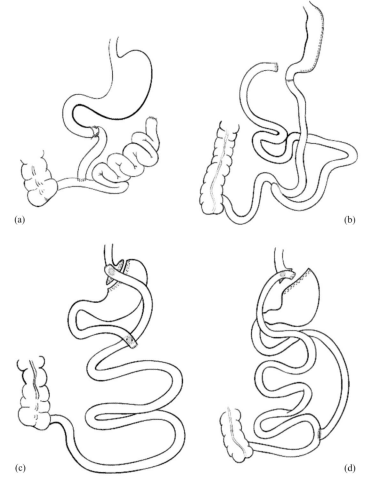

(a)

(b)

(c)

(d)

Figure 10.1 Bariatric surgical procedures.
(a) Jejunoileal bypass
(b) Biliopancreatic diversion
(c) Roux-en-Y gastric bypass
(d) Distal gastric bypass

more significant is the progression of steatohepatitis to fibrosis and irreversible liver failure. The increasing recognition of this problem and the number of deaths from liver failure led to the opinion that intestinal bypass was not an appropriate operation for morbidly obese patients.

Weight loss from these procedures is approximately 70% of excess weight. Weight drops precipitously in the first few months but plateaus during the second postoperative year. Both structural and functional adaptation of the in-continuity segment occurs during this period [4]. Long-term follow-up suggests that weight loss following JIB is not durable, with a significant increase after 10 years.

There has been recent interest in JIB as the first step of a staged approach to high-risk bariatric patients [5,6]. Reversal of the JIB with conversion to a gastric bypass is planned within 12 months of the initial procedure and before the development of irreversible complications. During this interval, patients require careful follow-up for metabolic complications.

Although this operation has largely been abandoned, many patients still have an intact bypass. Reversal of intestinal bypass procedures continues to be an important clinical issue [7]. Metabolic problems account for one-half of conversions. Renal disease and hepatic dysfunction account for approximately one fourth each. An estimated 25% of patients undergoing JIB have required reversal. Furthermore, the risk of complications, particularly renal disease continues to increase with time. Liver disease is progressive and

liver transplantation has been performed more than 20 years after the initial bypass [8]. Reversal of the JIB should be considered at the time of liver transplantation, or soon after recovery, as recurrent steatotic liver disease can occur in the transplanted liver in the presence of an intact bypass [9]. Although reversal can generally be accomplished without significant morbidity, the mortality of reversal for liver disease is approximately 20%. The majority of patients will regain their excess weight if they don't undergo conversion to a gastric restrictive procedure.

All patients with a JIB should be followed closely by a physician knowledgeable about the procedure and its sequelae (Figure 10.2). Reversal should be undertaken before irreversible organ injury results. It should be considered in patients with severe diarrhea, recurrent nephrolithiasis or renal insufficiency, and hepatic dysfunction. The issue of prophylactic reversal remains controversial. A simultaneous or delayed gastric restrictive procedure should be considered to prevent weight regain after reversal.

Biliopancreatic diversion

Biliopancreatic diversion (BPD) was developed because of the disappointing results with the JIB [10]. It allows reversible shortening of the alimentary tract without the side effects of a nonfunctional bypassed portion. The alimentary and biliary limbs both have either intraluminal nutrients or pancreaticobiliary secretions that appears to prevent many of the complications related

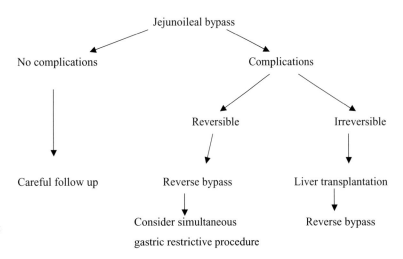

Figure 10.2 Management of the patient with jejunoileal bypass.

to the bypassed segment. Gastric resection is performed to reduce gastric acidity and restrict intake. The long Roux-en-Y reconstruction delays the mixing of food and pancreaticobiliary secretions, which reduces digestion and intestinal absorption of nutrients. Early after the procedure, there is significant malabsorption and weight loss which stabilizes with time. Weight maintenance relates to the ongoing selective malabsorption of fat and starch. The procedure has evolved to include a common channel (mixing of nutrients and pancreatobiliary secretions) of 100 cm, compared to the initial 50 cm. The concept of a sleeve gastrectomy with duodenal switch was developed in the 1990s to accomplish the decrease in size of the stomach and prevent peptic ulceration, while preserving more physiologic gastric emptying and digestion [11]. The greater curve of the stomach is resected longitudinally leaving the lesser curve and pylorus intact. The duodenum is divided and the proximal end anastomosed to the ileum. The remaining duodenum and jejunum (the biliary limb) is anastomosed to the alimentary limb to form the common channel (Figure 10.1). However, there appears to be no significant difference in postoperative gastrointestinal or nutritional side effects with this modification if a similar common channel length is employed [12].

BPD results in 70% excess weight loss, which is stable beyond 10 years [13]. Flatulence and malodorous stools are frequent long-term problems. Two-thirds of patients have persistent diarrhea. Protein malnutrition requiring treatment with parental nutrition occurs in 12% of patients. This occurs during the first year in most cases but may develop later [13]. Approximately one-half of these patients will manifest a nutrient or vitamin deficiency, particularly of fat-soluble vitamins [12]. Liver disease appears to be less frequent than with JIB, but sporadic cases have been reported. If irreversible liver failure occurs, lengthening of the common channel should be performed at the time of liver transplantation [14].

Revisional procedures for malabsorptive complications are required in 4 to 5% of patients after BPD [12,13]. This generally involves lengthening the common channel but restoration of gastrointestinal continuity may also be performed. Revision may be required up to 5 years after the initial operation and usually results in approximately 10–20% increase in excess body weight. BPD continues to be an acceptable bariatric procedure but patients require careful follow-up.

Distal gastric bypass

Standard Roux-en-Y gastric bypass (GBP) is a generally safe and effective operation for weight loss and has a negligible incidence of hypoproteinemia. The Roux limb is generally 60 to 100 cm in length (Figure 10.1). However, this procedure often leads to unsatisfactory weight loss in super obese (body mass index >50 kg/m^2) individuals. Distal gastric bypass (DGBP) has been performed both as a primary procedure in this group of patients and for revision of a failed short limb GBP [15–17]. The Roux limb of a primary DGBP is greater than 250 cm in length with a 30–60 cm biliary limb and a 100 cm common channel (Figure 10.1) [15]. Revisional procedures may have a variety of configurations, but the Roux limb is greater than 150 cm and the common channel is usually 100 cm [16–17].

Weight loss after DGBP is significantly greater at 6 months compared to shorter Roux limbs of the standard GBP and is also maintained long term [17]. However, metabolic abnormalities are more frequent after DGBP. One-third of patients have persistent diarrhea. Approximately 10% of DGBP patients have persistent hypoproteinemia and 4% require parenteral nutrition support. Overall, the metabolic effects are very similar to BPD [15].

Approximately 15% patients undergoing GBP will fail to lose a satisfactory amount of weight with resultant recurrence of obesity-related comorbidity [16]. In the absence of obvious technical failures, these patients have been considered for malabsorptive revision. Typically, this involves lengthening the Roux limb to 150 cm and creating a 100–150 cm common channel. A shorter 50 cm common channel is almost uniformly associated with protein-calorie malnutrition in these patients and may lead to hepatic failure [16]. 15% patients with the revised 150 cm common channel have required limb lengthening [16]. Malnutrition in these patients with malabsorptive procedures will often require parenteral nutrition support before reversal procedures.

Short bowel syndrome resulting from bariatric procedures

Bariatric patients are at risk for a variety of postsurgical complications that can lead to resection and, in

Table 10.2 Causes of short bowel syndrome in bariatric patients.

Obstruction due to adhesions
Internal hernias and volvulus
Incarcerated incisional hernia
Mesenteric ischemia
Complications in bypassed intestine

some cases, the SBS [18]. These patients develop incisional hernias, postoperative adhesions, mesenteric ischemia, and internal hernias (Table 10.2). The increasing number of these procedures being performed have made bariatric procedures an important cause of postoperative SBS [19]. However, the incidence of this complication after bariatric procedures is quite low. Although some of these postoperative complications may be related to any intra-abdominal procedure, there are several problems that are more specific to bariatric procedures.

Internal hernias are a specific concern in patients undergoing bariatric procedures [20–21]. These are detected in approximately 5% of patients undergoing GBP [22]. They generally occur either through the transverse mesocolon defect of a retrocolic Roux limb, through the mesenteric defect of the jejunojejunostomy, or posterior to the Roux limb mesentery (Petersen's hernia). Internal hernias are more common after laparoscopic procedures because fewer adhesions are formed [21]. Internal hernias are difficult to diagnose clinically and radiographically, which can lead to catastrophic results. Both the herniated intestinal segment and the intestine bordering the defect are at risk for ischemia. Fortunately, the incidence of irreversible ischemia and SBS is low [22–24]. Pregnant patients may be particularly prone to this complication and several massive resections and deaths have been reported [22,23]. Closure of the defects at the time of operation and expeditious abdominal exploration in patients with suspicious symptoms are important aspects of management.

Mesenteric ischemia can occur after bariatric procedures and there are several potential mechanisms. Splanchnic vein thrombosis has been described after several laparoscopic procedures, including more recently, laparoscopic gastric bypass [25–26]. This appears to be related, in part, to the hemodynamic effects of pneumoperitoneum. Intraoperative vascular injury can also occur. Direct portal vein injury has been described in a few cases as a result of distorted anatomy [27]. Hypercoagulability is responsible for some instances.

The bypassed segment of a JIB is at risk for resection due to either inflammation or mechanical problems e.g. volvulus or intussusception. Bypass enteritis may be associated with pneumatosis cystoides [1]. Hocking [2] reported 2 incidences of intussusception in 100 patients with JIB undergoing long-term follow-up. This can be a challenging clinical and radiologic diagnosis. These complications may result in resection of the involved, bypassed segment.

We recently analyzed the outcome of 11 patients developing SBS after bariatric procedures (18). Nine (82%) occurred after GBP and two (18%) after JIB. Two of the procedures were performed laparoscopically. Two patients were undergoing revision of their initial bariatric procedure. One-third of the patients had an abdominal catastrophe in the first 30 days. Another third developed the complications between 1 and 2 years after operation. The rest of the patients developed the SBS more than 10 years after their initial bariatric procedure. Five patients had an internal hernia, four patients had mesenteric ischemia, and two patients required multiple resections for obstruction. Gastrointestinal reconstructive procedures were performed in five patients and intestinal transplantation in one.

The management of the SBS after bariatric procedures often involves reversal of the bariatric procedure. The reconstruction required will depend on the initial operation. A gastrogastrostomy, restoring continuity with the distal stomach, will improve nutrient intake after a previous gastric bypass. Takedown of the Roux limb with restoration of intestinal continuity will maximize absorptive capacity. A distal intestinal anastomosis can be moved to a more proximal location. Any bypassed intestinal segments should be recruited into continuity. These maneuvers will be important in optimizing nutrient intake and absorption in these challenging patients.

Patients developing SBS after bariatric surgery may have several special considerations. If SBS develops early after the operation, the patients will still be morbidly obese. This may cause difficulty in care, for example, in vascular access. The surgical alteration in the gastrointestinal tract will influence nutritional support and reversal procedures may be required, as described earlier. These patients may be at an increased risk for liver disease because steatohepatitis may already be present. These observations are speculative and will require further evaluation in this growing group of SBS patients.

References

1 Griffen WO, Bivins BA, Bell RM. The decline and fall of the jejunoileal bypass. *Surg Gynecol Obstet* 1983;157:301–330.

2 Hocking MP, Duerson MC, O'Leary JP, Woodward ER. Jejunoileal bypass for morbid obesity: Late follow up in 100 cases. *N Engl J Med* 1983;308:995–999.

3 Kirkpatrick JR. Jejunoileal bypass. A legacy of late complications. *Arch Surg* 1987;122:610–614.

4 Dudrick SJ, Daly JM, Castro G, Akhtar M. Gastrointestinal adaption following small bowel bypass for obesity. *Ann Surg* 1977;185:646–647.

5 Grant JP. Duke Procedure for super obesity: Preliminary report with 3.5 year—follow up. *Surgery* 1994;115:718–726.

6 Arteaga JR, Huerta S, Basa N, Livingston EH. Interval Jejunoileal bypass reduces the morbidity and mortality of Roux-en-Y gastric bypass in the super obese. *Am Surg* 2003;69:873–878.

7 Requarth JA, Burchard KW, Colaccio TA, et al. Long term morbidity following jejunoileal bypass: The continuing need for surgical reversal. *Arch Surg* 1995;130:318–325.

8 Lowell JA, Shenoy S, Ghalib R, et al. Liver transplantation after jejunoileal bypass for morbid obesity. *J Am Coll Surg* 1997;185:123–127.

9 D'souza-Gburek SM, Batts KP, Nikias GA, et al. Liver Transplantation for jejunoileal bypass associated cirrhosis: allograft histology in the setting of an intact bypassed limb. *Liver Transpl Surg* 1997;3:23–27.

10 Scopinaro N, Gravetti E, Civarelli D, et al. Two years of clinical experience with biliopancreatic bypass for obesity. *Am J Clin Nutr* 1980;33:506–514.

11 Marceau P, Biron S, Bourque RA, et al. Biliopancreatic diversion with a new type of gastrectomy. *Obes Surg* 1993;3:29–35.

12 Dolan K, Hatzifotis M, Newbury L. A clinical and nutritional comparison of biliopancreatic diversion with and without duodenal switch. *Ann Surg* 2004;240:51–56.

13 Scopinaro N, Gianetta E, Adami GF, et al. Biliopancreatic diversion for obesity at 18 years. *Surgery* 1996;119:261–268.

14 Castillo J, Fabvegn Z, Escalante CF, et al. Liver transplantation in a case of steatohepatitis and subacute hepatic failure after biliopancreatic diversion for morbid obesity. *Obes Surg* 2001;11:640–642.

15 Murr MM, Balsiger BM, Kennedy FP, Mai JL, Sarr MB. Malabsorptive procedures for severe obesity: Comparison of pancreaticobiliary bypass and very long Roux-en-Y bypass. *J Gastrointest Surg* 1999;3:607–612.

16 Sugarman HJ, Kellum JM, DeMaria EJ. Conversion of proximal to distal gastric bypass for failed gastric bypass in super obesity. *J Gastrointest Surg* 1997;1:517–526.

17 Brolin RE, Lemarca LB, Keuler HA, et al. Malabsorptive gastric bypass in patients with super obesity. *J Gastrointest Surg* 2002;6:195–205.

18 McBride CL, Dabney A, Sudan D, Thompson JS. Short bowel syndrome following bariatric surgical procedures. *Am J Surg* 2006;192:828–832.

19 Thompson JS, DiBaise JK, Iyer KR, et al. Short bowel syndrome as a postoperative complication. *J Am Coll Surg* 2005;201:85–89.

20 Garza E, Kuhn J, Arnold D, et al. Internal hernias after laparoscopic Roux-en-Y gastric bypass. *Am J Surg* 2004;188:796–800.

21 Higa KD, Ho T, Boone KB. Internal hernias after laparoscopic Roux-en-Y gastric bypass: incidence, treatment, and prevention. *Obes Surg* 2003;13:350–354.

22 Carmody B, Demaria EJ, Jamal M, et al. Internal hernia after laparoscopic roux en Y gastric bypass. *Surg Obes Relat Disease* 2005;1:543–548.

23 Charles A, Domingo S, Goldfadden A, et al. Small bowel ischemia after Roux en Y Gastric Bypass complicated by pregnancy: A case report. *Am Surg* 2005;71:231–234.

24 Champion JK, Williams M. Small bowel obstruction and internal hernias after laparoscopic Roux en Y Gastric Bypass. *Obes Surg* 2003;13:596–600.

25 Denne JL, Kowalski C. Portal vein thrombosis after laparoscopic gastric bypass. *Obesity Surgery* 2005;15:885–889.

26 Johnson CM, de la Torre RA, Scott JS, Johansen T. Mesenteric venous thrombosis after laparoscopic Roux-en-Y gastric bypass. *Surg Obes Rel Dis* 2005;1:580–583.

27 Livingston EH. Complications of bariatric surgery. *Surg Clin North Am* 2005;85:853–868.

11 Inflammatory Bowel Disease and the Short Bowel Syndrome

Ramsey K. Umar and Alan L. Buchman

Key points

- Severe inflammatory bowel disease contributing to short bowel syndrome primarily applies to Crohn's disease.

- The management of Crohn's disease in the context of short bowel syndrome is similar to standard therapy.

- Newer therapies (namely anti-TNF-α drugs) have reduced morbidity and surgical bowel resections associated with moderate–severe Crohn's disease but no controlled data exists in the postoperative setting.

- Nutritional deficiencies seen in short bowel syndrome with superimposed Crohn's disease must be addressed and treated.

Introduction

Short bowel syndrome (SBS), defined as having less than 200 cm of small intestine, is caused by a variety of conditions as detailed in earlier chapters. Crohn's disease, an inflammatory bowel disease that may afflict any part of the intestinal tract, is a cause of SBS that must be treated aggressively. By comparison, ulcerative colitis affects only the large intestine and does not directly contribute to the causes of SBS. Mesenteric vein thrombosis due to hypercoagulable states seen in ulcerative colitis or Crohn's disease may result in SBS, but this is rare [1,2].

The development of SBS within Crohn's disease typically occurs as a complication of Crohn's disease. When

Intestinal Failure: Diagnosis, Management and Transplantation.
Edited by Alan N. Langnas, Olivier Goulet, Eamonn M.M. Quigley and Kelly A. Tappenden. © 2008 Blackwell Publishing. ISBN 978-1-4051-4637-1.

Crohn's disease is severe, the development of fistulas, obstruction, abscesses, or perforations frequently necessitate surgical resection of diseased small bowel with the subsequent shortening of available small intestine [3]. The appropriate use of available immunosuppressive and anti-inflammatory therapies is required to minimize the activity of Crohn's disease in the small bowel, and hence reduce the need for small bowel resection [4]. Additionally, the use of less invasive surgeries such as stricturoplasty has decreased the development of SBS as a result of Crohn's disease [5,6].

This chapter will focus on the management of previously diagnosed Crohn's disease in the SBS patient. The approach to management will be based on the assumption that patients with known Crohn's disease underwent bowel resection surgery, leading to the complication of SBS.

Diagnosis

The initial presentation of Crohn's disease is variable. Medical management of recurrent Crohn's disease is essentially the same as standard Crohn's disease with a few exceptions. Given the focus of this chapter, the reader will be referred to the following sources for further understanding of the diagnosis and initial management of Crohn's disease [7–9].

Detection of recurrent Crohn's disease

Resection of small bowel in the setting of Crohn's disease is not a curative procedure. Crohn's disease may recur at the site of a surgical anastomosis, within a stoma, or within a previously unaffected area of small

Table 11.1 Crohn's disease recurrence rates after surgery.

Author	Number of patients followed	Follow-up time	% disease recurrence (per patient cohort)
Pritchard et al.	13	median 24 months	69% at 2 years range 0.5 to 7 years
Hurst et al.	57	mean 38 months (range 2–5 years)	15% +/− 6% at 2 years and 22% +/− 10% at 5 years
Stebbing et al.	52	median 49.5 months	36% at 1–57 months
Serra et al.	43	mean 54.4 months range 4–108 months	32.5% at 2.4 years
Fazio et al.	452	median 3 years	24% at 3 years
Yamamoto et al.	111	median 107 months	54% at 107 months
Spencer et al.	244	3 years	20% at 3 years
Tonelli et al.	44	47.8 months +/− 42.4 months range 3–132 months	22.7% at 50 months range, 18–89 months

bowel [10,11]. Recurrence of Crohn's disease is common and unpredictable. Although endoscopic recurrence of Crohn's disease may be as high as 74–93% within 1 year of operation, it has been shown that clinical presentation may be only as low as 5–20%. Factors influencing recurrence include disease activity, the indication for surgery, and the number of prior surgical resections. Surgical resections for fistulizing disease or abscess tend to have higher postoperative Crohn's disease recurrence rates than surgeries performed for structure alone [12]. Stricureplasty surgeries, typically performed for symptomatic obstructive symptoms, are not curative and recurrence after these operations are common (see Table 11.1) [13–20]. Recurrent disease may be difficult to detect. Elevated serum C-reactive protein and decreased serum albumin concentrations may be seen in the setting of recurrent Crohn's disease, but these are nonspecific findings [21]. Fecal alpha-1 antitrypsin (a marker for protein losing enteropathy) is a surrogate marker of intestinal inflammation. Measurement of fecal alpha-1 antitrypsin has been evaluated in recurrent Crohn's ileitis and it demonstrates a sensitivity of 75%, specificity of 85% and negative predictive value of 94% [22].

Other markers have been examined for the detection of active Crohn's disease including calprotectin and lactoferrin. However, as opposed to fecal alpha-1 antitrypsin, these markers have not been studied specifically in postoperative recurrence. Calprotectin, a protein released from the cytoplasm of neutrophils, has been found to have a sensitivity and specificity of nearly 80% when tested in patients with active Crohn's disease. A limitation for this test is the lack of correlation with clinical presentation or with disease activity scores such as the CDAI (Crohn's Disease Activity Index). Lactoferrin, another protein released from white blood cells, has been found to have a similar sensitivity and specificity [23,24].

Table 11.2 Most common medication regimens for recurrent Crohn's disease.

Medication Class/Name	Dosage	Efficacy
Aminosalicylates		
Mesalamine	2.4–4.8 g/daily	Limited benefit, if any
Sulfasalazine	2–4 g/daily	
Steroids		
Prednisone	40–60 mg/daily	Helpful for short-term reduction of Crohn's flares
Hydrocortisone (IV)	300 mg/daily (12.5 mg/hr)	
Antibiotics		
Ciprofloxacin	500 mg/day	Useful in mild-moderate Crohn's disease.
Metronidazole	500 mg TID-QID	Limited data for benefit in recurrent disease
Thiopurines		
Azathioprine	2.5 mg/kg/day	Reasonable data conferring benefit in recurrent
6-MP	1.5 mg/kg/day	disease
TNF-α inhibitors		
Infliximab	5–10 mg/kg at time 0, 2 weeks, every 6 weeks	Efficacious in Crohn's flares and maintenance
Adalimumab	80–160 mg SC every 2 weeks	therapy. Data lacking in postoperative recurrent disease.
Methotrexate	12.5–25 mg IM weekly	No proven efficacy in postoperative disease. Not used postoperatively.

Endoscopy (ileoscopy) or radiographic studies (such as small bowel follow through or CT scan) are helpful for evaluation of recurrent disease, but positive findings seem to precede symptomatic disease. Additionally, early mild asymptomatic disease recurrence detected by endoscopy or radiography tends to remain asymptomatic [25]. Ultimately, prompt recognition of disease recurrence and subsequent medical therapy (see Table 11.2) has been shown to improve perioperative outcomes [26].

Medical therapy for recurrent Crohn's disease

Aminosalicylates

5-aminosalicylic acid (5-ASA) compounds have been used for the maintenance of Crohn's disease for over 20 years with minimal efficacy. As opposed to therapy in acute ulcerative colitis, 5-ASA compounds appear to be most helpful in the maintenance of otherwise quiescent mild Crohn's colitis [27,28].

The data for use of 5-ASA compounds in recurrent small bowel Crohn's disease is even less encouraging. Earlier studies demonstrated modest improvements in outcome in recurrent Crohn's disease with the use of 5-ASA compounds. However, when tested in randomized controlled trials, the benefits were not apparent [29] or very small (10% reduced risk of recurrence) [30]. As in nearly all the drugs to be discussed in this chapter, 5-ASA drugs were not specifically evaluated with controlled trials in SBS patients with recurrent Crohn's disease. The overall use of 5-ASA in recurrent Crohn's disease, although likely not to cause harm, is of limited benefit.

Antibiotics

In animal models, intestinal bacteria appear to play a role in Crohn's activity. This may be related to bacterial influence on chronic immune-mediated intestinal inflammation. In Crohn's disease, the use of ciprofloxacin and metronidazole have been shown to be effective in achieving remission in mild-moderate Crohn's ileitis and Crohn's colitis [31–33]. Advantages of this regimen include efficacy in patients with abscesses or fistulizing disease. It is important to note that many patients with SBS with Crohn's no longer have ileum present, and hence this data is extrapolated to Crohn's jejeunitis.

Antibiotics are also helpful in recurrent Crohn's disease. The use of metronidazole in recurrent Crohn's disease for three months after ileal resection with ileocolonic anastamosis has been shown to reduce the incidence of recurrent Crohn's disease [34]. This benefit was not conferred after one year; patient dropout rates were high related to medication side effects including gastrointestinal intolerance, metallic taste, and limb paresthesias. Another nitroimidazole antibiotic with a better side-effect profile, ornidazole, has been evaluated in a randomized controlled trial in the postoperative Crohn's setting. Significant improvement was seen at one year post-therapy, however, dropout rates were still higher than placebo [35]. No controlled data exists for ciprofloxacin in the postoperative setting, with only a single case report in the literature that suggested benefit in severe recurrent Crohn's disease at the ileocolonic anastomosis site [36].

Corticosteroids

With the widening use of immunomodulator therapy, reliance on corticosteroids for the management of Crohn's has lessened. In fact, use of steroids has been limited to the management of acute flares of Crohn's disease as a result of the consequences of long-term steroid dependence, including osteoporosis, glucose intolerance, and poor wound healing.

Ultimately, corticosteroids are used for short-term control of Crohn's flares [37]. Budesonide is an oral steroid formulation that is favored because of its limited systemic effects as a result of a high first-pass metabolism. This medication typically exerts its effects in the distal small bowel and very proximal colon, making it an effective directed therapy for mild-moderate small bowel Crohn's disease [38]. Budesonide has demonstrated efficacy in the maintenance of remission of Crohn's disease for up to 6 months, although this may be of minimal clinical significance [38,39]. Furthermore, when examined in the postoperative setting, budesonide does not prevent disease recurrence and is not recommended [40,41].

Azathioprine and 6-mercaptopurine

The thiopurine class of immunosuppressants is effective in the management of Crohn's disease. 6-MP molecules are converted into active 6-thioguanine compounds (6-TG) by one pathway or into inactive 6-methylmercaptopurine by the thiopurine methyltransferase (TPMT) enzyme by another pathway. Less than 1% of the population appears to have complete TPMT deficiency, which results in significant leukopenia as a result of overdosing of active metabolites. Patients with SBS have varying abilities to absorb medications because of rapid intestinal transit times and decreased absorptive surface area and are at risk for underdosing of medication. Measurement of 6-MP metabolites may therefore be helpful in clinical management. Diligent follow-up of complete blood counts (CBC) to evaluate for leukopenia is necessary, with weekly CBCs for 2–3 weeks, followed by gradual lengthening of laboratory intervals not to exceed 6–8 weeks.

Present et al. performed the first randomized placebo controlled-trial testing the use of 6-MP in Crohn's disease with significant benefits against placebo (67% vs. 8%) [42]. Since that time, use of both 6-MP and azathioprine have been used as mainstays of steroid-sparing therapy in Crohn's disease [43]. Azathioprine differs from 6-MP in that it requires nonezymatic breakdown to form the 6-MP metabolite. Dosing is different, with 6-MP requiring 1–1.5 mg/kg/day compared to azathioprine requiring 2–2.5 mg/kg/day. Optimal duration of therapy with 6-MP compounds is unclear although more recent data suggests that once a patient is committed to this regimen, length of therapy is generally greater than 3 years, and may be lifelong [44].

Use of azathioprine and 6-MP have been examined in recurrent disease in the postoperative setting

[45,46]. Limitation of these trials include dosing regimens [46], varying available endoscopic data documenting mucosal improvement and lack of blinding in the study published by Ardizzone et al. [45] Despite these limitations, these trials do support the use of 6-MP/azathioprine in Crohn's disease in the postoperative setting and do confer a benefit over 5-ASA compounds.

Infliximab

Much has been learned about tumor necrosis-factor alpha (TNF-α) inhibitors in the management of Crohn's disease. TNF-α stimulates the production of cytokines by T-helper cells, which is thought to play a major role in the inflammatory process behind Crohn's disease. Infliximab is a chimeric antibody (part mouse, part human) that inhibits TNF-α. As a result, the formation of antibodies against infliximab with the clinical consequences of infusion reactions and loss of efficacy has complicated the use of this medication. Premedication with corticosteroids, 6-MP/azathioprine or methotrexate has been helpful in decreasing antibody formation, although it does not eliminate this phenomenon [47,48]. New fully humanized TNF-α inhibitors are being tested such as adalimumab and certolizumab and integrin-inhibitors such as natalizumab are being evaluated, which may prove to be effective while having lower rates of immunogenicity [49–51].

In Crohn's disease, an induction dosing regimen was defined by Hanauer et al. in the ACCENT I trial, using a dose of 5 mg/kg at time 0, followed by an infusion at 2 weeks and again at 6 weeks. Maintenance of remission was confirmed by repeat dosing of 5 mg/kg every 8 weeks for 46 weeks [48]. Infliximab is also beneficial in fistulizing Crohn's disease, with improvements in nearly two-thirds of treated patients compared to 26% in a placebo group [52], with sustained closure rates seen during maintenance therapy [53]. The growing use of this medication has been important in avoiding or delaying bowel resection related to severe Crohn's disease [54]. Notably, some early data exists showing that patients with established short bowel syndrome may be at higher risk of relapse through infliximab therapy [55]. Controlled data demonstrating the efficacy of TNF-α inhibitors are lacking in the management of postoperative Crohn's disease.

Nutrition in Crohn's disease

Although control of active Crohn's disease is critical, it is important to optimize nutritional status. Patients with ileal Crohn's disease (or status-post ileal resection) are frequently deficient in vitamin B12 as well as deficient in fat soluble vitamins (A, D, E, K) related to bile salt malabsorption [56]. Iron deficiency may be seen as a result of duodenal inflammation or may be a result of poor nutritional intake [57]. Selenium deficiency may be seen in Crohn's patients related to chronic TPN requirements. Manifestations of this may included macrocytosis, discoloration of the nail beds or muscle weakness [58]. Zinc may also be deficient in small bowel or Crohn's colitis related to diarrhea. Side effects such as retinal dysfunction improve with repletion of serum zinc [59]. The testing and treatment of nutritional deficiencies in Crohn's disease is vitally important in the management of these patients.

References

1 Fichera A, Cicchiello LA, Mendelson DS, et al. Superior mesenteric vein thrombosis after colectomy for inflammatory bowel disease: a not uncommon cause of postoperative acute abdominal pain. *Dis Colon Rectum* 2003;46:643–648.

2 Novotny DA, Rubin RJ, Slezak FA, Porter JA. Arterial thromboembolic complications of inflammatory bowel disease. Report of three cases. *Dis Colon Rectum* 1992;35:193–196.

3 Agwunobi AO, Carlson GL, Anderson ID, et al. Mechanisms of intestinal failure in Crohn's disease. *Dis Colon Rectum* 2001;44:1834–1837.

4 Krupnick AS, Morris JB. The long-term results of resection and multiple resections in Crohn's disease. *Semin Gastrointest Dis* 2000;11:41–51.

5 Sampietro GM, Cristaldi M, Maconi G, et al. A prospective, longitudinal study of nonconventional stricture-plasty in Crohn's disease. *J Am Coll Surg* 2004;199:8–20;discussion-2.

6 Sampietro GM, Cristaldi M, Porretta T, et al. Early perioperative results and surgical recurrence after strictureplasty and miniresection for complicated Crohn's disease. *Dig Surg* 2000;17:261–267.

7 Lichtenstein GR, Abreu MT, Cohen R, Tremaine W. American Gastroenterological Association Institute medical position statement on corticosteroids, immunomodulators, and infliximab in inflammatory bowel disease. *Gastroenterology* 2006;130:935–939.

8 Stange EF, Travis SP, Vermeire S, et al. European evidence based consensus on the diagnosis and management of Crohn's disease: definitions and diagnosis. *Gut* 2006;55(Suppl 1):1–15.

9 Travis SP, Stange EF, Lemann M, et al. European evidence based consensus on the diagnosis and management of Crohn's disease: current management. *Gut* 2006;55(Suppl 1):16–35.

10 Sagar PM, Dozois RR, Wolff BG. Long-term results of ileal pouch-anal anastomosis in patients with Crohn's disease. *Dis Colon Rectum* 1996;39:893–898.

11 Olaison G, Smedh K, Sjodahl R. Natural course of Crohn's disease after ileocolic resection: endoscopically visualised ileal ulcers preceding symptoms. *Gut* 1992;33:331–335.

12 Rutgeerts P, Geboes K, Vantrappen G, et al. Predictability of the postoperative course of Crohn's disease. *Gastroenterology* 1990;99:956–963.

13 Fazio VW, Tjandra JJ, Lavery IC, et al. Long-term follow-up of strictureplasty in Crohn's disease. *Dis Colon Rectum* 1993;36:355–361.

14 Hurst RD, Michelassi F. Strictureplasty for Crohn's disease: techniques and long-term results. *World J Surg* 1998;22:359–363.

15 Pritchard TJ, Schoetz DJ, Jr, Caushaj FP, et al. Strictureplasty of the small bowel in patients with Crohn's disease. An effective surgical option. *Arch Surg* 1990;125:715–717.

16 Serra J, Cohen Z, McLeod RS. Natural history of strictureplasty in Crohn's disease: 9-year experience. *Can J Surg* 1995;38:481–485.

17 Spencer MP, Nelson H, Wolff BG, Dozois RR. Strictureplasty for obstructive Crohn's disease: the Mayo experience. *Mayo Clin Proc* 1994;69:33–36.

18 Stebbing JF, Jewell DP, Kettlewell MG, Mortensen NJ. Recurrence and reoperation after strictureplasty for obstructive Crohn's disease: long-term results [corrected]. *Br J Surg* 1995;82:1471–1474.

19 Tonelli F, Ficari F. Strictureplasty in Crohn's disease: surgical option. *Dis Colon Rectum* 2000;43:920–926.

20 Yamamoto T, Bain IM, Allan RN, Keighley MR. An audit of strictureplasty for small-bowel Crohn's disease. *Dis Colon Rectum* 1999;42:797–803.

21 Moran A, Jones A, Asquith P. Laboratory markers of colonoscopic activity in ulcerative colitis and Crohn's colitis. *Scand J Gastroenterol* 1995;30:356–360.

22 Biancone L, Fantini M, Tosti C, et al. Fecal alpha 1-antitrypsin clearance as a marker of clinical relapse in patients with Crohn's disease of the distal ileum. *Eur J Gastroenterol Hepatol* 2003;15:261–266.

23 Gaya DR, Lyon TD, Duncan A, et al. Faecal calprotectin in the assessment of Crohn's disease activity. *Qjm* 2005;98:435–441.

24 D'Inca R, Dal Pont E, Di Leo V, et al. Calprotectin and lactoferrin in the assessment of intestinal inflammation and organic disease. *Int J Colorectal Dis* 2006; 13.

25 McLeod RS, Wolff BG, Steinhart AH, et al. Risk and significance of endoscopic/radiological evidence of recurrent Crohn's disease. *Gastroenterology* 1997;113:1823–1827.

26 Tay GS, Binion DG, Eastwood D, Otterson MF. Multivariate analysis suggests improved perioperative outcome in Crohn's disease patients receiving immunomodulator therapy after segmental resection and/or strictureplasty. *Surgery* 2003;134:565–572; discussion 72–3.

27 de Franchis R, Omodei P, Ranzi T, et al. Controlled trial of oral 5-aminosalicylic acid for the prevention of early relapse in Crohn's disease. *Aliment Pharmacol Ther* 1997;11:845–852.

28 Hanauer SB, Krawitt EL, Robinson M, et al. Long-term management of Crohn's disease with mesalamine capsules (Pentasa). Pentasa Crohn's Disease Compassionate Use Study Group. *Am J Gastroenterol* 1993;88:1343–1351.

29 Lochs H, Mayer M, Fleig WE, et al. Prophylaxis of postoperative relapse in Crohn's disease with mesalamine: European Cooperative Crohn's Disease Study VI. Gastroenterology. 2000;118:264–273.

30 Caprilli R, Cottone M, Tonelli F, et al. Two mesalazine regimens in the prevention of the post-operative recurrence of Crohn's disease: a pragmatic, double-blind, randomized controlled trial. *Aliment Pharmacol Ther* 2003;17:517–523.

31 Greenbloom SL, Steinhart AH, Greenberg GR. Combination ciprofloxacin and metronidazole for active Crohn's disease. *Can J Gastroenterol* 1998;12:53–56.

32 Ishikawa T, Okamura S, Oshimoto H, Kobayashi R, Mori M. Metronidazole plus ciprofloxacin therapy for active Crohn's disease. *Intern Med* 2003;42:318–321.

33 Prantera C, Zannoni F, Scribano ML, et al. An antibiotic regimen for the treatment of active Crohn's disease: a randomized, controlled clinical trial of metronidazole plus ciprofloxacin. *Am J Gastroenterol* 1996;91:328–332.

34 Rutgeerts P, Hiele M, Geboes K, et al. Controlled trial of metronidazole treatment for prevention of Crohn's recurrence after ileal resection. *Gastroenterology* 1995;108:1617–1621.

35 Rutgeerts P, Van Assche G, Vermeire S, et al. Ornidazole for prophylaxis of postoperative Crohn's disease recurrence: a randomized, double-blind, placebo-controlled trial. *Gastroenterology* 2005;128:856–861.

36 Elliott PR, Moore GT, Bell SJ, Connell WR. Severe recurrent Crohn's disease of the ileocolonic anastomosis disappearing completely with antibacterial therapy. *Gut* 2005;54:1818–1819.

37 Smith RC, Rhodes J, Heatley RV, et al. Low dose steroids and clinical relapse in Crohn's disease: a controlled trial. *Gut* 1978;19:606–610.

38 Greenberg GR, Feagan BG, Martin F, et al. Oral budesonide as maintenance treatment for Crohn's disease: a placebo-controlled, dose-ranging study. Canadian Inflammatory Bowel Disease Study Group. *Gastroenterology* 1996;110:45–51.

39 Sandborn WJ, Lofberg R, Feagan BG, et al. Budesonide for maintenance of remission in patients with Crohn's disease in medically induced remission: a predetermined pooled analysis of four randomized, double-blind, placebo-controlled trials. *Am J Gastroenterol* 2005;100:1780–1787.

40 Ewe K, Bottger T, Buhr HJ, et al. Low-dose budesonide treatment for prevention of postoperative recurrence of Crohn's disease: a multicentre randomized placebo-controlled trial. German Budesonide Study Group. *Eur J Gastroenterol Hepatol* 1999;11:277–282.

41 Hellers G, Cortot A, Jewell D, et al. Oral budesonide for prevention of postsurgical recurrence in Crohn's disease. The IOIBD Budesonide Study Group. *Gastroenterology* 1999;116:294–300.

42 Present DH, Korelitz BI, Wisch N, et al. Treatment of Crohn's disease with 6-mercaptopurine. A long-term, randomized, double-blind study. *N Engl J Med* 1980;302:981–987.

43 Candy S, Wright J, Gerber M, et al. A controlled double blind study of azathioprine in the management of Crohn's disease. *Gut* 1995;37:674–678.

44 Lemann M, Mary JY, Colombel JF, et al. A randomized, double-blind, controlled withdrawal trial in Crohn's disease patients in long-term remission on azathioprine. *Gastroenterology* 2005;128:1812–1818.

45 Ardizzone S, Maconi G, Russo A, et al. Randomised controlled trial of azathioprine and 5-aminosalicylic acid for treatment of steroid dependent ulcerative colitis. *Gut* 2006;55:47–53.

46 Hanauer SB, Korelitz BI, Rutgeerts P, et al. Postoperative maintenance of Crohn's disease remission with 6-mercaptopurine, mesalamine, or placebo: a 2-year trial. *Gastroenterology* 2004;127:723–729.

47 Farrell RJ, Alsahli M, Jeen YT, et al. Intravenous hydrocortisone premedication reduces antibodies to infliximab in Crohn's disease: a randomized controlled trial. *Gastroenterology* 2003;124:917–924.

48 Hanauer SB, Feagan BG, Lichtenstein GR, et al. Maintenance infliximab for Crohn's disease: the ACCENT I randomised trial. *Lancet* 2002;359:1541–1549.

49 Ghosh S, Goldin E, Gordon FH, et al. Natalizumab for active Crohn's disease. *N Engl J Med* 2003;348:24–32.

50 Sandborn WJ, Colombel JF, Enns R, et al. Natalizumab induction and maintenance therapy for Crohn's disease. *N Engl J Med* 2005;353:1912–1925.

51 Hanauer SB, Sandborn WJ, Rutgeerts P, et al. Human anti-tumor necrosis factor monoclonal antibody (adalimumab) in Crohn's disease: the CLASSIC-I trial. *Gastroenterology* 2006;130:323–333; quiz 591.

52 Present DH, Rutgeerts P, Targan S, et al. Infliximab for the treatment of fistulas in patients with Crohn's disease. *N Engl J Med* 1999;340:1398–1405.

53 Sands BE, Anderson FH, Bernstein CN, et al. Infliximab maintenance therapy for fistulizing Crohn's disease. *N Engl J Med* 2004;350:876–885.

54 Lichtenstein GR, Yan S, Bala M, Hanauer S. Remission in patients with Crohn's disease is associated with improvement in employment and quality of life and a decrease in hospitalizations and surgeries. *Am J Gastroenterol* 2004;99:91–96.

55 Kohgo Y, et al. Short Residual Intestine of Postsurgical CD Patients is a Risk for Earlier Relapse of Infliximab Adminstration. DDW 2006 (Abstract).

56 Kastin DA, Buchman AL. Malnutrition and gastrointestinal disease. *Curr Opin Clin Nutr Metab Care* 2002;5:699–706.

57 Lomer MC, Kodjabashia K, Hutchinson C, et al. Intake of dietary iron is low in patients with Crohn's disease: a case-control study. *Br J Nutr* 2004;91:141–148.

58 Ishida T, Himeno K, Torigoe Y, et al. Selenium deficiency in a patient with Crohn's disease receiving long-term total parenteral nutrition. *Intern Med* 2003;42:154–157.

59 Myung SJ, Yang SK, Jung HY, et al. Zinc deficiency manifested by dermatitis and visual dysfunction in a patient with Crohn's disease. *J Gastroenterol* 1998;33:876–879.

12 Motility Disorders

Hayat Mousa and Carlo Di Lorenzo

Key points

- Motility disorders are associated with substantial morbidity.
- Motility disorders are mostly restricted to the gut when primary, and associated with systemic involvement when secondary to other diseases.
- Motility disorders present with symptoms that are related to the extent and severity of the enteric muscle and nerve involvement.
- In their most severe forms, motility disorders may require intestinal transplantation as the only option for a cure.

Spectrum of gastrointestinal motility disorders

Gastrointestinal (GI) motility disorders are extremely common. Motility abnormalities have been identified in prevalent, benign conditions, such as gastroesophageal reflux and childhood constipation, and in more severe but less frequent entities, such as chronic intestinal pseudo-obstruction (CIP) and Hirschsprung's disease. Abnormal motility, either as a baseline dysfunction or as an exaggerated or blunted response to physiologic events, has also been demonstrated in children with a variety of functional gastrointestinal disorders (FGID), such as irritable bowel syndrome and functional dyspepsia [1–3]. GI dysmotility adds considerable co-morbidity to gastrointestinal structural anomalies such as intestinal atresia, stenosis,

Intestinal Failure: Diagnosis, Management and Transplantation.
Edited by Alan N. Langnas, Olivier Goulet, Eamonn M.M. Quigley and Kelly A. Tappenden. © 2008 Blackwell Publishing.
ISBN 978-1-4051-4637-1.

gastroschisis, or short gut syndrome secondary to volvulus, necrotizing enterocolitis, or trauma. Gastrointestinal motility disorders account for up to 15% of pediatrics intestinal failure cases. Motility disorders may involve only part of the GI tract:

1 When limited to the stomach, they present with gastric failure. Gastric pacing may be necessary in the most severe forms.

2 Isolated small bowel dysmotility may lead to a critical reduction in functioning gut, leading to intestinal failure.

3 Isolated colonic dysmotility causes defecatory disorders with refractory constipation and possible compromise in small bowel function (with the colon acting as an outlet obstruction).

4 Generalized foregut and hindgut motility disorders usually present with the phenotype of CIP.

Pediatric motility disorders have been classified as either congenital or acquired, depending on the presence or absence of symptoms at birth [4]. Congenital disorders usually cause symptoms within the first two months of life and can be sporadic or familial. Acquired motility disorders present later in life and can be secondary to a variety of insults, such as infections and adverse reactions to medications [5]. Based on histopathology and patterns of motility abnormalities, motility disorders have traditionally been classified as a visceral myopathy or a visceral neuropathy [5]. Neuropathic disorders are more common but myopathies are usually associated with more severe symptoms [4,5]. The role of genetic mutations in visceral myopathies or neuropathies has not yet been thoroughly elucidated and their mode of inheritance cannot be predicted at this time [6]. Intrauterine ischemic insults and exposure to amniotic fluid and to transplacental alcohol have been linked to CIP [7–10].

Delayed maturation of either the enteric nervous system or the interstitial cells of Cajal is also associated with abnormal motility [11]. Inflammation within the myenteric ganglia has been described to cause severe progressive neuropathic CIP in conjunction with autoimmune disease and circulating antienteric neuronal antibodies [12]. Mitochondrial myopathies are known to be associated with a variety of clinical syndromes including CIP [13]. Patients with mitochondrial neurogastrointestinal encephalomyopathy (MNGIE) have GI dysmotility, peripheral neuropathy, ophthalmoparesis, and muscle biopsy shows histological features of mitochondrial myopathy [14,15]. Other individuals who initially presented with signs of GI dysmotility were later found to have a disorder of the mitochondrial electron transport chain enzymes [16]. In this chapter, we will discuss only the motility disorders that are likely to be complicated by intestinal failure and/or a need for intestinal transplantation:

1 Chronic intestinal pseudoobstruction
2 Hirschsprung's disease

Chronic intestinal pseudoobstruction

CIP is a rare syndrome caused by a heterogeneous group of enteric nerve and muscle diseases characterized by chronic or repetitive episodes of bowel obstruction in the absence of a lumen-occluding lesion [4,17–20]. CIP often results in intestinal failure and requires life-long medical care [4,18–22]. Data from the American Pseudo-obstruction and Hirschsprung's Society suggested that approximately 100 infants with CIP are born each year in the United States [18]. The most common symptoms include vomiting, abdominal distension, and constipation [4,17–19]. Other symptoms are the result of complications: diarrhea from bacterial overgrowth and urinary voiding disorders caused by involvement of the nerves and muscles of the urinary tract [4]. Patients may present with overlapping phenotypic features of mitochondrial myopathy, encephalopathy, lactic acidosis, and stroke-like episodes (MELAS) and MNGIE [15] or with different mitochondrial deficiencies [23–27]. Megacystis microcolon intestinal hypoperistalsis syndrome (MMIHS) (Figure 12.1) is a rare, congenital, and often fatal disease characterized by a distended, nonobstructed urinary bladder microcolon, incomplete intestinal rotation, hypoperistalsis in the entire GI tract, and failure to pass meconium. Berdon et al. [28] first

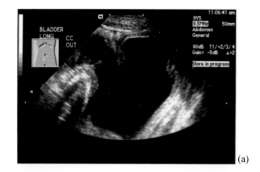
(a)

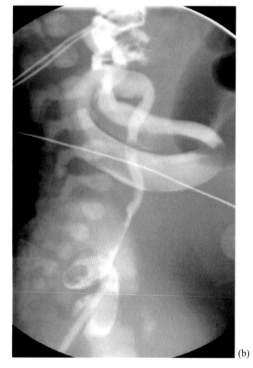
(b)

Figure 12.1 (a) Prenatal ultrasound demonstrating a megacystis in a child with megacystis microcolon intestinal hypoperistalsis syndrome. (b) Barium enema in a newborn with megacystis microcolon intestinal hypoperistalsis syndrome.

described this syndrome in 1976 and since then the number of newly diagnosed MMIHS cases has been steadily increasing. Enlarged bladder is the earliest and most frequent defect detected (88%), followed by hydronephrosis (53%), polyhydramniosis (34%), and oligohydramniosis (10%). Other associated problems include prematurity and cleft palate. Although the advent of total parenteral nutrition (TPN) has extended the lives of patients with CIP [4,29], complications related to TPN, including central venous catheter–associated sepsis, cholestasis, and end-stage liver disease, are now major contributing factors to CIP mortality and morbidity [4,29].

CIP may also arise acutely in adults (Ogilvie's syndrome), concurrent with nongastrointestinal disorders such as myocardial infarction, pneumonia, or fractured hip [30]. Typically, there is acute colonic dilatation, with pain and abdominal distension. Ogilvie's syndrome is thought to be caused by an imbalance of extrinsic autonomic nerves innervating the gut, with excessive sympathetic inhibitory activity or diminished prokinetic cholinergic drive. It can be managed by colonic decompression or the acute use of an anticholinesterase such as neostigmine. The chronic type of CIP in adults is mostly secondary to neuromuscular diseases, such as scleroderma, systemic sclerosis, bronchial carcinoma, or amyloidosis [31]. More rarely, it is primary, with the disease usually selectively affecting either intestinal smooth muscle or enteric nerve plexuses [30]. These myopathies or neuropathies can be either degenerative or inflammatory.

A number of important etiological factors have emerged over recent years. The use of immunohistochemical techniques has allowed the identification of biochemical abnormalities in some patients, whereas previously only structural or morphological diagnosis was possible. An abnormality of enteric smooth muscle alpha actin has been identified in a patient with normal histology [32]. Epstein-Barr virus has been identified on polymerase chain reaction and in situ hybridization, localized to the myenteric plexus, in a patient with CIP as a result of inflammatory plexitis [33].

Adults with CIP and irreversible intestinal failure are at high risk for major fluid/electrolyte imbalances associated with proximal gastrointestinal stomas or fistula, extreme bowel dilatation with bacterial overgrowth, intractable abdominal pain, and frequent central venous catheter infections as a result of multidrug-resistant organisms, with high risk for metastatic abscesses, infective myocarditis, and multiorgan failure [34].

Systemic abnormalities associated with CIP

Intestinal malrotation is common in children with congenital CIP. Twenty-eight to 40% of children presenting at birth with either myopathic or neuropathic congenital CIP are diagnosed with intestinal malrotation [4].

The incidence of *urological involvement* in children with CIP varies form 33% to 92%, and includes megacystis, hydronephrosis, urinary retention, and infection [35–37]. Children with CIP have hypocontractile detrusor with large bladder capacity and high compliance [37]. Bladder biopsies usually show a thinned and fibrosed detrusor. When associated with ureterohydronephrosis, megacystis proves to be a significant risk factor for the development of febrile urinary tract infections, increasing morbidity as they are often associated with synchronous gastrointestinal decompensation.

Hirschsprung's disease

Hirschsprung's disease is a disorder once thought to exclusively involve the aganglionic segment of the distal colon. Recent evidence suggests that it affects also the motor function of other areas of the gut. Recognizable abnormalities in esophageal motility are common, and duodenal motor dysfunction is present in 48% of patients [5,38]. Miele et al found that all transit measurements (gastric, colonic, total gut) were prolonged in patients with HD [39].

Diagnosis

Manometric assessment is the gold standard for establishing the diagnosis and in particular to differentiate CIP from severe FGID.

Manometry

Contractions of the antrum, duodenum, and colon are measured using catheters with sensors spaced 3–5 cm apart in the stomach and small bowel, and 10–15 cm apart in the colon. Guidelines to conduct and analyze manometric studies are well established [40,41]; their implementation is necessary to ensure optimal diagnostic and prognostic outcomes. Motility studies are also helpful in mapping the gastrointestinal tract to localize the functioning or diseased areas before performing decompressing ileostomy, colostomy, or colectomy. Evaluation of colonic function before reconnective surgery is another indication for performing motility studies on children with congenital CIP. A manometry showing nearly normal results is not consistent with a diagnosis of CIP and should raise the possibility of an emotional or factitious disorder.

Gastric emptying studies

Direct noninvasive measurements of liquid or solid gastric emptying can be performed by means of scintigraphy, stable isotope breath tests, ultrasonography, and magnetic resonance imaging [42–44].

Histology

Full thickness biopsies and advanced techniques in histopathology allow for better understanding of abnormalities in the enteric nervous system and deficiencies in neuropeptides and neurotransmitters. In particular, full thickness biopsies are beneficial toward establishing the diagnosis of autoimmune or mitochondrial etiology for pseudo-obstruction.

Differential diagnosis

a *Functional gastrointestinal disorders*: The symptoms of the FGIDs are derived from a combination of (1) increased motor reactivity, (2) enhanced visceral hypersensitivity, (3) altered central nervous system or enteric nervous system regulation [45]. Establishing the diagnosis of FGID depends on symptom-based diagnostic criteria. A manometry showing minor baseline abnormalities is consistent with a diagnosis of FGID.

b *Narcotic Bowel Syndrome (NBS)*: This should be suspected in patients who are referred for signs of delayed gastrointestinal transit time with nausea, bloating, constipation, associated with chronic or frequently recurring abdominal pain that is treated with acute high dose or chronic narcotics. Pain in NBS worsens or incompletely resolves with continued or escalating dosages of narcotics [46]. There is also marked worsening of pain when the narcotic dose wanes and improvement when narcotics are reinstituted.

Management

The management goals of CIP are to restore proper nutrition and fluid balance, relieve symptoms, improve intestinal motility, and treat complications.

1 *Nutritional support*: The majority of patients with CIP require nutritional support and almost half of the affected individuals are dependent on TPN. Dependency on artificial feedings is significantly higher in patient with onset of symptoms at birth, those with megacystis, and in those who undergo repeated surgical interventions.

2 *Prokinetics and antibiotics*: Prokinetics like erythromycin, cisapride, octreotide, tegaserod, or bethanechol are used in the majority of patients with variable efficacy. Nonabsorbable antibiotics and probiotics are used in more than third patients to treat bacterial overgrowth.

3 *Surgical approaches*: When medical management is unsuccessful, then "shortening the gut" by feeding distal to the stomach and diverting the fecal stream proximal to the colon with the creation of an ileostomy are recommended. Decompressing the bowel through a gastrostomy or jejunostomy is reported to be the most beneficial intervention in patients with CIP [22]. Gastrostomies and jejunostomies are also used for drip feeding prior to resorting to TPN. When constipation is the predominant symptom, then use of antegrade enemas through a cecostomy or an appendicostomy may also be beneficial. Every patient with pseudo-obstruction should have a trial of jejunal feeding and receive an ileostomy before considering intestinal transplantation. Closure of a decompressing ileostomy after clinical improvement is generally discouraged. However, in rare patients with clear clinical improvement after ileostomy placement and who have demonstrated an ability to tolerate enteral feeding without symptom exacerbation for more than 2 years, total colectomy and ileo-rectal anastomosis may be considered [22].

4 *Small bowel transplantation*: Patients with gastrointestinal motility disorders are considered candidates for small bowel transplantation, if they are need TPN and have recurrent episodes of sepsis, limited intravenous access or impending liver failure [47–49]. Pseudoobstruction comprised 9% and other motility disorders 2% of the International Intestinal Transplant Registry (children and adults) as of May 2003 [48]. Careful mapping of gut dysfunction is mandated before transplantation. Factors peculiar to patients with motility disorders that need to be addressed before intestinal transplantation include the evaluation of the presence of gastric or colonic dysfunction, with the difficult decision or whether to proceed with an isolated or a multivisceral transplantation. The presence of bladder

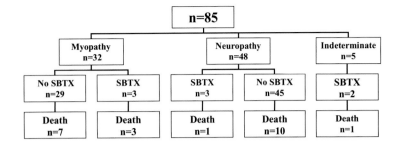

Figure 12.2 Long term outcome of congenital pseudo-obstruction in children. (Data from Mousa et al. [4].)

dysfunction may lead to repeated episodes of urosepsis in a heavily immunosuppressed individual. Chronic visceral pain may make weaning from narcotics very challenging in the postoperative period. The decision of whether *and* when to list for intestinal transplantation a patient with a motility disorder is one of the most challenging that physicians, patients and their families face.

Guidelines for intestinal transplantation in children [47] and adults [50] are well defined in the literature. Waiting times for intestinal transplantation are still long. Patients with intestinal failure and life-threatening complications should be identified before they become critically ill. Death resulting from complications of liver failure is especially common during the waiting period for a combined liver and intestinal transplant, and survival following combined liver and intestinal transplant is probably lower than following an isolated intestinal transplant [47]. Interdigestive motor activity with normal manometric characteristics is found in the small bowel allograft in 62% of patients and may be recognized as early as 3 months post-transplant. Propagated clusters of contractions persist after feeding in the allograft bowel and may partially responsible for the diarrhea which often complicates the post-transplant course [51].

Morbidity

Cholelithiasis (6%), hematemesis (5%), diversion colitis (4%) and stoma prolapse (4%) have been described in CIP [4,5,21,22]. In patients with multiple endocrine neoplasias, hypersecretion with excessive water and electrolyte losses and medullary thyroid carcinoma may develop. Recurrent pancreatitis, gastric bezoar, gastric perforation, and gastric volvulus on gastrostomy are also reported.

Mortality

The long-term outcome of intestinal failure secondary to congenital CIP is described in Figure 12.2. In another review by Vargas et al. [20], one-third of all congenital CIP patients died in the first year of life as a result of malnutrition, infections, or fluid and electrolyte imbalance [20]. Neonatal onset, urinary tract involvement, acute onset, and requirement for surgery indicate poor prognosis [8]. Most cases can only be cured by isolated small bowel or multivisceral transplantation. Dependency on parenteral nutrition to provide more than 50% of caloric needs increases mortality significantly with the 5 years survival rate of 50% compared to 100% if enteral feeds are used to provide >50% of caloric needs [4].

Health and economic impact

Although carefully designed studies are lacking in pediatrics, health care costs of motility disorders can be substantial. Each year, every child with CIP using TPN accounts for more than $50,000 in nutritional costs alone. The medical consequences of prolonged TPN in infants and children with long-segment Hirschsprung's disease and CIP include hospitalizations and medical and surgical care for repeated catheter-related sepsis and liver disease. Feeding intolerance occurs in 50% to 70% of preterm infants. Thus, approximately 20,000 infants are affected each year in the United States. A reduction by 1 week in the use of TPN use in preterm infants would save an estimated $1 billion annually in the United States alone.

Quality of daily life

A study by Schwankovsky et al. [17] found that children with CIP had less freedom from pain, depression, and anxiety than healthy children. In addition, parents of children with CIP had poorer emotional status than parents of healthy children. Appropriate treatment of chronic visceral pain, including a multidisciplinary approach using medications and psychological interventions to teach pain and stress management, may improve the QOL for patients with CIP and their families.

References

1 Van Ginkel R, Voskuijl WP, Benninga MA, et al. Alterations in rectal sensitivity and motility in childhood irritable bowel syndrome. *Gastroenterology* 2001;120:287–290.

2 Chitkara DK, Di Lorenzo C. From the bench to the "crib"-side: implications of scientific advances to paediatric neurogastroenterology and motility. *Neurogastroenterol Motil* 2006;18:251–262.

3 Guarino A, De Marco G, Italian National Network for Pediatric Intestinal Failure. Natural history of intestinal failure, investigated through a national network-based approach. *J Pediatr Gastroenterol Nutr* 2003;37:136–141.

4 Mousa H, Hyman PE, Cocjin J, et al. Long-term outcome of congenital intestinal pseudoobstruction. *Dig Dis Sci* 2002;47:2298–2305.

5 Connor FL, Di Lorenzo C. Chronic intestinal pseudo-obstruction: assessment and management. *Gastroenterology* 2006;130:S29–S36.

6 Guze CD, Hyman PE, Payne VJ. Family studies of infantile visceral myopathy: a congenital myopathic pseudo-obstruction syndrome. *Am J Med Genet* 1999;82:114–122.

7 Srinathan SK, Langer JC, Blennerhassett MG, et al. Etiology of intestinal damage in gastroschisis III: morphometric analysis of the smooth muscle and submucosa. *J Pediatr Surg* 1995;25:1122–1126.

8 Simmons M, Georgeson KE. The effect of gestational age at birth on morbidity in patients with gastroschisis. *J Pediatr Surg* 1996;31:1060–1062.

9 Uc A, Vasiliauskas E, Piccoli DA, et al. Chronic intestinal pseudoobstruction associated with fetal alcohol syndrome. *Dig Dis Sci* 1997;42:1163–1167.

10 Heneyke S, Smith W, Spitz L, et al. Chronic intestinal pseudoobstruction: treatment and long term follow up of 44 patients. *Arch Dis Child* 1999;81:21–27.

11 Kenny SE, Vanderwinden JM, Rintala RJ, et al. Delayed maturation of the interstitial cells of Cajal: a new diagnosis for transient neonatal pseudo-obstruction: report of two cases. *J Pediatr Surg* 1996;33:94–98.

12 Schappi MG, Smith VV, Milla PJ, et al. Eosinophilic myenteric ganglionitis is associated with functional intestinal obstruction. *Gut* 2003;52:752–755.

13 Wedel T, Tafazzoli K, Sollner S, et al. Mitochondrial myopathy (complex I deficiency) associated with chronic intestinal pseudo-obstruction. *Eur J Pediatr Surg* 2003;13:201–205.

14 Hirano M, Silvestri G, Blake DM, et al. Mitochondrial neurogastrointestinal encephalomyopathy (MNGIE)—clinical, biochemical, and genetic features of an autosomal recessive mitochondrial disorder. *Neurology* 1994;44:721–727.

15 Chang TM, Chi CS, Tsai CR, et al. Paralytic ileus in MELAS with phenotypic features of MNGIE. *Pediatr Neurol* 2004;31:374–377.

16 Chitkara D, Nurko S, Shoffner J, et al. Abnormalities in gastrointestinal motility are associated with diseases of oxidative phosphorylation in children. *Am J Gastroenterol* 2003;98:871–877.

17 Schwankovsky L, Mousa H, Rowhani A, et al. Quality of life outcomes in congenital chronic intestinal pseudo-obstruction. *Dig Dis Sci* 2002:47:1965–1968.

18 Rudolph CD, Hyman PE, Altschuler SM, et al. Diagnosis and treatment of chronic intestinal pseudo-obstruction in children: report of consensus workshop. *J Pediatr Gastroenterol Nutr* 1997;24:102–112.

19 Di Lorenzo C. Pseudo-obstruction: current approaches. *Gastroenterology* 1999;116:980–987.

20 Vargas JH, Sachs P, Ament ME. Chronic intestinal pseudoobstruction syndrome in pediatrics. *J Pediatr Gastroenterol Nutr* 1988;7:323–332.

21 Faure C, Goulet O, Ategbo S, et al. Chronic intestinal pseudoobstruction syndrome: clinical analysis, outcome, and prognosis in 105 children. French-Speaking Group of Pediatric Gastroenterology. *Dig Dis Sci* 1999;44:953–959.

22 Goulet O, Jobert-Giraud A, Michel JL, et al. Chronic intestinal pseudo-obstruction syndrome in pediatric patients. *Eur J Pediatr Surg* 1999;9:83–89.

23 Mori O, Yamazaki M, Ohaki Y, et al. Mitochondrial encephalomyopathy with lactic acidosis and stroke like episodes (MELAS) with prominent degeneration of the

intestinal wall and cactus-like cerebellar pathology, *Acta Neuropathol* 2000;100:712–717.

24 Lowsky R, Davidson G, Wolman S, et al. Familial visceral myopathy associated with a mitochondrial myopathy. *Gut* 1993;34:279–283.

25 Hom XB and Lavine JE. Gastrointestinal complications of mitochondrial disease. *Mitochondrion* 2004;4:601–607.

26 Slama A, Lacroix C, Plante-Bordeneuve V, et al. Thymidine phosphorylase gene mutations in patients with mitochondrial neurogastrointestinal encephalomyopathy syndrome. *Mol Genet Metab* 2005;87:326–331.

27 Said G, Lacroix C, Plante-Bordeneuve V, et al. Clinicopathological aspects of the neuropathy of neurogastrointestinal encephalomyopathy (MNGIE) in four patients including two with a Charcot-Marie-Tooth presentation. *J Neurol* 2005;252:655–662.

28 Berdon WE, Baker DH, Blanc WA, et al. Megacystis microcolon intestinal hypoperistalsis syndrome: A new cause of intestinal obstruction in the newborn. Report of radiological findings in five newborn girls. *AJR* 1976;126:957–964.

29 Hyman PE. Chronic intestinal pseudo-obstruction in childhood: progress in diagnosis and treatment. *Scand J Gastroenterol* 1995;213:39–46.

30 Kamm MA. Primary and secondary disorders of gut muscle and nerve. *Scand J Gastroenterol* 1996;31:3191–3193.

31 Mann SD, Debinski HS, Kamm MA. Clinical characteristics of chronic idiopathic intestinal pseudo-obstruction in adults. *Gut* 1997;41:675–681.

32 Smith VV, Lake BD, Kamm MA, et al. Intestinal pseudo-obstruction with deficient smooth muscle alpha actin. *Histopathology* 1992;21:535–542.

33 Debinski HS, Kamm MA, Talbot IC, et al. DNA viruses in the pathogenesis of sporadic chronic idiopathic intestinal pseudo-obstruction (CIIP). *Gut* 1997;41:100–106.

34 Masetti M, Di Benedetto F, Cautero N, et al. Intestinal transplantation for chronic intestinal pseudo-obstruction in adult patients. *Am J Transplant* 2004;5:826–829.

35 Higman D, Peters P, Stewart M, et al. Familial hollow visceral myopathy with varying urological manifestations. *Br J Urol* 1992;70:435–480.

36 Ghavamian R, Wilcox DT, Duffy PG, et al. The urological manifestations of hollow visceral myopathy in children. *J Urol* 1997;158:286–290.

37 Lapointe SP, Rivet C, Goulet O, et al. Urological manifestations associated with chronic intestinal pseudo-obstructions in children. *J Urol* 2002;168:1768–1770.

38 Li BUK, Altschuler SM, Berseth CL, et al. Research agenda for pediatric gastroenterology, hepatology and nutrition: motility disorders and functional gastrointestinal disorders: report of the North American Society for Pediatric Gastroenterology, Hepatology and Nutrition for the Children's Digestive Health and Nutrition Foundation. *J Pediatr Gastroenterol Nutr* 2002;35:S263–S267.

39 Miele E, Tozzi A, Staiano A, et al. Persistence of abnormal gastrointestinal motility after operation for Hirschsprung's disease. *Am J Gastroenterol* 2000;95:1226–1230.

40 Tomomasa T, Di Lorenzo C, Morikawa A, et al. Analysis of fasting antroduodenal manometry in children. *Dig Dis Sci* 1996;41:2195–2203.

41 Di Lorenzo C, Flores AF, Reddy SN, et al. Colonic manometry in children with chronic intestinal pseudo-obstruction. *Gut* 1993;34:803–807.

42 Akkermans, LMA, Van Isselt, JW. Gastric motility and emptying studies with radionuclides in research and clinical settings. *Dig Dis Sci* 1994;39:95.

43 Hussain S, Di Lorenzo C. Motility disorders: diagnosis and treatment for the pediatric patient. *Pediatr Clin North Am* 2002;49:27–51.

44 Braden B, Adams S, Duan LP, et al. 13C-acetate breath test accurately reflects gastric emptying of liquids in both liquid and semi-solid test meals. *Gastroenterol* 1995;108:1048–1055.

45 Drossman D, Dumitrascu D. Rome III: New Standard for Functional Gastrointestinal Disorders. *J Gastrointestin Liver Dis* 2006;15:237–241.

46 Grunkemeier D, Cassara JE, Dalton CB, Drossman DA. The narcotic bowel syndrome: clinical features, pathophysiology, and management. *Clin Gastroenterol Hepatol* 2007; 5:1126–1139.

47 Kaufman SS, Atkinson JB, Bianchi A, et al. Indications for pediatric intestinal transplantation: a position paper of the American Society of Transplantation. *Pediatr Transplant* 2001;5:80–87.

48 Grant D. Report of the International Intestinal Transplant Registry, VIII International Small Bowel Transplant Symposium. Stockholm (2003).

49 Abu-Elmagd K, Bond G, Reyes J, et al. Intestinal transplantation: a coming of age. *Adv Surg* 2002;36:65–101.

50 Pironi L, Spinucci G, Paganelli F, et al. Italian guidelines for intestinal transplantation: potential candidates among the adult patients managed by a medical referral center for chronic intestinal failure. *Transplant Proc* 2004;3:659–661.

51 Mousa H, Bueno J, Griffiths J, et al. Intestinal motility after small bowel transplantation. *Transplant Proc* 1998;30:2535–2536.

4 Assessment and General Management of Intestinal Failure

13 Assessment of Intestinal Failure Patients

Clarivet Torres

Key points

- Short bowel syndrome is a complex condition which requires a multidisciplinary approach.
- The intrinsic characteristics of the remaining intestine after small bowel resection are crucial in determining the functional ability of the bowel.
- To determine the anatomy and the intestinal length of the remaining bowel, review surgical records and obtain radiological studies such as barium enema, upper gastrointestinal and small bowel examination (UGI and SBS). These may be followed with esophagogastroduodenoscopy and colonoscopy.
- At the end of the initial assessment, the physician should understand the cause of the intestinal failure, the reasons for feeding intolerance, the likelihood of intestinal anatomy, the patient's nutritional status, and also recognize any acute or chronic complications.

Introduction

Intestinal failure (IF) results from surgical resection, congenital defect, or disease associated loss of absorption and is characterized by the inability to maintain protein-energy, fluid, electrolyte or micronutrient balances when on a normal diet [1]. The causes of IF can be separated by pathogenesis into three different groups: anatomic reduction of the gut length, short bowel syndrome (SBS), the most common cause; neuromuscular diseases involving the GI tract; and congenital diseases of the intestinal epithelium (Table 13.1). Intestinal adaptation, the progressive recovery from IF that follows a loss of intestinal length, usually allows the restoration of adequate intestinal function within several weeks to months. Only in a small number of children is adaptation inadequate; these continue to be dependent on parenteral nutrition (PN).

The likelihood that a patient with SBS will reestablish enteral autonomy is influenced by the length, location, and function of the remaining bowel. Regardless of multiple attempts to describe this syndrome on the basis of intestinal length alone, it appears that no minimum length of small bowel can be used reproducibly to define the short bowel syndrome. The essential defect is the lack of an adequate mucosal surface to permit enteral nutrition autonomy [2,3]. The purpose of this article is to discuss strategies for the initial assessment of an intestinal failure patient and focuses on the SBS while endeavoring to define the optimal approach for each individual patient.

Assessment

SBS is a complex condition which requires a multidisciplinary approach including a gastroenterologist, surgeon, nurse practitioner/coordinator, dietitian, as well as a psychological evaluation. To determine the most appropriate therapy, a comprehensive evaluation is necessary. An experienced physician taking care of patients with IF should supervise and guide

Intestinal Failure: Diagnosis, Management and Transplantation.
Edited by Alan N. Langnas, Olivier Goulet, Eamonn M.M. Quigley and Kelly A. Tappenden. © 2008 Blackwell Publishing.
ISBN 978-1-4051-4637-1.

Table 13.1 Causes of intestinal failure.

1 Anatomic reduction of the gut length: SBS the most common cause.
- Normal GI anatomy: Necrotizing enterocolitis, gastroschisis (as a result of resection), multiple resections of Crohn's disease, volvulus, mesenteric arterial embolism, venous thrombosis, volvulus trauma, or tumor resections.
- Congenital anomalies: intestinal atresia, shortened small bowel at birth.

2 Neuromuscular diseases involving the GI tract: Total aganglionosis (long segment Hirschsprung's disease) or chronic intestinal pseudoobstruction.

3 Diseases of the intestinal epithelium: Microvillus atrophy, intestinal epithelial dysplasia, tufting enteropathy, autoimmune enteropathy, radiation enteritis.

the management of these complex patients. Treatment options for SBS in children include long-term PN, intestinal rehabilitation, and/or intestinal transplantation. The components of an initial evaluation are identified in Table 13.2.

History and physical evaluation

Evaluating a neonate who has recently suffered from an anatomic reduction of the gut with subsequent SBS

Table 13.2 Components of an initial evaluation.

1 History and physical evaluation
2 Determine the anatomy and bowel length
- Upper GI and small bowel series.
- Barium enema.
- Endoscopic studies: to rule out intestinal stricture/obstruction, to obtain tissue for histology studies, and duodenal fluid for bacterial overgrowth.
3 Ultrasound of the abdomen with Doppler evaluation of hepatic vessels and upper extremities (to determined vascular access).
4 Liver biopsy, if liver disease is associated.
5 Chest X-ray.
6 Bone age.
7 Nutritional assessment.
8 Psychological evaluation.
9 Laboratory exams: See Table 13.3.

is not as difficult as evaluating a patient with a long history of multiple enterotomies and complications.

Important components of the initial history include:
1 A thorough review and summary of past medical record.
2 The cause of SBS, the anatomy and length of the intestine, including a detailed review of prior surgical procedures and any related complications.
3 The number of central lines and the reasons they were changed.
4 The causal microorganism of any prior central line infections (bacteria/fungus) and the clinical consequences associated with each infection (sepsis, thrombosis), including whether intensive care or mechanical ventilation were required.
5 Nutritional assessment.
6 A detailed vaccination status.
7 A complete physical exam (PE) emphasizing hydration and nutritional status (weight, height, basal metabolic index), type of central line, signs of vascular thrombosis, cardiovascular status, dermatologic examination including diaper rash and signs of chronic liver disease.

Bowel anatomy

The intrinsic characteristics of the remaining intestine after small bowel resection are crucial in determining the functional ability of the bowel. Most nutrient absorption occurs within the initial two-thirds of the small bowel. There are three major types of bowel anatomy in SBS: jejunocolic anastomosis, end-jejunostomy, and jejunoileal anastomosis. The third is the least common, but is associated with the best overall prognosis [4]. In general, a jejunal resection is better tolerated, as the ileum can replace the absorptive capacity of the jejunum through adaptation. However, the jejunum cannot adapt the ileal functions. Vitamin B12 and bile acids are exclusively absorbed in the distal ileum [2,4]. In SBS patients, the colon becomes an important digestive organ by absorbing sodium, water, some amino acids, and short chain fatty acids used as energy substrates [2].

The remaining bowel length necessary to prevent PN dependence in adults is approximately 100 cms in the absence of intact and functional colon or 60 cm in the presence of complete functional colon; however, the degree of adaptation and PN dependence is highly individualized. Adult patients at the greatest nutritional risk are those with a duodenostomy or with a jejunoileal anastomosis with <35 cm of residual small bowel, a jejunocolic or ileocolic anastomosis with <60 cm of residual small intestine, or an end jejunostomy with <115 cm of residual small bowel [5]. Children with <30 cm of jejunum-ileum, lack of enterocolonic continuity, and lack of feeding tolerance early after birth are associated with failure of weaning from PN [6]. Forty percent of children with <40 cm of residual small bowel and without an ICV remain dependent on parenteral nutrition after 8 years [3].

It is sometimes difficult to determine the anatomy and the intestinal length of the remaining bowel. A good approach is to start by reviewing surgical records and obtaining radiological studies (Table 13.2). If the previous steps are combined with an esophagogastroduodenoscopy (EGD) and a colonoscopy, it is possible to define the anatomy, histology and any anomalies of the remnant intestine. In a recent review of the outcomes of IF, it was observed that 58% of the patients with intestinal stricture/obstruction were misdiagnosed by an UGI and SBS and correctly diagnosed by endoscopic procedures [7].

Nutritional assessment

Nutritional assessment begins with a detailed history of a patient's weight, and parenteral and enteral nutrition intake, either by tube or oral feeding (fluids/kg, calories/kg, macro and micronutrients components). Questions related to bowel functions include diarrhea, nausea, vomiting, bloating, and other factors affecting appetite. Referral to a dietitian for estimation of the type and amount of daily food is appropriated. The physical exam should begin with accurate height and weight measurements, calculating the body mass index. Poor dentition, loss of subcutaneous fat and loss of temporal muscle mass are other signs of weight loss and inadequate nutrition. Measurement of triceps skinfold thickness and midarm circumference may also be followed. Laboratory tests including serum electrolytes, albumin level, prothrombine time, Vitamin B12, and fat soluble vitamins are important.

Evaluation of the small bowel absorptive capacity with functional assays such as D Xylose and 3-O-methylglucose absorption test 6 and 7 and net digestive ratio of nutrients have been developed, but these methods are time consuming and complicated to analyze, more suited for research than for medical screening. Monitoring of weight gain and growth is the most beneficial tool to evaluate nutritional status and nutrition absorption. Efforts to identify malabsorbed nutrients in the stool are not helpful.

Biological assessment of intestinal failure

Serum citrulline, a nonessential amino acid synthesized exclusively in small intestinal enterocytes, was recently found to be a reliable biochemical marker of small bowel enterocyte mass. Plasma citrulline correlated with remnant small bowel length and net digestive absorption of fat and protein in patients with SBS, villous-atrophy associated small bowel disease or during intestinal graft rejection with subsequently villous atrophy [8,9]. Citrulline is a marker of small bowel absorptive capacity independent of intestinal inflammation [10]. Whether citrulline levels are predictive of intestinal recovery or not has to be confirmed.

Assessment of complications

It is important to assess the acute and chronic complications to determine prognosis and future management. The most common problems in the acute or chronic stages of IF are diarrhea, fluid and electrolyte abnormalities and nutrient loss. Many of the chronic complications come from the use of PN, including central venous catheter (CVC) infections, central venous thrombosis (CVT), pulmonary embolism (PE), intestinal failure associated-liver disease (IFALD), metabolic complications, anemia, bone demineralization and rickets. Complications not related to PN include bacterial overgrowth, nutritional deficiencies and renal stones [11].

CVC infections and IFALD are a major cause of morbidity and mortality of patients with IF. CVC may be suspected if a patient develops clinical signs of fever, metabolic acidosis, thrombocytopenia, fluctuations in serum bilirubin, glucose instability, or a new onset of recurrent vomiting. Blood cultures taken from both peripheral and central sites are imperative in the presence

Table 13.3 Laboratory exams.

Day 1:
1 CBC with differential and platelet count. Comprehensive metabolic panel, GGT, phosphorous, magnesium, PT/PTT, cholesterol, triglycerides, urinalysis.

Day 2: For patients with concomitant liver disease.
2 HIV1/HIV2 antibody screen
3 Hepatitis Panel: HB/SAG and AB, HCAB, HepA
4 Alpha fetoprotein.
5 Alpha 1 antitrypsin.

Day 3:
Carnitine free and total, zinc, selenium, copper, Vitamin D250H, Vitamin A and E, Vitamin B12.
If liver disease coexists:
For children under 1:
  1 CMV DNA
  2 EBV DNA
  3 CMV IgG, IgM
For children over 1:
  1 EBV DNA
  2 EBV antibodies
  3 CMV IgG, IgM

Table 13.4 Indications for intestinal transplantation [14].

1 Imminent or evident liver failure as a result of TPN-induced liver injury. A total bilirubin of more than 7 mg/dL, stage 2 fibrosis, or portal hypertension have been recognize as clear indications for liver/intestinal transplantation.
2 Thrombosis of two or more central veins.
3 The development of two or more episodes of systemic sepsis secondary to line infection per year that require hospitalization.
4 A single episode of line-related fungemia, septic shock, or acute respiratory distress.
5 Frequent episodes of severe dehydration despite intravenous fluid supplementation in addition to PN.

the patient's nutritional status and also recognize any acute or chronic complications. In this way, one can choose the best management approach intestinal rehabilitation or liver small bowel transplantation (Table 13.4).

of any of these symptoms. Although CVT is a common sequel of central venous catheterization, the majority of patients remain asymptomatic. Clinical symptoms of CVT are swelling in the neck, face, or limbs, prominent superficial veins or pain on starting PN. CVT is confirmed by Echocardiography Doppler Ultrasound, CT scan, and/or venography. Spiral computed tomography is a safe stand-alone test for the diagnosis of PE [12].

Early hepatic dysfunction is asymptomatic, but jaundice is an obvious sign of cholestasis. Clinical signs of advanced IFALD are jaundice, hepatosplenomegaly, collateral vessels, ascites, and signs of coagulopathy. Despite fairly extensive hepatic fibrosis and splenomegaly, esophageal varices are uncommon in SBS patients. The development of hepatic dysfunction should be strongly investigated for other causes of liver disease before assuming the diagnosis of IFALD with specific tests described in Table 13.3, as well as liver ultrasound and liver biopsy [11,13].

At the end of the initial assessment, the physician should understand the cause of IF, the reasons for feeding intolerance, the likelihood of intestinal anatomy,

References

1 O'Keefe SJ, Buchman AL. Short bowel syndrome and intestinal failure: consensus definitions and overview. *Clin Gastroenterol Hepatol* 2006;4:6–10.
2 Torres C, Vanderhoof JA. Short bowel syndrome. In Rolandelli RH et al. (eds). *Clinical Nutrition, Enteral and Tube Feedings*, 4th edn. Philadelphia, PA: Elsevier Saunders 2005; pp. 451–453.
3 Goulet O, Ruemmele F. Causes and management of intestinal failure. *Gastroenterology* 2006;130:516–528.
4 DiBase JK, Young RJ. Intestinal rehabilitation and the short bowel syndrome: part 1. *Am J Gastroenterol* 2004;99:1386–1395.
5 AGA technical review on short bowel syndrome and intestinal transplantation. *Gastroenterology* 2003;124:1111–1134.
6 Pharaon I, Despres C, Aigrain Y, et al. Long-term parenteral nutrition in children who are potentially candidates for small bowel transplantation. *Transplant Proc* 1994;26:1442.
7 Torres C, Sudan D. The role of an intestinal rehabilitation program in the treatment of advanced intestinal failure. *J Pediatr Gastroenterol Nutr* 2007;45:204–212.
8 Crenn P, Vahedi K, Lavergne-Slove A, et al. Plasma citrulline: A marker of enterocyte mass in villous

atrophy-associated small bowel disease. *Gastroenterology* 2003;124:1210–1219.

9 Pappas PA, Saudubray JM, Tzakis AG, et al. Serum citrulline and rejection in small bowel transplantation: a preliminary report. *Transplantation* 2001;72:1212–1216.

10 Papadia C, Sherwood RA, Kalantzis C, et al. Plasma citrulline concentration: a reliable marker of small bowel absorptive capacity independent of intestinal inflammation. *Am J Gastroenterol* 2007;102:1474–1482.

11 Torres C, Vanderhoof JA. Chronic complications of short bowel syndrome. *Current Paediatrics* 2006;16:291–297.

12 Koletzko B, Goulet O. Guidelines on paediatric parenteral nutrition. *J Pediatr Gastroenterol Nutr* 2006;41:S76–S83.

13 Kelly DA. Intestinal failure-associated liver disease: what do we know today? *Gastroenterology* 2006;130(2 Suppl 1):S67–69.

14 Health Care Financing Administration (HCFA), Program Memorandum Intermediaries/Carriers. Intestinal Transplantation 2000. December. Issuance AB–00-130.

14 Guidelines for Home Parenteral Nutrition Support in Chronic Intestinal Failure Patients

Bernard Messing, Francisca Joly and Virginie Colomb

Key points

- Parenteral nutrition (PN) is the gold standard treatment for chronic intestinal failure (CIF).

- In SBS patients, the minimal lengths of remnant "normal" postduodenal small bowel required to achieve independence from PN are greater than 100 cm, 60 cm, and 35 cm, respectively, for end-jejunostomy (type I, no colon in continuity), jejuno-colonic anastomosis (type II, part of the colon in continuity) or jejuno-ileal (type III, the full colon in continuity) anastomosis.

- In SBS, a postabsorptive plasma level of citrulline lower than 20 µmol/1 (half the normal value in adult controls) is significantly associated with permanent CIF, when measured past the adaptive 2-year period following the reestablishment of bowel continuity.

- The goal to be reached, for each patient, is the minimum required level of PN dependence. Exclusive or total PN should be avoided. A high degree of PN dependence is a risk factor for the occurrence of metabolic complications, including liver.

- A specialized NST, covering and integrating expertise in all medical and surgical aspects of CIF treatment, is a prerequisite for running HPN programs.

- The management of HPN should be an integrated part of the management of the underlying CIF disease.

Intestinal Failure: Diagnosis, Management and Transplantation.
Edited by Alan N. Langnas, Olivier Goulet, Eamonn M.M. Quigley and Kelly A. Tappenden. © 2008 Blackwell Publishing. ISBN 978-1-4051-4637-1.

Introduction

Parenteral nutrition (PN) is the gold standard treatment for chronic intestinal failure (CIF), when nutritional requirements are not accomplished by oral or enteral feeding [1].

CIF results either from removal, or severe disease of the small intestine leading to very short bowel syndrome (SBS), or when the gut is intact but impossible to use by enteral support even when accessed through gastrostomy or jejunostomy (e.g. chronic intestinal pseudo-obstruction or diseases involving extensive villous atrophy) [2,3].

Home PN (HPN) is the only alternative to prolonged hospitalization and is recognized as the best option for improving the quality of life of these patients and their families [4].

Learning objectives

Guidelines for the use of (H)PN in adults and children have been published recently [1,5–7]. Guidelines for HPN in adults are summarized in Table 14.1.

1 This chapter focuses on nutritional support of HPN patients in a tertiary care centre in the setting of CIF, especially patients with SBS, and excluding cancer patients [8]. We wish to consider, first, CIF, PN dependency, and HPN management, and, second, practical aspects of HPN by addressing the two following questions:

- What are their nutritional needs?
- How will the individual needs of a given patient best be covered?

Table 14.1 Practice Guidelines (A.S.P.E.N.): monitoring efficacy for SNS including HPN.

Nutrition and outcome goals should be stated in the nutrition assessment prior to the initiation of Specialized Nutrition Support (SNS)	C
Nutritional and outcome parameters should be measured serially during SNS therapy	B
Periodic comparison of nutritional and outcome measures with SNS goals should occur to monitor efficacy of therapy	C

The authors used the AHRQ criteria to classify the strength of the evidence supporting each guideline statement. The evidence supporting each statement is classified as follows 1:

A: There is good research-based evidence to support the guideline (prospective, randomized trials)

B: There is fair research-based evidence to support the guideline (well-designed studies without randomization)

C: The guideline is based on expert opinion and editorial consensus

Chronic intestinal failure in SBS patients and probability of PN dependency

CIF is a reduction in functioning gut mass below the minimal amount necessary for adequate digestion and absorption of nutrients. SBS accounts for nearly 80% of CIF leading to long-term HPN in adults [8–10] and for about 50% in children [11–15].

Three (two clinical and one biochemical) parameters have been shown to delineate transient from permanent, or indefinite, CIF in SBS, in adults [16–20].

1 The length of small bowel remnant required to achieve weaning from PN varies according to the anatomical type of SBS [16–18], whether end-jejunostomy (type I, no colon in continuity), jejuno-colonic anastomosis (type II, part of the colon in continuity) or jejuno-ileal (type III, the full colon in continuity) anastomosis (Figure 14.1). The minimal lengths of remnant "normal" small bowel required to achieve independence from PN are 100 cm, 60 cm, and 35 cm, respectively, for these three variants [16–18].

2 The probability of weaning off PN drops below 10%, if weaning has not been achieved over the first 2 years of HPN [17–18].

3 A postabsorptive plasma level of citrulline lower than 20 μmol/1 (half the normal value in adult controls) is significantly associated with permanent intestinal failure, when measured past the adaptive 2-year period following the reestablishment of bowel continuity after extensive small bowel resection [19]. This biochemical marker, if renal function is normal, is highly correlated to remnant small bowel length and absorptive capacity. In adults, it is more predictive of permanent CIF (negative and positive predictive values at 86% and 95% respectively) than the length of remnant small bowel within the three anatomical SBS types.

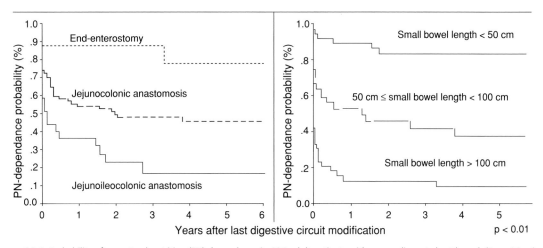

Figure 14.1 Probability of parenteral nutrition (PN) dependency in 124 adult patients with non-malignant short bowel. (From Messing [18], with permission from Elsevier.)

Similarly, in children, recent pediatric studies have demonstrated that the duration of HPN and the probability of weaning off PN depend on the length of remnant bowel (especially expressed as percentage of the expected small bowel length for age in neonates [20]), the presence of the colon and of the ileocaecal valve [20–22]. Plasma citrulline seems also to be a reliable marker of intestinal function [23].

The combination of the length of remnant bowel plus the plasma citrulline level helps to identify appropriate HPN candidates for either complementary (pharmacological trophic gut factors or reconstructive surgery) or alternative treatments of permanent intestinal failure [8].

PN dependence and HPN management

In adult patients, the primary disease causing SBS and the remnant anatomy are also important to consider in order to assess survival probability [18] (Figure 14.2). The goal to be reached, for each patient, is the minimum required level of PN dependence. Exclusive or total PN should be avoided, and enteral feeding should be implemented, as much as possible, because it has been demonstrated that a high degree of PN dependence is a risk factor for the occurrence of metabolic complications, that is, liver failure in both adults and children (see Chapter 21) [24–28].

The length and function of the intestinal remnant are the main parameters which determine PN dependence. It has been shown that a functioning and accessed short gut has a better prognosis than a longer but nonfunctioning gut [9]. The prognosis of HPN adult patients is significantly better in patients without bowel obstruction than in patients with chronic obstruction (Figure 14.3A) (e.g. Crohn's or radiation enteritis patients). This provides the rationale for:

1 Reestablishing colonic continuity in SBS patients whatever the age or the percentage of remaining colon [29–32], providing anal sphincter functioning is sufficient.

2 Performing bowel resection, extensive if necessary, in patients with multifocal obstructive disease [9].

As well as knowing the probability of HPN weaning (see previous paragraph), it is also important to assess the food intake of each patient with CIF, and the absorptive capacity of the remnant gut (under optimal therapy, including dietary counselling) [32–35], to set up a minimum level of PN dependence which may be defined as the minimal complementary water, minerals (Na, K, Mg) and macronutrients which need to be provided through the IV route.

Insufficient oral intake—not directly dependent upon the intestinal condition—might compromise intestinal autonomy and may also induce a higher than needed PN supply. In that circumstance, apart from psychological evaluation, a period of nasogastric tube feeding may be used in order to properly evaluate the absorptive capacity of the remnant gut. Indeed, the macronutrient absorption of a very short remnant bowel is never negligible and the net absorptive balance increases in parallel with the increase in food intake as large as threefold the patient's Resting Energy Expenditure (REE) [19,32]. Hyperphagia should be encouraged and futile food restrictions discouraged since it promotes the physiological adaptive intestinal process [32] and gives some patients with a "borderline" length of remnant gut a full oral nutritional autonomy [33–35].

Therefore, HPN management in a patient with CIF might be described as a two-stage process:

1 The first goal is to restore a low-normal BMI in underweight patients, is the implementation of a 6-cycles per week-PN regimen, with a PN-free night (water and electrolytes only if necessary), each cycle supplying no more than 1.3-fold the REE in adults [24] together with a free intake of oral solids as long as intestinal obstruction is not present [32].

2 The second goal is to maintain a near normal nutritional status, is a progressive decrease of PN supply [36], in order to reach, step by step, a minimum number of PN cycles per week, water-electrolytes needs being dissociated from energy-protein needs, especially in SBS patients type I, where the fluid balance is more difficult to achieve than the energy balance. Indeed, it has been shown that 20% of these adult patients may require only a water-electrolyte supply [17,34].

General HPN guidelines

Nutrition support teams (NST) [37,38] are required to manage HPN safely. They include physicians and surgeons trained in both nutrition and gastroenterology, as well as a specialized nurse, dietician and pharmacist,

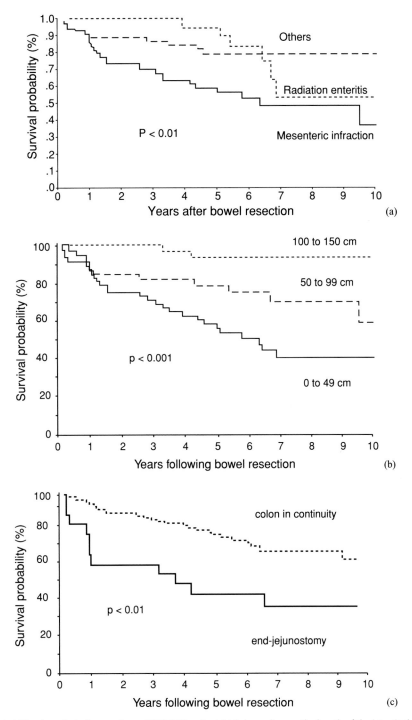

Figure 14.2 Probability of survival of nonmalignant SBS (124 patients) (a) depending on the length of the intestinal remnant, (b) depending on whether or not the colon remained in situ, and (c) according to main types of primary disease. (From Messing [18], with permission from Elsevier.)

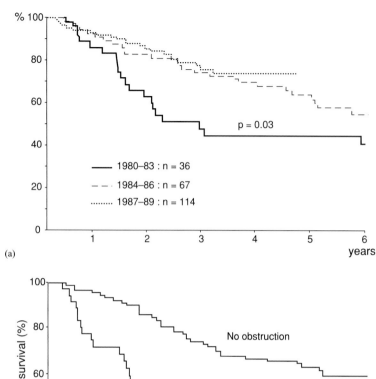

(a)

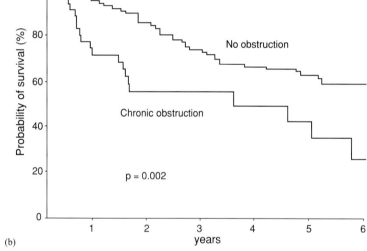

(b)

Figure 14.3 Overall prognosis on HPN for patients with non malignant disease 1980–89 (n = 217 patients). (a) HPN prognosis 1980–89 depending on whether or not chronic obstruction was present. (b) HPN prognosis: 1980–89. Probability of survival according to date of inclusion. (From Messing [9], with permission from Elsevier.)

plus a social worker, care giver for materials needed to establish Home PN and general practitioner, with the patient and their family being at the centre of the medical sphere. The NST has to:

1 identify candidates for HPN,

2 develop a nutritional plan of care agreeable to the patient and care-givers,

3 make an appropriate prescription for home setting, and

4 properly train the patient/care-giver.

According to ASPEN, the standard but "minimally required" care for HPN patients is a standardized

method for "ordering and monitoring HPN support": this is necessary because physicians with various degrees of training may order HPN.

The use of "disease specific pathways" is also highly recommended to organize the patient's clinical and biological follow-up and formal communication between the NST and the general practitioner [38].

A French survey in adult HPN centers has shown a significant increase in the probability of survival according to the date of inclusion in the HPN program, mortality being higher during a 3-year run-in period than in the two following 3-year periods [9]

(Figure 14.3B). Therefore, a specialized NST, covering and integrating expertise in all medical and surgical aspects of CIF treatment, is a prerequisite for running HPN programs.

Nutritive mixtures

Nutritive mixtures, apyrogenic and sterile, are compounded under the supervision of hospital pharmacists in single bags called "all-in-one" bags—sometimes bi-partite (the second compartment containing lipid emulsion is opened and mixed with other components immediately before its use). Bags are made of phtalate-free multilayered ethyl vinyl acetate plastic (EVA). The use of all-in-one bags facilitates the practice of cyclic (nocturnal) PN which is the main mode of HPN therapy in children and adults [39–41,11–14].

Total (H)PN means that PN must be "complete" for each cycle of infusion and should include adequate amounts of amino-acids and glucose, a maximum of 30% of total non-protein energy being furnished as lipids, which provide variable amount of polyunsaturated essential fatty acids. "Complete" PN should include the 35 essential nutrients (amino-acids, electrolytes, vitamins, trace elements...) and should be tailored according to the individual status of the patient. All nutrients, of which excess and deficit should be avoided, play a major role in nutritional efficiency and, along with energy, in nitrogen retention.

A separate sheet for PN prescription should be used to avoid any omission.

The use of nutritive mixtures compounded by pharmaceutical companies in HPN patients increases the risk of deficiencies (vitamins are usually absent from these mixtures) and imbalances (e.g. electrolytes, minerals, excess fat/glucose ratio). These necessary supplements when added to the bag at home either by a nurse, care givers or the patients themselves, bring, despite aseptic techniques, an additional risk of infection. The stability of the mixture might also be compromised by inappropriate supplementation. Thus, the best possible-HPN care is still not provided to all the patients after more than a 30-year experience [42–44].

Therefore, for each HPN patient, a cyclic nocturnal infusion of an "all-in-one" complete nutritive mixture should be tailored according to the specific type of CIF, in terms of volume, infusion duration (10 to 16 h) and, if the patient is not totally dependent on PN, in the number of cycles per week.

Conclusion

The management of HPN should be an integrated part of the management of the underlying CIF disease.

Along with medical therapy, dietary management of CIF, especially as a result of very short bowel, is essential to reduce PN dependence to its lowest possible level, therefore, decreasing the risk of the complications associated with long-term HPN.

Indeed, HPN for intestinal failure should not be viewed as "hyperalimentation" but, rather, as a complete nutritional support for each PN cycle with a minimum number of nocturnal cycles per week. This is better observed in patients in which hyperphagia develops. Then, HPN is, in most cases, a complementary mode of nutritional support.

References

1 Guidelines for the use of parenteral and enteral nutrition in adult and pediatric patients. *JPEN J Parenter Enteral Nutr* 2002;26:1SA–138SA.

2 Nightingale JM. Introduction: definition and classification of intestinal failure. In: Nightingale JMD, ed. *Intestinal Failure*. London, San Francisco: GMM, 2001: XIX–XX.

3 Goulet O, Ruemmele F, Lacaille F, Colomb V. Irreversible intestinal failure. *J Pediatr Gastroenterol Nutr* 2004;38:250–269.

4 Gottrand F, Staszewski P, Colomb V, et al. Satisfaction in different life domains in children receiving home parenteral nutrition and their families. *J Pediatr* 2005;146:793–797.

5 Klein S, Kinney J, Jeejeebhoy K, et al. Nutrition support in clinical practice: review of published data and recommendations for future research directions. National Institutes of Health, American Society for Parenteral and Enteral Nutrition, and American Society for Clinical Nutrition. *JPEN J Parenter Enteral Nutr* 1997;21:133–156.

6 Evans-Stoner N. Guidelines for the care of the patient on home nutrition support. An appendix. *Nurs Clin North Am* 1997;32:769–775.

7 Home parenteral nutrition in children. Guidelines on paediatric parenteral nutrition of the European Society

of Paediatric Gastroenterology, Hepatology and Nutrition (ESPGHAN) and the European Society for Clinical Nutrition and Metabolism (ESPEN). *J Pediatr Gastroenterol Nutr* 2005;41:S70–S75.

8 Buchman AL, Scolapio J, Fryer J. AGA technical review on short bowel syndrome and intestinal transplantation. *Gastroenterology* 2003;124:1111–1134.

9 Messing B, Lemann M, Landais P, et al. Prognosis of patients with nonmalignant chronic intestinal failure receiving long-term home parenteral nutrition. *Gastroenterology* 1995;108:1005–1010.

10 Bakker H, Bozzetti F, Staun M, et al. Home parenteral nutrition in adults: a european multicentre survey in 1997. ESPEN-Home Artificial Nutrition Working Group. *Clin Nutr* 1999;18:135–140.

11 Vargas JH, Ament ME, Berquist WE. Long-term home parenteral nutrition in pediatrics: ten years of experience in 102 patients. *J Pediatr Gastroenterol Nutr* 1987;6:24–32.

12 Ricour C, Gorski AM, Goulet O, et al. Home parenteral nutrition in children: 8 years of experience with 112 patients. *Clin Nutr* 1990;9:65–71.

13 Bisset WM, Stapleford P, Long S, et al. Home parenteral nutrition in chronic intestinal failure. *Arch Dis Child* 1992;67:109–114.

14 Puntis JWL. Home parenteral nutrition. *Arch Dis Child* 1995;72:186–190.

15 Guarino A, De Marco G, for the Italian National Network for Pediatric Intestinal Failure. Natural history of intestinal failure, investigated through a national network-based approach. *J Pediatr Gastroenterol Nutr* 2003;37:136–141.

16 Carbonnel F, Cosnes J, Chevret S, et al. The role of anatomic factors in nutritional autonomy after extensive small bowel resection. *JPEN J Parenter Enteral Nutr* 1996;20:275–280.

17 Ingham Clark CL, Lear PA, Wood S, et al. Potential candidates for small bowel transplantation. *Br J Surg* 1992;79:676–679.

18 Messing B, Crenn P, Beau P, et al. Long-term survival and parenteral nutrition dependence in adult patients with the short bowel syndrome. *Gastroenterology* 1999;117:1043–1050.

19 Crenn P, Coudray-Lucas C, Thuillier F, et al. Postabsorptive plasma citrulline concentration is a marker of absorptive enterocyte mass and intestinal failure in humans. *Gastroenterology* 2000;119:1496–1505.

20 Spencer AU, Neaga A, West B, et al. Pediatric short bowel syndrome. Redefining predictors of success. *Ann Surg* 2005;242:403–412.

21 Goulet O, Baglin-Gobet S, Talbotec C, et al. Outcome and long-term growth after extensive small bowel resection in the neonatal period: a survey of 87 children. *Eur J Pediatr Surg* 2004;14:000A–000G.

22 Colomb V, Dabbas-Tyan M, Taupin P, et al. Long-term outcome of children on home parenteral nutrition. The 20 year-experience of a single center in 302 patients. *J Pediatr Gastroenterol Nutr* 2006: in press.

23 Rhoads JM, Plunkett E, Wu G, et al. Serum citrulline correlates with enteral tolerance and bowel length in infants with short bowel syndrome. *J Pediatr* 2005;146:542–547.

24 Cavicchi M, Beau P, Crenn P, et al. Prevalence of liver disease and contributing factors in patients receiving home parenteral nutrition for permanent intestinal failure. *Ann Intern Med* 2000;132: 525–532.

25 Stanko RT, Nathan G, Mendelow H, Adibi SA. Development of hepatic cholestasis and fibrosis in patients with massive loss of intestine supported by prolonged parenteral nutrition. *Gastroenterology* 1987;92:197–202.

26 Meehan JJ, Georgeson KE. Prevention of liver failure in parenteral nutrition-dependent children with short bowel syndrome. *J Pediatr Surg* 1997;32:473–475.

27 Kaufman SS. Prevention of parenteral nutrition-associated liver disease in children. *Pediatr Transplantation* 2002;6:37–42.

28 Colomb V, Jobert-Giraud A, Lacaille F, et al. Role of lipid emulsions in cholestasis associated to long term parenteral nutrition in children. *JPEN J Parenter Enteral Nutr* 2000;24:345–350.

29 Cummings JH, James WP, Wiggins HS. Role of the colon in ileal-resection diarrhoea. *Lancet* 1973;1:344–347.

30 Harig JM, Soergel KH, Komorowski RA, Wood CM. Treatment of diversion colitis with short-chain-fatty acid irrigation. *N Engl J Med* 1989;320:23–28.

31 Kelly DA. Liver complications of pediatric parenteral nutrition-Epidemiology. *Nutrition* 1998;14:153–157.

32 Crenn P, Morin MC, Joly F, Penven S, Thuillier F, Messing B. Net digestive absorption and adaptive hyperphagia in adult short bowel patients. *Gut* 2004;53:1279–1286.

33 Messing B, Pigot F, Rongier M, Morin MC, Ndeindoum U, Rambaud JC. Intestinal absorption of free oral hyperalimentation in the very short bowel syndrome. *Gastroenterology* 1991;100:1502–1508.

34 Jeppesen PB, Mortensen PB. Intestinal failure defined by measurements of intestinal energy and wet weight absorption. *Gut* 2000;46:701–706.

35 Jeejeebhoy KN. Short bowel syndrome: a nutritional and medical approach. *CMAJ* 2002;166:1297–1302.

36 Dibaise JK, Matarese LE, Messing B, Steiger E. Strategies for parenteral nutrition weaning in adult patients with short bowel syndrome. *J Clin Gastroenterol* 2006;40 (5 suppl 2):S94–S98.

37 Agostoni C, Axelson I, Colomb V, et al; ESPGHAN Committee on Nutrition; European Society for Paediatric Gastroenterology Hepatology and Nutrition. The need for nutrition support teams in pediatric units: a commentary by the ESPGHAN committee on nutrition. *J Pediatr Gastroenterol Nutr* 2005;41:8–11. Erratum in: *J Pediatr Gastroenterol Nutr* 2005;41: 267–271.

38 Ireton-Jones C, Orr M, Hennessy K. Clinical pathways in home nutrition support. *J Am Diet Assoc* 1997;97: 1003–1007.

39 Messing B, Hebuterne X, Nightingale JM. Home enteral and parenteral nutrition in adults. In Nightingale JMD,

ed. Intestinal Failure. London, San Francisco: GMM, 2001:407–430.

40 Van Gossum A, Peeters I, Lievin V. Home parenteral nutrition in adults: the current use of an experienced method. *Acta Gastroenterol Belg* 1999;62:201–209.

41 Pichard C, Muhlebach S, Maisonneuve N, Sierro C. Prospective survey of parenteral nutrition in Switzerland: a three-year nation-wide survey. *Clin Nutr* 2001;20:345–350.

42 Allwood NC, Lee MJ. Formulation of parenteral feeds. In Nightingale JMD, ed. Intestinal Failure. London, San Francisco: GMM, 2001:351–362.

43 Catania PN, Ogbru O. Sterility of intravenous therapy in home care settings. *Home Care Provid* 1999;4:19–20.

44 Howard L, Hassan N. Home parenteral nutrition. 25 years later. *Gastroenterol Clin North Am* 1998;27:481–512.

15 Home Parenteral Nutrition: Complications, Survival, Costs and Quality of Life

John K. DiBaise

Key points

- Home parenteral nutrition (PN) has evolved to become a successful treatment in the management of intestinal failure yet continues to be associated with significant morbidity. In many instances, the separation of the effects of PN from the patient's underlying disease or state of intestinal failure is difficult.

- A number of factors, some that can be modified, have been demonstrated to influence outcome in home PN patients, the most important being the patient's underlying disease/primary diagnosis.

- Most patients with intestinal failure are able to be weaned from PN within 2 years. For those with permanent intestinal failure, particularly those with complications of PN, other treatment options should be considered to facilitate PN weaning such as the use of trophic factors, autologous gastrointestinal reconstruction, or intestinal transplantation.

- Home PN is associated with a number of factors that, when combined with effects from their underlying disease process, may result in a restriction of activities and deleteriously impact daily life. With time and experience, most home PN patients can modify their lifestyles to minimize the impact of this therapy.

- The expense of home PN tends to be offset by its lifesaving nature and the likelihood of recovery of intestinal function.

- The management of PN by a nutrition support team reduces PN-related morbidity and may reduce costs associated with PN use. Because chronic intestinal failure is an uncommon condition and clinical expertise in its management is not widely available, the referral of these patients to experienced centers for periodic assessment should be encouraged.

Introduction

The development and introduction of parenteral nutrition (PN) almost 40 years ago has led to substantial contributions to the lives of patients with intestinal failure, particularly in terms of survival. With increased experience and knowledge, PN has become an effective and relatively safe therapy. Nevertheless, the provision of PN remains intrusive, expensive and continues to be associated with significant morbidity. This chapter will describe PN-related complications and review what is currently known regarding the impact of this therapy on survival and quality of life. Finally, the costs related to PN use at home will also be reviewed. Whereas some of the information presented may be applicable to the pediatric patient, the focus of this review is on the adult population.

Parenteral nutrition-related complications

PN-related complications can be categorized into three groups: catheter-related, metabolic and organ dysfunction [1]. Catheter-related complications occur most

---

Intestinal Failure: Diagnosis, Management and Transplantation.
Edited by Alan N. Langnas, Olivier Goulet, Eamonn M.M. Quigley and Kelly A. Tappenden. © 2008 Blackwell Publishing. ISBN 978-1-4051-4637-1.

commonly and include infection, occlusion, mechanical problems, and central vein thrombosis. Improvements in catheter design and aseptic placement techniques have resulted in a reduction of septic complications [2]. The clinical recognition, management and prevention of catheter-related complications are described further in Chapter 16. The focus of this chapter will be on metabolic complications and effects of PN on organ function. Importantly, in many instances, the separation of the effects of PN from the patient's underlying cause of intestinal failure is difficult if not impossible.

The administration of excessive or insufficient fluid, macronutrients or micronutrients can result in significant morbidity. Over the years, refinements in parenteral solutions (see Chapter 14), which have taken into account an improved understanding of energy, fluid, and micronutrient requirements, and careful prescribing and monitoring have reduced but not eliminated metabolic complications and organ dysfunction.

Metabolic complications

Fluid and electrolytes

Although fluid and electrolyte disturbances are common during the first few weeks following massive bowel resection, these problems occur less commonly in those on long-term home PN. Exceptions may include patients with a high output end-jejunostomy or enterocutaneous fistula both of whom will require additional water and electrolytes and more rigorous monitoring. Additionally, the short bowel patient with compensatory hyperphagia may also develop large enteric losses resulting in fluid and electrolyte disturbances [3]. Chronic dehydration may result in renal problems and fatigue. In contrast, sodium and water retention may occur in malnourished patients, particularly when the energy component of the parenteral formula consists mainly of carbohydrate, and could contribute to postoperative respiratory problems when administered preoperatively [4].

In the acute setting, initiation of parenteral nutrition in the severely malnourished patient may result in rapid, intracellular shifts of magnesium, potassium and phosphate leading to severe and potentially dangerous hypophosphatemia and hypokalemia, a condition referred to as the "refeeding syndrome" [5]. An increased need for thiamine and folate can also be present in this situation. These problems should be anticipated and prevented by adequate monitoring, parenteral formula prescribing, and electrolyte/thiamine replacement prior to commencing PN. Although these problems are uncommon in the long-term home PN patient, fluid and electrolyte problems can still occur, particularly in patients with large enteric losses, such as can occur in the short bowel patient, which may result in difficult to replete hypokalemia, hypomagnesemia, and hypocalcemia. In the setting of the short bowel syndrome, home PN patients should be instructed on the measurement of daily input and output as periodic assessment of these parameters can help to guide fluid needs; with adequate hydration being based on a goal urine output of >1 L/day. This becomes particularly useful in the patient who is being weaned from PN [6]. Occasionally, parenteral fluids without macronutrients may be useful in those patients who require the fluid but not the calories.

Macronutrients and micronutrients

Hyperglycemia may occur in long-term PN patients, particularly in diabetic and septic patients. The administration of excess glucose in the PN leads to lipogenesis and is associated with increased respiratory demands, hepatic steatosis, and other untoward effects of hyperinsulinemia. Glucose administration should be limited to 4 mg/kg/min in the critically ill patient in order to avoid hyperglycemia [7]. The goal nonprotein energy needs in most stable adults is between 25 and 35 kcal/kg/day (infants and children may have higher needs). In general, 40 kcal/kg should not be exceeded in the adult PN patient and, for reasons discussed previously, nonprotein energy should be administered below the estimated needs when initiating PN in the severely malnourished patient [8]. Hypoglycemia is unusual in the home PN patient unless the PN infusion is stopped abruptly; a problem that can be avoided by tapering the infusion before the end of the cycle. Blood sugars should be monitored at least daily with a goal level <200 mg/dl. The simultaneous infusion of lipids with other macronutrients provides a number of advantages such as allowing adequate energy needs with less carbohydrate infusion, supplying essential fatty acids, reducing water and electrolyte retention, and reducing the likelihood of hypoglycemia following cessation of the PN infusion.

Generally, intravenous lipids should provide 20–30% of infused PN calories; however, a greater percentage of lipids may be preferred in the patient with significant glycemic control and/or fluid management problems. Disadvantages of lipid infusions include concerns about immunosuppressive effects, effects on respiratory function, central venous catheter occlusion, stability/shelf-life, and cost. In general, these concerns have either been shown not to be clinically significant or can be prevented by not exceeding the recommended rates of infusion [9,10]. The potential role of lipids on the development of liver disease is discussed in Chapter 21.

Since the introduction of home PN infusions, commercially available lipid, multivitamin, and trace element preparations have undergone substantial modifications in order to provide the 35 essential nutrients (electrolytes, minerals, vitamins, and trace elements) and reduce the potential for micronutrient deficiencies. As a consequence, micronutrient deficiencies described in the early years of PN such as iron, selenium, copper, zinc, thiamine, copper, vitamin A, vitamin E, vitamin D, and essential fatty acid are now rare [3]. However, when home PN patients are completely or incompletely weaned from PN, they are at risk for developing deficiencies as determined by their underlying bowel condition and clinical status [11] and lifelong oral supplementation and monitoring of micronutrient levels is necessary [6,12]. Importantly, most commercial trace element solutions only provide the estimated daily nutrient need without consideration of replacement of deficient micronutrient stores and additional supplementation may be necessary [13]. In addition, degradation of certain vitamins may occur during the infusion, either as a consequence of sunlight (e.g. vitamins A and C) or PN compounding with amino acid solutions that contain sulfite as an antioxidant (e.g. thiamine and vitamin E) [14].

Syndromes reflecting the accumulation of excess micronutrients have also been described. These are typically seen in cases of inadequate excretion rather than administration of excessive amounts, although the latter can occur as well. For example, manganese, like copper, is excreted via the biliary system and can accumulate in the presence of significant cholestatic liver disease. Recent reports have demonstrated manganese deposition in the basal ganglia of home PN patients presenting with Parkinsonian-like features

Table 15.1 Potential effects of parenteral nutrition on organ function.

Organ	Effect
Bone	Osteomalacia, osteopenia, osteoporosis
Gallbladder	Sludge, cholelithiasis, hypocontractility, acalculous disease
Immune system	Immunosuppression
Intestine	Bacterial overgrowth, increased permeability, bacterial translocation
Kidney	Chronic renal insufficiency, hyperoxaluria, nephrolithiasis
Liver	Steatosis, cholestasis, fibrosis, cirrhosis, portal hypertension
Neurologic	Memory disturbance

and subsequent improvement in magnetic resonance imaging findings after reduction in manganese intake [15].

Organ dysfunction

PN can have deleterious effects, either directly or indirectly, on a variety of organ systems (Table 15.1). Although the clinical significance of many of these effects remains uncertain, there has been particular interest and more evidence available on long-term PN effects on hepatobiliary and bone disease.

Hepatobiliary

Liver disease is a well-recognized complication in long-term PN patients and remains an important life-threatening complication and indication for combined liver and small bowel transplantation [16–18]. However, it often remains difficult to assign blame solely to the effects of PN because of the presence of a number of conditions in these patients that may also be associated with hepatic dysfunction [19,20]. Intestinal failure-associated hepatobiliary diseases and

Table 15.2 Risk factors for metabolic bone disease in home parenteral nutrition patients.

Patient-related

Malabsorption syndromes
Chronic inflammatory conditions
Chronic liver disease
Corticosteroid use
Heparin use
Female gender
Increasing age
Menstrual status
Thin body habitus
Tobacco use
Excessive alcohol use
Sedentary lifestyle
Reduced sunlight exposure

Parenteral Nutrition–related

Aluminum toxicity
Excessive vitamin D
Acidosis
Excessive amino acid infusion
Calcium deficiency
Magnesium deficiency
Copper deficiency
Hypercalciuria

suggestions for their management and prevention are discussed in detail in Chapter 21.

Skeletal

A spectrum of metabolic bone disease, including osteomalacia, osteoporosis, osteopenia, and secondary hyperparathyroidism, may occur in home PN patients. As with PN-associated hepatobiliary diseases, extricating the effects of the PN from those of underlying patient factors (Table 15.2) is problematic [21]. Although the prevalence and clinical significance of bone disease in home PN patients is poorly understood, a recent study of 165 patients who had received home PN for at least 6 months and had undergone bone mineral density measurements using dual-energy X-ray absorptiometry (DXA) demonstrated a T-score < −1 in 84% (< −2.5 in 41%) [22]. Furthermore, bone pain occurred in 35% and bone fracture in 10% of patients. The prevalence of bone disease did not differ among the various underlying diseases; however, the dura-

tion of time receiving home PN and body mass index were associated with lower Z-scores. In a follow-up to this study, these investigators performed a second DXA scan on 65 of the original patients after a period of 18.1 ± 5.5 months and found that home PN was not associated with a further decrease in bone mineral density in most patients [23]. In addition, Z-score variations seen were related to general risk factors for bone disease rather than PN, showing a negative correlation with age and female gender.

Current evidence suggests that in patients on home PN for intestinal failure, bone turnover undergoes variations that appear to relate to the duration of PN treatment with increased bone resorption during the early treatment period and a low bone-formation rate being a characteristic feature of long-term PN use [24,25]. Patients receiving long-term PN may develop a restructuring osteopathy, particularly involving the lower extremities, characterized by joint pains, hypercalciuria, and low bone formation rate. Factors present in PN formulations that may contribute to bone disease include aluminum and vitamin D. Aluminum contamination of the PN formula with aluminum accumulation at the bone mineralization front was a serious problem in the early years of this therapy [24]. The replacement of casein hydrolysates with synthetic amino acid solutions has reduced but not eliminated this problem [26]. A toxic effect of vitamin D associated with long-term PN use in the setting of low serum levels of parathyroid hormone (PTH) and $1,25 \, (OH)_2$ vitamin D and resulting in low bone turnover has been suggested although not proven [27]. It has also been suggested that long-term PN may alter the balance of the effect of PTH so that resorption is favored over formation and higher levels of PTH are needed to reverse this imbalance [28]. Finally, in some patients, there is an excessive excretion of calcium and phosphorus which may reflect acidosis associated with too rapid nutrient infusion. An increase in phosphorus in the PN formula may improve calcium balance by enhancing renal tubular calcium absorption [29].

An assessment of bone density should be undertaken in all chronic intestinal failure patients regardless of the need of PN and repeated every 2–3 years. The identification of significant bone disease should lead to an assessment of calcium, phosphorus, magnesium, vitamin D, and PTH status. In addition, an assessment of the PN formula and additives is warranted. Management includes exercise, sunlight exposure, minimizing alcohol use, and eliminating tobacco use. Calcium, magnesium, and vitamin D replacement should be provided as needed. Estrogen replacement may be considered in postmenopausal women without other risk factors for hypercoagulability. The withdrawal of heparin from the PN bag or flushes should be considered; however, the risk of catheter-related central venous thrombosis needs to be considered. Additional study is needed on the role of intravenous bisphosphonate therapy in home PN patients [30].

Survival, quality of life and cost issues

Factors influencing survival

As most home PN patients resume full oral nutrition and some die, less than 20% of patients who begin home PN ultimately require it long term and the majority do not require PN for more than 1 year [31,32]. A 94% probability of requiring home PN permanently has been demonstrated in those patients who are unable to be weaned within 2 years of its initiation [32]. A number of factors, some that can be modified, have been demonstrated to influence outcome in home PN patients (Table 15.3). Studies from both the United States and Europe have shown that the most important factor influencing home PN survival is the patient's underlying disease/primary diagnosis (Table 15.4) [31,33–35]. Indeed, death occurs relatively uncommonly as a consequence of a PN complication, particularly in those requiring PN for less than a year (e.g. cancer patients) [31]. In contrast, for those patients who require home PN over a much longer time period (e.g. nonmalignant causes of short bowel syndrome), a 10–15% risk of mortality from a PN-related complication (e.g. line sep-

Table 15.3 Factors influencing survival in long-term parenteral nutrition patients.

Primary diagnosis
Age
Remnant bowel length
Type of remaining bowel
Experience of the supervising clinician
Narcotic use (?)
Social support (?)

Table 15.4 Survival on home parenteral nutrition according to primary diagnosis [31,36].

Diagnosis	% Survival		
	1 year	3 year	5 year
Crohn's disease	96	84	82
Mesenteric ischemia	87	84	56
Radiation enteritis	87	58	52
Motility disorder	87	62	—
Congenital bowel defects	94	80	—
Chronic bowel obstruction	83	40	—
Cancer	*20*	—	—

Modified from Howard [62].

sis, liver failure, loss of vascular access) exists [31–36]. Younger home PN patients have lower mortality rates than older home PN patients [37]; however, because the underlying diseases across the ages tend to be very different, the overall influence of age on survival becomes less clear [36]. Nevertheless, it has been demonstrated that when patients of varying age but similar diagnoses are compared, survival is still better in the younger patients; a finding that is independent of the expected higher mortality in the geriatric population (Figure 15.1) [31]. In addition, younger patients tend to be more likely to regain nutritional autonomy and achieve greater rehabilitation. Despite the decreased overall survival, older home PN patients do not seem to experience more PN-related complications. Indeed, younger patients appear to have a 50% greater likelihood of requiring hospitalization for sepsis. Therefore, it has been suggested that age should not, in and of itself, disqualify anyone from home PN therapy so long as there is adequate support at home to provide the necessary assistance [31].

The length of the remaining bowel is closely linked to both the probability of regaining nutritional autonomy and survival [32,38]. In adult short bowel patients, a remnant small bowel length of <100 cm was found to be highly predictive of permanent intestinal failure [32]. Survival was inversely correlated to the presence of an end-jejunostomy and a remnant small bowel length of <50 cm (Figure 15.2). Cut-off values for remnant small bowel lengths separating transient from permanent intestinal failure/PN dependence were 100, 65 and 30 cm in end-jejunostomy, jejunocolic, and

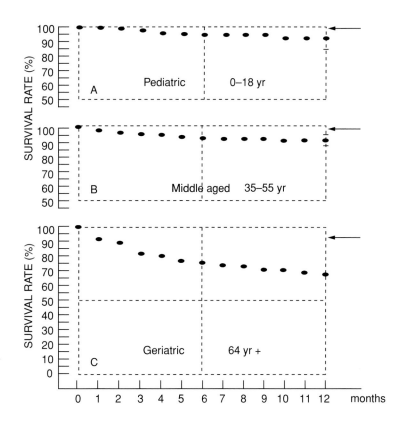

Figure 15.1 Survival according to age at start of home parenteral nutrition. The arrows indicate the expected mortality rate in the general population. (From Howard et al. [31], with permission from American Gastroenterological Association.)

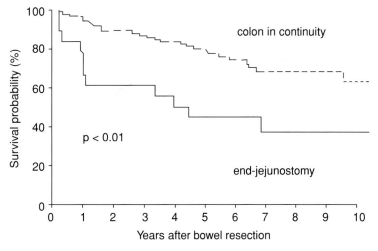

Figure 15.2 Survival according to presence or absence of an end-jejunostomy. (From Messing et al. [32], with permission from American Gastroenterological Association.)

jejunoileocolic bowel anatomies, respectively. These results are virtually identical to those obtained by others [39] and underscore the important contributions provided by the colon and distal ileum with regard to both weaning from PN and survival.

It is worth highlighting a recent report in which the outcome of 80 infants with SBS was reviewed and predictors of survival and successful PN weaning determined [40]. Over a mean follow-up of 5.1 years, a survival of 72.5% and PN weaning success of 64% were

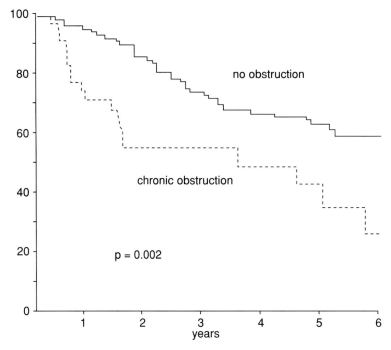

Figure 15.3 Survival according to presence or absence of chronic intestinal obstruction. (From Messing et al. [36], with permission from American Gastroenterological Association.)

found. Cholestasis (conjugated bilirubin ≥2.5 mg/dL) and age-adjusted small bowel length (<10% of normal length) were the major predictors of mortality, whereas age-adjusted small bowel length (≥10% of normal length) and the presence of the ileocecal valve were major predictors of PN weaning.

The presence of chronic mechanical bowel obstruction has been shown to worsen survival in home PN patients, with a relative risk of death of 2.6 (95% confidence interval, 1.1–5.8) (Figure 15.3) [36]. These patients are also at higher risk for hospitalization as a result of sepsis [31]. There appears to be a relationship between sepsis and survival in patients with chronic intestinal obstruction [36].

The experience of the clinician caring for the home PN patient also appears to influence survival. This is highlighted in a study from France in which mortality was shown to be considerably higher in patients started on home PN in the early years at designated home PN centers (relative risk of 5.6 [95% confidence interval, 2.4–21]) [36]. Additional support of the importance of clinician experience comes from a comparison of mortality rates of 407 home PN patients with Crohn's dis-

ease cared for at large teaching programs versus smaller non-teaching programs (5.2% vs. 12.5%, respectively) [41].

Two additional factors that influence the risk for complication and, as a consequence, have been suggested to influence survival of home PN patients are narcotic dependence and participation in peer support organizations. Narcotic-dependent patients have been shown to require more hospitalizations and have a higher frequency of sepsis when compared to home PN patients not using narcotics [42]. Finally, in a case-controlled study conducted in the United States, participation in a home PN support organization was shown to be associated with a reduction in septic events [43].

Quality of life on home PN

In addition to overall survival, quality of life (QoL), taking into account physical, psychosocial and emotional functioning, is an important factor when determining the effectiveness of health care interventions. The transition of parenteral support from the hospital

Table 15.5 Factors affecting home parenteral nutrition patients' quality of life.

Inconvenience
Expense
Interference with social and leisure activities
Altered body image/disfigurement
Parenteral nutrition-related complications
Emotional strain
Pain
Lack of employment or lowered status at work
Loss of income
Decreased social interaction
Loss of independence
Loss of control of bodily functions
Inability to eat normally
Sexual functioning

to the home has been shown to lead to significant improvements in patients' QoL [44]. However, home PN is associated with a number of factors that, particularly when combined with effects from their underlying disease process, may result in a restriction of activities and deleteriously impact daily life (Table 15.5). A number of studies, using a variety of instruments to measure QoL have demonstrated that home PN patients have lower QoL than the general population [31,44–48]. In one of the few studies that has compared QoL in home PN (n = 49) patients versus non-home PN (n = 36) patients with short bowel syndrome, home PN patients scored worse overall on both the nondisease specific sickness impact profile and disease-specific inflammatory bowel disease questionnaire, two validated QoL questionnaires [49]. Female home PN patients and home PN patients >45 years of age scored worse. Home PN also appeared to worsen QoL in patients with a stoma, whereas a stoma did not reduce QoL in non-home PN patients. It was felt that the impairment in QoL in the home PN patients was related to all the factors required to provide PN rather than the inconveniences and bowel symptoms that accompany intestinal failure.

With time and experience, patients on home PN can modify their lifestyles to minimize the impact of this therapy (e.g. infuse PN overnight, travel with help from home health care company and support groups, modify diet and leisure activities). This would expect

to be reflected as an improvement in QoL. Indeed, home PN patients tend to have the lowest QoL during the first year on PN, particularly if the patient was previously healthy (e.g. mesenteric infarct). Importantly, the QoL of the patient prior to requiring home PN plays a significant role in determining the level of QoL achieved afterwards, particularly during the early period [3,46,50]. In general, after the first year on home PN, the QoL slowly improves until about 4 to 5 years on PN [43].

There have been conflicting findings with regards to the effect of patient age on QoL [51]. Nevertheless, in general, younger patients seem to report a better QoL than those over 55 years of age [46]. The lower QoL in older home PN patients may, in part, reflect the increased incidence of catheter infections occurring in older patients [52]. Interestingly, younger home PN patients with the highest QoL have also been shown to be more interested in intestinal transplantation than older patients, a finding that may indicate an unwillingness to accept permanent home PN [47]. Currently, QoL appears to be similar in those who have undergone a successful intestinal transplant compared to stable patients on home PN [53,54]. Certainly, as survival and overall QoL following intestinal transplantation improves (see Chapter 40), recommendations for transplantation versus home PN may change [55,56].

In addition to its adverse effect on morbidity and mortality, chronic narcotic use also has deleterious effects on home PN patients' QoL [42]. In general, sexual functioning decreases in most home PN patients [50]. Approximately 5–20% of home PN patients remain in full-time employment [46,47,49]. Although a 52% employment rate was reported in a European multicenter survey, 20% worked only part-time [57]. The reason for lack of employment is likely multifactorial but may reflect physical limitations and, importantly, illness-related financial benefits/disincentives. Finally, factors that seem to favor a better QoL in home PN patients include a strong self-esteem and good family/social support [43,58].

Cost of home PN

Similar to the increasingly common use of QoL measurements in assessing outcomes of a treatment, economic appraisals are also being increasingly reported.

The rise in popularity of these appraisals is undoubtedly related to current demands on healthcare resources. Surprisingly, given the expense of long-term PN, there are few economic analyses reported in the literature [44,59–61]. Although practice variations, patient heterogeneity, and uncertainty regarding outcomes pose methodological problems, economic evaluations of home PN in intestinal failure have shown that PN at home is up to 75% more cost-effective than keeping patients in the hospital [44,46]. In addition, home PN costs less in long-term users (>1 year of use) and in younger patients (<44 years of age) [47,59].

Direct costs associated with home PN include the nutrient solution, administration sets, infusion pump, and catheter dressing kits. In a report using 1992 dollars, these costs were estimated to range from $238 to $390 per day, which translated into $86,000 to $140,000 per year [31,62]. Importantly, these costs do not include fees associated with medical visits, laboratory monitoring, home nursing support, or hospitalizations for complications of PN. Nor do they include the numerous indirect costs incurred by home PN patients such as missed work by the patient or other family members and home alterations to support home PN therapy. A recent report estimated the annual cost/patient/year of home PN at $55,193 ± $30,596 plus $0 to $140,220 for rehospitalization (63). While clearly an extremely expensive therapy, the expense of home PN tends to be offset by its lifesaving nature and the likelihood of recovery of intestinal function.

In the United States, Medicare is the primary payer for 25% of all new home PN patients and eventually covers the costs for more than 60% [62]. In comparison, in many European countries, the direct costs related to home PN use are borne by a national health program. Periodic assessment of compliance, appropriateness of formulation, infusion regimen and status of intestinal adaptation/ability to wean PN is critically important in order to provide the most cost-effective care for the home PN patient [64].

Conclusion

Home PN has evolved to become a very successful, life-saving treatment in the management of intestinal failure. Nevertheless, the provision of PN remains intrusive, expensive and continues to be associated with significant morbidity. The separation of the effects of PN from the patient's underlying cause of intestinal failure is often difficult if not impossible. A number of factors, some that can be modified, have been demonstrated to influence outcome in home PN patients, the most important being the patient's underlying disease/primary diagnosis. Fortunately, most patients with intestinal failure are able to be weaned from PN within 2 years. For those with permanent intestinal failure, other treatment options should be considered to facilitate PN weaning such as the combination of recombinant human growth hormone, glutamine and a modified diet [65], autologous gastrointestinal reconstruction [66], or intestinal transplantation [55]. Although home PN is associated with a number of factors that, particularly when combined with effects from their underlying disease process, may result in a restriction of activities and deleteriously impact daily life, with time and experience, patients on home PN can modify their lifestyles to minimize the impact of this therapy. The management of PN by a nutrition support team that optimally includes, at a minimum, an experienced clinician, nurse specialist, dietitian, and pharmacist, reduces PN-related morbidity and may reduce costs associated with its use. Because chronic intestinal failure is an uncommon condition and clinical expertise in its management is not widely available, the referral of these patients to experienced centers for periodic assessment should be encouraged (67). While clearly an expensive therapy, the expense of home PN tends to be offset by its lifesaving nature and the likelihood of recovery of intestinal function.

References

1 Buchman AL. Complications of long-term home total parenteral nutrition: their identification, prevention and treatment. *Dig Dis Sci* 2001;46:1–18.

2 Pironi L, Paganelli F, Labate AM, et al. Safety and efficacy of home parenteral nutrition for chronic intestinal failure: a 16-year experience at a single centre. *Dig Liver Dis* 2003;35:314–324.

3 Howard L, Ashley L. Management of complications in patients receiving home parenteral nutrition. *Gastroenterology* 2003;124:1651–1661.

4 Gil MJ, Franch G, Guirao X, et al. Response of severely malnourished patients to preoperative parenteral

nutrition: a randomized clinical trial of water and sodium restriction. *Nutrition* 1997;13:26–31.

5 Solomon SN, Kirby DS. The refeeding syndrome: a review. *JPEN J Parenter Enteral Nutr* 1990;1:90–95.

6 DiBaise JK, Matarese LE, Messing B, Steiger E. Strategies for weaning parenteral nutrition in adult patients with short bowel syndrome. *J Clin Gastroenterol* 2006;40:S94–S98.

7 Rosmarin D, Wardlaw G, Mirtallo J. Hyperglycemia associated with high, continuous infusion rates of total parenteral nutrition dextrose. *Nutr Clin Pract* 1996;11:151–156.

8 Kraft MD, Btaiche IF, Sacks GS. Review of the refeeding syndrome. *Nutr Clin Pract* 2005;20:625–633.

9 Ota DM, Jessup JM, Babcock GF, et al. Immune function during intravenous administration of a soybean oil emulsion. *J Parent Enteral Nutr* 1985;9:23–27.

10 Askanazi J, Nordenstrom J, Rosenbaum SH, et al. Nutrition for the patient with respiratory failure: glucose vs. fat. *Anaesthesiology* 1981;54:373–377.

11 Jeppesen PB, Hoy CE, Mortensen PB. Deficiencies of essential fatty acids, vitamin A and E and changes in plasma lipoproteins in patients with reduced fat absorption and intestinal failure. *Eur J Clin Nutr* 2000;54:632–642.

12 Falk A. Evaluating the effectiveness of a micronutrient assessment tool for long-term total parenteral nutrition patients. *Nutr Clin Pract* 2002;17:240–245.

13 Malone M, Shenkin A, Fell GS, Irving MH. Evaluation of a trace element preparation in patients receiving home intravenous nutrition. *Clin Nutr* 1989;8:307–312.

14 La France RJ, Miyagawa CI. Pharmaceutical considerations in total parenteral nutrition. In: Fischer JE, ed., *Total Parenteral Nutrition*, 2nd ed. Boston: Little Brown, 1991, pp. 57–92.

15 Kafrisa Y, Fell J, Long S, et al. Long term outcome of brain manganese deposition in patients on home parenteral nutrition. *Arch Dis Child* 1998;79:263–265.

16 Buchman AL, Iyer K, Fryer J. Parenteral nutrition-associated liver disease and the role for isolated intestine and intestine/liver transplantation. *Hepatology* 2006;43:9–19.

17 Chan S, McCowen KC, Bistrian BR, et al. Incidence, prognosis, and etiology of end-stage liver disease in patients receiving home total parenteral nutrition. *Surgery* 1999;126:28–34.

18 Cavicchi M, Beau P, Crenn P, et al. Prevalence of liver disease and contributing factors in patients receiving home parenteral nutrition for permanent intestinal failure. *Ann Intern Med* 2000;132:525–532.

19 Quigley EMM, Marsh MN, Shaffer JL, Markin RS. Hepatobiliary complications of total parenteral nutrition. *Gastroenterology* 1993;104:286–301.

20 Kelly DA. Intestinal failure-associated liver disease: what do we know today? *Gastroenterology* 2006;130:S70–S77.

21 Epstein S, Traberg H, Levine G, et al. Bone and mineral status of patients beginning total parenteral nutrition. *JPEN J Parenter Enteral Nutr* 1986;10:263–264.

22 Pironi L, Labate AMM, Pertkiewicz M, et al. Prevalence of bone disease in patients on home parenteral nutrition. *Clin Nutr* 2002;21:289–296.

23 Pironi L, Tjellesen L, De Francesco A, et al. Bone mineral density in patients on home parenteral nutrition: a follow-up study. *Clin Nutr* 2004;23:1288–1302.

24 Shike M, Harrison JE, Sturtridge WC. Metabolic bone disease in patients receiving long-term total parenteral nutrition. *Ann Intern Med* 1980;92:343–350.

25 Pironi L, Zolezzi C, Ruggeri E, et al. Bone turnover in short-term and long-term home parenteral nutrition for benign disease. *Nutrition* 2000;16:272–277.

26 Davis A, Spillane R, Zublena L. Aluminum: a problem trace metal in nutrition support. *NCP Nutr Clin Pract* 1999;14:227.

27 Verhage AH, Cheong WK, Allard JP, Jeejeebhoy KN. Increase in lumbar spine bone mineral content in patients on long-term parenteral nutrition without vitamin D supplementation. *JPEN J Parent Enteral Nutr* 1995;19:431–436.

28 Jeejeebhoy KN. Metabolic bone disease and total parenteral nutrition: a progress report. *Am J Clin Nutr* 1998;67:186–187.

29 Wood RJ, Sitrin MD, Cusson CJ, Rosenberg IH. Reduction of total parenteral nutrition induced urinary calcium loss by increasing the phosphorus in the TPN prescription. *JPEN J Parenter Enteral Nutr* 1986;10:188–190.

30 Haderslev KV, Jiellesen L, Sorensen HA, et al. Effect of cyclical intravenous clodronate therapy on bone mineral density and markers of bone turnover in patients receiving home parenteral nutrition. *Am J Clin Nutr* 2002;76:482–488.

31 Howard L, Ament M, Fleming CR, et al. Current use and clinical outcome of home parenteral and enteral nutrition therapies in the United States. *Gastroenterology* 1995;109:355–365.

32 Messing B, Crenn P, Beau P, et al. Long-term survival and parenteral nutrition dependence in adult patients with the short bowel syndrome. *Gastroenterology* 1999;117:1043–1050.

33 Van Gossum A, Bakker H, Bozzetti F, et al. Home parenteral nutrition in adults: a European multicenter survey in 1997. *Clin Nutr* 1999;18:135–140.

34 Scolapio JS, Fleming CR, Kelly DG, et al. Survival of home parenteral nutrition-treated patients: 20 years of experience at the Mayo Clinic. *Mayo Clin Proc* 1999;74:217–222.

35 Colomb V, Dabbas-Tyan M, Taupin P, et al. Long-term outcome of children receiving home parenteral nutrition: a 20-year single-center experience in 302 patients. *J Pediatr Gastroenterol Nutr* 2007;44:47–353.

36 Messing B, Lemann M, Landais P, et al. Prognosis of patients with nonmalignant chronic intestinal failure receiving long-term home parenteral nutrition. *Gastroenterology* 1995;108:1005–1010.

37 Howard L, Heaphey LL, Fleming CR, et al. Four years of North American Registry home parenteral nutrition: outcome data and their implications for patient management. *JPEN J Parenter Enteral Nutr* 1991;15:384–394.

38 Jeppesen PB, Mortensen PB. Significance of a preserved colon for parenteral energy requirements in patients receiving home parenteral nutrition. *Scand J Gastroenterol* 1998;33:1175–1179.

39 Carbonnel R, Cosnes J, Chevret S, et al. The role of anatomic factors in nutritional autonomy after extensive small bowel resection. *JPEN J Parenter Enteral Nutr* 1996;20:275–280.

40 Spencer AU, Neaga A, West B, et al. Pediatric short bowel syndrome: redefining predictors of success. *Ann Surg* 2005;242:403–412.

41 Howard L, Hassan N. Home parenteral nutrition—25 years later. *Gastroenterol Clin North Am* 1998;

42 Richards DM, Scott NA, Shaffer JL, et al. Opiate and sedative dependence predicts poor outcome for patients receiving home parenteral nutrition. *JPEN J Parenter Enteral Nutr* 1997;21:336–338.

43 Smith CE, Curtas S, Werkonitch M, et al. Home parenteral nutrition: does affiliation with a national support and education organization improve patient outcome? *JPEN J Parenter Enteral Nutr* 2002;26:159–163.

44 Detsky AS, McLaughlin JR, Abrams HB, et al. Quality of life of patients on long-term total parenteral nutrition at home. *J Gen Intern Med* 1986;1:26–33.

45 Ladefoged K. Quality of life in patients on home parenteral nutrition. *JPEN J Parenter Enteral Nutr* 1981;5:132–137.

46 Richards DM, Irving MH. Assessing the quality of life of patients with intestinal failure on home parenteral nutrition. *Gut* 1997;40:218–222.

47 Carlson GL, Maguire G, Williams N, et al. Quality of life on home parenteral nutrition and attitudes toward intestinal transplantation. A single centre study of 37 patients. *Clin Nutr* 1995;14:219–228.

48 Pironi L, Paganelli F, Mosconi P, et al. The SF-36 instrument for the follow-up of health-related quality-of-life assessment of patients undergoing home parenteral nutrition for benign disease. *Transplant Proc* 2004;36:254–258.

49 Jeppesen PB, Langholz E, Mortensen PB. Quality of life in patients receiving home parenteral nutrition. *Gut* 1999;44:844–852.

50 Price BS, Levine EL. Permanent TPN, psychological and social responses to the early stages. *JPEN J Parenter Enteral Nutr* 1979;3:49–52.

51 Burnes JU, O'Keefe SJD, Fleming CR. Home parenteral nutrition: a 3-year analysis of clinical and laboratory monitoring. *JPEN J Parenter Enteral Nutr* 1992;16:327–332.

52 Williams N, Carlson GL, Scott NA, Irving MH. Incidence and management of catheter-related sepsis in patients receiving home parenteral nutrition. *Br J Surg* 1994;81:392–394.

53 DiMartini A, Rovera GM, Graham TO, et al. Quality of life after small intestinal transplantation among home parenteral nutrition patients. *JPEN J Parenter Enteral Nutr* 1999;22:357–362.

54 Pironi L, Paganelli F, Lauro A, et al. Quality of life on home parenteral nutrition or after intestinal transplantation. *Transplant Proc* 2006;88:1673–1675.

55 Grant D, Abu-Elmagd K, Reyes J, et al.; on behalf of the Intestine Transplant Registry. 2003 report of the intestine transplant registry: a new era has dawned. *Ann Surg.* 2005;241:607–613.

56 Pironi L, Hebuterne X, Van Gossum A, et al. Candidates for intestinal transplantation: a multicenter survey in Europe. *Am J Gastroenterol* 2006;101:1633–1643.

57 Messing B, Landais P, Goldfarb B, et al. Home parenteral nutrition in adults. A multicenter survey in Europe. *Clin Nutr* 1989;8:3–9.

58 Smith CE. Quality of life in long term TPN patients and their family caregivers. *JPEN J Parenter Enteral Nutr* 1993;17:501–506.

59 Richards FM, Irving MH. Cost-utility analysis of home parenteral nutrition. *Br J Surg* 1996;83:1226–1229.

60 Dzierba SH, Mirtallo JM, Grauer DW, et al. Fiscal and clinical evaluation of HPN. *Am J Hosp Pharm* 1984;41:285–291.

61 Wateska LP, Sattler LL, Steiger E. Cost of a HPN program. *JAMA* 1980;244:2303–2304.

62 Howard L. Home parenteral nutrition: survival, cost, and quality of life. *Gastroenterology* 2006;130:S52–S59.

63 Reddy P, Malone M. Cost and outcome analysis of home parenteral and enteral nutrition. *JPEN J Parenter Enteral Nutr* 1998;22:302–310.

64 Baptista RJ, Lahey MA, Bistrian BR, et al. Periodic reassessment for improved, cost-effective care in HPN: a case report. *JPEN J Parenter Enteral Nutr* 1984;8:708–710.

65 Byrne TA, Wilmore DW, Iyer K, et al. Growth hormone, glutamine, and an optimal diet reduces parenteral nutrition in patients with short bowel syndrome. A prospective, randomized, placebo-controlled, double-blind clinical trial. *Ann Surg* 2005;242:655–661.

66 Sudan D, DiBaise J, Torres C, et al. A multidisciplinary approach to the treatment of intestinal failure. *J Gastrointest Surg* 2005;9:165–177.

67 DiBaise JK, Young RM, Vanderhoof JA. Intestinal rehabilitation and the short bowel syndrome. Part 2. *Am J Gastroenterol* 2004;99:1823–1832.

16 Vascular Access, Including Complications

Sanja Kolaček and Julije Meštrović

Key points

- Patients on long-term parenteral nutrition require central venous access.

- The superior vena cava is the preferred insertion site and the central venous catheter (CVC) tip should be positioned outside the heart outline on the postprocedure chest X-ray.

- When intestinal transplantation can be anticipated as a future therapeutic option, inferior vena cava as the central tip position should be avoided as excessive thrombotic complications may impede the procedure and graft survival.

- Single lumen tunnelled cuffed silicon catheter, dedicated to parenteral nutrition only, is the optimal choice for long-term/home PN.

- Inexperienced physician, large diameter of the CVC, perpendicular position of the tip and femoral insertion site, all increase the frequency of mechanical complications.

- Insertion site hygiene, aseptic placement and catheter maintenance, performed by a dedicated team, are the most important measures in the prevention of CVC related infections.

- When CVC-related bacteriemia is suspected in patients with chronic intestinal failure, broad spectrum antibiotic treatment should be commenced, leaving the catheter *in situ*. If the condition does not improve after 48 hours of appropriate antibiotic treatment, if there is a subcutaneous tunnel infection, or if sepsis is caused by fungi, the CVC should be removed.

Intestinal Failure: Diagnosis, Management and Transplantation.
Edited by Alan N. Langnas, Olivier Goulet, Eamonn M.M. Quigley and Kelly A. Tappenden. © 2008 Blackwell Publishing.
ISBN 978-1-4051-4637-1.

Introduction

Inherent to the definition of chronic intestinal failure is the requirement for parenteral nutrition. To deliver it, vascular access becomes a "conditio sine qua non," and the patient's life literally depends on its safety [1]. However, the widespread use of venous catheters has been accompanied by an increased frequency of complications, both hazardous to the patient and expensive for the health provider. The purpose of this chapter is to provide an updated review on the key issues concerning vascular access in patients on PN, including the most common complications associated with their use.

Selection of the route

Phlebitis of a peripheral vein can be expected to occur when the osmolality exceeds 600 mOsm. As PN solutions are mostly hyperosmolar, access through peripheral veins is limited to short-term and partial nutritional support, and will not be further described here. Prolonged PN requires central venous access defined as placement of a catheter tip into the superior or inferior vena cava or into the right atrium. When considering such placement, it is necessary to differentiate between catheters inserted through subcutaneous peripheral veins (PICC—peripherally inserted central catheters), and central venous catheters (CVCs) which enter via deep veins such as the jugular, subclavian, or femoral. The placement of PICC is relatively safe and easy, and carries a lower risk of complications but they are more easily displaced, with a median survival of two weeks, thereby, limiting their application in long-term PN [2].

CVCs can be non-tunnelled, inserted directly into the deep vein, or tunnelled with an extravascular portion of the catheter running subcutaneously before exiting the skin, where it terminates in two possible ways: cuffed catheters surrounded by a Dacron cuff, providing fixation and a barrier against microorganisms; and ports, where the catheter ends into a small reservoir completely implanted in the region of the pectoralis major muscle. Compared to nontunnelled CVCs, tunnelled Dacron cuffed silicon catheters (e.g. Broviac, Hickman, Groshong) have a fivefold increased life span as they are less prone to infection and to accidental removal, and are, therefore, the first choice for patients on long-term and home PN [3]. Totally implanted devices (e.g. Port-a-Cath, Mediport, Vascuport), which, for entry, require a percutaneous puncture with a special needle, are ideal for long-term but intermittent vascular access, and their use for PN is limited. More details regarding the practical aspects of the techniques required may be found elsewhere [4].

Selection of the CVC (Table 16.1)

Ideally, the catheter material should be flexible and soft, nontrombogenic, biologically inert, stiff enough for easy insertion, radio-opaque, and with anti-infective properties (Table 16.1). Because no such product is readily available, silicon elastomer is the current material of choice, and polyurethane coated with hydromers its first alternative [4,5] (Table 16.1). A sound recommendation for patients on long-term PN is to use a single lumen CVC dedicated for PN only, and to allow blood sampling from it, provided that the procedure is strictly aseptic. Although multilumen catheters are associated with an increased risk of infectious complications, they are sometimes necessary for critically ill patients with poor venous access who need PN, as well as frequent monitoring and a variety of intravenous medications. When a multilumen CVC is used, a reasonably safe compromise is to designate one port exclusively for PN solutions [6–11].

As will be discussed later, catheter-related infection is common and a very serious complication. Many studies have shown that an effective method for reducing the risk of infection is the use of antimicrobial impregnated CVCs [7,12], such as antiseptic chlorhexidin/silver sulfadiazine and antibiotic minocycline/rifampicin impregnated catheters, with the latter being more effective [13]. For patients requiring long-term PN the important concerns in relation to such catheters are the duration of antimicrobial activity and the possible emergence of antibiotic-resistant strains of bacteria [14]. Present guidelines recommend their use in settings associated with a high rate of catheter-related infections [6,8,11,15].

Table 16.1 Properties of catheter material (based on [4,5]).

Catheter	Advantages	Disadvantages	Long-term use
Polyethylene	Easy to insert	Very stiff and thrombogenic, increased microorganism adherence	Not appropriate
Polyvinyl-cloride	Easy to insert	Very stiff and thrombogenic, bendy, may fracture, increased adhearance of microorganisms	Not appropriate
Polyurethane	Easy to insert	Slightly thrombogenic	Suitable
Polyurethane-coated with Hydromers	Best surface properties, least thrombogenic	Easily damaged during insertion	Alternative material of choice
Silicon elastomer	Superior mechanical properties, nonthrombogenic	Difficult to insert	Material of choice

Selection of insertion site and positioning of the tip (Figure 16.1, Table 16.2)

Four main central venous routes (Figure 16.1) can be used as an insertion site for the CVC: subclavian, external jugular, internal jugular, and femoral vein. Each of them is associated with particular risks for mechanical, thrombotic, and infectious complications. Based on frequency of complications, presented in Table 16.2, and following the recently published guidelines in children [6,7] and in adults [5,8,11], the subclavian vein can be recommended as the preferred site for adult patients and older children because of less patient discomfort, and the lowest risk for infection and thrombosis. In children, femoral catheters have not been associated with the significantly increased incidence of mechanical or infectious complications seen in adults, and femoral access has the advantage of easily identifiable landmarks, which are usefull if rapid vascular access in a non-sedated child is required [6,7,16]. However, when intestinal transplantation can be anticipated as a future therapeutic option, preservation of the inferior

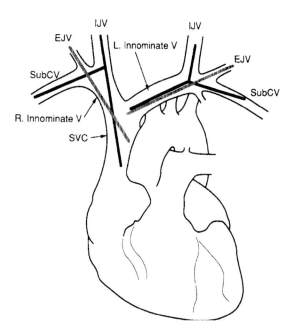

Figure 16.1 Various venous approaches to the superior vena cava. EJV: external jugular vein IJV: internal jugular vein SubCV: subclavian vein SVC: superior vena cava (Reproduced from Jones [35], with permission from Elsevier.)

vena cava becomes a necessary prerequisite as extensive thrombosis may impede the procedure and graft survival [17]. In assessing vascular patency different methods, such as Doppler ultrasound, angio CT scan, MRI, could be applied.

During central venous cannulation maximal sterile barrier precautions are to be observed. For skin preparation, 2% chlorhexidine is preferred as an antiseptic solution [6]. Both the sterile approach and skin hygiene during CVC placement reduce the risk of catheter-related infectious complications. The same is true for antibiotic (vancomycin or teicoplanin) administration prior to catheter insertion [8,11,18], but potential benefits need to be weighed against the possibility of the emergence of antibiotic resistant organisms.

The two available methods of insertion (percutaneous and surgical cut-down) are equally effective, but the latter is associated with an increased risk of permanent vein damage [5,6]. In adults, the procedure is usually performed under local anesthesia, while in paediatric patients general anesthesia and correct positioning of the child are the optimal conditions for CVC placement, particularly for tunnelled catheters [16]. Studies have shown that the frequency of mechanical complications is significantly increased by failed previous insertions, prior catheterization at the same site and multiple attempts [19]. An experienced physician, who has performed 50 or more catheterizations, is twice as likely to be successfull in avoiding mechanical complications, compared to one with less experience [20].

As stated above, central venous access is obtained by advancing the catheter into the superior or inferior vena cava or right atrium. However, if the tip of the CVC lies within the heart outline on chest X-ray, there is an increased risk of serious complications such as severe arrhythmia and pericardial tamponade. Therefore, the postprocedure chest radiograph, though not recommended by all authors [5], is useful in assessing the position of the catheter, at least in children [6,16]. In the latest guidelines [6], it is recommended that, on the chest X-ray, the CVC tip should preferably be 0.5 cm outside the heart outline in small infants, 1.0 cm in older infants and above the carina in adults and older children. For femoral catheters, the tip should lie above the renal veins [21]. Some other techniques may be helpful in inserting and positioning the CVC, for example, Doppler ultrasound for the cannulation of

Table 16.2 Selection of CVC insertion site.

	Ext. jugular	Inter. jugular	Subclavian	Femoral
Features				
Ease of venepuncture	+++	+	+	+++
Central placement success	++ (only with J wire)	+++	+++	++
Suitable for rapid procedure	++	+++	+	+++
Suitable for long-term PN	+	++	+++	+
Other	Tortuous	Right side preferred—ductus thoracus left	Left side preferred—missplacement more frequent right	Discomfort for patient
Mechanical complications				
Serious complications (haemotorax, pnemotorax.)	+	++	+++	+
Arterial puncture		++	+	+++
Thrombotic complications*	+	++	+	+++
Infectious complications*		++	+	+++

*In children, frequency of mechanical and thrombotic complications of femoral vein comparable to jugular and subclavian sites [6,15]. (Adapted from [5,7,8,15,16]).

the jugular veins and ECG for verifying the tip position [22].

CVC maintenance

The duration of catheterization is an important risk factor for CVC-related complications, particularly after the 5th to 7th day. Despite this, routine replacement does not prevent catheter-related bloodstream infection [8,11], and the CVC should be removed promptly when no longer needed. In the case of a malfunctioning nontunnelled CVC, exchange over a guidewire lowers the risk of mechanical complications, but is not advised in the presence of bacteraemia or in patients with catheter-related bloodstream infections [6,11].

Studies on systemic antibiotic prophylaxis and antibiotic lock, designed to prevent infectious complications (using mainly vancomycin), have been performed. Some preventive effects were shown in children and in adults, but the prophylactic use of vancomycin is an independent risk factor for the acquisition of resistant enterococcus [23].

The second most frequent clinically significant complication associated with a CVC is thrombosis. Moreover, thrombus may serve as a nidus for bacterial colonization. Though heparin has been advocated in an attempt to prolong catheter life, evidence of efficacy as well as current prescribing habits, vary widely. According to the recently published pediatric guidelines, the routine use of heparin for the prevention of thrombotic occlusion of CVCs in regular use can not be recommended. However, to maintain the patency of a CVC that is not in constant use, it is advisable to flush it once to twice weekly with 5 to 10 U/ml of heparinized saline [6].

Insertion site hygiene

Nursing care and a dedicated team approach, particularly with respect to skin preparation before catheter insertion and during subsequent care, are considered to be among the most important measures for prevention of complications [12,24], and are described in detail in recently published guidelines [6,11]. Before insertion of an intravascular device and for the postinsertion care, the skin should be cleaned and disinfected with 2% chlorhexidin, which is more effective than either povidone-iodine or 70% alcohol. Organic solvents or topical antibiotic ointments should not be routinely applied to the skin, as they may promote fungal infection, antimicrobial resistance and damage the surface of the catheter. Dressings provide protection from external contamination and help to prevent catheter dislodgement or trauma. Traditionally, a dry sterile gauze and tape have been used, but different forms of transparent polyurethane film dressings, enabling visibility of the insertion site, have recently been promoted. There are concerns that these may increase skin humidity and result in increased microbial colonization, thereby increasing the risk of catheter-related infections. In a Cochrane systematic review, Gillies et al. failed to demonstrate any advantage for one method over another and it is, therefore, recommended that either may be used, based on the patient's preference [25]. The dressing should be replaced when damp, loose, or when the inspection is necessary. Routinely, for nontunnelled CVCs, gauze and tape should be replaced every two days, and the polyurethane film dressing at least once a week. For tunnelled or implanted devices, dressings need to be changed once per week until the insertion site has healed [11], and even then it is useful to have them covered, particularly in a mobile and inquisitive child [6].

Complications

Central venous access is indispensible for long term PN, but is also associated with numerous complications. Based on a Medline search, during almost 40 years of their use (1966–2004) more than 900 articles dealt with the adverse effects of CVCs in paediatric patients alone [26]. Up to 15% of patients will experience some form of complication, with infection, mechanical complications and thrombosis accounting for the great majority. Intravenous hyperalimentation is considered to be a risk factor itself, but the frequency of complications is lower with home, compared with in-hospital PN [27]. Risk factors for complications can be further devided into those related to the catheter itself, to the patient (including the site used for the insertion), and finally to subsequent catheter and insertion site care,

and have already been described in the text and in Tables 16.1 and 16.2.

Thrombosis (Figure 16.2)

CVC-related thrombosis has been described in 1%—60% of patients. This wide variation reflects different methods of diagnosis, and whether all patients or only those with clinical signs of thrombosis are included. Although thrombosis in as many as 80% of patients may remain subclinical, manifestations may be devastating, such as thrombosis of the central veins (Figure 16.2) and right atrium, or pulmonary embolism. Thrombus within the catheter lumen may cause occlusion or serve as the nidus for bacterial growth. Fibrin can be deposited around or inside the catheter, at its tip as a fibrin "tail", or inside the vessel as a layer (mural thrombus). Increased risk is related to longer indwelling time, a more peripheral location in the central vein, repeated and complicated insertions, larger diameter of the CVC, or small diameter of the vessel, perpendicular position of the tip in relation to the vessel wall, catheter material (Table 16.1), a femoral insertion site (Table 16.2), and patient conditions such as cancer, haemodialysis or coagulopathies [5,8,16,26]. Acute symptomatic thrombosis is treated with thrombolytic agents and anticoagulants, whereas their use as a preventive measure has been disputed and is already disscused in the text above. Prophylaxis with low molecular heparin or vitamin K antagonists appears to be a sound measure in patients on long-term PN with additional risk factors for thrombosis or with a history of previous thromboembolism [6,28].

CVC occlusion (Figure 16.3)

Intraluminal fibrin deposition is the most common cause of the CVC occlusion. It may develop either suddenly, or by a slow progression from an increasing infusion pressure, through withdrawal occlusion (blood aspiration not possible), to complete cessation of flow. A safe and effective strategy, which re-establishes patency in over 75% of thrombosed catheters, is thrombolysis with agents such as urokinase, streptokinase, or more recently alteplaze [29]. A CVC may also be

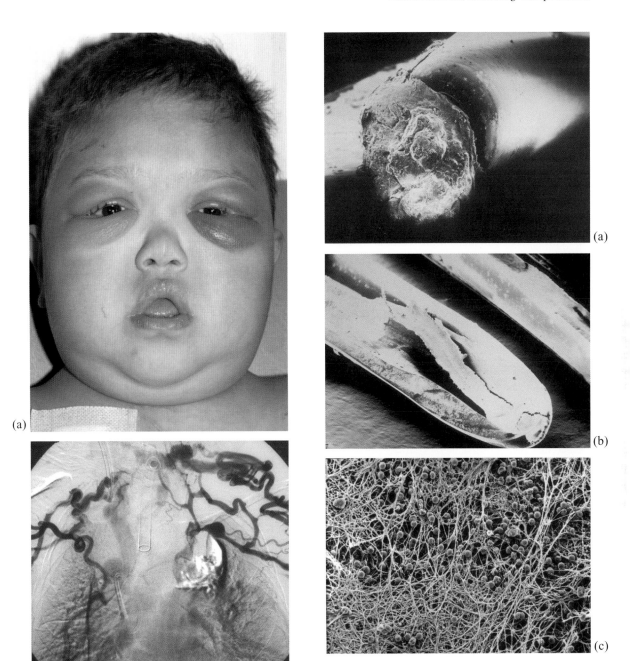

(a)

(b)

(a)

(b)

(c)

Figure 16.2 Superior vena cava thrombosis. (a) Clinical photograph of patient showing severe facial congestion. (b) Bilateral simultaneous arm venogram showing occlusion of both subclavian veins, with numerous collaterals. (Reproduced from Peters [36], with permission from the BMJ Publishing Group.)

Figure 16.3 Occluded CVCs (a) CVC occluded by a fibrin plug. (b) Sliced open CVC with "biofilm" on the internal lumen. (c) High power CVC internal surface showing fibronectin strands with "planktonic" organisms, most probably coagulase-negative *Staphyloccocus*. (Courtesy of Dr. J.W.L. Puntis, Leeds, UK.)

blocked with elements from PN solutions (e.g. calcium phosphate precipitates), or from drug precipitates, particularly when administration is not followed by flushing (Figure 16.3). When chemical/drug precipitates are suspected, and external mechanical pressure or thrombotic occlusion have been ruled out, 0.1 N hydrochloric acid can be used for flushing the line. Finally, a waxy lipid cast has been found in the catheters of patients receiving PN with lipids (Figure 16.3); in this situation, the treatment of choice is to fill the catheter with 70% ethanol solution, leave it inside for one hour and then aspirate. To prevent occluding episodes, CV lines are flushed with sodium chloride 0.9% between all therapies and blood samplings, while terminal in-line filters trap debris or precipitates from PN solutions. More about the etiology and management of occluded CVCs may be found elsewhere [5,29,30].

CVC-related infections

Infection is the second most common complication associated with catheterization (after occlusion), and the primary cause of nosocomial bloodstream infection in general. CVC-related infection can refer to the skin around the insertion site, the tunnel itself, or to bacteremia (with positive blood culture) when associated with clinical manifestations of infection, and when no other source can be identified. More detailed and precise definitions of CVC-related infections may be found elsewhere [11,31]. The inconsistencies in definitions and in presentation of data result in wide variations in incidence rates, but in general, CVC-related bacteremia occurs 3–5 times per 1,000 catheter days in adult hospitalized patients, and the rate is 5–7 per 1,000 catheter days in paediatric intensive care units. The rates are highest for infants weighing <1,000 g and in burn patients [11,19]. In addition to underlying patient conditions, other potentially important factors determining the risk for infection may be catheter related and include: the nature of the material from which it is made, indwelling time, insertion site and the number of lumens. Also, uncomplicated and aseptic placement and subsequent catheter maintenance and hygiene are important variables for infection prevention. Parenteral nutrition, in general (particularly in the first 2 years), and the lipid component, in particular, have been related to increased infection rate, whereas home

treatment decreases the rates of septic episodes by some 50% to 80% [32].

The single most common organism isolated, particularly in patients on home PN, is coagulase-negative *Staphylococcus* accounting for 35%–40% of bacteriemias (up to 60% on home PN). It is followed by *Enterococcus*, *Staphylococcus aureus*, and *Candida sp* (10%–15% each), with Gram-negative bacteria accounting for some 14%–25% of infections [11,16,21]. The emergence of the antibiotic resistant strains such as vancomycin resistant enterococci, methicillin resistant staphylococci, ESBL *Enterobacteriaceae*, and fluconazole resistant candida present a particularly serious problem.

Early catheter infections (within 45 days of insertion) are mostly caused by skin organisms migrating from the insertion site into the cutaneous track up to the CVC tip. Long-term catheters are more frequently infected through the lumen, beginning from the catheter hub. Hematogenous spread from another focus, or infusate contamination are also potential pathogenetic pathways, but are much less frequently involved. Fibrin deposited on the internal and external CVC surface facilitates bacterial adhearance. Moreover, some species such as coagulase-negative staphylococci, or candida spp, produce a polysaccharide often referred to as fibroglycocalyx or slime, which increases their resistance to phagocytosis and antibacterial treatment [11,18].

In all patients with unexplained fever and/or other signs of catheter-related infection, a blood culture should be taken from the CVC [30]. Simultaneous peripheral blood cultures are useful if a semi-quantitative or quantitative culture technique is used, and are recommended in various guidelines [8,11,16], stressing the fact that a single positive blood culture could indicate either contamination or colonization. The often recommended technique of over-the-guide wire CVC replacement and catheter tip culture [8] is not particularly relevant to patients with chronic intestinal failure, who depend upon long term vascular accesses. In these patients, when CVC-related bacteremia is suspected, a broad spectrum antibiotic treatment should be commenced promtly, leaving the catheter in place. The choice of antimicrobial drugs depends on local epidemiological information, but vancomycin in combination with an antibiotic covering gram-negative bacteria, given via the CVC, is the most appropriate intial strategy, changed to a narrower-spectrum agent when the infecting micro-organism and its resistance are identified. Such a strategy of CVC salvage is justified by the fact that about 80% of sacrificed catheters, implicated as the source of sepsis, are in fact sterile [29,33], and only about 20% of colonized catheters will eventually lead to bacteremia [16]. However, the CVC should be removed if the patient's condition does not improve after 48 hours of appropriate antibiotic treatment and in all episodes caused by fungi. Septic emboli, subcutaneous tunnell infection or continuing positive blood cultures, despite appropriate antibiotics, are seen as additional reasons for removing infected CVCs [6,16]. Last but not least, the importance of the dedicated team approach cannot be overemphasized, both for hospitalized patients and for patients on long-term home PN [34].

References

1 Pironi L, Paganelli F, Labate AMM, et al. Safety and efficacy of home parenteral nutrition for chronic intestinal failure: a 16-year experience at a single centre. *Digestive and Liver Disease* 2003;35:314–324.

2 Forbes A. Achieving and maintaining venous access for home parenteral nutrition. *Curr Opin in Clin Nutr Metab Care* 2005;8:285–289.

3 Latto IP, Ng SW, Jones PL, Jenkins B (eds). *Percutaneous Central Venous and Arterial Catheterisation*, 3rd edn. London: WB Saunders, 2000.

4 Ng SW. Choosing the equipment. In: Latto IP, Ng SW, Jones PL, Jenkins B (eds) *Percutaneous Central Venous and Arterial Catheterisation*, 3rd edn. London: WB Saunders, 2000:13–31.

5 Polderman KH, Girbes ARJ. Central venous catheter use. Part 1: Mechanical complications. *Intensive Care Med* 2002;28:1–17.

6 Koletzko B, Goulet O, Hunt J, et al. Guidelines on paediatric parenteral nutrition of the ESPGHAN and ESPEN, supported by the ESPR. Venous access. *J Pediatr Gastroenterol Nutr* 2005;41:S54–S62.

7 Kline AM. Pediatric catheter-related bloodstream infections: Latest strategies to decrease risk. *AACN Clinical Issues* 2005;185–198.

8 McGee D, Gould MK. Preventing complications of central vein catheterization. *N Engl J Med* 2003;16:1123–1133.

9 Dimick JB, Swoboda S, Talamini MA, et al. Risk of colonization of central venous catheters: catheters for total parenteral nutrition vs other catheters. *Am J Crit Care* 2003;12:328–335.

10 Desphande KS. Total parenteral nutrition and infections associated with use of central venous catheters. *Am J Crit Care* 2003;12:326–327.

11 O'Grady NP, Alexander M, Dellinger EP, et al. Guidelines for the prevention of intravascular catheter-related infections. *Pediatrics* 2002;110:1–24.

12 Alonso-Echanove J, Edwards JR, Richards MJ, et al. Effect of nurse staffing and antimicrobial-impregnated central venous catheters on the risk for bloodstream infections in intensive care units. *Infect Control Hosp Epidemiol* 2003;24:916–925.

13 Darouiche RO, Raad II, Heard SO, et al. Comparison of two antimicrobial-impregnated central venous catheters: catheter study group. *N Engl J Med* 1999; 340:1–8.

14 Theaker C. Infection control issues in central venous catheter care. *Intensive Crit Care Nurs* 2005;21:99–109.

15 Latto P. Choosing the vein. In: Latto IP, Ng SW, Jones PL, Jenkins B, eds. *Percutaneous Central Venous and Arterial Catheterization*, 3rd edn. London; WB Saunders, 2000:3–11.

16 de Jonge RCJ, Polderman KH, Gemke RJBJ. Central venous catheter use in the pediatric patient: Mechanical and infectious complications. *Pediatr Crit Care Med* 2005;6:329–339.

17 Kaufman SS, Atkinson JB, Bianchi A, et al. Indications for pediatric intestinal transplantation: A position paper of the American Society of Transplantation. Pediatr Transplantation 2001;5:80–87.

18 van de Wetering MD, van Woensel JBM, Kremer LCM, Caron HN. Prophylactic antibiotics for preventing early Gram-positive central venous catheter infections in oncology patients, a Cochrane systematic review. *Cochrane Database Syst Rev* 2003;CD003295.

19 Johnson EM, Saltzman DA, Suh G, et al. Complications and risks of central venous catheter placement in children. *Surgery* 1998;124:911–916.

20 Sznajder JI, Zveibil FR, Bitterman H, et al. Central vein catheterization: failure and complication rates by three percutaneous approaches. *Arch Intern Med* 1986;146:259–261.

21 Fletcher SJ, Bodeham AR. Safe placement of central venous catheters: where should the tip of the catheter lie? *Br J Anaesth* 2000;85:188–191.

22 Ng WS. Practical aspects of technique. In: Latto IP, Ng WS, Jones PL, Jenkins BJ (eds). Percutaneous central venous and arterial catheterization, 3rd edn. London: WB Saunders 2000;33–56.

23 CDC. Recommendations for preventing the spread of vancomycin resistance. Recommendations of the

Hospital Infection Control Practices Advisory Board. *MMWR Recomm Rep.* 1995;44(No. RR-12):1–13.

24 Sutton CD, Garcea G, Pollard C, et al. The introduction of a nutrition clinical nurse specialist results in a reduction in the rate of catheter sepsis. *Clin Nutr* 2005;24:220–223.

25 Gillies O, O'Riordan L, Carr D, et al. Gauze and tape and transparent polyurethane dressings for central venous catheters. *Cochrane Database Syst Rev* 2003;CD3827.

26 Garden AL, Laussen PC. An unending supply of "unusual" compliations from central venous catheters. *Pediatr Anesthesia* 2004;14:905–909.

27 Colomb V, Febairo M, Dabbas M, et al. Central venous catheter related infections on long-term home parenteral nutrition: Incidence and risk factors. *Clin Nutr* 2000;19:355–362.

28 Klerk CPW, Smorenburg SM, Buller HR. Thrombosis prophylaxis in patient populations with a central venous catheter. *Arch Intern Med* 2003;163:1913–1921.

29 Hardy G, Ball P. Clogbusting: time for a concerted approach to catheter occlusion. *Curr Opin in Clin Nutr Metab Care* 2005;8:277–283.

30 Koletzko B, Goulet O, Hunt J, et al. Guidelines on paediatric parenteral nutrition of the ESPGHAN and ESPEN, supported by the ESPR. *Complications.* 2005;41:S76–S84.

31 Randolph A, Brun-Buisson C, Goldmann D. Identification of central venous catheter-related infections in infants and children. *Pediatr Crit Care Med* 2005;6:S19–S24.

32 Melville CA, Bisset WM, Long S, et al. Counting the cost: hospital versus home central venous catheter survival. *J Hosp Infect* 1997;35:197–205.

33 Dobbins BM, Kite P. Endoluminal brushing in catheter-related sepsis: a sweeping statement. *Nutrition* 1999;15:66–67.

34 Messing B, Joly F. Guidelines for management of home parenteral support in adult chronic intestinal failure patients. *Gastroenterology* 2006;130:S43–S51.

35 Jones PL. Choosing the vein. In: Latto IP, Ng SW, Jones PL, Jenkins B (eds). *Percutaneous Central Venous and Arterial Catheterisation*, 3rd edn. London: WB Saunders, 2000:227–231.

36 Peters M, Beath SV, Puntis JWL, John P. Superior vena cava thrombosis causing respiratory obstruction successfully resolved by stenting in a small bowel transplant candidate. *Arch Dis Child* 2000:163–164.

17 Enteral Support for Children with Intestinal Failure

Daniel S. Kamin and Christopher Duggan

Key points

- Enteral nutrition is vital for normal intestinal growth and function.
- Adaptation—the physical and physiological processes by which the intestine compensates for loss of intestinal length or function—is optimized with the provision of enteral nutrition.
- Multiple mechanisms—direct contact with nutrients, pancreaticobiliary secretions, neurohormal factors—may explain how enteral nutrition promotes adaptation.
- Observational studies have identified early enteral nutrition, dietary intake of breastmilk, and use of amino acid- and long chain fat-containing formulas as correlates of earlier weaning from parenteral nutrition in children with IF. Few randomized trials have been performed.
- Multiple methods (gastric, trans-pyloric) and modes (bolus, continuous, both) of providing enteral nutrition allow for the nutritional support of most infants with intestinal failure.

Introduction

By definition, patients with intestinal failure (IF) do not tolerate enteral nutrition to adequately support basic metabolic/physiologic functions and many therefore require prolonged courses of parenteral nutrition.

Intestinal Failure: Diagnosis, Management and Transplantation.
Edited by Alan N. Langnas, Olivier Goulet, Eamonn M.M. Quigley and Kelly A. Tappenden. © 2008 Blackwell Publishing.
ISBN 978-1-4051-4637-1.

Clinical experience and some scientific data support the concept that both the composition and administration of enteral nutrition in pediatric IF have a critical impact on outcomes in these patients. This has long been known to be the case in short bowel syndrome (SBS), the most common cause of IF in children, and emerging data support the importance of enteral nutrition in other diseases of the small intestine, including disorders of epithelial structure and function, motility, and autoimmunity (causes of IF in children, Table 17.1). We review the rationale for enteral nutrition in pediatric IF, with specific recommendations regarding formula composition, route, and methods for enteral advancement.

Rationale for enteral nutrition

Intestinal adaptation refers to the gross anatomic, histologic, and functional changes that occur after significant intestinal resection. These adaptive changes begin 12–24 hours after massive intestinal resection and will continue for a year or longer after resection [1]. Villi lengthen, the intestinal absorptive surface area increases, and absorptive function gradually improves. It should be noted, however, that the full phenotype of intestinal adaptation in humans has not been fully described (e.g. changes in intestinal motility, commensal microbiota, and barrier function, to name a few), nor have molecular mechanisms of intestinal adaptation been well defined (see Chapter 5).

Enteral nutrition is critical for successful intestinal adaptation. Animal [2–4] and human [5] data suggest that enteral, and not parenteral, nutrition maintains normal intestinal structure and function, even

Table 17.1 Causes of intestinal failure in children.

Category	Disorder	
Short Bowel Syndrome	*Infant* • Gastroschisis • Necrotizing enterocolitis • Small intestinal atresia • Malrotation with volvulus	*Older Child* • Crohn's Disease • Mesenteric infarction • Radiation enteritis • Tumors • Trauma
Motility	• Hirschsprung's disease • Pseudo-obstruction • Neuronal intestinal dysplasia	
Mucosa	*Primary epithelial* • Microvillus inclusion disease • Tufting enteropathy	*Immune-mediated* • Autoimmune enteropathy • Immunodeficiency syndromes
Miscellaneous	• Enteroendocrine cell hypoplasia	

(Adapted from Gupte et al. *Arch Dis Child* 2006;259–64, with permission from the BMJ Publishing Group Ltd.)

in the absence of intestinal resection. Enteral nutrition promotes mucosal hyperplasia and enhanced nutrient absorption via direct mucosal contact [6] and release of humoral [7,8] and pancreaticobiliary [9] factors. Candidate hormones and other humoral factors are discussed in Chapter 25.

Studies of children with protracted diarrhea and SBS additionally support the primacy of enteral nutrition in maintaining intestinal function. Greene et al. [10] gave 16 infants with protracted diarrhea either total parenteral nutrition (PN) followed by semi-elemental oral formula (n = 10), or dilute PN and continuous enteral feeding with elemental formula (n = 6). After 2–3 weeks of treatment, sucrase and maltase activity in jejunal biopsies improved in both groups, but to the normal range only in the group that received early enteral nutrition, and hospital stay was significantly shorter in this group. Orenstein [11] later extended these findings by studying 13 infants with intractable diarrhea, malnutrition, and malabsorption. The severe

group (defined as D-xylose <10 mg/dl, n = 8) was randomized to receive continuous enteral nutrition (EN) using semi-elemental formula or parenteral nutrition for 3–4 weeks followed by EN. Diarrhea resolved more quickly among those receiving EN versus those who received PN, while the resolution of malabsorption, assessed by achieving D-xylose >15 mg/dl, also occurred sooner among those receiving EN.

The role of enteral nutrition in infants with SBS was first noted by Sondheimer et al. [12], who reported that a greater percentage of calories received enterally at 12 weeks adjusted age was correlated with weaning from PN. Other groups have confirmed this finding [13].

What to feed

Although the general role of enteral nutrition in intestinal function and structure is well-supported, the specific composition, especially in IF syndromes, has been less well delineated.

Breast milk: Breast milk's special immunologic and anti-infective properties ought to be especially advantageous to infants with IF. Breast milk contains growth factors, nucleotides, long chain fatty acids, glutamine, and other amino acids that may promote intestinal adaptation. In addition, breast-feeding has been associated with improved immune function, as well as the genesis of a fecal microbiota rich in lactobacilli and bifidobacteria, both of which might improve IF prognosis. By contrast, breast milk contains lactose, which is sometimes not well tolerated in patients with reduced intestinal surface area. In a population of 30 infants with SBS (defined as more than 90 days of dependency on PN), we found that the percentage of days that infants received breast milk was strongly correlated with fewer days of PN use (r = −0.821, p < .03) [13]. As a result of these theoretical and practical data, our practice is to use breast milk, if available, for most infants with IF receiving enteral support.

Enteral formulas: For infants with SBS for whom breast milk is not available, the choice of enteral formulas is controversial. On the one hand, the "functional workload" presented by complex nutrients may promote mucosal cell proliferation [14], via direct contact with disaccharides [15] or indirectly, whereby distal small intestinal or colonic exposure to luminal nutrients promotes release of trophic factors that stimulate small bowel adaptation [16,17]. On the other hand, the presence of a limited mucosal surface area can lead to lactose, protein, and long-chain fatty acid malabsorption. If this malabsorption is severe, fluid, electrolyte, and metabolic balance can be difficult to achieve.

Carbohydrates may be poorly tolerated by patients with IF, as they are broken down by gastrointestinal bacteria into small, osmotically active organic acids that can present a major osmotic load to the distal small intestine and colon [18]. For this reason, carbohydrate content should generally not exceed 40% of calories, and formulas given to IF patients are usually lactose-free. Although lactase activity is significantly lower in the jejunum as compared with sucrase-isomaltase and maltase-glucoamylase activity [19], unless there is an extensive jejunal resection, most infants and children with SBS will tolerate small to moderate amounts of lactose [1].

Fiber supplementation may be helpful in the older child with SBS with intact colon. Colonic bacterial fermentation of the unabsorbed fiber produces short-chain fatty acids, such as butyrate, which appears to induce trophic changes in animal small intestinal mucosa [20,21]. Moreover, pectin, a fermentable but nondigestable oligosaccharide, increased nitrogen absorption and decreased transit time in a child with SBS [22], whereas supplementation improved electrolyte absorption and mucosal permeability for infants with protracted diarrheal illnesses [23].

Although fat tends to be poorly absorbed in SBS, it is a dense energy source relative to carbohydrate or protein. Considering the relatively greater adverse effect of carbohydrate on osmotic diarrhea, it is usually advantageous for patients with SBS to include at least moderate amounts of fat in their diets.

Medium chain triglycerides (MCTs) may be more reliably absorbed than long chain triglycerides (LCTs). MCTs are efficiently hydrolyzed by gastric and pancreatic lipases, giving rise to relatively water-soluble component fatty acids and monoglycerides, which readily diffuse into enterocytes and enter the portal blood directly [24]. This is relevant because infants with dysmotility or SBS often have dilated, poorly motile segments of intestine, conditions which encourage small intestinal bacterial overgrowth [25]. Bacteria metabolize and inactivate bile acids, preventing the solubilization necessary for LCT digestion and absorption. By contrast, excessive provision of MCT oil can cause diarrhea and ketosis, whereas MCTs do not provide essential fatty acids. Thus, MCT content should not be the sole source of dietary lipid.

Moreover, free fatty acids derived from hydrolyzed LCTs may have strong trophic effects on small intestinal mucosa [26,27]. Specific fatty acids may influence intestinal adaptation, as animal data suggest that Omega-3-, Omega-6- [28,29], and polyunsaturated fatty acid- [30] supplemented diets promote mucosal growth or function.

An ideal protein source for infants with IF has not yet been determined. Protein itself may have trophic properties. Colostrum protein concentrate improved weight gain and morphometric measures of intestinal adaptation in a piglet model of SBS using polymeric diet plus colostrum versus polymeric diet alone [31].

Nevertheless, is not yet clear if the type of protein in infant formulas influences outcomes. Bines et al. [32] reported a series of four SBS patients with persistent feeding intolerance. After receiving an elemental amino acid based-formula, all four patients discontinued PN within 15 months. In addition, histologic and physiologic measures of small bowel function improved concurrently. Our retrospective review also found better outcomes (shorter duration of PN dependency) with the use of an amino-acid based formula [13].

Hydrolyzed protein formulas have also been evaluated clinically. Intact protein infant formula was compared to hydrolyzed protein formula in a crossover study of 60 days duration in 10 infants with SBS [33]. No effect of formula type was observed on growth, nitrogen absorption, or mucosal permeability. An earlier study in adult jejunostomy patients produced similar findings [34]. However, Cosnes et al. [35] found that six adults patients with jejunosomies who received alternating intact or hydrolyzed protein formula every 3 days had improved nitrogen assimilation for periods over which the hydrolyzed formula was given. It is worth noting that the Cosnes et al. study followed few patients for a limited time, preventing clear application of their findings.

Glutamine (Gln) is a nonessential amino acid that plays an important role in energy metabolism for

Table 17.2 Formulas used for enteral nutrition in the child with intestinal failure.

Product	Kcal/ml	Osm (mOsm/kgH2O)	Carb (% calories)	Pro (% calories)	Fat (% calories)	MCT/LCT ratio	Comment
Infant							
Human Milk	0.67	255	Lactose (38)	Whey and casein/5	Long-chain fatty acids high in palmitic, linoleic, and linolenic acids (55)	5:95	Preferred nutrition for infants with IF
EleCare (Ross)	0.67	335	Corn syrup solids (43)	Free amino acids (15)	Safflower, MCT, soy (42)	33:66	Preferred for infants with SBS and fat malabsorption
Neocate (SHS)	0.67	375	Corn syrup solids (47)	Free amino acids (12)	Safflower, coconut, soy oils (41)	5:95	CHB standard formula for infants with IF when BM not available
Pregestimil* (Mead Johnson)	0.67	320	Corn syrup solids, modified cornstarch (41)	Casein hydrolysate (11)	MCT, soy, safflower (41)	55:45	Standard formula choice as MCT-predominant, semi-elemental
Nutramigen** LIPIL (Mead Johnson)	0.67	270	Corn syrup solids, modified corn starch (41)	Casein hydrolysate, amino acids (11)	Palm, soy, sunflower oils (48)	0:100	No MCT—poor choice for infant with fat malabsorption
Alimentum*** Advance (Ross)	0.67	370	Corn maltodextrin, sucrose, modified tapioca starch (41)	Casein hydrolysate, amino acids (11)	Safflower, MCT, soy oil (50)	33:66	Appropriate choice for infant on formula and mild fat malabsorption
Toddler/child							
EleCare (Ross)	1.0	551	Corn syrup solids (43)	Free amino acids (15)	Safflower, MCT, soy (42)	33:66	Same product as for infant but higher energy density
Neocate 1+ (SHS)	1.0	610–835	Corn syrup solids (58)	Free amino acids (10)	MCT, canola, safflower, coconut (32)	35:65	High carbohydrate MCT-containing product
Neocate Junior (SHS)	1.0	607–690	Corn syrup solids (42)	Free amino acids (12)	Coconut, MCT, canola, safflower (46)	35:65	
Pediatric Peptinex DT (Novartis)	1.0	460	Maltodextrin, modified food starch (65)	Casein hydrolysate, amino acids (20)	MCT, soybean oil (15)	50:50	Choice for fat malabsorption, high protein requirement, and osmolality sensitivity
Peptamen Junior (Nestle)	1.0	260–360	Maltodextrin, cornstarch (55)	Hydrolyzed whey (12)	MCT, soy, canola (33)	60:40	Appropriate for fat malabsorption and osmolality sensitivity
Pediatric E028 (SHS)	1.0	820	Maltodextrin, sucrose (58)	Free amino acids (10)	Coconut, canola, safflower, MCT oil (32)	35:65	Relatively high osmolality because of disaccharide
Pepdite One+ (SHS)	1.0	430–440	Corn syrup solids (35)	Free amino acids, hydrolyzed pork and soy (12)	MCT, coconut, canola, safflower (46)	35:65	Choice for fat malabsorption, osmolality sensitivity, and severe protein allergy
Vivonex Pediatric (Novartis)	0.8	360	Maltodextrin, modified starch (63)	Free amino acids (12)	MCT, soy (30)	68:32	

Abbreviation: CHB Children's Hospital Boston

* made also as LIPIL version, with 2.5% of fat blend as docosahexaenoic acid (DHA) and arachidonic acid (ARA);

** only made as LIPIL version, with 2.5% of fat blend as DHA and ARA;

*** 2% fat blend is DHA and ARA

Table 17.3 Devices.

Devices	Indications	Contraindications	Advantages	Disadvantages
Gastric feeding				
Naso-gastric	Nutritional support <3 months	Severe GE reflux, aspiration, slow gastric emptying	Easy to place at home	Frequent dislodgements, nasal symptoms
Percutaneous endoscopic gastrostomy (PEG)	Nutritional support >3 months	History of abdominal surgery, abnormal abdominal anatomy, portal hypertension with dilated abdominal vessels	Fewer occlusions with larger bore, one-step low profile devices available	
Surgical gastrostomy	Nutritional support >3 months and higher risk for injury to abdominal organs	Coagulopathy, poor candidate for surgery (cardiac or respiratory insufficiency)	Immediate placement of low-profile device, direct visualization of stomach	Open surgery
Trans-pyloric feeding				
Gastro-jejunal (GJ)	Longer-term enteral nutrition for patients with severe GERD, gastric dysmotility or need for gastric decompression	Recent proximal surgical anastamoses	Radiologic placement, transpyloric tube can be passed through existing gastrostomy tube	Requires healing of gastrostomy tract prior to replacement with GJ, intussception around tube, frequent occlusions of jejunal port
Naso-jejunal	Short term nutritional support for patients with severe GERD, gastric dysmotility, pancreatitis	Recent proximal surgical anastamoses	Radiologic or bedside placement techniques, noninvasive	Frequent dislodgements, intussception, nasal symptoms
Jejunal	Long-term enteral nutrition for patients with severe GERD, upper intestinal dysmotility	Generalized dysmotility, poor wound healing	Direct access to small intestine	Open surgical procedure, mechanical problems

gastrointestinal epithelia and other rapid turnover tissues. We performed a randomized, controlled, pilot study of glutamine-supplemented enteral nutrition in infants who were at risk for intestinal failure [36]. Twenty infants were randomly assigned to receive Gln (n = 9) or an iso-nitrogenous mix of amino acids (n = 11). Median (IQR) days of PN duration was 39 (12–99) in the Gln group and 21 (6–59) in the control group (p = .201). There were no differences in the occurrence of infections between the groups. We concluded that enteral Gln supplementation was well tolerated among infants with surgical gastrointestinal disease, but that this study, admittedly limited in power, did not detect a significant difference in clinical outcomes. Larger, multi-center trials are needed to evaluate new nutritional therapies in infants with IF.

Concern for the development of non-IgE mediated sensitization and allergic enteritis has favored the use of protein hydrolysate or amino-acid based formulas for children with IF. Noninfectious colitis has been

Table 17.4 Enteral advancement methodology.

A. Feeding initiation

Absent bowel sounds?

Contraindications?*

Yes, then continue IVF/PN/NPO

No, then start feeds (NG/NJ/G-tube/J-tube)

Day 1: Breastmilk (full strength) or formula (20 cal/oz) @10–20 ml/kg/d continuously** × 24 h

Contraindications to enteral feeding:

1) paralytic or drug-induced ileus
2) grossly bloody stools or ostomy output and/or radiological changes of intestinal ischemia
3) shock/poor perfusion due to cardiac or respiratory insufficiency
4) bilious and/or persistent vomiting (defined as more than 3 episodes of emesis in 12 h)
5) clinical suspicion of obstruction or ileus (severe abdominal distension, decreased ostomy or stool output, and/or radiologic changes of obstruction or ileus)
6) electrolyte instability
7) ostomy or stool volumes >3 ml/kg/hr

**Oral feeds may be offered as follows:

1) infant is developmentally able to feed by mouth (po)
2) *one hour's* worth of continuous feeds may be offered PO QD-TID after 5 days of continuous feeds. During this time, tube feeds should be held
3) *more than one hour's* worth of continuous feeds may be offered PO once the infant has reached full volume of feeds by continuous route *OR* at least seven days have passed on the feeding advancement protocol

B. Feeding Advancement

Principle 1: Quantify feeding intolerance primarily by stool or ostomy output and secondarily by reducing substances. Persistent vomiting may also be indication of intolerance.

Principle 2: Tolerance assessed no more than twice per 24 h. No more than one advance per 24 h period.

Principle 3: Ultimate goals: 150–200 mL/kg/d, 100–140 kcal/kg/d

Principle 4: If ostomy/stool output precludes advancement at 20 cal/oz for 7 days, then increasing caloric density of the formula can be performed.

Principle 5: Isocaloric reductions in PN support should be undertaken simultaneous with feeding advancement.

1. Stool output

If <10 g/kg/d or <10 stools/d————> advance rate by 10–20 mL/kg/d

If 10–20 g/kg/d or 10–12 stools/d————> no change

If > 20 g/kg/d or > 12 stools/d————> reduce rate or hold feeds*

2. Ileostomy output

If < 2 g/kg/h————————> advance rate by 10–20 mL/kg/d

If 2–3 g/kg/h————————> no change

If > 3 g/kg/h————————> reduce rate or hold feeds*

3. Stool reducing substances

If < 1%————————————> advance feeds per stool or ostomy output

If = 1%————————————> no change

If > 1%————————————> reduce rate or hold feeds*

*feeds should generally be held for 8 h, then restarted at 3/4 the previous rate

(Adapted from Utter S, Duggan C. Short bowel syndrome. In Hendricks KM, Duggan C (eds.), *Manual of Pediatric Nutrition*, 4th ed., BC Decker, Inc. 2005, with permission from BC Decker, Inc.)

reported in patients with SBS [37]. Allergy may occur in children with IF because of sensitization associated with abnormal mucosal permeability. Increased small intestinal mucosal permeability occurs in the context of intestinal inflammation [32], oftentimes a complication of small intestinal bacterial overgrowth [38]. As noted earlier, dilated, poorly motile segments of small bowel in close proximity to colon are common in patients with SBS and dysmotility, and the stagnation and contamination that results promotes abnormal growth of bacteria in small intestine [39].

In summary, animal and some human data support an important role of enteral nutrition in children with SBS/IF. Modest data support the use of protein hydrolysate or amino acid-based formulas. Most formulas are lactose-free and many include a portion of their fat source as MCTs. Infants with diarrhea and protein losing enteropathies may require formulas with enhanced protein content. Table 17.2 provides important details on enteral products used in infants and children with IF.

Supplementary fluids, electrolytes, and micronutrients. Excess fluid and electrolyte losses may complicate the management of IF patients, particularly in patients with high output jejunostomies, in pseudo-obstruction patients who incur large gastric/duodenal fluid losses, or in those with persistent secretory diarrhea. Glucose-containing electrolyte solutions (also called oral rehydration solutions) with sodium concentrations of 75–90 mEq/L are typically used to replace jejunostomy and diarrheal losses. Replacement fluids, be they enteral or intravenous, may be adjusted based on electrolyte concentration of the lost fluids. The intravenous route should be used when there is still net loss of fluid following enteral replacement. Monitoring urine sodium concentration for excessive retention (<10 mEq/L) may indicate the need to provide more sodium, even if serum values are near normal. Excessive magnesium losses can occur with large ostomy volumes, and appropriate magnesium replacement may also improve calcium nutriture [40].

Zinc [41] and selenium [42] losses increase with watery diarrhea and high ostomy output. Zinc supplements are often used empirically, given that serum values do not reliably reflect body stores. Fat-soluble vitamin supplements should be considered, as fat malabsorption is common when absorptive surface area or micellar function is limited. Vitamin B12 monitoring

or parenteral supplementation is necessary for infants with ileal resection or diversion.

How to feed

Continuous enteral feeding via a nasogastric or gastrostomy tube is advantageous in the patient with SBS or diarrhea [11,43], as this permits constant saturation of carrier transport proteins, thus taking full advantage of the available absorptive surface area. A controlled study of intragastric feeds in infants with chronic diarrhea or SBS found that continuous feeding was associated with improved nutrient balance and weight gain, as compared to intermittent feeding [44].

Devices. Most centers recommend percutaneous enteral access for children who will require enteral nutrition for greater than 3 months. Nevertheless, most infants start with nasogastric or nasoenteric (transpyloric) feedings. Table 17.3 displays the methods, contraindications, and important features of enteral feeding strategies.

Methods for advancement. Our protocol for enteral advancement in SBS, or in IF in general, is outlined in Table 17.4. Strict adherence to an ostomy/stool output maximum is unwise, and enteral advancement can occur so long as fluid and electrolyte balance is maintained. Small quantities of oral feedings should be introduced in infants two or three times a day to stimulate sucking and swallowing and to minimize the chances of feeding aversion in the future. Frequent setbacks are not unusual. Enteral feedings may eventually be transitioned to oral/bolus feedings, or oral/bolus and nocturnal feedings, to allow more freedom from the feeding pump.

Prognosis

The transition from IF to adequate intestinal function can take weeks, months, and sometimes years. The infant with SBS is at an advantage for improvements in bowel function over time as compared to the adult, due to the opportunity for further intestinal growth. Provision of enteral nutrition plays a major role in the management of any child with intestinal failure, even for those in whom complete weaning from PN seems unlikely.

References

1 American Gastroenterological Association medical position statement: short bowel syndrome and intestinal transplantation. *Gastroenterology* 2003;124:1105–1110.

2 Levine GM, Deren JJ, Steiger E, Zinno R. Role of oral intake in maintenance of gut mass and disaccharide activity. *Gastroenterology* 1974;67:975–982.

3 Castillo RO, Feng JJ, Stevenson DK, Kwong LK. Altered maturation of small intestinal function in the absence of intraluminal nutrients: rapid normalization with refeeding. *Am J Clin Nutr* 1991;53:558–561.

4 Liu X, Nelson DW, Holst JJ, Ney DM. Synergistic effect of supplemental enteral nutrients and exogenous glucagon-like peptide 2 on intestinal adaptation in a rat model of short bowel syndrome. *Am J Clin Nutr* 2006;84:1142–1150.

5 Sullivan PB, Marsh MN. Small intestinal mucosal histology in the syndrome of persistent diarrhoea and malnutrition: a review. *Acta Paediatr Suppl* 1992;381:72–77.

6 Menge H, Robinson JW. Functional and structural characteristics of the rat intestinal mucosa following ileojejunal transposition. *Acta Hepatogastroenterol (Stuttg)* 1978;25:150–154.

7 Dworkin LD, Levine GM, Farber NJ, Spector MH. Small intestinal mass of the rat is partially determined by indirect effects of intraluminal nutrition. *Gastroenterology* 1976;71:626–630.

8 Martin GR, Wallace LE, Hartmann B, et al. Nutrient-stimulated GLP-2 release and crypt cell proliferation in experimental short bowel syndrome. *Am J Physiol Gastrointest Liver Physiol* 2005;288:G431–G438.

9 Altmann GG. Influence of bile and pancreatic secretions on the size of the intestinal villi in the rat. *Am J Anat* 1971;132:167–177.

10 Greene HL, McCabe DR, Merenstein GB. Protracted diarrhea and malnutrition in infancy: Changes in intestinal morphology and disaccharidase activities during treatment with total intravenous nutrition or oral elemental diets. *J Pediatr* 1975;87:695–704.

11 Orenstein SR. Enteral versus parenteral therapy for intractable diarrhea of infancy: a prospective, randomized trial. *J Pediatr* 1986;109:277–286.

12 Sondheimer JM, Cadnapaphornchai M, Sontag M, Zerbe GO. Predicting the duration of dependence on parenteral nutrition after neonatal intestinal resection. *J Pediatr* 1998;132:80–84.

13 Andorsky DJ, Lund DP, Lillehei CW, et al. Nutritional and other postoperative management of neonates with short bowel syndrome correlates with clinical outcomes. *J Pediatr* 2001;139:27–33.

14 Bines JE, Taylor RG, Justice F, et al. Influence of diet complexity on intestinal adaptation following massive small bowel resection in a preclinical model. *J Gastroenterol Hepatol* 2002;17:1170–1179.

15 Weser E, Babbitt J, Hoban M, Vandeventer A. Intestinal adaptation. Different growth responses to disaccharides compared with monosaccharides in rat small bowel. *Gastroenterology* 1986;91:1521–1527.

16 Williamson RC, Buchholtz TW, Malt RA. Humoral stimulation of cell proliferation in small bowel after transection and resection in rats. *Gastroenterology* 1978;75:249–254.

17 Tappenden KA, Thomson AB, Wild GE, McBurney MI. Short-chain fatty acids increase proglucagon and ornithine decarboxylase messenger RNAs after intestinal resection in rats. *JPEN J Parenter Enteral Nutr* 1996;20:357–362.

18 Jirapinyo P, Young C, Srimaruta N, et al. High-fat semielemental diet in the treatment of protracted diarrhea of infancy. *Pediatrics* 1990;86:902–908.

19 Gray G, Santiago N. Disaccharide absorption in normal and diseased human intestine. *Gastroenterology* 1966;51:489.

20 Koruda MJ, Rolandelli RH, Bliss DZ, et al. Parenteral nutrition supplemented with short-chain fatty acids: effect on the small-bowel mucosa in normal rats. *Am J Clin Nutr* 1990;51:685–689.

21 Pirman T, Ribeyre MC, Mosoni L, et al. Dietary pectin stimulates protein metabolism in the digestive tract. *Nutrition* 2007;23:69–75.

22 Finkel Y, Brown G, Smith HL, et al. The effects of a pectin-supplemented elemental diet in a boy with short gut syndrome. *Acta Paediatr Scand* 1990;79:983–986.

23 Rabbani GH, Teka T, Saha SK, et al. Green banana and pectin improve small intestinal permeability and reduce fluid loss in Bangladeshi children with persistent diarrhea. *Dig Dis Sci* 2004;49:475–484.

24 Jeppesen PB, Mortensen PB. Colonic digestion and absorption of energy from carbohydrates and medium-chain fat in small bowel failure. *JPEN J Parenter Enteral Nutr* 1999;23(5 suppl):S101–S105.

25 Quigley EM, Quera R. Small intestinal bacterial overgrowth: roles of antibiotics, prebiotics, and probiotics. *Gastroenterology* 2006;130(2 suppl 1):S78–S90.

26 Jenkins AP, Thompson RP. Trophic effect of Efamol on the rat small-intestinal mucosa. *Clin Sci (Lond)* 1989;77:555–559.

27 Maxton DG, Cynk EU, Jenkins AP, Thompson RP. Effect of dietary fat on the small intestinal mucosa. *Gut* 1989;30:1252–1255.

28 Vanderhoof JA, Blackwood DJ, Mohammadpour H, Park JH. Effect of dietary menhaden oil on normal

growth and development and on ameliorating mucosal injury in rats. *Am J Clin Nutr* 1991;54:346–350.

29 Kollman KA, Lien EL, Vanderhoof JA. Dietary lipids influence intestinal adaptation after massive bowel resection. *J Pediatr Gastroenterol Nutr* 1999;28:41–45.

30 Sagher FA, Dodge JA, Moore R, et al. Modulation of fluid absorption and the secretory response of rat jejunum to cholera toxin by dietary fat. *Gut* 1990;31:1256–1261.

31 Nagy ES, Paris MC, Taylor RG, et al. Colostrum protein concentrate enhances intestinal adaptation after massive small bowel resection in juvenile pigs. *J Pediatr Gastroenterol Nutr* 2004;39:487–492.

32 Bines J, Francis D, Hill D. Reducing parenteral requirement in children with short bowel syndrome: impact of an amino acid-based complete infant formula. *J Pediatr Gastroenterol Nutr* 1998;26:123–128.

33 Ksiazyk J, Piena M, Kierkus J, Lyszkowska M. Hydrolyzed versus nonhydrolyzed protein diet in short bowel syndrome in children. *J Pediatr Gastroenterol Nutr* 2002;35:615–618.

34 McIntyre PB, Fitchew M, Lennard-Jones JE. Patients with a high jejunostomy do not need a special diet. *Gastroenterology* 1986;91:25–33.

35 Cosnes J, Evard D, Beaugerie L, et al. Improvement in protein absorption with a small-peptide-based diet in patients with high jejunostomy. *Nutrition* 1992;8:406–411.

36 Duggan C, Stark AR, Auestad N, et al. Glutamine supplementation in infants with gastrointestinal disease: a randomized, placebo-controlled pilot trial. *Nutrition* 2004;20:752–756.

37 Taylor SF, Sondheimer JM, Sokol RJ, et al. Noninfectious colitis associated with short gut syndrome in infants. *J Pediatr* 1991;119(Pt 1):24–28.

38 Vanderhoof JA, Young RJ. Hydrolyzed versus nonhydrolyzed protein diet in short bowel syndrome in children. *J Pediatr Gastroenterol Nutr* 2004;38:107.

39 O'Keefe SJ. Bacterial overgrowth and liver complications in short bowel intestinal failure patients. *Gastroenterology* 2006;130(2 suppl 1):S67–S69.

40 Buchman AL. Etiology and initial management of short bowel syndrome. *Gastroenterology* 2006;130(2 suppl 1):S5-S15.

41 Hambidge KM. Zinc and diarrhea. *Acta Paediatr Suppl* 1992;381:82–86.

42 Rannem T, Hylander E, Ladefoged K, et al. The metabolism of [75Se]selenite in patients with short bowel syndrome. *JPEN J Parenter Enteral Nutr* 1996;20:412–416.

43 Weizman Z, Schmueli A, Deckelbaum RJ. Continuous nasogastric drip elemental feeding. Alternative for prolonged parenteral nutrition in severe prolonged diarrhea. *Am J Dis Child* 1983;137:253–255.

44 Parker P, Stroop S, Greene H. A controlled comparison of continuous versus intermittent feeding in the treatment of infants with intestinal disease. *J Pediatr* 1981;99:360–364.

18 The Use of Enteral Nutrition in the Adult with Intestinal Failure

Khursheed N. Jeejeebhoy

Key points

- Fluid and electrolyte losses are the main limitation to successful oral-enteral nutrition after intestinal resection.

- Rehydration with isotonic oral rehydration solution and avoidance of excessive free water intake and hypertonic drinks are crucial to maintenance of hydration.

- Hyperphagia with a mixed fat/carbohydrate diet to maximize protein-energy intake and the avoidance of restrictive diets are crucial to maintenance of nutrition. Exception is the role of low fat diets in patients with <150 cm of isolated ileal resection.

- Supplements are necessary for the provision of magnesium, potassium, fat-soluble, and B12 vitamins.

Introduction

The short bowel syndrome refers to the clinical effects of extensive small bowel resection. It includes diarrhea, fluid and electrolyte disturbances, and malabsorption associated with malnutrition. The consequences of a short bowel depend on the extent of resection, site of resection, and presence or absence of a colon.

Despite loss of a major part of the small bowel it is possible to maintain nutrition by the oral-enteral route. The majority of patients with a short bowel can be fed by voluntary oral nutrition and rarely require tube feeding. The subject of enteral nutrition in the adult encompasses a vast area from ICU nutrition to feeding unconscious neurologically injured patients. This chapter will be restricted to the use of the oral-enteral route of nutrition in the short bowel patient.

The rational formulation of successful use of the oral-enteral route in the short bowel patient requires an understanding of the physiological principles of gastrointestinal handling of oral-enteral nutrients and the changes resulting from small bowel resection.

Physiological considerations

Gastric emptying

The rate at which a meal enters the intestine is regulated by the rate of gastric emptying. Gastric emptying of liquids depends on their osmolarity. For digestible solids, the rate of emptying is regulated by particle size. However, of greater importance in relation to the short bowel syndrome, is the fact that chyme entering the distal intestine inhibits gastric emptying [1]. Hence, a distal resection results in rapid, unregulated gastric emptying, and hypersecretion of acid.

Small bowel transit

Motility of the small bowel is three times slower in the ileum than in the jejunum [2]. In addition, the ileocecal valve may slow transit, especially when the ileum has been resected [3].

The adult small bowel absorbs most of the 5–6 liters of endogenous secretions and 2–3 liters of exogenous fluids, which are presented to it each day. The amount reabsorbed in the small intestine depends upon the nature of the meal [4]. With a low osmotic meal of

Intestinal Failure: Diagnosis, Management and Transplantation.
Edited by Alan N. Langnas, Olivier Goulet, Eamonn M.M. Quigley and Kelly A. Tappenden. © 2008 Blackwell Publishing. ISBN 978-1-4051-4637-1.

meat and salad, most of the fluid is absorbed in the jejunum, whereas with a high osmotic meal of milk and doughnuts less is absorbed proximally and more distally. The net absorption of intestinal fluids is less in the jejunum as compared with the ileum. These differences depend partly on the nature of the electrolyte transport processes and partly on the permeability of the intercellular junctions. In general, water absorption is a passive process resulting from the active transport of nutrients and electrolytes. In the jejunum and ileum, the transport of sodium drives the uptake of carbohydrates and amino acids across the intestinal mucosa. In addition, in the ileum there is neutral sodium/chloride absorption. However, net absorption depends, in addition, to the extent of back diffusion of the transported material back into the intestinal lumen through "leaky" intercellular junctions. In the jejunum these junctions are very leaky and thus jejunal contents are always isotonic. Fluid absorption in this region of the bowel is very inefficient when compared with the ileum. It has been estimated that the efficiency of water absorption is 44% and 70% of the ingested load in the jejunum and ileum, respectively. For sodium, the corresponding estimates are 13% and 72%. Hence the ileum is important in the conservation of fluid and electrolytes.

Colon

The colon has the slowest transit, varying between 24 and 150 hours. The intercellular junctions are the tightest in this part of the bowel and the efficiency of water and salt absorption in the colon exceeds 90% [5]. In addition, carbohydrate is fermented in the colon to short-chain fatty acids (SCFAs) which have two important actions. First, SCFAs enhance salt and water absorption [6]. Second, the energy content of malabsorbed carbohydrates is salvaged by being absorbed as SCFAs. Our recent data suggest that in short bowel patients this salvage may be greater than in normals [7]. Thus, the colon becomes an important organ for fluid and electrolyte conservation and for the salvage of malabsorbed energy substrates in patients with a short bowel.

Unique functions of the ileum

The ileum uniquely absorbs vitamin B12 and bile salts. Bile salts are essential for the efficient absorption of fats and fat soluble vitamins. Normally, 90% of the bile salt content of bile is maintained by recycling through the ileum. With ileal resection recycling of bile salts is reduced, the bile salt pool is depleted and fat absorption is reduced. In addition, unabsorbed bile salts, due to ileal insufficiency, reduce the ability of the colon to reabsorb salt and water resulting in diarrhea. If more than 100 cm of the ileum is removed, there is also fat malabsorption and fatty acids entering the colon increase water secretion and diarrhea.

Effects of intestinal resection

Motility

Gastric motility is enhanced following small bowel resection. Although proximal resection does not increase the rate of intestinal transit [8], ileal resection significantly accelerates intestinal transit [9]. In this situation, the colon aids in slowing intestinal transit so that in patients with a short bowel without a colon, a marker fed by mouth was completely excreted in a few hours [10].

Absorption of fluid and electrolytes

The effect of intestinal resection depends upon the extent and site of resection. Proximal resection results in no bowel disturbance because the ileum and colon absorb the increased fluid and electrolyte load efficiently. The remaining ileum continues to absorb bile salts and thus there is little reaching the colon to impede salt and water reabsorption. In contrast, when the ileum is resected, the colon receives a much larger load of fluid and electrolytes and also receives bile salts which reduce its ability to absorb salt and water, resulting in diarrhea. If the colon has also been resected in addition to the ileum, the ability to maintain fluid and electrolyte homeostasis is severely impaired [11].

Absorption of nutrients

Absorption of nutrients occurs throughout the small bowel and the removal of the jejunum alone results in the ileum taking over most of the lost function. In this situation, there is no malabsorption [12]. In contrast even a loss of a 100 cm of ileum causes steatorrhea [13]. The degree of malabsorption increases with the length of resection and the variety of nutrients malabsorbed increases [14,15]. Balance studies of energy absorption showed that the absorption of fat and carbohydrate are equally reduced to between 50% and 75% of intake [16]. However, nitrogen absorption is reduced to a lesser extent than carbohydrates and fats, namely, to 81% of intake.

The data taken as a whole suggest that it is easier to meet needs for energy and nitrogen by increasing oral intake than the needs for electrolytes and divalent ions. A review of the literature prior to the availability of parenteral nutrition showed that resections of up to 33% result in no malnutrition and those up to 50% could be tolerated without special aids but those in excess of 75% required parenteral support to avoid severe malnutrition. In addition to malabsorption, diarrhea results in excessive losses of zinc and selenium, but not copper. Zinc losses have caused immune deficiency and selenium losses have resulted in cardiomyopathy.

Implications for management of short bowel syndrome

Jejunal resection with intact and disease-free ileum and colon

Patients in this category can be fed orally immediately and rarely have any problems. However, disease in the ileum and colon may cause the same loss of function as a resection of these segments of the bowel.

Ileal resection of less than 100 cm with colon largely intact

Patients in this category have so-called bile salt-induced diarrhea, and are best helped by the administration of 4 g of cholestyramine three times a day to bind bile salts left unabsorbed by the resected ileum. Vitamin B12 absorption should be measured and if low supplemental B12 should be provided by intramuscular injection in a dose of 200 ug per month.

Ileal resection of more than 100 to 150 cm with colon largely intact

This group of patients has little difficulty in maintaining nutrition with an oral diet, but has fatty acid diarrhea. For such a patient, fat restriction is mandatory. With this larger resection, the bile salt pool is depleted and cholestyramine is no longer beneficial. Parenteral vitamin B12 replacement is required.

Resection in excess of 150 cm of small bowel and lesser resection with associated colectomy

Patients of this class require the graduated adaptation program as indicated below.

Resection leaving less than 60 cm small bowel or only duodenum: massive bowel resection

Patients in this category need supplemental or total parenteral nutrition at home indefinitely. However many patients, even in this category, may show a surprising degree of adaptation and require less parenteral nutrition and benefit from orally absorbed nutrients. The indication to reduce parenteral nutrition is weight gain beyond the desired limit and the fact that a reduced rate of infusion does not cause electrolyte imbalance and dehydration.

Nutritional treatment

Initial treatment after resection

Control of diarrhea

Diarrhea is caused by a combination of increased secretions, increased motility and osmotic stimulation of water secretion caused by malabsorption of luminal contents. Initially, diarrhea is controlled by keeping the patient nil per os (NPO) to reduce any osmotic component. Gastric hypersecretion can be controlled by the continuous infusion of appropriate doses of proton pump inhibitors such as pantaprazole. In addition, loperamide can be used to slow gastric and intestinal transit. If loperamide does not work, then codeine or phenoxylate may be tried.

Intravenous fluids

In the immediate postoperative period all patients will require intravenous fluids and electrolytes to replace losses. Sodium and potassium chloride as well as magnesium are the most important ions to be replaced and plasma levels of these ions should be monitored frequently. Fluid is infused according to measured losses and to maintain an adequate urine output. The infusion is tapered as oral intake is increased.

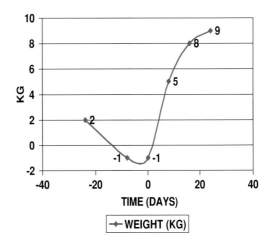

Figure 18.1 Weight gain with nocturnal enteral nutrition. Pattern of weight gain among a group of patients who were unable to maintain weight on oral diet and who developed severe diarrhea on meal feeding. Note weight gain following institution of nocturnal enteral nutrition (time 0). (Data from McIntyre et al. [20].)

Liquid formula diets and tube feeding

It is common practice to start patients who have developed a short bowel acutely on parenteral nutrition and then transition to enteral nutrition rather than progressive oral feeding.

There have been case reports showing that dilute enteral formulations, infused slowly are efficiently absorbed by the short bowel patients. Patients with a short bowel can avoid parenteral nutrition and be able to meet their nutritional needs by the continuous infusion of dilute enteral feeding [17].

In other series, the same objective has been attained by feeding a viscous liquid containing polysaccharides, protein hydrolysate, and tapioca starch [18]. In a study comparing liquid diets of different composition, it was shown that high fat diets reduce water losses from the intestine [19]. However, the question that remains is whether any liquid formula is better than an oral solid diet. In a controlled study in which patients with a very short bowel were fed four different preparations, McIntyre and colleagues [20] have shown that liquid formula diets are not absorbed better than a normal solid diet taken by mouth. Hence, most patents can start oral feeds with a solid diet at an early stage while reducing parenteral infusions. However, if after following the plan indicated below, patients remain malnourished, then nocturnal nasogastric feeding, followed by removal of the tube during the day for ambulation allows nutritional rehabilitation [21] (Figure 18.1).

Oral feeding (Figure 18.2)

Jejunal resection with intact ileum and colon

The next consideration is to determine the nature of oral feeds. In patients who have more than 100 cm of jejunum left, refeeding should be progressive with a view, ultimately, to feeding a normal oral diet. These patients do not need any special diet or formal enteral nutrition.

Ileal resection <150 cm

These patients have diarrhea from bile salt loss into the colon together with diarrhea due to undigested fatty acids entering the colon. These patients need a low fat <30 g/day diet with the addition of cholestyramine 4 g/day to three times a day and supplements of fat-soluble vitamins as given in Table 18.1.

Ileal resection >= 150 cm, with/without colonic resection

These patients malabsorb carbohydrates and fats to the same extent and the problem is mainly inability to maintain fluid and magnesium balance. If they take hypotonic fluids (plain water), they wash out salt from the body and if they take hypertonic fluids (juices), they lose water. Hence, there is the paradox that the more they drink hypo- or hypertonic fluids the more they dehydrate and become thirsty. They do, however, absorb isotonic fluids very well and can avoid

OVERVIEW OF TREATMENT OF SHORT BOWEL

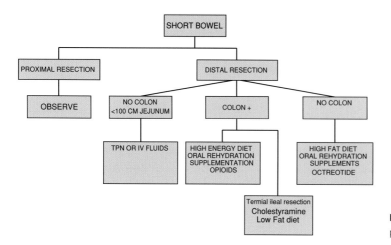

Figure 18.2 Algorithm for management of patients after intestinal resection.

parenteral infusions to maintain hydration by taking isotonic fluids [22]. The initial objective should be small volume isotonic feeds containing a glucose-electrolyte content similar to the oral rehydration solution. The composition of this solution should be glucose 100 mmol/L with sodium chloride 60 mmol/L, sodium citrate 60 mmol/L. In these patients, it has been shown that fluid absorption improves with increasing sodium concentration to a maximum of 120 mmol/L [23]. In addition to providing sufficient sodium to absorb dietary carbohydrate, it is necessary to ingest 10–15 g of sodium chloride as tablets with meals. Such a regimen avoids osmotic stimulation of secretion and yet stimulates the bowel to absorb, thus promoting adapta-

tion. For those with intermediate lengths of remaining bowel, progressive feeding should be attempted with the following plan:

The same carbohydrate/electrolyte feeds, as above, should be started. A mixture of a similar composition has been shown to be well absorbed by patients with massive resection who have previously been dependent on intravenous fluids [22]. The diet should be lactose-free since lactase levels in such patients are reduced [24]. Vitamin B12 absorption should be measured and, if subnormal, injections of 200 micrograms per month should be started. Recently it has been shown that very high dose oral vitamin B12 will maintain normal levels, even in patients with malabsorption. The daily oral dose is 3 mg.

Early observations had suggested that a low fat diet with added medium chain triglyceride (MCT), together with a high carbohydrate content, was better for patients with a short bowel. The theory behind these suggestions was the finding that malabsorbed long chain fatty acids (LCT) can cause colonic water secretion resulting in higher fecal output with steatorrhea and consequently greater loss of divalent ions. However, such studies were not controlled and MCT can also cause osmotic diarrhea. Using a controlled cross-over design in two studies [10,16], we showed that a high-fat diet was comparable to a high-carbohydrate diet in regard to total fluid, energy, nitrogen, sodium, potassium, and divalent ion absorption. We, therefore, recommend a

Table 18.1 Supplements required in patients with intestinal resection.

- Zinc and Selenium losses are high
- Zinc Gluconate 100 mg/d
- Selenium 60–100 g/d
- Malabsorption of Fat soluble vitamins
- Vitamin A 10,000 IU/d
- 1,25 OH Vitamin D 0.25–0.5 g/d
- Vitamin E 1200 IU/d
- Calcium gluconate 1500 mg/d
- Severe osteoporosis
- Pamidronate 30 mg IV/every 3 months

low lactose diet containing high calories from both fat and carbohydrate and a high nitrogen intake. In adults who require about 30 kcals/kg/day, we aim to increase intake gradually to about 60 kcals/kg/day to provide sufficient absorbed calories despite malabsorption. The rationale for this approach is discussed by Woolf et al. [16]. In summary, the diet should be palatable rather than restricted to promote hyperphagia. The key to nutritional success is hyperphagia so as to overcome reduced absorption and allow adequate net absorption of energy and protein.

Micronutrient supplementation

Supplements of potassium, magnesium, and zinc are given while monitoring serum levels. In particular, potassium as gluconate may be added to a concentration of 12 mmol/L in the carbohydrate-electrolyte fluid. In addition, we have found that magnesium glucoheptonate is especially useful as a supplement to correct hypomagnesemia without causing diarrhea. Again, 30 mmol/L is added to the glucose-electrolyte mixture and sipped over the day. In addition, these patients benefit from oral supplementation of vitamins (Table 18.1).

Conclusion

The short bowel syndrome is a very variable condition that can be as mild as that following terminal ileal resection to a very debilitating condition that follows total ileal and colonic resection with an end-jejunostomy. Management varies according to the extent and site of resection and the degree of adaptation of the remaining bowel.

References

1 Malagelada J-R. Gastric, pancreatic and biliary response to a meal. In: Johnson LR, ed. *Physiology of the Gastrointestinal Tract*. New York: Raven Press, 1981.

2 Summers RW, Kent TH, Osborne JW. Effects of drugs, ileal obstruction and irradiation on rat gastrointestinal propulsion. *Gastroenterology* 1970;59:731–739.

3 Ricotta J, Zuidema GD, Gadacz TR, et al. Construction of an ileocecal valve and its role in massive resection

of the small intestine. *Surg Gynecol Obstet* 1981;152:310–314.

4 Fordtran JS, Locklear TW. Ionic constituents and osmolality of gastric and small-intestinal fluids after eating. *Am J Dig Dis* 1966;11:503–521.

5 Powell DW. Intestinal water and electrolyte transport. In: Johnson LR, ed. *Physiology of the Gastrointestinal Tract*. 2nd ed. New York: Raven Press, 1987.

6 Binder HJ, Mehta, P. Short-chain fatty acids stimulate active sodium and chloride absorption in vitro in the rat distal colon. *Gastroenterology* 1989;96:989–996.

7 Royall D, Wolever TMS, Jeejeebhoy KN. Evidence for colonic conservation of malabsorbed carbohydrate in short bowel syndrome. *Am J Gastroenterol* 1992;87:751–756.

8 Nylander G. Gastric evacuation and propulsive intestinal motility following resection of the small intestine in the rat. *Acta Chir Scand* 1967;133:131–138.

9 Reynell PC, Spray GH. Small intestinal function in the rat after massive resections. *Gastroenterology* 1956;31:361–368.

10 Woolf GM, Miller C, Kurian R, Jeejeebhoy KN. Diet for patients with a short bowel: High fat or high carbohydrate? *Gastroenterology* 1983;84:823–828.

11 Cummings JH, James WPT, Wiggins HS. Role of the colon in ileal-resection diarrhea. *Lancet* 1973;1:344–347.

12 Booth CC, Aldis D, Read AE. Studies on the site of fat absorption. 2. Fat balances after resection of varying amounts of small intestine in man. *Gut* 1961;2:168–174.

13 Hoffman AF, Poley JR. Role of bile acid malabsorption in the pathogenesis of diarrhea and steatorrhea in patients with ileal resection. I. Response to cholestyramine or replacement of dietary long-chain triglycerides by medium-chain triglycerides. *Gastroenterology* 1972;62:918–934.

14 Hylander E, Ladefoged K, Jarnum S. Nitrogen absorption following small intestinal resection. *Scand J Gastroenterol* 1980;15:853–858.

15 Ladefoged K, Nicolaidou P, Jarnum S. Calcium, phosphorus, magnesium, zinc and nitrogen balance in patients with severe short bowel syndrome. *Am J Clin Nutr* 1980;33:2137–2144.

16 Woolf GM, Miller C, Kurian R, Jeejeebhoy KN. Nutritional absorption in short bowel syndrome: evaluation of fluid, calorie, and divalent cation requirements. *Dig Dis Sci* 1987;32:8–15.

17 Christie DL, Ament ME. Dilute elemental diet and continuous infusion technique for management of short bowel syndrome. *J Pediatr*. 1975;87:705–708.

18 Levy E, Frileux P, Sandrucci S, et al. Continuous enteral nutrition during the early adaptive stage of

the short bowel syndrome. *Br J Surg* 1988;75:549–553.

19 Simko V, Linscheer WG. Absorption of different elemental diets in a short-bowel syndrome lasting 15 years. *Am J Dig Dis* 1976;21:419–425.

20 McIntyre PB, Fitchew M, Lennard-Jones JE. Patients with a high jejunostomy do not need a special diet. *Gastroenterology* 1986;91:25–33.

21 McIntyre PB, Wood SR, Powell-Tuck J, Lennard-Jones JE. Nocturnal nasogastric tube feeding at home. *Postgrad Med J* 1983;59:767–769.

22 Griffin GE, Fagan EF, Hodgson HJ, Chadwick VS. Enteral therapy in the management of massive gut resection complicated by chronic fluid and electrolyte depletion. *Dig Dis Sci* 1982;27:902–908.

23 Lennard-Jones JE. Oral rehydration solutions in short bowel syndrome. *Clin Ther* 1990;12(suppl A):12129–12137.

24 Richards AJ, Condon JR, Mallinson CN. Lactose intolerance following extensive small intestinal resection. *Br J Surg* 1971;58:493–494.

19

The Enteric Flora in Intestinal Failure

Small Intestinal Bacterial Overgrowth and Gut-Derived Sepsis

Eamonn M.M. Quigley, Rodrigo Quera and Ahmed Abu-Shanab

Key points

- The enteric flora influences a variety of intestinal functions, including the development and maturation of the mucosal barrier and the mucosal immune system.

- Several factors intrinsic to disorders that commonly lead to the development of intestinal failure predispose to bacterial overgrowth and explain its high prevalence in this patient population.

- Bacterial overgrowth may significantly compromise digestive and absorptive functions in intestinal failure and may delay or prevent weaning from TPN.

- Traditional clinical tests for overgrowth may be unreliable in intestinal failure and a therapeutic trial of antibiotic therapy is advocated as a first-line approach.

- Antibiotics remain the foundation of therapy for overgrowth; other approaches, including probiotics, offer potential based on experimental evidence but lack sufficient data from human studies.

The normal flora: a key factor in gut homeostasis

The human gastrointestinal microflora (or microbiota) is a complex ecosystem of approximately 300–500

Intestinal Failure: Diagnosis, Management and Transplantation.
Edited by Alan N. Langnas, Olivier Goulet, Eamonn M.M. Quigley and Kelly A. Tappenden. © 2008 Blackwell Publishing.
ISBN 978-1-4051-4637-1.

bacterial species and comprising nearly two million genes (the "microbiome") [1]. Indeed, the number of bacteria within the gut is about 10 times that of eukaryotic cells in the human body [2,3]. At birth, the entire intestinal tract is sterile; bacteria enter the gut with the first feed. Following infancy, the composition of the intestinal microflora remains relatively constant thereafter.

Because of peristalsis and the antimicrobial effects of gastric acid, the stomach and proximal small intestine contain relatively small numbers of bacteria in healthy subjects; jejunal cultures may not detect any bacteria in as many as 33%. When bacterial species are present, they are usually lactobacilli, enterococci, oral streptococci, and other gram-positive aerobic or facultative anaerobes reflecting the bacterial flora of the oropharynx; coliforms rarely exceed 10^3 CFU/mL in jejunal juice. The microbiology of the terminal ileum represents a transition zone between the jejunum, containing predominantly aerobic species, and the dense population of anaerobes found in the colon (Figure 19.1). Bacterial colony counts may be as high as 10^9 CFU/mL in the terminal ileum immediately proximal to the ileocecal valve, with a predominance of gram-negative organisms and anaerobes. On crossing into the colon, the bacterial concentration and variety of the enteric flora changes dramatically. Concentrations as high as 10^{12} CFU/mL may be found; comprised mainly of anaerobes such as bacteroides, porphyromonas, bifidobacterium, lactobacillus, and clostridium, with anaerobic bacteria outnumbering aerobic bacteria by a factor of 100–1000:1 [2]. At any given level of the gut, the composition of the flora also demonstrates variation along the diameter of the gastrointestinal

The Normal flora

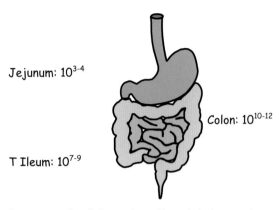

Jejunum: 10^{3-4}

Colon: 10^{10-12}

T Ileum: 10^{7-9}

Figure 19.1 The relative numbers of bacteria in the normal intestine.

tract with certain bacteria tending to be adherent to the mucosal surface while others predominate in the lumen.

The normal enteric bacterial flora influences a variety of intestinal functions and plays a key role in nutrition and angiogenesis as well as in maintaining the integrity of the epithelial barrier and the development of mucosal immunity. Unabsorbed dietary sugars, such as lactose, and alcohols are salvaged by bacterial dissacaridases, converted into short-chain fatty acids (SCFAs) and used as an energy source by the colonic mucosa. SCFAs promote the growth of intestinal epithelial cells and control their proliferation and differentiation. Nutrients and vitamins, such as folate and vitamin K, are produced by enteric bacteria. The relationship between the host's immune system and nonpathogenic flora is important in protecting the host from colonization by pathogenic species. In this regard, intestinal bacteria produce a variety of substances, ranging from relatively nonspecific fatty acids and peroxides to highly specific bacteriocins, which can inhibit or kill other, potentially pathogenic, bacteria. Bacterial metabolism of some medications (such as sulfasalazine), within the intestinal lumen, is essential for the release of their active moieties [4]. Given the critical role of the colonic flora, by virtue of their numbers and diversity, in these homeostatic functions, one

can appreciate the potential impact of colectomy to the individual with compromised small intestinal function; similarly in the patient with an intact colon one should always strive not to disturb the indigenous colonic flora.

In order to achieve the above-mentioned functions, the bacterial flora provides regulatory signals that condition the development and function of the gut [5,6]. In germ-free animals, villi are longer and more uniform and crypts shorter than normal, digestive enzyme activity and local cytokine production are reduced and the development of the mucosa- or gut-associated lymphoid tissue (MALT or GALT), lamina propria cellularity and mucosal vascularity are impaired [7].

The delicate balance between host and luminal environment is central to intestinal homeostasis. The intestinal epithelium is exposed, on a daily basis, to the bacterial antigens of the commensal microflora, which, in turn, induce a state of controlled inflammation. This, physiological, response to bacterial antigens is not harmful to the host and generates both the induction of immune tolerance [8,9] and the secretion of immunoglobulin A (IgA). Antibodies produced against antigenic components of the normal flora are sometimes referred to as "natural" antibodies. In disease states, a pro-inflammatory response to these same luminal antigens leads to the development of such disorders as celiac sprue and inflammatory bowel disease. Through interactions with the host immune system, the flora promotes an appropriate response to antigenic stimuli; in this manner, the enteric flora has also been proposed to assist in preventing allergies [10].

Small intestinal bacterial overgrowth: definition, pathogenesis and prevalence

SIBO is usually defined as an overgrowth of $>10^5$ colony forming units (CFUs) per mL of bacteria in the proximal small bowel [11,12]. Other authors have entertained the diagnosis of SIBO in the presence of lower colony counts ($>10^3$ CFU/mL), provided that the species of bacteria isolated from the jejunal aspirate are those that normally colonize the large bowel or providing that the same species are absent from saliva

Table 19.1 Etiological factors associated with small bowel bacterial overgrowth.

Disordered anatomy
- Diverticula
- Surgical blind loops
- Small bowel obstruction
- Intestinal resection with dilatation
- Loss of ileocolonic (ileocecal) valve (sphincter)
- Enterocolic fistula
- Stricture(s)

Motor disorders
- Chagasic megacolon
- Chronic intestinal pseudo-obstruction
- Autonomic neuropathy
- Amyloidosis
- Hypothyroidism
- Scleroderma
- Vagotomy effects on motility

Immunological factors
- Immunodeficiency
- Malnutrition
- Iatrogenic
  - Corticosteroids
  - Antibiotics
  - Oral contraceptives

Non-immune mechanisms
- Achlorhydria/hypochlorhydria
- Exocrine pancreatic insufficiency
- Bile salt deficiency
- Malabsorption syndromes

and gastric juice. [12] Contaminating flora in small intestinal bacterial overgrowth (SIBO) commonly feature both oropharyngeal and colonic-type bacteria, including streptococci (71%), escherichia coli (69%), staphylococci (25%), micrococci (22%), and klebsiella (20%) [13,14]. One or more of the mechanisms that normally prevent overgrowth (Table 19.1) is often compromised in patients with intestinal failure [15,16]. In a rat model, Nieuwenhuijs and colleagues reported that the migrating motor complex (MMC), often referred to as the housekeeper of the gut, was critical to the prevention of bacterial overgrowth in the

upper small bowel [17]. Disruption of the MMC appears to be the main factor leading to the development of SIBO in patients with radiation enteropathy and acute pancreatitis [18,19]. Although motor adaptation does occur in the shortened intestine, motility remains abnormal [20] and may contribute to overgrowth. Although the ileocecal valve forms a physical barrier to reflux of colonic material from the colon into the small bowel, results from both experimental animal models [21,22] and human studies [23] have failed to identify a major effect on either bacterial translocation or SIBO following resection of the valve. It would appear that specialized motor patterns in the distal ileum, and not the valve itself, are the critical elements in sustaining the propulsive functions of this region [24,25]. SIBO has also been well documented as a cause of diarrhea and malnutrition among apparently healthy elderly subjects [26–28]. Diseases that commonly result in intestinal failure such as radiation enteritis [18], Crohn's disease [29], and scleroderma [30] are associated with SIBO. The prevalence of SIBO in the short bowel syndrome has varied considerably [21,22,31,32], depending on whether or not the colon remained in continuity [31], the terminal ileum [21], or the ileocecal valve had been resected [22] or whether or not distal intestinal obstruction was present [32].

Diagnosis

Although aspiration and direct culture of jejunal contents are regarded by many as the gold standards for the diagnosis of SIBO [33], these methods have several limitations, such as the potential for contamination by oropharyngeal bacteria during intubation, and may lead to an over diagnosis of SIBO syndrome in older, asymptomatic, subjects. By contrast, bacterial overgrowth may be patchy and thus missed by a single aspiration. Overall, the reproducibility of jejunal aspiration and culture has been reported to be as low as 38%, in comparison to 92% for breath tests. In addition, intubation methods may be regarded as cumbersome and invasive for patients with nonspecific symptoms or for those who may require repeated testing. As a result of these limitations, the use of breath tests has largely replaced jejunal aspiration, in clinical practice.

These, noninvasive, tests are largely based on the excretion, in exhaled breath, of hydrogen generated by the metabolism of carbohydrate by luminal bacteria [34,35]. Sensitivities for breath tests, in the diagnosis of SIBO, range from 70 to 90%, specificities have been less consistent, ranging from as low as 40 to as high as 100%. In general, it is believed that the glucose hydrogen breath test has a higher sensitivity than the lactulose breath test. Glucose is readily absorbed in the small bowel and, therefore, does not reach the colon; the diagnostic confusion caused, in the interpretation of the lactulose breath test by accelerated small intestinal transit, can thus be avoided [34–40]. In these breath tests, the diagnosis of SIBO is usually established when the exhaled breath H_2 increases by more than 10, or 12 [34], parts per million (ppm) over baseline on two consecutive samplings. A fasting breath hydrogen level that exceeds 20 ppm is also considered suggestive of SIBO. Indeed, the reliability of these diagnostic techniques has been criticized in patients with intestinal failure, and especially those with short bowel syndrome, because of the rapid intestinal transit that accompanies these disorders. For this reason, the combination of lactulose breath test with scintigraphy has been advocated and while this approach may increase test specificity to 100%, sensitivity remains low at 38.9% [40].

Although bacterial overgrowth is, undoubtedly, common in intestinal failure, its diagnosis may be difficult. For example, the interpretation of breath tests may be complicated, in patients with short bowel syndrome, not only by rapid transit but also by carbohydrate malabsorption and a resultant premature delivery of unabsorbed carbohydrate to the colon where it will undergo fermentation. Again, any condition that impairs the digestion or absorption of sugars and carbohydrates in the small intestine can produce an abnormal hydrogen breath test when dietary sugars, that is, glucose, are used for testing. Therefore, conditions other than SIBO, such as pancreatic insufficiency and celiac sprue, can result in abnormal breath tests.

It must also be borne in mind that false-negative or "flat" responses to lactulose administration may be found among those whose bacterial flora has been altered by antibiotic therapy or diarrhea or in whom motility disorders coexist; situations commonly present in patients with intestinal failure. Finally, between 15 and 27% of the population do not generate hydrogen, following the ingestion of lactulose but, rather, produce methane; the measurement of hydrogen alone will clearly underestimate the prevalence of SIBO among such individuals. The combined measurement of hydrogen and methane will, in contrast, permit the detection of those who harbor Methanobrevibacter smithii [41–43].

The presence of SIBO is suggested by an acidic stool pH, the development of D-lactic acidosis, increased levels of SCFAs or keto-bile acids in duodenal fluid or elevated urinary concentrations of 4-hydroxyphenylacetic acid; none of these assays has become a part of the routine diagnostic assessment of SIBO. Imaging studies, and especially radiographic studies of the small intestine, do not diagnose SIBO but play an important role in the definition of underlying predisposing causes of SIBO, such as strictures, malrotation, diverticulosis, fistulae and pseudo-obstruction.

An alternative approach to the diagnosis of SIBO is the therapeutic trial. Initial studies employing this strategy suggested that patients with SIBO should demonstrate a symptomatic response within one week of therapy with tetracycline administered in a dose of 250 mg four times a day [16]. More recent studies indicate that as many as 60% will not respond to this particular regime; other antibiotics (detailed later) may prove more effective though few, if any, have been critically assessed in this context. Nevertheless, given the technical and interpretative difficulties, described earlier, associated with current diagnostic techniques, it should come as no surprise that many advocate the therapeutic trial as a viable alternative to diagnostic testing [44].

The diagnostic approach to SIBO should be based, first and foremost, on clinical assessment: does the patient have symptoms, signs, or clinical findings that suggest SIBO, or, as is commonly the case, is this simply an instance of small intestinal bacterial contamaination without clinical consequences? If the former is suspected, culture of intestinal contents remains the test of choice in the context of intestinal failure. Because of the risks, such as C difficile infection, attendant on unnecessary courses of antibiotic therapy, empriric use of antibiotics should be resisted in this patient population.

Consequences of small intestinal bacterial overgrowth

Morphological and metabolic effects

SIBO may influence gut function through direct and indirect mechanisms. Deconjugation of bile acids in the proximal small bowel will disrupt fat digestion and lead to the production of lithocholic acid, which is poorly absorbed and may be directly toxic to enterocytes [45]. Biopsies from the descending duodenum may reveal reductions in villus height, crypt depth and total mucosal thickness and increased intra-epithelial lymphocytes; abnormalities that are reversible following successful therapy. Morphological changes may also occur secondary to cobalamin deficiency [46]. Enterocyte injury leads to both a loss of activity of brush border disaccharidases and altered permeability [47], the latter predisposing to the development of a protein-losing enteropathy [48].

Bacteria may compete with the host for protein and lead to the production of ammonia [49]. In the context of an impaired mucosal barrier, encephalopathy may result, as suggested by the recently reported case of recurrent encephalopathy, in an intestinal transplant recipient, which resolved following resection of an intestinal stricture [50], which, presumably, led to the eradication of SIBO. Moreover, short bowel syndrome patients, especially those with an intact colon, may suffer D-lactic acidemia and encephalopathy, on administration of enteral nutrition, as a result of the production of D-lactic acid by gram-positive anaerobes [51,52]. The development of neurological symptoms, such as somnolence, ataxia or altered behavior in a patient with short bowel syndrome should lead one suspect D-lactic acidosis [53].

Nutritional consequences

The syndrome of SIBO is characterized, in its florid form, by diarrhea and weight loss. Malabsorption of nutrients and some vitamins commonly occurs. Fat malabsorption that, in turn, will further delay oro-cecal transit through the activation of the "ileal brake" [54] leads to steatorrhea and deficiencies in fat-soluble vitamins. Carbohydrate malabsorption, consequent on SIBO, can contribute to diarrhea due to metabolism of malabsorbed carbohydrates by bacteria to form SCFAs that, in turn, increase the osmolarity of intestinal fluid. Although some degree of hypoproteinemia is common in SIBO, severe malnutrition is rare, in the absence of other intestinal disease. Cobalamin (vitamin B_{12}) deficiency occurs commonly in SIBO as a result of utilization of the vitamin by anaerobic bacteria; the only bacteria that can utilize vitamin B_{12} once coupled to intrinsic factor. SIBO also may also result in a reduction in bone mineral density, especially in vulnerable age groups [55,56]. Levels of both folate and vitamin K are, however, usually normal or elevated in the context of SIBO as a result of bacterial synthesis of these vitamins. The clinical and nutritional consequences of SIBO in short bowel syndrome depend on the clinical context; in the patient with a remnant, which is marginal for independent existence or in whom adaptation has been compromised [57], the superimposition of SIBO may prove nutritionally devastating.

Immunological effects

SIBO, not surprisingly, may exert immune effects: luminal concentrations of IgA_2, IgM and interleukin-6, but not IFN-γ and TNF-α and lamina propria IgA plasma cell and intra-epithelial lymphocyte counts are increased in the proximal small intestine [58,59]. Lamina propria T- and B-cell populations are unaltered [14,60]. Of interest, given reported overlap between SIBO and celiac sprue [61,62], elevated luminal levels of IgA anti-gliadin antibodies were documented, in one study, in 6 of 17 patients with SIBO [63].

SIBO may also be associated, locally, with defective complement activation [64] and with decreased circulating levels of IgG_3 [65]. Through dysfunctional interactions between the flora and the host immune system, the intestinal flora is also known to play an important role in the pathogenesis of inflammatory bowel disease [66], an important cause of intestinal failure in the adult.

Bacterial translocation and gut-derived sepsis

The possible contributions of SIBO to bacterial translocation and sepsis are key issues in intestinal failure, a disorder where sepsis is an important cause of morbidity and mortality, as bacterial migration to extraintestinal sites is regarded as central to the development of gut-derived sepsis.

Bacterial translocation is defined as the passage of viable bacteria from the gastrointestinal tract to extraintestinal sites, such as the mesenteric lymph node complex, liver, spleen, kidney, and bloodstream [67]. Although the traditional definition of bacterial translocation has been based on the culture of viable bacteria from mesenteric lymph nodes, more recent studies have shown that intestinal bacterial translocation can be detected by the polymerase chain reaction [68,69], which recognizes bacterial DNA alone. The presence of bacterial DNA in serum and ascitic fluid has recently been proposed as a relatively non-invasive surrogate marker of bacterial translocation in the clinical setting [70,71]. Moreover, Albillos and colleagues reported that, in their cirrhotic patients, endotoxin from nonviable bacteria promoted many of the pathophysiological mechanisms previously attributed to the translocation of live bacteria [72].

Experimental animal models have shown that bacterial translocation may be promoted by mucosal inflammation, intestinal obstruction, ischemia and hypo-perfusion injury, acute pancreatitis, prematurity, burns, trauma, and liver disease. Several studies confirm a high prevalence of translocation in the context of cirrhosis, a disorder that frequently complicates or accompanies intestinal failure, and even in the early stages of the disease, before the development of ascites [73–78].

In SIBO, increased intestinal permeability and impaired host immune defense are considered to be the primary mechanisms which promote bacterial translocation [7]. However, experimental and human studies have failed to confirm a relationship between bacterial translocation and intestinal permeability [79–81]. These observations imply, instead, a role for a distinct, presumably transcellular [79], mechanism of transport for bacteria across the intestinal barrier. It is evident that rates of translocation for the various constituents of the indigenous flora vary considerably, with pseudomonas aeruginosa, klebsiella pneumoniae, escherichia coli, and proteus mirabilis demonstrating the greatest aptitude for traversing the intestinal epithelium [82]. In healthy individuals, bacterial translocation and transference occur continuously; translocated bacteria and their particulate products being phagocytosed by the gut-associated lymphoid tissue. However, when the intestine is diseased or anatomically changed, as is the case in most patients with intestinal failure, the host could, in theory, be overwhelmed by the sheer concentration of organisms which may translocate from the contaminated intestine.

The term gut-derived sepsis is used to describe a state of systemic inflammation and organ dysfunction associated with severe catabolic stress; it has been hypothesized that this syndrome is initiated and perpetuated by the intestinal microflora. Although the gut plays a role in the development of sepsis syndrome and multiple organ failure, recent studies have shown that gut-derived-bacteremia, even when caused by potent nosocomial pathogens, is an event of low pro-inflammatory potential and is, of itself, an insufficient stimulus for the systemic inflammatory response and organ failure state typically seen after severe and prolonged catabolic stress [83]. This is not to dismiss a role for the intestinal flora but to state that their role in the pathophysiology of this syndrome may have more to do with bacteria-induced alterations in the immune function of the gut and consequent interactions between the gut-associated immune tissue and the rest of the body [83,84], rather than to direct translocation [85,86]. The status of translocation in man, as distinct from experimental animal models, remains to be defined.

Central venous infection is the most prevalent infectious complication among patients with intestinal failure on total parenteral nutrition (TPN) [87]. Although catheter sepsis is often associated with the isolation of enteric organisms, skin commensals are also prevalent [88]. Moreover, the presence of enteric organisms in the bloodstream does not necessarily impugn bacterial overgrowth and translocation; diarrhea, so common in this population, may lead to the colonization of skin by enteric flora [15]; of interest, it has been shown that a prior episode of translocation could generate an effective host defense response against a second episode

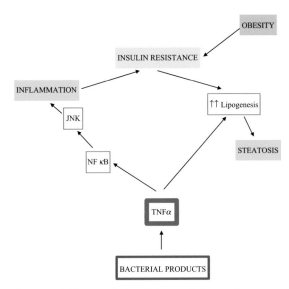

Figure 19.2 The contribution of the enteric flora to the pathogenesis of Non-Alcoholic Fatty Liver Disease (NAFLD). Note: This figure illustrates the main components of Non-Alcoholic Steatohepatitis (NASH) in the obese individual: inflammation and lipogenesis, secondary to insulin resistance.

The role of the enteric flora is though to be mediated through the generation of Tumor Necrosis Factor alpha (TNF α) which, acting through intermediaries NF κB and JNK, not only promotes inflammation in the liver, but also contributes to lipogenesis, the other hallmark of this condition.

of translocation induced by intestinal overgrowth with the same bacterial strain [89].

Systemic consequences

The enteric flora may also play a role in the pathogenesis of the liver abnormalities that frequently complicate parenteral nutrition-dependent intestinal failure, such as non-alcoholic fatty liver disease (NAFLD) [90,91]. Indeed, tumor necrosis factor α, whose release may be triggered by translocating bacteria, has been implicated in the pathogenesis of NAFLD [90–94]. (Figure 19.2) Furthermore, endogenous production of ethanol and lipolysaccharidases (LPS), by intestinal bacteria, may activate hepatic macrophages through the toll-like receptor (TLR) 4 [95], leading to the release of hepatotoxic factors, such as tumor necrosis factor α [96,97]. These observations may have therapeutic implications, given the recent observation, in both an experimental animal model [98] and an uncontrolled

human study [99], that the administration of probiotics and prebiotics may ameliorate the hepatic injury associated with NAFLD and the earlier observation of the amelioration of this syndrome, in intestinal failure, by the administration of antibiotics [100], perhaps medicated through a reduction in translocation [101].

The clinical features of SIBO

The principal symptoms of SIBO are diarrhea, steatorrhea, abdominal bloating and distension (often exacerbated by the intake of sugars, other carbohydrates and fiber), abdominal pain, flatulence and fatigue. These symptoms are non-specific and may enjoy a wide differential diagnosis in the intestinal failure patient; that SIBO can contribute to symptomatology in this patient population is supported by the demonstration of a parallel improvement in gastrointestinal symptoms and breath tests after antibiotic therapy, among intestinal failure patients with positive breath tests [29,31].

Management of small intestinal bacterial overgrowth in intestinal failure

The approach to the management of SIBO may be summarized under three headings [102]:
1 Reversal or removal of any predisposing condition(s).
2 Appropriate nutritional support/replacement.
3 Suppression or eradication of the contaminating bacterial flora.

Reversal or removal of any predisposing condition(s)

Clearly, the primary goal of therapy in intestinal failure and SIBO should be the treatment or correction of any underlying disease or defect when possible. Unfortunately, for many patients with intestinal failure, reversibility is simply not possible. Of the various surgical approaches advocated to improve digestive function in the short-bowel syndrome, such as the creation of reversed bowel segments, intestinal tapering and lengthening, or the construction of valves or recirculating loops, few, if any, have been shown to confer long-term benefit [103]. Some, indeed, may result in short-term impairments in motor and absorptive function [104]. Many promote stasis and may, therefore, lead to bacterial overgrowth.

Intestinal transplantation is the one therapeutic option that could entirely restore intestinal function to the patient with intestinal failure. As detailed elsewhere in this volume, rejection and sepsis, often inextricably linked, remain the major causes of morbidity and mortality among graft recipients. The enteric flora is frequently implicated; it has been suggested, for example, that rejection-induced changes in intestinal permeability promote bacterial translocation thus leading to systemic sepsis [105]. Here again, bacterial contamination, if present, could set the stage for the precipitation of sepsis. Apart from those that can be addressed surgically, underlying or exacerbating conditions that may prove amenable to reversal or treatment include intestinal infectious, hypothyroidism, inflammatory bowel disease, immunodeficiency states, and the use of gastric acid suppressants [37].

For those in whom intestinal stasis is present and, especially, where intestinal dysmotility is a prominent factor, as in chronic intestinal pseudo-obstruction, prokinetic agents would appear to offer considerable therapeutic potential. Although there is some evidence for efficacy for prokinetics, such as cisapride and erythromycin in particular, in chronic intestinal pseudo-obstruction [106–108], the ability of these agents to reduce bacterial contamination in this disorder, has been scarcely studied. In one small study, the somatostatin analog, octreotide, which induces migrating motor complex-like activity in the small intestine [109–111], was shown to reduce symptoms and breath-hydrogen excretion in patients with scleroderma [112]; a subsequent study, in an experimental animal model, failed to replicate this effect [113]. This may be explained by the observation that the net effect of this agent, in man, is to delay, and not accelerate, transit [111]. Both animal and human studies have demonstrated the ability of cisapride to reduce bacterial overgrowth in another context: chronic liver disease [76,114–116]; this agent is, however, no longer available.

Appropriate nutritional support/replacement

SIBO is an important determinant of nutritional status in intestinal failure. Kaufman and colleagues found that bacterial contamination was one of the predictors of failure to wean children with short-bowel syndrome off TPN; among seven patients who remained dependent on TPN, all had SIBO, whereas only 23 of 42 children who were successfully weaned from TPN had evidence of overgrowth [117]. It must be conceded, however, that as overgrowth is more likely among those with the shortest intestinal remnants, this latter factor, rather than SIBO, may have been the determinant of inability to come off TPN. The management of the patient with SIBO, in any context, must include the correction of any nutritional deficiencies. Among those with intestinal failure this is usually achieved by TPN; among those being weaned from TPN, or who acquire <75% of their nutritional requirements from TPN, the addition of supplemental fat-soluble vitamins, vitamin B_{12}, and certain minerals may be indicated, in the presence of SIBO.

In terms of enteral feeding, consideration needs to be given, not only to the correction of deficiencies but also to the use of those nutrients that will minimize symptoms and losses from diarrhea. Given the effects of SIBO on brush border enzymes, a strict grain-free, lactose- and sucrose-free diet may be of benefit. Fat and calorie intake can be optimized by the use of medium-chain triglycerides.

Suppression or eradication of the contaminating bacterial flora

Antibiotic therapy

The objective of antibiotic therapy in SIBO is not so much to eradicate the bacterial flora but rather to modify it in a manner that results in symptomatic improvement. Although, ideally, the choice of antimicrobial agent should reflect in vitro susceptibility testing, this is usually impractical as many different bacterial species, with different antibiotic sensitivities, typically coexist [13]. Antibiotic treatment remains, therefore, primarily empirical. The polymicrobial nature of the contaminating flora usually requires the administration of broad-spectrum antibiotics [102],

Table 19.2 Antibiotic therapy for SIBO.

- Amoxicillin-clavulanic acid (500 mg TID)
- Ciprofloxacin (250 mg BID)
- Chloramphenicol (250 mg QID)
- Doxycycline (100 mg BID)
- Metronidazole (250 mg TID)
- Neomycin (500 mg BID)
- Norfloxacin (800 mg/day)
- Tetracycline (250 mg QID)
- Trimethroprim-sulfamethoxazole (1 double-strength tablet BID)
- Rifaxamin (400 mg TID)

which can cover both aerobic and anaerobic enteric bacteria [37,102,118,119]. Various regimes have been proposed and are listed in Table 19.2.

Bouhnik and colleagues showed that amoxicillin-clavulanic acid and cefoxitin were effective against over 90% of isolated species in SIBO, indicating that they were suitable candidates for first line therapy [13]. Although a single, short (7- to 10-day) course of an antibiotic has been shown to improve symptoms for up to several months in between 46 and 90% and render breath tests negative in 20–75% of all patients with SIBO, those in whom SIBO complicates intestinal failure may prove more refractory to antibiotic therapy and may require either repeated (e.g. the first 5 to 10 days out of every months) or continuous courses of antibiotic therapy [120]. For the latter, rotating antibiotic regimens are recommended, in order to prevent the development of resistance. Where small bowel abnormalities cannot be rectified, rotating courses of antibiotics are often employed [11]. More recently, the introduction of broad-spectrum, poorly absorbable antibiotics, such as rifaximin, has presented a safe and effective alternative to the treatment of SIBO with a low risk of causing microbial resistance [121].

Decisions on management should be individualized and must consider such risks of long-term antibiotic therapy as diarrhea, clostridium difficile infection, intolerance, and bacterial resistance, as well as cost. For these reasons, norfloxacin, amoxicillin-clavulanic acid and metronidazole are excellent options. Despite their narrow antibacterial spectrum, fluoroquinolones are

effective against overgrowth by aeroanaerobic rods [122], thus supporting the hypothesis that anaerobic growth in the proximal intestine is, in turn, regulated by the aerobic flora [123]. In one of only a few randomized studies of antibiotic therapy for bacterial overgrowth in short bowel patients, Attar and colleagues found both norfloxacin and amoxicillin-clavulanic acid to be effective in improving diarrhea and reducing breath-hydrogen excretion. It was interesting to note, however, that despite this excellent symptomatic response, not all patients normalized breath hydrogen excretion [124]. Among patients with the short bowel syndrome antibiotic therapy may fail completely, indicating a need for alternative strategies in this clinical context [125]. Antibiotic therapy may also prove effective in the prevention or therapy of complications of SIBO such as liver disease [126] and D-lactic acidosis [127,128]. Whether antibiotic therapy, or even bowel decontamination, can prevent overgrowth, translocation and related sepsis following intestinal transplantation remains to be defined [129,130]. Selective decontamination, an approach that attempts to suppress gram-negative and pathogenic flora and fungi by using antibiotic and antifungal combinations, has been employed in an attempt to prevent sepsis of gastrointestinal origin in relation to neturopenia [131], critical illness [132,133], cirrhosis [134], liver failure [135], pancreatitis [136,137] and transplantation [138]. Although this approach has resulted in the expected bacteriological changes, the impact on the prevalence of clinical infections has been more variable and concerns have also been raised regarding the potential for the development of rebound colonization and antibiotic resistance [139]. Although this approach has not been tested in a prospective or randomized manner in the context of intestinal failure, it would appear to be a reasonable strategy in those in whom symptoms and signs can be attributed to SIBO and in whom mono-therapy has failed.

Prebiotics and synbiotics

Prebiotics are defined as nondigestible but fermentable foods that beneficially affect the host by selectively stimulating the growth and activity of one species, or a limited number of species, of bacteria in the colon [140] (Table 19.3). Compared with probiotics, which introduce exogenous bacteria into the human colon,

Table 19.3 Prebiotic oligosaccharidases.

- Fructo-oligosaccharidases
- Galacto-oligosaccharidases
- Gentio-oligosaccharidases
- Inulin
- Isomalto-oligosaccharidases
- Lactulose
- Lactosucrose
- Soybean oligosaccharidases
- Xilo-oligosaccharidases

Table 19.4 Microorganisms used as probiotics agents.

Lactobacillus species
- L. acidophilus
- L. bulgaricus
- L. casei (rhamnosus)
- L. johnsonii
- L. lactis
- L. plantarum
- L. reuteri

Bifidobacterium species
- B. adolescentis
- B. bifidum
- B. breve
- B. infantis
- B. lactis
- B. longum

Other species
- Bacillus cereus
- Enterococcus faecalis
- Escherichia coli
- Saccharomyces boulardii
- Saccharomyces cerevisiae
- Streptococcus thermophilus

prebiotics stimulate the preferential growth of a limited number of health-promoting commensal flora, especially, but not exclusively, lactobacilli and bifidobacteria [141–143]. The oligosaccharides in human breast milk are considered the prototypic prebiotics as they facilitate the preferential growth of bifidobacteria and lactobacilli in the colon in exclusively breast-fed neonates [144,145].

There is little or no data on their use in either intestinal failure or SIBO. However, evidence accumulates to support a role for prebiotics, either alone, or in combination with a probiotic (a synbiotic), in the prevention of translocation and sepsis in liver disease and hepatic encephalopathy [78,146–149].

Probiotics

Probiotics, derived from the Greek and meaning "for life," are defined as live organisms that, when ingested in adequate amounts, exert a health benefit on the host [150]. The most widely available probiotics are lactic acid bacteria and nonpathogenic yeasts (Table 19.4). Although probiotics have been proposed for use in inflammatory, infectious, neoplastic and allergies disorders, the ideal probiotic strain for any one of these indications has yet to be defined [151]. Although probiotic "cocktails" have also been advocated to maximize effect, it needs to be noted that some probiotic combinations have been shown to prove antagonistic in certain situations [152,153]. Guidelines for routine clinical use of probiotics are confounded by insufficient data to guide optimum strain selection, dose, mode of delivery, and methods for monitoring efficacy [153]. Experimental studies have revealed several potential mechanisms of action for probiotics.

Thus, competition with pathogens, production of bacteriocins, inhibition of bacterial translocation, enhancement of mucosal barrier function, and signaling between the luminal bacterium, the intestinal epithelium and the immune system have all been reported as possible modes of action for a number of probiotic strains [153–160]. Probiotics have been shown to enhance epithelial barrier function through both direct effects on mucin expression, proteins of the cytoskeleton and intercellular tight junctions and indirect effects emanating from the interactions between the bacterium, the mucosa and the mucosa-associated lymphoid tissue [161–163]. Any one, or all, of the above probiotic effects could be of benefit to the patient with SIBO and/or intestinal failure. In experimental models of the short bowel syndrome, bifidobacterium lactis reduced the rate of translocation [164,165].

Although evidence for efficacy for probiotics in various diseases, including necrotizing enterocolitis in infants [166–168] continues to accumulate, data in intestinal failure is scanty. Based on their study in children with bacterial overgrowth associated with short bowel syndrome, Young and Vanderhoof suggested that lactobacillus plantarum 299v may either prevent or delay symptom recurrence following antibiotic therapy [169]. In one randomized, double-blind trial among 12 patients with bacterial overgrowth-related chronic diarrhea, both Lactobacillus casei and acidophilus strains cerela proved effective [170], in others, lactobacillus fermentum [171] and saccharomyces boulardii [124] proved ineffective.

Probiotics may also be beneficial for those with complications related to SIBO in intestinal failure: the combination of a probiotic and kanamycin proved effective in a case of recurrent encephalopathy caused by D-lactic acidosis [172] and experimental models have suggested a role for probiotics in NAFLD [98].

Could probiotics have a role in the prevention of sepsis related to surgery or even intestinal transplantation in the patient with intestinal failure? Direct studies are lacking on this issue; whereas experimental animal studies indicate a potential for the administration of a variety of probiotics to reduce translocation and even sepsis associated with a variety of surgical procedures [173–175], limited studies in man have produced conflicting findings [176–178]. Probiotics are, for the most part, well tolerated [179], with infection rates as low as 0.05% to 0.4% being reported in relation to the administration of lactobacillus and bifidobacterium species [180,181].

Probiotics appear, therefore, to possess a number of properties that could be of benefit in bacterial overgrowth and intestinal failure; their introduction into the therapeutic armamentarium must await, however, the results of well-conducted clinical trials.

Acknowledgment

Supported by grants from Science Foundation Ireland (SFI).

References

1 Xu J, Gordon JI. Honor thy symbionts. *Proc Natl Acad Sci USA* 2003;100:10452–10459.

2 Simon GL, Gorbach SL. The human intestinal microflora. *Dig Dis Sci* 1986;31:147–162.

3 Bengmark S. Ecological control of the gastrointestinal tract. The role of probiotic flora. *Gut* 1998;42:2–7.

4 Guarner F, Malagelada JR. Gut flora in health and disease. *Lancet* 2003;361:512–519.

5 Neish AS. The gut microflora and intestinal epithelial cells: a continuing dialogue. *Microbes Infect* 2002;4:309–317.

6 Rakoff-Nahoum S, Paglino J, Eslami-Varzaneh F, et al. Recognition of commensal microflora by toll-like receptors is required for intestinal homeostasis. *Cell* 2004;118:229–241.

7 Shanahan F. The host-microbe interface within the gut. *Best Pract Res Clin Gastroenterol* 2002;16:915–931.

8 Weiner HL. Oral tolerance, an active immunologic process mediated by multiple mechanisms. *J Clin Invest* 2000;106:935–937.

9 Sartor RB. Mucosal immunology and mechanisms of gastrointestinal inflammation. In: Feldman M, Friedman LS, Brandt LJ, eds. *Sleisenger and Fordtran's Gastrointestinal and Liver Disease: Pathophysiology, Diagnosis, Management.* 8th ed. Philadelphia: WB Saunders Co, 2006;27–66.

10 Björkstén B, Sepp E, Julge K, et al. Allergy development and the intestinal microflora during the first year of life. *J Allergy Clin Immunol* 2001;108:516–520.

11 Singh VV, Toskes PP. Small bowel overgrowth: Presentation, diagnosis, and treatment. *Curr Treat Options Gastroenterol* 2004;7:19–28.

12 Bauer TM, Steinbrückner B, Brinkmann FE, et al. Small intestinal bacterial overgrowth in patients with cirrhosis: prevalence and relation with spontaneous bacterial peritonitis. *Am J Gastroenterol* 2001;96:2962–2967.

13 Bouhnik Y, Alain S, Attar A, et al. Bacterial populations contaminating the upper gut in patients with small intestinal overgrowth syndrome. *Am J Gastroenterol* 1999;94:1327–1331.

14 Riordan SM, McIver CJ, Wakefield D, et al. Small intestinal mucosal immunology and morphometry in luminal overgrowth of indigenous gut flora. *Am J Gastroenterol* 2001;96:494–500.

15 Vanderhoof JA, Langnas AN. Short-bowel syndrome in children and adults. *Gastroenterology* 1997;113:1767–1778.

16 Gregg CR, Toskes PP. Enteric bacterial flora and small bowel bacterial overgrowth syndrome. In: Feldman M, Friedman LS, Sleisenger MH, eds. *Sleisenger and Fordtran's Gastrointestinal and Liver Disease. Pathophysiology/Diagnosis/Management.* 7th ed. Philadelphia: WB Saunders Co, 2002;1783–1793.

17 Nieuwenhuijs VB, Verheem A, van Duijvenbode-Beumer H, et al. The role of interdigestive small bowel motility in the regulation of gut microflora, bacterial overgrowth, and bacterial translocation in rats. *Ann Surg* 1998;228:188–193.

18 Husebye E, Skar V, Hoverstad T, et al. Abnormal intestinal motor patterns explain enteric colonization with gram-negative bacilli in late radiation enteropathy. *Gastroenterology* 1995;109:1078–1089.

19 Van Felius ID, Akkermans LM, Bosscha K, et al. Interdigestive small bowel motility and duodenal bacterial overgrowth in experimental acute pancreatitis. *Neurogastroenterol and Motil* 2003;15:267–276.

20 Quigley EMM, Thompson JS. The intestinal motor response to resection. *Gastroenterology* 1993;105:791–798.

21 Schimpl G, Feierl G, Linni K, et al. Bacterial translocation in short-bowel syndrome in rats. *Eur J Pediatr Surg* 1999;9:224–227.

22 Asensio AB, Garcia-Urkia N, Aldazabal P, et al. Incidence of bacterial translocation in four different models of experimental short bowel syndrome. *Cir Pediatr* 2003;16:20–25.

23 Maestri L, Fava G, Fontana M, et al. Small bowel overgrowth: a frequent complication after abdominal surgery in newborns. *Pediatr Med Chir* 2002;24:374–376.

24 Quigley EMM, Phillips SF, Dent J. Distinctive patterns of interdigestive motility at the canine ileocolonic junction. *Gastroenterology* 1984;87:836–844.

25 Quigley EMM, Borody TJ, Phillips SF, et al. Motility of the terminal ileum and ileocecal sphincter in healthy man. *Gastroenterology* 1984;87:857–866.

26 Hoffmann JC, Zeitz M. Small bowel disease in the elderly: Diarrhoea and malabsorption. *Best Pract Res Clin Gastroenterol* 2002;16:17–36.

27 Mitsui T, Kagami H, Kinomoto H, Kondo T, Shimaoka K: Small bowel bacterial overgrowth and rice malabsorption in healthy and physically disabled older adults. *J Hum Nutr Diet* 2003;16:119–122.

28 Mitsui T, Shimaoka K, Goto Y, et al. Small bowel bacterial overgrowth is not seen in healthy adults but is in disabled older adults. *Hepatogastroenterology* 2006;53:82–85.

29 Castiglione F, Del Vecchio Blanco G, Rispo A, et al. Oro-cecal transit time and bacterial overgrowth in patients with Crohn's disease. *J Clin Gastroenterol* 2000;31:63–66.

30 Madrid AM, Soto L, Defilippi C, et al. Gastrointestinal motor involvement in scleroderma and its clinical correlation. *Gastroenterol Latinoam* 2002;13:381.

31 Justino SR, Goncalves Dias MC, Maculevicius J, et al. Fasting breath hydrogen concentration in short bowel syndrome patients with colon in continuity before and after antibiotic therapy. *Nutrition* 2004;20:187–191.

32 O'Boyle CJ, MacFie J, Mitchell CJ, et al. Microbiology of bacterial translocation in humans. *Gut* 1998;42:29–35.

33 Corazza GR, Menozzi MG, Strocchi A, et al. The diagnosis of small bowel bacterial overgrowth. *Gastroenterology* 1990;98:302–309.

34 Romagnuolo J, Schiller D, Bailey RJ. Using breath tests wisely in a gastroenterology practice: an evidence-based review of indications and pitfalls in interpretation. *Am J Gastroenterol* 2002;97:1113–1126.

35 Clinically relevant breath tests in gastroenterological diagnositics-recommendations of the German Society for Neurogastroenterology and Motility as well as the German Society for Digestive and Metabolic Diseases. *Z Gastroenterol* 2005;43:1071–1090.

36 Stotzer PO, Kilander AF: Comparison of the 1-gram ^{14}C-D-xylose breath test and the 50 gram hydrogen glucose breath test for diagnosis of small intestinal bacterial overgrowth. *Digestion* 2000;61:165–171.

37 Elphick DA, Chew TS, Higham SE, et al. Small bowel bacterial overgrowth in symptomatic older people: can it be diagnosed earlier? *Gerontology* 2005;51:396–401.

38 Thomas PD, Forbes A, Green J, et al: Guidelines for the investigation of chronic diarrhoea. *Gut* 2003;52(suppl V):v1–v15.

39 Ghoshal UC, Ghoshal U, Das K, Misra A. Utility of hydrogen breath tests in diagnosis of small intestinal bacterial overgrowth in malabsorption syndrome, and its relationship with oro-cecal transit time. *Indian J Gastroenterol* 2006;25:6–10.

40 Riordan SM, MacIver CJ, Walker BM, et al. The lactulose breath hydrogen test and small intestinal overgrowth. *Am J Gastroenterol* 1996;9:1795–1803.

41 Levitt MD, Ingelfinger FJ. Hydrogen gas and methane production in man. *Ann NY Acad Sci* 1965;150:75–81.

42 Melcher EA, Levitt MD, Slavin JL. Methane production and bowel function parameters in healthy subjects on low- and high-fiber diets. *Nutr Cancer* 1991;16:85–92.

43 Strocchi A, Levitt MD. Factors affecting hydrogen production and consumption by human fecal flora. The

critical roles of hydrogen tension and methanogenesis. *J Clin Invest* 1992;89:1304–1311.

44 Gregg CR. Enteric bacterial flora and bacterial overgrowth syndrome. *Semin Gastrointest Dis* 2002;13:200–209.

45 Wanitschke R, Ammon HV. Effects of dihydroxy bile acids and hydroxy fatty acids on the absorption of oleic acid in the human jejunum. *J Clin Invest* 1978;61:178–186.

46 Saltzman JR, Russell RM. Nutritional consequences of intestinal bacterial overgrowth. *Comp Ther* 1994;20:523–530.

47 Riordan SM, McIver CJ, Thomas DH, et al. Luminal bacteria and small-intestinal permeability. *Scand J Gastroenterol* 1997;32:556–563.

48 King CE, Toskes PP. Protein-losing enteropathy in the human and experimental rat blind loop syndrome. *Gastroenterology* 1981;80:504–509.

49 Varcoe R, Haliday D, Tavill AS. Utilization of urea nitrogen for albumin synthesis in the stagnant loop syndrome. *Gut* 1974;15:898–902.

50 Shah SM, Roberts PJ, Watson CJ, et al. Relapsing encephalopathy following small bowel transplantation. *Transplant Proc* 2003;35:1565–1566.

51 Gurevitch J, Sela B, Jonas A, et al. D-lactic acidosis: a treatable encephalopathy in pediatric patients. *Acta Paediatr* 1993;82:119–121.

52 Angelet P, Compte MT, Cid JL, et al. Recurrent episodes of acidosis with encephalophaty in a hemodialysis program patient with short bowel syndrome. *Nefrologia* 2002;22:196–198.

53 Soler Palacin P, Garzon Lorenzo P, Castilla Fernandez Y, et al. D-lactic acidosis in an 11-year-old patient with short bowel syndrome. *An Pediatr (Barc)* 2006;64:385–387.

54 Ghoshal UC, Ghoshal U, Ayyagari A, et al. Tropical sprue is associated with contamination of small bowel with aerobic bacteria and reversible prolongation of orocaecal transit time. *J Gastroenterol Hepatol* 2003;18:540–547.

55 Stotzer PO, Johansson C, Mellstrom D, et al. Bone mineral density in patients with small intestinal bacterial overgrowth. *Hepatogastroenterol* 2003;50:1415–1418.

56 Mitsui T, Shimaoka K, Takagi C, et al. Small bowel bacterial overgrowth may not affect bone mineral density in older people. *Clin Nutr* 2005;24:920–924.

57 Carbonnel F, Cosnes J, Chevret S, et al. The role of anatomic factors in nutritional autonomy after extensive small bowel resection. *JPEN* 1996;20:275–280.

58 Riordan SM, McIver CJ, Wakefield D, et al. Mucosal cytokine production in small-intestinal bacterial overgrowth. *Scand J Gastroenterol* 1996;31:977–984.

59 Kett K, Baklien K, Bakken A, et al. Intestinal B-cell isotype response in relation to local bacterial load: evidence for immunoglobulin A subclass adaptation. *Gastroenterology* 1995;109:819–825.

60 Riordan, McIver CJ, Wakefield D, et al. Luminal immunity in small intestinal bacterial overgrowth and old age. *Scand J Gastroenterol* 1996;31:1103–1109.

61 Ghoshal UC, Ghoshal U, Misra A, Choudhuri G. Partially responsive coeliac disease resulting from small intestinal bacterial overgrowth and lactose intolerance. *BMC Gastroenterology* 2004;4:10.

62 Tursi A, Brandimarte G, Giorgetti GM. High prevalence of small intestinal bacterial overgrowth in celiac patients with persistence of gastrointestinal symptoms after gluten withdrawal. *Am J Gastroenterol* 2003;98:839–843.

63 Riordan, McIver CJ, Wakefield D, et al. Luminal antigliadin antibodies in small intestinal bacterial overgrowth. *Am J Gastroenterol* 1997;92:1335–1338.

64 Riordan, McIver CJ, Wakefield D, et al. Local and systemic complement activity in small intestinal bacterial overgrowth. *Dig Dis Sci* 1997;42:1128–1136.

65 Riordan SM, McIver CJ, Wakefield D, et al. Serum immunoglobulin and soluble IL-2 receptor levels in small intestinal bacterial overgrowth with indigenous gut flora. *Dig Dis Sci* 1999;44:939–944.

66 Marteau P, Shanahan F. Basic aspects and pharmacology of probiotics: an overview of pharmacokinetics, mechanisms of action and side-effects. *Best Pract Res Clin Gastroenterol* 2003;17:725–740.

67 Berg RD. Bacterial translocation from the gastrointestinal tract. *Adv Exp Med Biol* 1999;473:11–30.

68 Kane TD, Johnson SR, Alexander JW, et al. Detection of intestinal bacterial translocation using PCR. *J Surg Res* 1996;63:59–63.

69 Kazez A, Saglam M, Doyzmaz MZ, et al. Detection of bacterial translocation during intestinal distention in rats using the polymerase chain reaction. *Pediatr Surg Int* 2001;17:624–627.

70 Such J, Frances R, Munoz C, et al. Detection and identification of bacterial DNA in patients with cirrhosis and culture-negative, nonneutrocytic ascites. *Hepatology* 2002;36:135–141.

71 Frances R, Munoz C, Zapater P, et al. Bacterial DNA activates cell mediated immune response and nitric oxide overproduction in peritoneal macrophages from patients with cirrhosis and ascites. *Gut* 2004;53:860–864.

72 Albillos A, de la Hera, Gonzalez M, et al. Increased lipopolysaccharide binding protein in cirrhotic patients with marked immune and hemodynamic derangement. *Hepatology* 2003;37:208–217.

73 Sánchez E, Casafont F, Guerra A, et al. Role of intestinal bacterial overgrowth and intestinal motility in bacterial translocation in experimental cirrhosis. *Rev Esp Enferm Dig* 2005;97: 805–814.

74 Wiest R, Garcia-Tsao G. Bacterial translocation (BT) in cirrhosis. *Hepatology* 2005;41:422–433.

75 Zhang S, Wang W, Ren W, et al. Effects of lactulose on intestinal endotoxin and bacterial translocation in cirrhotic rats. *Chin Med J* 2003;116:767–771.

76 Zhang SC, Wang W, Ren WY, et al. Effects of cisapride on intestinal bacterial and endotoxin translocation in cirrhotic rats. *Zhonghua Ganzangbing Zazhi* 2003;11:539–541.

77 Perez-Paramo M, Munoz J, Albillos A, et al. Effect of propranolol on the factors promoting bacterial translocation in cirrhotic rats with ascites. *Hepatology* 2000;31:43–48.

78 Almeida J, Galhenage S, Yu J, et al. Gut flora and bacterial translocation in chronic liver disease. *World J Gastroenterol* 2006;12:1493–1502.

79 O'Boyle C, MacFie J, Dave K, et al. Alterations in intestinal barrier function do not predispose to translocation of enteric bacteria in gastroenterological patients. *Nutrition* 1998;14:358–362.

80 O'Brien DP, Nelson LA, Kemp CJ, et al. Intestinal permeability and bacterial translocation are uncoupled after small bowel resection. *J Pediatr Surg* 2002;37:390–394.

81 Riordan SM, McIver CJ, Thomas DH, et al. Luminal bacteria and small-intestinal permeability. *Scand J Gastroenterol* 1997;32:556–563.

82 Steffen EK, Berg RD, Deitch EA. Comparison of translocation rates of various indigenous bacteria from the gastrointestinal tract to the mesenteric lymph node. *J Infect Dis* 1988;157:1023–1028.

83 Alverdy JC, Laughlin RS, Licheng W. Influence of the critically ill state on host-pathogen interactions within the intestine: gut-derived sepsis redefined. *Crit Care Med* 2003;31:598–607.

84 Alverdy J, Holbrook C, Rocha F, et al. Gut-derived sepsis occurs when the right pathogen with the right virulence genes meets the right host: evidence for in vivo virulence expression in Pseudomonas aeruginosa. *Ann Surg* 2000;232:480–489.

85 Ferri M, Gabriel S, Gavelli A, et al. Bacterial translocation during portal clamping for liver resection. A clinical study. *Arch Surg* 1997;132:162–165.

86 Kanwar S, Windsor AC, Welsh F, et al. Lack of correlation between failure of gut barrier function and septic complications after major upper gastrointestinal surgery. *Ann Surg* 2000;231:88–95.

87 Reimund JM, Arondel Y, Finck G, et al. Catheter-related infection in patients on home parenteral nutrition: results of a prospective survey: *Clin Nutr* 2002;21:33–38.

88 Catton JA, Dobbins BM, Wood JM, et al. The routine microbial screening of central venous catheters in home parenteral nutrition patients. *Clin Nutr* 2004;23:171–175.

89 Salzedas-Netto AA, Silva RM, Martins JL, et al. Can bacterial translocation be a beneficial event? *Transplant Proc* 2006;38:1836–1837.

90 Angulo P. Nonalcoholic fatty liver disease. *N Engl J Med* 2002;346:1221–1231.

91 Solga SF, Diehl AM. Non-alcoholic fatty liver disease: lumen–liver interactions and possible role for probiotics. *J Hepatol* 2003;38:681–687.

92 Wigg AJ, Roberts-Thomson IC, et al. The role of small intestinal overgrowth, intestinal permeability, endotoxemia, and TNF alpha in the pathogenesis of nonalcoholic steatohepatitis. *Gut* 2001;48:206–211.

93 Aguirre V, Uchida T, Yenush L, et al. The c-Jun NH(2)-terminal kinase promotes insulin resistance during association with insulin receptor substrate-1 and phosphorylation of Ser (307). *J Biol Chem* 2000;275: 9047–9054.

94 Solga SF, Diehl AM. Non-alcoholic fatty liver disease: lumen-liver interactions and possible role for probiotics. *J Hepatol* 2003;38:681–687.

95 Szabo G, Velayudham A, Romics L, Mandrekar P. Modulation of non-alcoholic steatohepatitis by pattern recognition receptors in mice (the role of toll-like receptors 2 and 4). *Alcohol Clin Exp Res* 2005;29:S140–S145.

96 Enotomo E, Ikejima K, Bradford BU, et al. Role of Kupffer cells and gut-derived endotoxins in alcoholic liver injury. *J Gastroenterol Hepatol* 2000;15:D20–25.

97 Cope K, Ribsy T, Diehl AM. Increased gastrointestinal ethanol production in obese mice. Implications for fatty liver pathogenesis. *Gastroenterology* 2000;119:1340–1347.

98 Li Z, Yang S, Lin H, et al. Probiotics and antibodies to TNF inhibit inflammatory activity and improve nonalcoholic fatty liver disease. *Hepatology* 2003;37:343–350.

99 Loguercio C, De Simone T, Federico A, et al. Gut-liver axis: a new point of attack to treat chronic liver damage. *Am J Gastroenterol* 2002;97:244–246.

100 Quigley EMM, Marsh MN, Shaffer JL, Markin RS. Hepatobiliary complications of total parenteral nutrition. *Gastroenterology* 1993;104:286–301.

101 Seehofer D, Rayes N, Schiller R, et al. Probiotics partly reverse increased bacterial translocation after simultaneous liver resection and colonic anastomosis in rats. *J Surg Res* 2004;117:262–271.

102 Di Stefano M, Miceli E, Missanelli A, Corazza GR. Treatment of small intestine bacterial overgrowth. *Eur Rev Med Pharmacol Sci* 2005;9:217–222.

103 Buchman AL, Scolapio J, Fryer J. AGA technical review on short bowel syndrome and intestinal transplantation. *Gastroenterology* 2003;124:1111–1134.

104 Thompson JS, Quigley EMM, Adrian TE. Effect of intestinal tapering and lengthening on intestinal structure and function. *Am J Surg* 1995;169:111–119.

105 Cicalese L, Sileri P, Green M, et al. Bacterial translocation in clinical intestinal transplantation. *Transplantation* 2001;71:1414–1417.

106 Di Lorenzo C, Reddy SN, Villanueva-Meyer J, et al. Cisapride in children with chronic intestinal pseudoobstruction. An acute, double-blind, crossover, placebo-controlled trial. *Gastroenterology* 1991;101:1564–1570.

107 Abell TL, Camilleri M, DiMango EP, et al. Long-term efficacy of oral cisapride in symptomatic upper gut dysmotility. *Dig Dis Sci* 1991;36:616–620.

108 Hyman PE, Di Lorenzo C, McAdams L, et al. Predicting the clinical response to cisapride in children with chronic intestinal pseudo-obstruction. *Am J Gastroenterol* 1993;88:832–836.

109 Verne GN, Eaker EY, Hardy E, Sninsky CA. Effect of octreotide and erythromycin on idiopathic and scleroderma-associated intestinal pseudoobstruction. *Dig Dis Sci* 1995;40:1892–1901.

110 Perlemuter G, Cacoub P, Chaussade S, et al. Octreotide treatment of chronic intestinal pseudoobstruction secondary to connective tissue diseases. *Arthritis Rheum* 1999;42:1545–1549.

111 Von der Ohe MR, Camilleri M, Thomforde GM, Klee GG. Differential regional effects of octreotide on human gastrointestinal motor function. *Gut* 1995;36:734–738.

112 Soudah HC, Hasler WL, Owyang C. Effect of octreotide on intestinal motility and bacterial overgrowth in scleroderma. *N Engl J Med* 1991;325:1461–1467.

113 Nieuwenhuijs VB, van Duijvenbode-Beumer H, Verheem A, et al. The effects of ABT-29 and octreotide on interdigestive small bowel motility, bacterial overgrowth and bacterial translocation in rats. *Eur J Clin Invest* 1999;29:33–40.

114 Zhang SC, Wang W, Ren WY, et al. Effect of cisapride on intestinal bacterial and endotoxin translocation. *World J Gastroenterol* 2003;9:543–548.

115 Pardo A, Bartoli R, Lorenzo-Zuñiga V, et al. Effect of cisapride on intestinal bacterial overgrowth and bacterial translocation in cirrhosis. *Hepatology* 2000;31:858–863.

116 Wang XD, Soltestz V, Andersson R. Cisapride prevents enteric bacterial overgrowth and translocation by improvement of intestinal motility in rats with acute liver failure. *Eur Surg Res* 1996;28:402–412.

117 Kaufman SS, Losecke CA, Lupo JV, et al. Influence of bacterial overgrowth and intestinal inflammation on duration of parenteral nutrition in children with short bowel syndrome. *J Pediatr* 1997;131:356–361.

118 Castiglione F, Rispo A, Di Girolama E, et al. Antibiotic treatment of small bowel bacterial overgrowth in patients with Crohn's disease. *Aliment Pharmacol Ther* 2003;18:1107–1112.

119 Di Steffano M, Malservisi S, Veneto G, et al. Rifaximin versus chlortetracycline in the short term treatment of small intestinal bacterial overgrowth. *Aliment Pharmacol Ther* 2000;14:551–556.

120 Kumar A, Forsmark CE, Toskes PP. The response of small bowel bacterial overgrowth to treatment: effects of coexisting conditions. *Gastroenterology* 1996;110:A340.

121 Cuoco L, Salvagnini M. Small intestine bacterial overgrowth in irritable bowel syndrome: retrospective study with rifaximin. *Minerva Gastroenterol Dietol* 2006;52:89–95.

122 Kaye SA, Lim SG, Taylor M, et al. Small bowel bacterial overgrowth in systemic sclerosis: detection using direct and indirect methods and treatment outcome. *Br J Rheumatol* 1995;34:265–269.

123 Goldstein F, Mandle RJ, Schaedler RW. The blind-loop syndrome and its variants. Microbiologic aspects of diagnosis and treatment. *Am J Gastroenterol* 1973;60:255–264.

124 Attar A, Flourié B, Rambaud JC, et al. Antibiotic efficacy in small intestinal bacterial overgrowth-related chronic diarrhea: a crossover randomized trial. *Gastroenterology* 1999;117:794–797.

125 Vanderhoof JA, Young RJ, Murray N, Kaufman SS. Treatment strategies for small bacterial overgrowth in short bowel syndrome. *J Pediatr Gastroenterol Nutr* 1998;27:155–160.

126 Kubota A, Okada A, Imura K, et al. The effect of metronidazole on TPN-associated liver dysfunction in neonates. *J Pediatr Surg* 1990;25:618–621.

127 Halperin ML, Kamel KS. D-lactic acidosis: turning sugar into acids in the gastrointestinal tract. *Kidney Int* 1996;49:1–8.

128 Bongaerts GP, Tolboom JJ, Naber AH, et al. Role of bacteria in the pathogenesis of short bowel syndrome-associated D-lactic academia. *Microb Pathog* 1997;22:285–293.

129 Jimenez Almonacid P, Calleja Kempin J, Vasquez Estevez J, et al. Bacterial translocation in intestinal transplant. *Cir Pediatr* 1999;12:56–60.

130 Biffi R, Privitera G, Matinato C, et al. Parenteral antibiotics and selective decontamination do not prevent enteric bacterial overgrowth or translocation observed in a swine model of small bowel transplantation. *J Surg Res* 1995;58:391–394.

131 Daxboeck F, Rabitsch W, Blacky A, et al. Influence of selective bowel decontamination on the organisms recovered during bacteremia in neutropenic patients. *Infect Control Hosp Epidemiol* 2004;25:685–689.

132 Bouter H, Schippers EF, Luelmo SA, et al. No effect of preoperative selective gut decontamination on endotoxemia and cytokine activation during cardiopulmonary bypass: a randomized, placebo-controlled trial. *Crit Care Med* 2002;30:38–43.

133 Lingnau W, Berger J, Javorsky F, et al. Changing bacterial ecology during a five-year period of selective intestinal decontamination. *J Hosp Infect* 1998;39:195–206.

134 Cirera I, Bauer TM, Navasa M, et al. Bacterial translocation of enteric organisms in patients with cirrhosis. *J Hepatol* 2001;34:32–37.

135 Rolando N, Wade JJ, Stangou A, et al. Prospective study comparing the efficacy of prophylactic parenteral antimicrobials, with or without enteral decontamination, in patients with acute liver failure. *Liver Transpl Surg* 1996;2:8–13.

136 Luiten EJ, Hop WC, Endtz HP, Bruining HA. Prognostic importance of gram-negative intestinal colonization preceding pancreatic infection in severe acute pancreatitis. Results of a controlled clinical trial of selective decontamination. *Intensive Care Med* 1998;24:438–445.

137 Dervenis C, Smailis D, Hatzitheoklitos E. Bacterial translocation and its prevention in acute pancreatitis. *J Hepatobiliary Pancreat Surg* 2003;10:415–418.

138 Kuo PC, Bartlett ST, Lim JW, et al. Selective bowel decontamination in hospitalized patients awaiting liver transplantation. *Am J Surg* 1997;174:745–748.

139 Tetteroo GW, Wagenvoort JH, Bruining HA. Bacteriology of selective decontamination: efficacy and rebound colonization. *J Antimicrob Chemother* 1994;34:139–148.

140 Gibson GR, Roberfroid MB. Dietary modulation of the human colonic microbiota: introducing the concept of prebiotics. *J Nutr* 1995;125:1401–1412.

141 Roberfroid MB. Prebiotics: preferential substrates for specific germs? *Am J Clin Nutr* 2001;73:406S–9.

142 Bouhnik Y, Flourie B, D'Agay-Abensour L, et al. Administration of transgalacto-oligosaccharides increases fecal bifidobacteria and modifies colonic fermentation metabolism in healthy humans. *J Nutr* 1997;127:444–448.

143 Duggan C, Gannon J, Walker WA. Protective nutrients and functional foods for the gastrointestinal tract. *Am J Clin Nutr* 2002;75:789–808.

144 Gnoth MJ, Kunz C, Kinne-Saffran E, Rudloff S. Human milk oligosaccharides are minimally digested in vitro. *J Nutr* 2000;130:3014–3020.

145 Dai D, Walker WA. Protective nutrients and bacterial colonization in the immature human gut. *Adv Pediatr* 1999;46:353–382.

146 Liu Q, Duan ZP, Ha da K, et al. Synbiotic modulation of gut flora: effect on minimal hepatic encephalopathy in patients with cirrhosis. *Hepatology* 2004;39:1441–1449.

147 Rayes N, Seehofer D, Theruvath T, et al. Supply of pre- and probiotics reduces bacterial infection rates after liver transplantation—a randomized, double-blind trial. *Am J Transplant* 2005;5:125–130.

148 Kanazawa H, Nagino M, Kamiya S, et al. Synbiotics reduce postoperative infectious complications: a randomized controlled trial in biliary cancer patients undergoing hepatectomy. *Langenbecks Arch Surg* 2005;390:104–113.

149 Bauer TM, Fernandez J, Navasa M, et al. Failure of Lactobacillus spp. to prevent bacterial translocation in a rat model of experimental cirrhosis. *J Hepatol* 2002;36:501–506.

150 Diplock AT, Aggett PJ, Ashwell M, et al. Scientific concepts of functional foods in Europe: consensus document. *Br J Nutr* 1999;81:s1–27.

151 Timmerman HM, Koning CJ, Mulder L, Rombouts FM, Beynen AC. Monostrain, multistrain and multispecies probiotics- a comparison of functionality and efficacy. *Int J Food Microbiol* 2004;96:219–233.

152 Murphy LM, Byrne FR, Collins K, et al. Evaluation and characterisation of probiotic therapy in the

CD45RB^HI transfer model of colitis. *Gastroenterology* 1999;116:A780.

153 Shanahan F. Probiotics: a perspective on problems and pitfalls. *Scand J Gastroenterol* 2003;38(suppl): 34–36.

154 Castagliuolo I, Riegler MF, Valenik L, La Mont JT, Pothoulakis C. Saccharomyces boulardii protease inhibits the effects of clostridium difficile toxins A and B in human colonic mucosa. *Infect Immun* 1999;67:302–307.

155 Madsen K, Cornish A, Soper P, et al. Probiotic bacteria enhance murine and human intestinal epithelial barrier function. *Gastroenterology* 2001;121:580–591.

156 Resta-Lenert S, Barrett KE. Live probiotics protect intestinal epithelial cells from the effects of infection with enteroinvasive Escherichia coli (EIEC). *Gut* 2003;52:988–997.

157 Akhtar M, Watson JL, Nazli A, McKay DM. Bacterial DNA evokes epithelial IL-8 production by a MAPK-dependent, NF-Kappa β-independent pathway. *FASEB J* 2003;17:1319–1321.

158 McCarthy J, O'Mahony L, O'Callaghan L, et al. Double blind, placebo controlled trial of two probiotic strains in interleukin 10 knockout mice and mechanistic link with cytokine balance. *Gut* 2003;52:975–980.

159 Rachmilewitz D, Katakura K, Karmeli F, et al. Toll-like receptor 9 signaling mediates the anti-inflammatory effects of probiotics in murine experimental colitis. *Gastroenterology* 2004;126:520–528.

160 Jijon H, Backer J, Diaz H, et al. DNA from probiotic bacteria modulates murine and human epithelial and immune function. *Gastroenterology* 2004;126:1358–1373.

161 Otte JM, Podolsky DK. Functional modulation of enterocytes by gram-positive and gram-negative microorganisms. *Am J Physiol Gastrointest Liver Physiol* 2004;286:G613–G626.

162 Heyman M, Ménard S. Probiotic microorganisms: how they affect intestinal pathophysiology. *Cell Mol Life Sci* 2002;59:1151–1165.

163 Ménard S, Heyman M. Modulation of epithelial cell function and local immune system by probiotics: mechanisms involved. In: Goktepe I, Juneja VK, Ahmedna M, eds. *Probiotics in Food Safety and Human Health*. Boca Raton, Florida: Taylor and Francis, 2006.

164 Eizaguirre I, Urkia NG, Asencio AB, et al. Probiotic supplementation reduces the risk of bacterial translocation in experimental short bowel syndrome. *J Pediatr Surg* 2002;37:669–702.

165 Garcia-Urkia N, Asensio AB, Zubillaga Aspiroz I, et al. Beneficial effects of bifidobacterium lactis in the prevention of bacterial translocation in experimental short bowel syndrome. *Cir Pediatr* 2002;15:162–165.

166 Li Y, Shimizu T, Hosaka A, et al. Effects of bifidobacterium breve supplementation on intestinal flora of low birth weight infants. *Pediatr Int* 2004;46:509–515.

167 Lin HC, Su BH, Chen AC, et al. Oral probiotics reduce the incidence and severity of necrotizing enterocolitis in very low birth weight infants. *Pediatrics* 2005;115:1–4.

168 Bin-Nun A, Bromiker R, Wilschanski M, et al. Oral probiotics prevent necrotizing enterocolitis in very low birth weight neonates. *J Pediatr* 2005;147:192–196.

169 Young RJ, Vanderhoof JA. Probiotic therapy in children with short bowel syndrome and bacterial overgrowth. *Gastroenterology* 1997;112:A916.

170 Gaon D, Garmendia C, Murrielo NO, et al. Effect of Lactobacillus strains (L. casei and L. acidophilus strains cerela) on bacterial overgrowth-related chronic diarrhea. *Medicina (B Aires)* 2002;62:159–163.

171 Stotzer PO, Blomberg L, Conway Pl, Henriksson A, Abrahamsson H. Probiotic treatment of small intestinal bacterial overgrowth by Lactobacillus fermentum KLD. *Scand J Infect Dis* 1996;28:615–619.

172 Uchida H, Yamamoto H, Kisadi Y, et al. D-lactic acidosis in short bowel syndrome managed with antibiotics and probiotics. *J Pediatr Surg* 2004;39:634–636.

173 Tsunoda A, Shibusawa M, Tsunoda Y, et al. Effect of Lactobacillus casei on a novel murine model of abdominal sepsis. *J Surg Res* 2002;107:37–43.

174 Gan BS, Kim J, Reid G, Cadieux P, Howard JC. Lactobacillus fermentum RC-14 inhibits Staphlococcus aureus infection of surgical implants in rats. *J Infect Dis* 2002;185:1369–1372.

175 Seehofer D, Rayes N, Schiller R, et al. Probiotics partly reverse increased bacterial translocation after simultaneous liver resection and colonic anastomosis in rats. *J Surg Research* 2004;117:262–271.

176 Rayes N, Seehofer D, Muller AR, et al. Influence of probiotics and fibre on the incidence of bacterial infections following major abdominal surgery-results of a prospective trial. *Z Gastroenterol* 2002;40:869–876.

177 McNaught CE, Woodcock NP, MacFie J, Mitchell CJ. A prospective randomized study of the probiotic Lactobacillus plantarum 299V on indices of gut barrier function in elective surgical patients. *Gut* 2002;51:827–831.

178 Anderson AD, McNaught CE, Jain PK, MacFie J. Randomised clinical trial of symbiotic therapy in elective surgical patients. *Gut* 2004;53:241–245.

179 Marteau P, Shanahan F. Basic aspects and pharmacology of probiotics: an overview of pharmacokinetics, mechanisms of action and side-effects. *Best Pract Res Clin Gastroenterol* 2003;17:725–740.

180 Borriello SP, Hammes WP, Holzapfel W, et al. Safety of probiotics that contain lactobacilli or bifidobacteria. *Clin Infect Dis* 2003;36:775–780.

181 Mäkeläinen H, Tahvonen R, Salminen S, Ouwehand AC. In vivo safety assessment of two Bifidobacterium longus strains. *Microbiol Immunol* 2003;47:911–914.

20 Management of Complex Fluid and Electrolyte Disturbances

Stuart S. Kaufman and Erin M. Fennelly

Key points

- Fluid depletion in patients with enterostomies is accompanied by sodium and chloride depletion and is generally exacerbated by increased oral intake.
- Fluid depletion in patients with anatomic continuity is often associated with metabolic acidosis and hypokalemia, usually in proportion to stool output.
- Clinicians should be alert to, and be prepared to manage aggressively, periodic occurrences of acute dehydration.
- Chronic dehydration and repeated episodes of acute dehydration increase risks of chronic renal disease, disorders of calcium and phosphorus metabolism, and growth failure (in pediatric patients).

Introduction

Maintenance of appropriate fluid and electrolyte balance is an essential component of the care of patients with intestinal failure. Both basic requirements and the impact of environmental stresses on the patient must be considered; each is influenced by alimentary tract anatomy. The challenge of maintaining optimal fluid and electrolyte status and the corollary, preventing or treating fluid and electrolyte disturbances, is considerable and often underappreciated in intestinal failure management. In this chapter, we shall describe

Intestinal Failure: Diagnosis, Management and Transplantation.
Edited by Alan N. Langnas, Olivier Goulet, Eamonn M.M. Quigley and Kelly A. Tappenden. © 2008 Blackwell Publishing.
ISBN 978-1-4051-4637-1.

the various derangements that commonly occur, the situations in which they typically arise, and methods of rectifying them.

Patients with an enterostomy

Background

Liquefaction of food must precede its digestion and absorption. This task is accomplished by the secretion of a large quantity of water into the upper gastrointestinal tract, up to 8 liters per day in adults [1]. Secretion of water from the duodenal and proximal jejunal epithelium is coupled to the isodirectional transport of electrolytes, mainly sodium and chloride, into the lumen. In contrast, the balance of electrolyte movement in most of the jejunum, ileum, and colon is absorptive, that is, directed from the gut lumen into enterocytes, as water passively follows [2]. Patients with a short bowel ending as a duodenostomy or jejunostomy, no more than 100–150 cm long in adults, have inadequate distal, absorptive bowel to compensate for the secretory, proximal small bowel. Those patients with a small bowel remnant in continuity with the rectum or with a short segment of sigmoid colon are in a similar situation; they can not maintain positive fluid balance without supplemental intravenous fluid irrespective of the magnitude of enteral fluid intake. In fact, food and fluid further increase stool output and the tendency for dehydration for at least three reasons. First, consumption of hypotonic fluids, especially water, produces a lumen-directed sodium gradient that also pulls water into the lumen. Second, additional luminal fluid is produced by the osmotic draw of unabsorbed nutrients. Third, food in the upper gastrointestinal tract stimulates the motility of the bowel remnant [3]. Adult patients with an enterostomy will only avoid supplemental intravenous fluid therapy if they have a net wet weight food absorption (weight of the oral intake—weight of stool) greater than or equal to 1.4 kg daily [4].

Management

Inconsistent intake of food and fluid, which is common in patients with intestinal failure, results in variable gastrointestinal fluid losses and correspondingly variable replacement fluid requirements. The practice of interrupting parenteral nutrition during the day, when oral intake and stoma output are at their peaks, increases the risk of dehydration. Traditional antiperistaltic drugs such as loperamide do not reduce intestinal fluid losses to a degree that precludes the need for intravenous fluid replacement in patients with a proximal enterostomy [5]. Clonidine administered transdermally (0.3 mg/day) may be somewhat more effective [6]. Therapy with the anti-secretory agent racecadotril, which is efficacious in treatment of acute diarrhea [7], alone or in combination with an antiperistaltic drug, might further reduce intestinal fluid losses in patients with high-output short bowel syndrome; no studies have been reported that support this possibility. Consequently, prevention of dehydration requires administration of appropriate quantities of intravenous crystalloid, either at the beginning, end, or between cycled parenteral nutrition infusions. A total daily intravenous fluid requirement ranging from 3.5 to 5.0 liters in older children and adults is not unusual, and the more proximal the stoma, the greater the volume that shall be needed. Because lumen sodium and potassium concentrations in the jejunum are about 90–110 and 10–15 mEq/L, respectively [8,9], normal saline is usually the best, readily available replacement fluid. A summary of luminal fluid electrolyte concentrations delineated by region is given in Table 20.1. It is noted, however, that patients with a high jejunostomy usually require little or no additional potassium, because adequate sodium replacement suppresses aldosterone secretion and urine potassium loss. The tendency for food and fluid-induced dehydration to occur can be minimized by a restriction of oral fluid intake to products with high sodium concentrations, that is, at least 90 mEq/L [4,10]. Fluid management in patients with an enterostomy is summarized in Table 20.2.

Table 20.1 Electrolyte concentrations of alimentary tract fluids by region.

Site	Sodium (mEq/L)	Potassium (mEq/L)	Chloride (mEq/L)	Bicarbonate (mEq/L)
Jejunum	90–110	10–15	100–120	10–20
Ileum	40–80	3–10	20–120	30–50
Colon	20–90	10–80	20–110	20–70

(Adapted from Benitz WE, Tatro DS. *The Pediatric Drug Handbook*. 3rd edn. St. Louis: Mosby, 1995:294; and Cima RK, Pemberton JH. Ileostomy, colostomy, and pouches. In: Feldman M, et al., eds., *Sleisenger and Fordtran's Gastrointestinal and Liver Disease*, 8th ed. St. Louis: WB Saunders, 2006:2550–2562.)

Patients in anatomic continuity

Background

Patients with remnant small bowel anastomosed to colon absorb substantially more calories than patients with an equal length of small bowel that ends as an enterostomy; for any given length of small bowel remnant the former group is more likely to be able to discontinue parenteral nutrition [11]. The water-conserving properties of the colon and ileum (when present) also provide partial protection against development of dehydration [2]. Similarly, sodium and chloride losses are usually diminished as a result of anatomic continuity,

Table 20.2 Fluid management in patients with an enterostomy.

- Parenteral nutrition volume calculated for maintenance based on weight or body surface area
- Extra daily intravenous crystalloid, usually normal saline, in proportion to prevailing stoma losses delivered either contiguous with, or separated from, nutrient admixture
- Oral rehydration solution in volume desired by patient with sodium concentration of at least 90 mEq/L
- Daily measurements of body weight and stoma output
- Weekly to monthly (based on clinical stability) determinations of plasma and urine electrolyte, hemoglobin, and albumin concentrations
- Anti-peristaltic agents relatively ineffective in reducing gut fluid losses

Table 20.3 Enteral hydration solutions.

Product	Sodium Concentration (mEq/L)	Potassium Concentration (mEq/L)	Chloride Concentration (mEq/L)	Citrate (Base) Concentration (mEq/L)	Glucose Concentration (g%)
Pedialyte®	45	20	35	30	2.5
Rehydralyte®	75	20	65	30	2.5
EqualYTE®	78.2	22.3	67.7	30.1	3.0*
Ceralyte 70®	70	20	60	30	4
Ceralyte 90®	90	20	80	30	4
WHO	90	20	80	30	2

*Glucose = 2.0 g% and fructooligosaccharides = 1.0 g%.

whereas bicarbonate and potassium losses are often increased (Table 20.1). Passage of stools via the rectum, however, may complicate estimation of fecal fluid losses, particularly in incontinent patients, as urine in a diaper may be impossible to distinguish from watery stool. In that event, subjective patient impressions of well-being and urine output and clinical assessment of hydration guide decision-making. As in patients with a terminal enterostomy, simple laboratory studies such as elevation of plasma urea nitrogen and albumin relative to the patient's established baseline or negligible urine sodium may reinforce clinical suspicion of acute or chronic dehydration.

Management

In contrast to patients with proximal enterostomies, patients in anatomic continuity (or very distal enterostomies) usually benefit from anti-peristaltic agents that prolong transit time such as loperamide (Imodium®), diphenoxylate-atropine (Lomotil®), and deodorized tincture of opium [12]. Effective doses are often considerably greater than those used for symptomatic treatment of acute gastroenteritis in otherwise healthy persons; daily doses of loperamide of 8 mg, in small children, and 24 mg, in adults, are common. Therapy is limited only by side effects, including abdominal distention, vomiting, and lethargy, all of which are unusual. Subcutaneous or intramuscular depot octreotide may be effective in some patients [13]. In contrast to patients with an enterostomy, the restriction of dietary lipid usually reduces gut fluid losses, because free long-chain fatty acids, not absorbed in the small bowel, stimulate colonocyte secretion [14]. In patients who continue to experience watery stools despite fat restriction, bile acid binding agents such as cholestyramine in doses of 2 (infants) to 12 g per day (adults) in 3 to 4 divided doses may further reduce colonic water loss, as fecal bile acids also induce water secretion by the colon [15].

Supplemental intravenous fluids are often necessary immediately following cessation of parenteral nutrition; they can be given as boluses over several hours during the day or night as convenient for the patient and family. As noted earlier, exchange of sodium for potassium and chloride for bicarbonate reduces the concentrations of sodium and chloride required compared to those needed by patients with an enterostomy, 50–75 mEq/L (one-third to one-half normal saline) [1,16,17]. Hypokalemia is avoided by the inclusion of potassium, 10–20 mEq/L, and metabolic acidosis is prevented by the substitution of half or more of chloride with bicarbonate. Later, supplemental enteral hydration becomes feasible, either by bolus during the day or by continuous infusion via tube at night. Table 20.3 lists proprietary products that can be used for this purpose. Fluid management in patients in anatomic continuity is summarized in Table 20.4.

Acute dehydration

Background

Despite ongoing intravenous fluid intake, patients with intestinal failure often have tenuous fluid balance that may become negative following minor increases in alimentary tract loss. Increased fecal losses are usually

Table 20.4 Fluid management in patients in anatomic continuity.

- Parenteral nutrition volume calculated for maintenance based on weight or body surface area
- Extra intravenous crystalloid, usually one-third to one-half normal saline, based on thirst, sense of patient well-being, and laboratory tests, and administered either with, or separate from, the nutrient admixture
- Oral rehydration proprietary solutions as desired with sodium concentration of about 50 mEq/L (see Table 20.3)
- Bi-weekly to bi-monthly (based on clinical stability) determinations of plasma and urine electrolyte, hemoglobin, and albumin concentrations
- Anti-peristaltic agents relatively effective in reducing gut fluid losses

the result of either drinking and/or eating in excess of tolerance or infectious enteritis. Many patients find it difficult or impossible to control binge eating or drinking that predictably results in dehydration. Dietary intake should be easier to regulate in infants than older children and adults. Preventive measures that reduce the frequency or severity of infectious enteritis such as rotavirus vaccination may be useful, although proof of efficacy for pediatric patients with short bowel syndrome has not been presented. An early clue to dehydration in infants, often apparent before appearance of characteristic physical features, is an unusual craving for fluid.

Management

Parenteral fluid-dependent patients who become acutely dehydrated generally require intravenous rehydration even if substantial quantities of enteral fluid are tolerated under stable conditions. Dehydration should be corrected rapidly, as delays may cause or contribute to other complications including hyperphosphatemia, which, in turn, leads to secondary hypocalcemia and tetany.

Free water replacement

Mild dehydration that is associated with thirst, lethargy, and reduced urine output may be corrected at home, particularly in adult patients. A fluid loss not exceeding 3% of total body weight, no more than 2 liters

in an adult, is to be expected, and rehydration can be accomplished in a few hours using normal saline or Ringer's lactate, depending on historical requirements for base, that is, acetate, in the parenteral nutrition admixture. More severe dehydration that produces an increase in heart rate or reduced blood pressure, combined with an obvious reduction in skin turgor, should be corrected in an Emergency Department or other acute care facility. The objective is the restoration of hemodynamic stability and urine output as quickly as possible. Tracking blood hemoglobin and plasma albumin concentrations as they fall to baseline values confirms the completion of rehydration. The duration of rehydration need not exceed 12 hours even when fluid loss amounts to 8 to 10% of body weight, provided that patients are monitored closely by experienced personnel. Ongoing vomiting and diarrhea must be factored into the volume of fluid to be replaced and the rate of replacement.

Electrolyte deficits

Acute dehydration in patients with intestinal failure tends to produce greater deficits of sodium and potentially potassium and base than dehydration in those with an anatomically normal gastrointestinal tract. Severe sodium depletion is particularly likely in the setting of a proximal, that is, sodium-secreting, enterostomy or jejunal anastomosis to a relatively short colonic remnant. In most of these patients, the presenting plasma sodium concentration will be normal or mildly reduced, usually no less than 128–130 mEq/L. Moderate to severe hyponatremia, [Na] ≤125–130 mEq/L, is unusual, unless mild hyponatremia was present before the onset of dehydration. In order to prevent the development of hyponatremia while restoring intravascular volume quickly, the initial rehydration fluid should generally be normal saline. In the rare event of a presenting plasma sodium concentration <120 mEq/L, the rise in plasma sodium under treatment should probably not exceed 8 to 10 mEq/L per 24 hours, in which case a change to half-normal saline, during the rehydration, is appropriate [18].

The presence of colon in continuity with the small bowel remnant conserves some sodium, generally at the cost of additional potassium and bicarbonate losses [19]. Most of these patients will present with a normal plasma sodium concentration; a few will be hypernatremic (plasma sodium concentration >150 mEq/L).

Extreme elevations of the serum sodium concentration that require slowing of rehydration to avoid iatrogenic cerebral edema are uncommon [20]. Base is needed roughly in proportion to the length of remnant colon or ileum in continuity with jejunum and is particularly necessary for correction of acidosis in patients with a maintenance requirement for base. Ringer's lactate or a solution consisting of half-normal saline plus up to 75 mEq/L of sodium bicarbonate is usually appropriate initially, and infusions should be adjusted based on repeated measurement of plasma electrolyte concentrations during rehydration.

Chronic dehydration

Background

The reality of intestinal failure is that many patients subsist in a state of protracted under-hydration, which results when fluid intake is just adequate to balance total body losses at the cost of chronically reduced urine volume. This relatively common situation develops as a result of a consistent underestimation of rectal (or stoma) output, leading to an overly optimistic estimate of enteral feeding tolerance and an underestimation of intravenous fluid needs. The prevention of chronic underhydration is essential because of the long-term risks of intravascular volume contraction, including chronic renal insufficiency complicated by nephrolithiasis and an exaggerated susceptibility to nephrotoxic drugs [21,22]. The main symptoms are usually protracted weakness and lethargy, and these symptoms often develop insidiously or may be mistaken for other medical disorders, for example, hypothyroidism. In fact, recognition of historical chronic dehydration may be apparent to the patient or family only following the improvement in well-being that accompanies correction. Similarly, a state of chronic dehydration may become apparent following occurrence of superimposed acute dehydration precipitated by stresses such as summer heat and increased physical activity. Suggestive physical findings include postural hypotension, tachycardia with weak pulse, and subtle reductions in skin turgor. Intermittent or consistent elevations of hematocrit, plasma urea nitrogen, and albumin, even if mild, as well as the presence of concentrated urine essentially devoid of sodium (in the absence of hyperbilirubinemia) are significant and easily obtainable laboratory findings.

Management

Increased fluid and sodium intake is titrated to improved clinical well-being and confirmed by improvements in the laboratory markers of hemoconcentration noted above; a falling plasma renin, plasma aldosterone, or urine sodium/potassium ratio provide supportive evidence in ambiguous situations [23]. Additional oral rehydration fluid may be practical for some patients with near-complete intestinal adaptation. For the remainder with substantial, ongoing parenteral caloric needs, the intravenous route should be employed. Supplemental intravenous fluid may be added either directly to the cycled, parenteral nutrition admixture, customarily at night, or separated from the parenteral nutrition infusion, often at mid-day. With the later practice 1 liter or more of one-half normal to normal saline may easily be infused over one-half to 1 hour daily.

References

1 Sundaram A, Koutkia P, Apovian CM. Nutritional management of short bowel syndrome in adults. *J Clin Gastroenterol* 2002;34:207–220.

2 Holtug K, Hansen MB, Skadhauge E. Experimental studies of intestinal ion and water transport. *Scand J Gastroenterol Suppl* 1996;216:95–110.

3 Lennard-Jones JE. Review article: practical management of the short bowel syndrome. *Aliment Pharmacol Ther* 1994;8:563–577.

4 Jeppesen PB, Mortensen PB. Intestinal failure defined by measurements of intestinal energy and wet weight absorption. *Gut* 2000;46:701–706.

5 Rodrigues CA, Lennard-Jones JE, Thompson DG, et al. The effects of octreotide, soy polysaccharide, codeine and loperamide on nutrient, fluid and electrolyte absorption in the short-bowel syndrome. *Aliment Pharmacol Ther* 1989;3:159–169.

6 Buchman AL, Fryer J, Wallin A, et al. Clonidine reduces diarrhea and sodium loss in patients with proximal jejunostomy: a controlled study. *J Parenter Enteral Nutr* 2006;30:487–491.

7 Nagpal J, Gogia S. Racecadotril. *Indian Pediatr* 2004;41:1218–1224.

8 Ladefoged K, Olgaard K. Fluid and electrolyte absorption and renin-angiotensin-aldosterone axis in patients

with severe short-bowel syndrome. *Scand J Gastroenterol* 1979;14:729–735.

9 Svaninger G, Nordgren S, Palselius IR, et al. Sodium and potassium excretion in patients with ileostomies. *Eur J Surg* 1991;157:601–605.

10 Cera Products [homepage on the Internet]. Columbia, MD: Cera Products, Inc; c1996–2006. Cera Products Nutritional Information. Available from: http://www.ceraproductsinc.com/productline/nutrition_cl.html.

11 Messing B, Crenn P, Beau P, et al. Long-term survival and parenteral nutrition dependence in adult patients with the short bowel syndrome. *Gastroenterology* 1999;117:1043–1050.

12 Awouters F, Megens A, Verlinden M, Schuurkes et al. Loperamide. Survey of studies on mechanism of its antidiarrheal activity. *Dig Dis Sci* 1993;38:977–995.

13 Nehra V, Camilleri M, Burton D, et al. An open trial of octreotide long-acting release in the management of short bowel syndrome. *Am J Gastroenterol* 2001;96:1494–1498.

14 Jeppesen PB, Mortensen PB. The influence of a preserved colon on the absorption of medium chain fat in patients with small bowel resection. *Gut* 1998;43:478–483.

15 Jacobsen O, Hojgaard L, Hylander Moller E, et al. Effect of enterocoated cholestyramine on bowel habit after ileal resection: a double blind crossover study. *Br Med J (Clin Res Ed)* 1985;290:1315–1318.

16 Ross Products [homepage on the Internet]. Abbott Park, IL: c 1999, 2006. Abbott Laboratories. Product Handbook. Pedialyte®. Available from: http://rpdcon40.ross.com/pn/PediatricProducts.NSF/web_Ross.com_XML_PediatricNutrition/CCF3870065DFF53585256A80007546E8?OpenDocument.

17 Ross Products [homepage on the Internet]. Abbott Park, IL: c 1999, 2006. Abbott Laboratories. Product Handbook. Rehydralyte®. Available from: http://rpdcon40.ross.com/pn/PediatricProducts.NSF/web_Ross.com_XML_PediatricNutrition/96A5745B1183947385256A80007546E5?OpenDocument.

18 Adrogué HJ, Madias NE. Hyponatremia. *N Engl J Med* 2000;342:1581–1589.

19 Ladefoged K, Olgaard K. Sodium homeostasis after small-bowel resection. *Scand J Gastroenterol* 1985;20:361–369.

20 Assadi F, Copelovitch L. Simplified treatment strategies to fluid therapy in diarrhea. *Pediatr Nephrol* 2003;18:1152–1156.

21 Schetz M, Dasta J, Goldstein S, et al. Drug-induced acute kidney injury. *Curr Opin Crit Care* 2005;11:555–565.

22 Manz F, Wentz A. The importance of good hydration for the prevention of chronic diseases. *Nutr Rev* 2005;63:S2–S5.

23 Lauverjat M, Hadj Aissa A, Vanhems P, et al. Chronic dehydration may impair renal function in patients with chronic intestinal failure on long-term parenteral nutrition. *Clin Nutr* 2006;25:75–81.

21 Intestinal Failure-Associated Liver Disease

Sue V. Beath and Jeremy M. Woodward

Key points

- Intestinal failure-associated liver disease (IFALD) is defined as a persistent (more than 2 weeks) elevation of liver function tests 1.5 times above the normal reference range.

- 50% of children and 30% adults have evidence of mild IFALD after 4–12 weeks of parenteral nutrition (PN).

- IFALD in children typically presents as cholestasis, whereas in adults steatosis is the usual underlying histopathology.

- Early detection of IFALD should prompt multi-professional review of the PN prescription, dietetic advice regarding enteral feeding, screening for infection and co-morbidity and focus efforts to achieve early discharge from hospital.

- Undernutrition, which normally defines severe liver disease, is masked by PN, frequently leading to an underestimation of IFALD severity.

- Persistent jaundice is a manifestation of advanced liver disease in the context of IFALD.

- When decompensation of IFALD occurs, it is often very rapid and accounts for the high mortality rate of patients awaiting liver and bowel transplants.

Introduction

Until the late 1960s, intestinal failure was incompatible with life. However, the dramatic improvement

Intestinal Failure: Diagnosis, Management and Transplantation.
Edited by Alan N. Langnas, Olivier Goulet, Eamonn M.M. Quigley and Kelly A. Tappenden. © 2008 Blackwell Publishing.
ISBN 978-1-4051-4637-1.

in life expectancy ushered in by the advent of parenteral nutrition (PN) resulted in the recognition of new metabolic complications of intestinal failure itself and of its treatment. Liver disease was quickly identified as one of the most significant among such problems and is now considered a major indication for intestinal transplantation [1]. Over recent years, it has become apparent that liver pathology associated with intestinal failure is expressed differently in adults and children, with the youngest patients demonstrating predominant cholestasis and more rapid progression to end stage liver disease [2], whereas steatosis is the principal lesion in adults [3].

Incidence and prevalence

There are wide variations in the numbers of patients with intestinal failure; in the late 1980s it was estimated that the prevalence was 2 patients on home PN (HPN) per million, whereas in France in 1995 the annual incidence was near 4 per million adults, and in the United States in 1995 use of HPN doubled between 1989 and 1992. In the United Kingdom, period prevalence varies from 4.5 per million population in Wales to 14.3 per million in Scotland, 12.5 per million in N Ireland and 9.5 per million in England [4]. This does not take account of the number of patients, especially children, who remain hospitalized for months or years, where the risk of intestinal failure-associated liver disease (IFALD), also known by the term parenteral nutrition associated cholestasis (PNAC), is higher. A 5-year pediatric study in Italy in 2003 identified 108 children with intestinal failure (22 new cases per year) for a population of 8 million children, giving an incidence of 2.5 per million children [5].

It has been reported consistently that around 50% of children on PN for 4–12 weeks have cholestasis [2,6,7], but in adults there is a much wider variation in the frequency of IFALD with around 30–50% having a mild disturbance of liver function tests and between 2% [8] and 30% [9] becoming cholestatic after a median of 6 months of PN. These variations in the incidence and subsequent natural history of IFALD reflect differences in case mix, health care systems, and the management of PN solutions, but it is reasonable to assume that one half of children and a third of adults on PN will develop mild liver disease with the potential to progress if not managed actively (see later in this chapter).

Definition

There are no consensus terminologies or diagnostic criteria for liver diseases associated with intestinal failure. In pediatrics, IFALD is commonly identified by the appearance of frank jaundice because this is very common in babies and can occur within weeks of commencing PN. In various studies of liver disease in pediatrics, researchers have defined IFALD in terms of a plasma bilirubin of 3, 4, 6, and 12 mg/dL (equivalent to 50, 70, 100, and 200 µmol/L). Using a serum bilirubin level of 50 mmol/L as a definition, up to 30–67% of infants aged less than 12 months develop IFALD [2,6,7,10]; in adults, jaundice is less common and takes longer to develop. However, using jaundice as the definition is far from satisfactory, as it represents a major disturbance of liver function and occurs after protracted and serious effects on hepatic structure and function have occurred. In common with adult practice, where jaundice is rarer, IFALD in children is defined in this chapter as liver function tests (that is alkaline phosphatase, gamma glutamyl transferase, aspartate transaminase, alanine transaminase) elevated to greater than 1.5 times the upper limit of the reference range, for at least 2 weeks, in the absence of another cause (e.g. drug-induced disease, viral hepatitis, biliary obstruction, metabolic disorder) [1,3]. This definition allows the problem of IFALD to be evaluated in a wider population of patients and at a potentially reversible stage.

Natural history of intestinal failure induced liver disease (see also Table 21.1)

IFALD encompasses both acute and chronic derangements of hepatobiliary function, as well as severe complications including fibrosis, cirrhosis, portal hypertension, and hepatocellular failure. The identification of IFALD relies on persistent elevations (i.e. for more than 2 weeks) of one or more liver enzymes or bilirubin in the peripheral blood, as liver biopsy is rarely performed in the early stages. However, the diagnosis can easily be confounded by alternative causes such as sepsis, drug toxicity and biliary obstruction.

Biochemistry

The earliest indications of IFALD are biochemical and include an elevation of serum alkaline phosphatase or gamma glutamyl transferase within 7–14 days of starting parenteral nutriton (PN). The hepatic transaminases also become elevated after 2–4 weeks to a lesser degree and, thereafter, the liver function tests may stabilize to within the normal range unless an event such as surgery or a catheter infection occurs. The next significant alteration in liver biochemistry is a rise in conjugated bilirubin concentration above 3 mg/dL (50 µmol/L), which heralds significant problems and is usually associated with changes in histology.

Histology

In young children, early changes include peri-portal inflammation and bile duct proliferation associated with peri-portal fibrosis. Ballooning hepatocyte necrosis is often present, but fatty change may be strikingly absent. Such changes may occur within 3 weeks in preterm infants requiring PN. Similar features may be found with biliary atresia, neonatal hepatitis or extrahepatic biliary obstruction. The fibrosis may be extensive (see Figure 21.1) but does not usually amount to cirrhosis, and cirrhosis is a relatively unusual and late event in IFALD [11]. There are no pathognomic features of IFALD and histologically the diagnosis is made by exclusion of other diseases and reference to the clinical context.

Steatosis in adults may occur rapidly on initiation of PN, and both macrovesicular and microvesicular fat loading may be apparent. This is an unusual pattern found otherwise only in association with fatty liver

Table 21.1 Clinical features of IFALD.

	Early	Established	Late
Clinical	Slightly enlarged liver (palpable 3 cm below right costal margin in young children)	Jaundice clearly discernible Spleen tip easily palpable Delayed developmental milestones	Intensely jaundiced, Marked hepato-splenomegaly Spider nevi, ascites Gastrointestinal bleeding
First line tests	Alkaline phophatase and γ-glutamyl transferase $\times$ 1.5 above upper limit reference range	Bilirubin 3–6 g/L Alkaline phophatase and γ-glutamyl transferase $\times$ 2–8 above normal range, alanine transaminase and aspartate transaminase $\times$ 2 above normal range Platelet count 100–150 $\times$ 10^9	Bilirubin more than 12 g/L, liver function tests $\times$ 3–5 above normal range, platelet count less than 100 $\times$ 10^9 INR worse than 1.5, unable to manage more than 2–4 hours off PN without hypoglycemia
Second line tests	Liver appears "echo-bright" 20% adult patients have ultrasound evidence of steatosis	Abdominal ultrasound shows enlarged spleen, biliary sludge +/− gallstones	Abdominal ultrasound shows grossly enlarged spleen, dampened portal vein flow and varices around gastro-esophageal junction, spontaneous porto-systemic shunts
Histology	Fatty changes	Fatty change, mild fibrosis	Extensive fibrosis, bile duct proliferation +/− plugs
Life expectancy pediatrics	As per underlying disease—70–90% five year survival if discharged home and no malignancy [22].	6–12 months* [17]	8 weeks* [11]
Life expectancy Adults	As per underlying disease and age 68% five year survival if no malignancy [24]	50–80% six year survival* [9]	100% mortality within 10–18 months of onset of jaundice* [22]

*For children and adults if remaining on unmodified PN regimen.

of pregnancy, Valproate or Tetracycline toxicity, or rare metabolic syndromes. The pattern of steatosis also helps to define the lesion, being predominantly periportal (see Figure 21.2), as with kwashiorkor or HIV-AIDS, rather than the pericentral steatosis seen with alcoholism, obesity, diabetes, or steroid therapy. Even quite marked elevations of liver enzymes may be associated with relatively bland steatosis, although steatohepatitis may occur, as with other conditions resulting in fatty liver, and result in periportal inflammation, hepatocyte necrosis, and pericellular fibrosis. Extensive fibrosis and progression to cirrhosis can occur with either predominant cholestatic or steatohepatitic lesions, but, generally, over a longer time course than in infants and then usually in association with steatosis.

Clinical

IFALD may become clinically apparent in infants after a septic event that precipitates jaundice, and can occur within days of commencing PN or after many months. Analysis of the pattern of IFALD in 70 neonates after surgery revealed an insidious rise in bilirubin until the onset of sepsis which heralded a rise to levels of 6–9 mg/dl (100–150 mmol/L). After one or two such episodes the bilirubin level fell to just above baseline, but jaundice generally persisted after further episodes, regardless of the resolution of infection, if PN feeding continued [6]. Hepatosplenomegaly may be present even in mildly jaundiced children and features of portal hypertension are generally more evident than the degree of histological fibrosis might suggest. Children may remain deceptively well despite being deeply

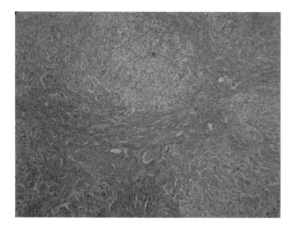

Figure 21.1 Light microscopy of liver biopsy magnified 100× to show extensive periportal fibrosis in a nine month infant who had received PN from birth because of short bowel syndrome secondary to multiple atresias. Masson trichrome high power. (Courtesy Dr Rachel Brown, consultant paediatric histopathologist, Birmingham Children's Hospital.)

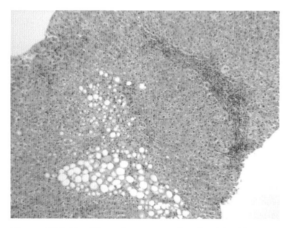

Figure 21.2 Liver biopsy from a young female adult with <20 cms of residual small intestine dependent on total parenteral nutrition. Features include zonal steatosis, which is of mixed type but predominantly macrovesicular, mild periportal inflammation, and fibrosis and ballooning hepatocyte degeneration. Hameatoxylin and eosin, medium power. (Courtesy Dr Susan Davies, consultant histopathologist, Addenbrooke's Hospital, Cambridge.)

jaundiced, as the parenteral nutrient supply masks the malabsorption and cachexia that would be expected to accompany severe liver disease. Progression to cirrhosis is relatively uncommon [11], but can occur after as short a period as 5 months on parenteral nutrition.

Decompensation occurs rapidly and accounts for the extremely high mortality rate of patients with end stage liver disease awaiting transplantation [12].

Progression to clinically overt liver disease in adults is insidious and until the onset of jaundice, the only symptom may be upper abdominal discomfort as a result of hepatic enlargement, and pruritus (often mild) as a result of cholestasis. Acute episodes of cholestasis, or more prolonged periods of chronic cholestasis can occur in adults with IFALD; in a study of 90 adults receiving home PN in France, 41.5% went on to develop more complicated liver disease, in which the bilirubin was greater than 60 µmol/L (3.5 g/L), in association with portal hypertension [9]. In contrast to children, the progression of IFALD was slower with a mortality of 22% for the group as a whole, with a 6-year survival of 84% in the patients aged less than 40 years and 53% 6-year survival for older patients. (See also Table 21.1.) In the United Kingdom, complicated IFALD in adults is uncommon with only around 2% of long-term PN patients becoming frankly jaundiced [8]. The reason for the difference in frequency of jaundice between different units is unclear but may reflect differences in exposure to intravenous lipid and the availability of Nutritional Support Teams. Cholelithiasis, however, has been frequently reported (45% of patients) and it is the practice of some centers to electively remove the gallbladder in patients who will remain on PN permanently [3].

Risk factors for the onset of IFALD

There is no single cause for the onset of IFALD, but the obvious differences in presentation and speed of progression between infants and adults strongly suggest that immaturity of the liver plays a major role. In addition there are probably a host of susceptibility genes yet to be discovered which interact with environmental triggers such as sepsis. The role of specific constituents in PN has been intensively studied, with associations between the onset and jaundice and excess exposure to phytosterols and lipid reported, although manganese seems to become a risk factor only once cholestasis is established [3,7]. Nevertheless, it is vital to screen for such toxic co-factors and reduce exposure to them, particularly if IFALD is developing. The relative lack of some conditionally essential substances such as

Table 21.2 Risk factors for IFALD.

Risk factor	Pediatrics	reference	Adults	reference
Age	Prematurity	6, 7, 10,	Older than 40 yrs Older than 50 yrs	12, 22
Co-morbidity	Loss of mucosal integrity	19	Malignancy Hepatitis C Crohn's disease	3, 9, 28
Short bowel syndrome	Lack of ICV* <25 cm	23, 2,	Lack of ICV* <100 cm	8
Catheter infections	>3 episodes	6	No definite association	13
Lipid	>3.5 g/kg/day	21	>1g/kg/day	9
Lack of staff trained in nutritional care	Infection rate reduced from 50% to 8%	16, 20		37
Lack of enteral stimulation	Biliary sludge	19	Decreased mucosal thickness and villus height Gallstones	3

* ICV = Ileo-cecal valve

taurine, carnitine, or glutamine should also be considered [1]. In children, catheter infections and other conditions that produce a systemic inflammatory response, such as necrotizing enterocolitis, are closely associated with IFALD, but in adults there is a much less clearly defined association with sepsis [13]. Table 21.2 summarizes risk factors which have been reported.

Pathophysiology

The liver receives around 25% of the cardiac output and much of that comes straight from the intestinal tract via the portal vein. Portal venous blood carries absorbed nutrients and a variety of hormones that modulate hepatocyte metabolism, especially insulin and glucagon. For example, the addition of glucagon to PN has been shown to prevent steatosis in parenterally fed rats [14]. The vascular route which nutrients follow may be important in the evolution of IFALD. For example, methionine metabolism differs significantly depending on whether it arrives via the systemic route (the hepatic artery) or via the portal vein. In the liver, methionine undergoes transulfuration, contributes to the methyl donor pathway that aids synthesis of choline and carnitine and is metabolized to substances such as cysteine, serine, and taurine. If delivered into the systemic circulation, this pathway is largely bypassed and hepatic metabolites such as cysteine may be undetectable and choline significantly reduced. Accordingly, serum methionine levels are increased in patients receiving PN, and as well as direct toxic effects, the relative deficiencies of taurine, serine and glutathione may increase the effect of endotoxin and so lead to IFALD [1].

Further evidence that the transulfuration pathway is important in IFALD comes from the observation that neonates, especially the premature infants who are most likely to develop IFALD, have an underdeveloped capacity for transulfuration for many weeks (in common with other enzyme systems such as conjugation of bilirubin with glucuronides) [15].

The role of sepsis in inducing cholestasis and parenchymal damage to the liver in children is very important particularly as in many cases it can be avoided with good line hygiene and monitoring by

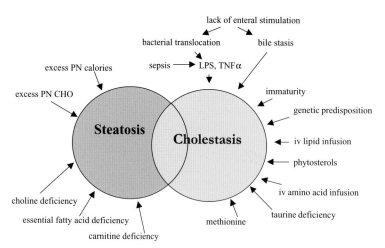

Figure 21.3 Some postulated mechanisms of IFALD.

the Nutritional Support Team [6,16,17]. The mechanism whereby septic episodes cause liver disease is via the cytokines and bacterial products, produced during infection, which have a direct effect on bilirubin metabolism. A summary of recent work has shown that endotoxin inhibits transcription of bile acid transporters located on the canalicular membrane and affects post transcriptional levels of Bsep and Ntep proteins as well [18].

Impaired bile acid recirculation caused by loss or disease to the distal ileum is another mechanism leading to IFALD. This is exacerbated by enteral starvation resulting in a lack of stimulation to bile flow and is considered to be a key reason for the development of biliary sludge and gall stones [3,19]. These mechanisms are illustrated in Figure 21.3.

Treatment

The treatment of IFALD requires a multiprofessional approach for children and adults. In children this should begin in the antenatal period with measures to reduce premature birth rates and identify congenital anomalies (e.g. gastroschisis) and continue through to coordinated monitoring of the infant by surgeons, pediatricians, nurses specializing in nutrition, dietitians, and pharmacists [20]. Although the prevention of IFALD must be the main goal, clearly many patients do unfortunately develop liver disease. As there are few good quality randomized trials and only a limited number of cohort and observational studies available (pre-

dominantly in the pediatric age group), preventative and therapeutic interventions for IFALD are mainly derived from expert opinion and are listed in Table 21.3.

A precise diagnosis for the cause of IFALD and persistent attempts to establish some enteral feeding should be made by the Nutrition Support Team in conjunction with a pathologist and radiologist (see Figure 21.4). Patients with chronic intestinal failure should be discharged home as soon as feasible as this has been shown to reduce the incidence of septic episodes, which have a close link with IFALD in children [16,17] (see also Chapter 14). Infections should be treated promptly and patients and their families advised on how to minimize the risk of catheter infections. Treatment with ursodeoxycholic acid and courses of metronidazole, for some patients with inflammatory lesions, have been shown to be helpful in a number of small studies [26–28]. Bacterial overgrowth leads directly to mucosal inflammation and indirectly to increase intestinal losses of bile by deconjugation of bilirubin, all of which seems to be a factor in prolonging dependency on PN [29]. Because an early introduction of lipid emulsions in pre-term infants was not associated with beneficial effects on growth, it has been suggested that starting lipid infusions should be delayed for some weeks, and that reduction or temporary cessation of intravenous lipid is now strongly recommended by several authorities [9,21,30] in patients with biochemical signs of liver dysfunction. The use of medium chain and long chain lipid emulsions should be considered as this mixture appears to enhance the incorporation of essential fatty

Table 21.3 Prevention and management of IFALD—summary of treatment recommendations based on expert opinion.

a) PATIENT RELATED

Modality	Comment
Stimulate entero-biliary axis	
a) commence enteral feeding to maximum tolerated	a) numerous cohort and case studies demonstrate benefits of enteral feeding on reduction in cholestasis [19,21,23].
b) supply choleretic agent e.g. ursodeoxycholic acid	b) ursodeoxycholic acid has minimal adverse effects and has been shown to improve liver function tests in neonates [26].
c) cholecystokinin	c) not been shown to be useful in neonates [33] (NB pancreatitis), but reversed cholestasis in an adult case report.
d) choline supplemented PN	d) in an RCT in adults was beneficial—reports from further studies are awaited [1].
Reduce impact of intestinal bacterial overgrowth	
a) metronidazole	a) retrospective study showing a link between inflammation and overgrowth, several studies (none RCT) showing improvements in liver function in metronidazole treated group [27–29].
b) avoid probiotics	b) caution advised in the use of probiotics for children with central venous lines because of risk of disseminated infection by probiotic [25].
Reduce intestinal stasis	
a) identify and treat strictures	a) reduces bacterial overgrowth and permits advances in enteral feeding [20,36].
b) consider tapering/plication for dilated dysmotile bowel	b) improves motility and reduces bacterial overgrowth [35].
Reduce impact of systemic sepsis	
a) antibiotic line locks	a) common practice in dialysis units but only marginal benefit in PN patients in one RCT—bigger studies needed [38].
b) nutritional support team (NST) to review sterile procedures for changing line	b) the role of NST in reducing sepsis rates is well described [16,17,21].
c) remove chronically infected line	
Improve absorptive function of intestinal tract	
a) tapering and lengthening surgery	a) several cohort studies with variable outcomes, delaying surgery until 12 months of age and focusing on optimising PN delivery seems to be an advantage [35].
b) re-establish continuity of intestine by taking down stomas	b) early reconnection or at least avoiding delay may be an advantage [20].
Isolated liver transplant (iLTx)	
Reserved for short bowel syndrome	iLTx has 60–80% 1-year survival in patients with short bowel who are progressing with weaning from PN before the onset of liver failure; avoid in patients with long-term need for PN especially if tolerance of enteral feed is poor (less than 50%) as IFALD recurs [34,36].

b) PARENTERAL NUTRITION RELATED

Modality	Comment
a) commence cyclical PN as soon as possible, i.e. from 3 months of age	a) cyclic PN is essential in avoiding a state of permanent hyperinsulinism caused by continuous infusion of glucose [21].
b) limit glucose intake to no more than 75% non protein calories	b) in infants glucose infusion should be no more than 1.2 g/kg/hour (20 mg/kg per minute) [21].
c) use pediatric amino acid solutions which provide additional taurine	c) Refs [21,32]
d) ensure manganese and aluminium content is minimized	d) managanese is neuro-toxic and concentra-tions rise in cholestasis because it is excreted in bile [7,19,21].
e) delay start of lipid in pre-term neonates	e) no adverse effect on growth compared with early introduction of lipid [30].
f) avoid more than 3.5 g/day lipid in infants and 1 g/kg/day lipid in adults	f) Refs [9,21].
g) consider using a mixture of medium and long chain triglyceride as lipid source	g) the addition of medium-chain triglyceride seems to enhance the incorporation of essential fatty acids and long-chain polyunsaturated fatty acids into circulating lipids [30].
h) consider using lipid emulsion enriched with alpha-tocopherol	h) in a short term RCT in intensive care setting patients receiving the alpha-tocopherol enriched emulsion had a smaller rise in plasma liver enzymes [31].

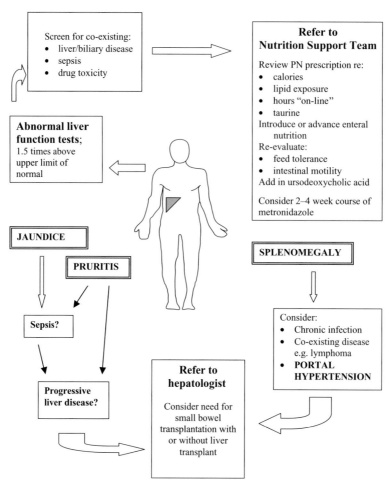

Figure 21.4 Algorithm for medical treatment options for IFALD.

acids and long chain polyunsaturated fatty acids into circulating liposomes compared with an emulsion containing only long chain triglyceride [30]. The addition of excess alpha-tocopherol to prevent peroxidation in lipid emulsions may protect against hepatic injury as suggested in a study of 20 adults in an intensive care setting [31]. Effective shielding of PN bags from light and their prompt use after addition of vitamins may also therefore be relevant. Taurine appears to be protective against IFALD in infants, especially those with a history of necrotizing enterocolitis [32] and is currently being evaluated in adults.

Steatosis rather than cholestasis is the key problem in adult IFALD, reducing total calories, or the carbohydrate:lipid ratio is an important part of clinical practice alongside the use of cyclical PN rather than continuous 24-hour infusions [3] in order to reduce circulating insulin levels. In pediatrics, it is recommended that glucose intake should usually cover 60–75% of non protein calories and that the maximal infusion rate should not exceed 1.2 g/kg per hour (20 mg/kg per minute) even during cyclical PN which is well tolerated from 3 months of age [21].

Cholecystokinin infusion has been demonstrated to reverse severe cholestasis and prevent IFALD, but a randomized placebo-controlled trial has demonstrated no benefit in neonates [33], and this treatment carries the risk of inducing acute pancreatitis. A well-conducted trial of choline-supplemented PN in long-term parenterally fed patients has demonstrated a reduction in steatosis and improvement in liver biochemistry [1].

Surgical treatment should also be considered carefully; routine cholecystectomy is practiced in some countries for patients who are clearly going to remain on PN for many years [3]. The decision to embark on further abdominal surgery in a child or adult with evolving liver failure is always a difficult one, but intestinal plication or tapering and lengthening operations for well selected patients with short bowel syndrome, can produce improvements in intestinal function and resolution of IFALD if the PN is, thereby, reduced or discontinued [20,34,35] (see also Chapter 26 of this volume for more detailed discussion of this important topic). The option of isolated liver transplant is available for patients (almost always young children aged less than 2 years with short bowel syndrome) with a good prognosis for future intestinal autonomy, but in whom liver failure has supervened [36]. The rehabilitation of these patients is more protracted than after small bowel transplantation so it is advisable to refer to an experienced unit [20,34].

Conclusion

Despite improvements in the type and mode of delivery of PN and the involvement of nutrition support teams, the occurrence of end-stage liver disease in IFALD is still relatively common [9,11,22]. Organ transplantation has an important role in treating end-stage liver disease, especially in young children, although a shortage of suitable donors means that the mortality remains high [12]. It is, therefore, vitally important for patients that the early signs of IFALD are recognized and treated, especially if sepsis is present at this is associated with progressive parenchymal damage to liver. Considerable advances have been made in our understanding of the genesis of IFALD; in particular, it seems clear that cholestatic presentations are largely related to prematurity and sepsis whereas steatosis is related to a suboptimal carbohydrate:lipid ratio. New therapies aimed at enhancing important metabolic pathways for methionine, choline, taurine, glutathione, and bile salts, optimizing the insulin and glucagon axis by modifying lipid and carbohydrate intake, and targeting harmful cytokine responses can be expected to reduce the severity and frequency of IFALD in future.

References

1 Buchman AL, Iyer K, Fryer J. Parenteral Nutrition-Associated Liver Disease and the role of Isolated intestine and Intestine/Liver Transplantation. *Hepatology* 2006;43:9–19.

2 Sondheimer JM, Asturias E, Cadnapaphornchai M. Infection and cholestasis in neonates with intestinal resection and long term parenteral nutrition. *J Pediatr Gastroenterol Nutr* 1998;6:131–137.

3 Nightingale JM. Hepatobiliary, renal and bone complications of intestinal failure. *Best Pract Res Clin Gastroenterol* 2003;17:907–929.

4 Home parenteral nutrition in the United Kingdom, a position paper prepared by BAPEN (2003) accessed on 27 March 2006 at http://www.bapen.org.uk/publications/homeparenteral nutrition.

5 Guarino A, De Marco G. Natural history of intestinal failure, investigated through a national network-based approach. *J Pediatr Gastroenterol Nutr* 2003;37:136–141.

6 Beath SV, Davies P, Papadopoulou A, et al. Parenteral nutrition related cholestasis in post surgical neonates: multivariate analysis of risk factors. *J Pediatr Surg* 1996;31:604–606.

7 Kelly DA. Liver complications of pediatric parenteral nutrition-epidemiology. *Nutrition* 1998;14:153–157.

8 Lumen W, Shaffer JL. Prevalence, outcome and associated factors of deranged liver function tests in patients on home parenteral nutrition. *Clin Nutr* 2002;21:337–343.

9 Cavicchi M, Beau P, Crenn P, et al. Prevalence of liver disease and contributing factors in patients receiving home parenteral nutrition for permanent intestinal failure. *Ann Intern Med* 2000;132:525–532.

10 Kubota A, Okada A, Nezu R, et al. Hyperbilirubinemia in neonates associated with total parenteral nutrition. *JPEN J Parenteral Enteral Nutr* 1988;12:602–606.

11 Beath SV, Needham SJ, Kelly DA, et al. Clinical features and prognosis of children assessed for isolated small bowel (ISBTx) or combined small bowel and liver transplantation (CSBLTx). *J Pediatr Surg* 1997;32:459–461.

12 Fryer J, Pellar S, Ormond D, et al. Mortality in candidates waiting for combined liver-intestine transplants exceeds that for other candidates waiting for liver transplants. *Liver Transpl* 2003;9:748–753.

13 Clarke PJ, Ball MJ, Kettlewell MG. Liver function tests in patients receiving parenteral nutrition. *JPEN J Parenter Enteral Nutr* 1991;15:54–59.

14 Li SJ, Nussbaum MS, McFadden DW, et al. Addition of glucagon to total parenteral nutrition (TPN) prevents hepatic steatosis in rats. *Surgery* 1988;104:350–357.

15 Vina J, Vento M, Garcia-Sala F, et al. L-cysteine and glutathione metabolism are impaired in premature infants due to cystathionase deficiency. *Am J Clin Nutr* 1995;61:1067–1069.

16 Puntis JWL, Holden CE, Smallman S, et al. Staff training: a key factor in reducing intravascular catheter sepsis. *Arch Dis Child* 1991;66:335–337.

17 Beath SV, Booth IW, Murphy MS, et al. Nutritional care and candidates for small-bowel transplantation. *Arch Dis in Child* 1995;73:348–350.

18 Trauner M, Boyer JL. Cholestatic syndromes. *Curr Opin Gastroenterol* 2003;19:216–231.

19 Kaufman SS. Prevention of parenteral nutrition-associated liver disease in children. *Pediatr Transplant* 2002;6:37–42.

20 Sudan D, DiBaise J, Torres C, et al. A multidisciplinary approach to the treatment of intestinal failure. *J Gastrointest Surg* 2005;9:165–176.

21 Guidelines on paediatric parenteral nutrition of the European Society of Paediatric Gastroenterlogy, Hepatology and Nutrition (ESPGHAN) and the European Society for Clinical Nutrition and Metabolism (ESPEN), supported by the European Society of Paediatric Research (ESPR). *J Pediatr Gastroenterol Nutr* 2005; suppl.

22 Chan S, McCowen KC, Bistrian BR, et al. Incidence, prognosis, and etiology of end-stage liver disease in patients receiving home total parenteral nutrition. *Surgery.* 1999;126:28–34.

23 Goulet O, Baglin-Gobet S, Talbotec C, et al. Outcome and long-term growth after extensive small bowel resection in the neonatal period: a survey of 87 children. *Eur J Pediatr Surg* 2005;15:95–101.

24 Pironi L, Paganelli F, Labate AM, et al. Safety and efficacy of home parenteral nutrition for chronic intestinal failure: a 16-year experience at a single centre. *Dig Liver Dis* 2003;35:314–324.

25 Michail S, Sylvester F, Fuchs G, Issenman R. Clinical practice guidelines on probiotics. *J Pediatr Gastroenterol Nutr* 2006;43:550–557.

26 Levine A, Maayan A, Shamir R, et al. Parenteral nutrition-associated cholestasis in pre-term infants: evaluation of urosdeoxycholic acid treatment. *J Pediatr Endocrinol Metab* 1999;12:549–553.

27 Kubota A, Okada A, Imura K, et al. The effect of metronidazole on TPN-associated liver dysfunction in neonates. *J Ped Surg* 1990;25:618–621.

28 Capron Jp, Herve MA, Gineston JL, Braillon A. Metronidazole in prevention of cholestasis associated with total parenteral nutrition. *Lancet* 1983;26:446–447.

29 Kaufman SS, Loseke CA, Lupo JV. Influence of bacterial overgrowth and intestinal inflammation on duration of PN in children with short bowel syndrome. *J Pediatr* 1997;131:356–361.

30 Krohn K, Koletzko B. Parenteral lipid emulsions in paediatrics. *Curr Opin Nutr Metab Care* 2006;9:319–323.

31 Antebi H, Mansoor O, Ferrier C, et al. Liver function and plasma antioxidant status in intensive care unit patients requiring total parenteral nutrition: comparisom of 2 fat emulsions. *JPEN J Parenter Enteral Nutr* 2004;28:142–148.

32 Spencer AU, Yu S, Tracy TF, et al. Parenteral nutrition-associated cholestasis in neonates: multivariate analysis of the potential protective effect of taurine. *JPEN J Parenter Enteral Nutr* 2005;29:337–343.

33 Teitelbaum DH, Tracy TF Jr, Aouthmany MM, et al. Use of cholecytokinin-octapeptide for the prevention of parenteral nutrition-associated cholestasis. *Pediatrics* 2005;115:1332–1340.

34 Hassan KO, Beath SV, McKiernan PJ, Kelly DA. Clarke SE, Pimpilwar A, Bianchi A, J de Ville de Goyet. Difficult management choices for infants with short bowel syndrome and liver failure. *J Ped Gastroenterol Nutr* 2002;35:1–3.

35 Bianchi A. From cradle to enteral autonomy: the role of autologous gastrointestinal reconstruction. *Gastroenterology* 2006;130:S138–S146.

36 Botha JF, Grant WJ, Torres C, et al. Isolated liver transplantation in infants with end-stage liver disease due to short bowel syndrome. *Liver Transpl* 2006;12:1062–1066.

37 Howard JP, Bruce J, Powell-Tuck J. Nutritional support: a course for developing multidisciplinary clinical teams. Education Committee, British Association for Parenteral and Enteral Nutrition. *JR Soc Med* 1997;90:675–678.

38 Rijnders BJ, Van Wijngaerden F, Vandecasteele SJ, et al. Treatment of long-term intravascular catheter-related bacteraemia with antibiotic lock: randomized, placebo-controlled trial. *J Antimicrob Chemother* 2005;55: 90–94.

22 Psychiatric Issues in the Assessment of the Patient with Intestinal Failure

James H. Sorrell

Key points

- Depression and anxiety are common psychiatric disorders seen in patients with intestinal failure and require aggressive treatment with consideration given to problems associated with poor enteral absorption of psychotropic medications.

- Chronic pain and narcotic dependence are frequent consequences of intestinal failure and efforts should be made to eliminate or substantially reduce the use of narcotic analgesia in this patient population.

- Psychiatric assessment and treatment of the child and adolescent with intestinal failure requires an understanding of normative developmental processes and family dynamics.

- Intestinal transplantation requires a thorough psychiatric assessment to determine a candidate's psychological suitability and areas of vulnerability that are amenable to intervention and treatment.

Introduction

Intestinal failure is a grave clinical outcome resulting from a wide variety of diseases and injuries in the widest assortment of patients. Although the severity of intestinal failure is often discussed in terms of bowel length, it is more properly understood as a functional disorder in which the remaining bowel lacks the integrity to support the nutritional and fluid requirements of the patient. Intestinal failure presents

Intestinal Failure: Diagnosis, Management and Transplantation. Edited by Alan N. Langnas, Olivier Goulet, Eamonn M.M. Quigley and Kelly A. Tappenden. © 2008 Blackwell Publishing. ISBN 978-1-4051-4637-1.

significant and even unique psychological challenges and social obstacles to the patient. The diversity of the patient population with intestinal failure, the host of associated psychiatric issues, and the ever-increasing sophistication of the medical care available, present, in turn, a formidable challenge to the medical team charged with their care. Nevertheless, there are few studies addressing these concerns.

The psychiatric consultant may be faced with a young child who has a history of necrotizing enterocolitis with growth and developmental delays and a family stretched to the end of their emotional and material resources. In contrast, he may be asked to evaluate a passive and sullen adolescent with short gut from a bullet wound who is non-adherent with his physician's recommendations. Likewise, he may be asked to address the issue of escalating opioid narcotic use in an adult woman with a history of Crohn's disease and multiple prior surgical interventions in the long course of her illness. These examples are merely a glimpse into breadth and depth of the intrapsychic and interpersonal dimensions of living with intestinal failure. The clinician needs to consider the developmental stage of the patient, issues of character and temperament, the different coping strategies utilized in managing the impact of a catastrophic acute injury, and the deforming effects of chronic illness and chronic pain. At the same time, the psychiatrist will be asked to treat psychiatric illnesses, mainly depression and anxiety, in patients with incompetent guts and evaluate and firmly confront substance dependence in persons at odds with, and risking alienation from, their medical team.

The present chapter will focus on just a few of the more common and pressing problems encountered in the care of patients with intestinal failure.

Depression and anxiety

It is increasingly recognized that depression is more common in patients with concomitant medical illnesses. Studies in heart disease, stroke, and diabetes have consistently demonstrated that the presence of depression worsens the course of the medical illness, increases the cost of care and is associated with excessive mortality. Although there are no studies devoted to patients with intestinal failure, patients with inflammatory bowel disease have been shown to have high rates of depression and anxiety with much of the risk occurring in the year following the diagnosis of their bowel disease [1]. Furthermore, the presence of depressed mood and anxiety correlated with earlier and more frequent relapse into active bowel disease [2]. Intestinal failure, like inflammatory bowel disease, involves multiple medical and surgical procedures, pain and incontinence, and disruption of social practices (e.g. eating), all of which can compromise quality of life and self-esteem and contribute to high rates of depression and anxiety. Given the high prevalence of depression seen in patients with intestinal failure, routine surveillance for symptoms of sadness and despair are warranted. Diagnosis can be enhanced with the use of standardized and well-validated screening instruments such as the Beck Depression and Anxiety inventories [3]. The clinician is strongly encouraged to avoid rationalizing or minimizing the depressive symptoms as "understandable" given the severity of the underlying clinical picture.

Once the diagnosis is made, aggressive treatment is necessary. In general, depression in the medically ill is associated with lower recovery rates and more chronicity. Adequate pharmacotherapy in patients with intestinal failure is limited by poor enteral absorption. The literature regarding clinical outcomes in depression in this patient group is limited to a handful of single case reports [4]. Most patients are initially treated with serotonin selective reuptake inhibitors (SSRIs) for depression and anxiety disorders. For those patients who fail to achieve a clinical remission after 4–8 weeks of drug therapy or who experience weight loss, diarrhea, or significant sexual dysfunction on these medications, an alternative strategy may include the use of the orally dissolvable agent, mirtazipine, or the use of a tricyclic antidepressant. Mirtazipine is less associated with weight loss and has fewest gastrointestinal side effects and the orally dissolved tablet may possibly facilitate some buccal and gastric absorption, thereby, increasing its bioavailability. Nortriptiline, a tricyclic antidepressant, is unique among antidepressants as it possesses a therapeutic window (50–150 ng/mL). The ability to determine blood levels can allow the clinician to determine if there is adequate absorption and guide dose titrations safely. Finally, a transdermal monamine oxidase inhibitor, selegiline, has just recently been released in the United States. This is the first commercially available antidepressant that bypasses the need for enteral absorption and may prove of great value in this patient population. The greatest drawback is the possibility of potentially dangerous drug interactions with this class of antidepressants with many of the drugs commonly used in patients with intestinal failure, and especially opioid narcotics. Finally, psychotherapeutic interventions should be utilized. Adult patients with recent acute or traumatic loss of their bowel are often overwhelmed and manifest significant anxiety about the powerlessness and loss of control they are experiencing. Psychological integrity can be threatened by the recent near-death experience and dramatic changes in body image. For the patient with a chronic illness that has progressed to intestinal failure, there may have been significant psychological adaptation, but this has often occurred at the expense of a rigid and overcontrolled coping style and diminished participation and satisfaction in important social functions. Individual therapy oriented toward personal insight and supportive group therapy with other patients with intestinal failure can make a significant improvement in understanding and agency. Furthermore, attention should be paid to the spouse or care partner who is often charged with significant clinical responsibilities and care-giving, but whose own emotional welfare may be threatened by the severity of their partner's illness and uncertainty regarding their future.

Chronic pain and substance abuse

Another recurring and particularly vexing problem in the care of the intestinal failure patient is the large number of these patients who rely on high levels of opioid narcotics. Most complain of chronic abdominal pain, others of back pain. Many are on extraordinary amounts of oral and transdermal narcotics. The literature on chronic pain in nonmalignant conditions demonstrates that there are high levels of opioid dependence and co-morbidity with depression and anxiety disorders in chronic pain patients. In the intestinal failure patient, there is often heavy reliance on sedative-hypnotics, primarily benzodiazepines. These co-dependent patients often experience worse opioid withdrawal symptoms compared to those patients on narcotics alone [5].

The impact of this chronic and often addictive use of opioids can be severe. In a study of quality of life among patients receiving home parenteral nutrition, the poorest scores were seen in patients dependent on narcotic drugs [6]. Another study compared outcomes for a group of narcotic-dependent home parenteral nutrition patients with a group of non-dependent patients over a 12-month period. The narcotic dependent patients had significantly more hospitalizations and complications, primarily as a result of a higher incidence of line sepsis [7].

Many patients receiving sustained-action narcotics have symptoms of fatigue, depression, diminished libido, and impaired sexual function associated with chronic narcotic use. Several studies have found frequent, sometimes profound, deficiencies in sex hormone levels in many men and women treated with narcotics [8]. The experience of pain is not merely one of sensory perception; it has a large emotional and evaluative component. These components are especially dominant in chronic pain. The experiences of uncertainty, fearful anticipation of further interventions, emotional suffering and a sense of loss of control can easily be constricted into the felt experience and language of "I am in pain." In turn, the clinician faced with the suffering and despondent patient may choose an unarticulated sense of his own discomfort to respond concretely with a prescription for a pain medication. A vicious cycle ensues; the opioid use leads to more sedation, apathy and inactivity, pain is reported to be unabated, dosages are escalated, clinical suspicion and resentment of addiction occur, and the physician-patient relationship is strained, often to a breaking point. This leads to a further loss of self-efficacy and control among both parties.

In light of the potential physical and psychological damage attributable to drug dependence in this patient population, one goal of the clinician and multidisciplinary team is the reduction and, preferably, elimination of these medications. Treatment of underlying psychiatric illnesses, referral to treatment programs for the selected patient with poly-substance abuse and efforts to bolster the patient's psychical activity and social functioning can be useful in reducing daily requirements of narcotics. Withdrawal is best achieved with a slow, yet predetermined, taper. Depending on the length of addiction, a decrease every 2–4 weeks of 10–25% of daily dosage can safely avoid severe withdrawal symptoms. For patients on shorter acting agents, a switch to longer acting narcotics, including methadone, can ease withdrawal. Subsequent use of pain medication following procedures or, as dictated by objective clinical findings, should be time-limited and closely monitored. The operative concern guiding the use of pain medications (as with any other clinical intervention we make) in this patient population should be to preserve health, facilitate independent functioning, and enhance well-being.

Special concerns in the care of the child and the adolescent

Intestinal failure, as in all chronic medical conditions, puts increased stress on the child and the child's parents and siblings. The clinical severity of the disorder is not generally the most significant factor predicting distress and the emergence of psychiatric illness. It is important to understand the developmental stage and cognitive capacities of the child and adolescent as they intersect with the particular stressors at that particular time. The child's resiliency depends, in large part, on the ability of the family to cope with the child's illness and preserve energy for their own self care and attention to the ill child's siblings. Clearly the burden of home parenteral nutrition taxes a family's resources. Sleep is disrupted, family rituals distorted and social activities curtailed [9]. Family dynamics in chronic illness become more regimented and less emotionally warm [10]. If the child is young, the mother often remains in hospital and care of the siblings fall to the father, who frequently copes less well and often utilizes avoidant coping behaviors [11]. Unfortunately, the reality of intentional illness creation by a parent (Munchhausen by proxy) in the child with intestinal failure must not be overlooked.

The expression that psychological distress takes depends on the child's cognitive, emotional and social development. In the face of significant clinical deterioration, a 9-year-old with intestinal failure may seem unaware of the growing concern for her health, yet at the same time her parents will hear from her school that they are witnessing a marked deterioration in her school work and previously unseen bullying behavior on the playground. By contrast, a 15-year-old may withdraw to his room, start wearing black exclusively, and start listening to music laden with themes of death and violence. This illustrates the need to understand normative development in order to identify an emergent clinical problem versus a developmentally appropriate coping response.

Of particular concern for the medical team is the appearance of nonadherence to their medical care in the adolescent patient. Addressing this potentially life-threatening behavior needs to be done in the full recognition of an adolescent's increasing need for autonomy and self-understanding. Simply "clamping down," as in requiring more parental supervision and less self-control, will only lead to more oppositional behavior and worse outcomes.

Assessment of the transplant candidate

Patients with intestinal failure are generally treated with home parenteral nutrition and/or attempts at bowel rehabilitation. Unfortunately, recurrent line infections and progressive liver disease can be life-threatening complications. The availability of intestinal transplantation, alone or in conjunction with liver transplantation, has the potential to be life-extending and significantly increase the quality of life of recipients [12,13]. The assessment of individual patients for intestinal transplantation includes an evaluation of their psychological suitability for the procedure.

The goals of a psychiatric assessment of the intestinal failure patient regarding transplantation are the identification and selection of the patients most likely to benefit from the procedure and the identification of areas of psychosocial concern that, unaddressed, might compromise survival and rehabilitation post transplantation. Much like the evaluation of any transplantation

candidate, the assessment should include a history of prior psychiatric illness, including suicidality, history of adherence or nonadherence to medical care, adaptation to past stressors, substance abuse history, and presence and quality of social support [14]. The use of a brief, standardized psychiatric interview, such as the Mini International Neuropsychiatric Interview, is recommended. In patients with co-morbid cirrhosis, a clinical interview and the use of neuropsychological screening instruments can identify subtle but problematic cognitive impairment (hepatic encephalopathy).

Depressive disorders should be treated aggressively as outlined here. For those patients living at a great distance from the transplant center, a psychiatrist should be identified in their own community who is comfortable with treating the medically ill patient and records of the transplantation evaluation and recommendations for treatment strategies should be sent to them. Narcotic dependent patients need tapering and preferably withdrawal from their opioid(s) before surgery. Doing so will dramatically simplify the management of their post operative pain. Finally, unrecognized or poorly treated psychiatric illness in the primary caregiver or partner should be addressed prior to placing a large burden of the post-transplant patient's care on their lap.

Conclusion

Uncertainty, intrusive medical care, loss of independence, and profound disturbances in bodily integrity and social functioning conspire to challenge and frequently undermine the psychological well-being of the patient with intestinal failure. Depression is a common clinical problem and treatment is problematic because of the severity of the underlying stressors and the difficulty of achieving therapeutic blood levels of antidepressants. Prior episodes of acute pain and a sense of interminable suffering can easily lead to a chronic pain syndrome. Narcotic analgesia offers relief but carries the real risk of addiction. Children and adolescents experience of illness is colored by their developmental stage and, subsequently, their experience of self is shaped by their illness and invalidism. Transplantation, which offers great promise, requires a commitment to lifelong immunosuppression and exposes the patient and their family to unique stresses. These are some of the major issues encountered that require psychiatric attention. The successful treatment of these difficulties can greatly enhance the quality of care of the patient with intestinal failure. The presence and participation of a psychiatrist as an active member of the treatment team will go far to achieving optimal outcomes for this challenging patient population.

References

1 Kurina LM, Goldacre MJ, Yeats D, Gill LE. Depression and anxiety in people with inflammatory bowel disease. *J Epidemiol Community Health* 2001;55:716–720.

2 Mittermaier C, Dejaco C, Waldhoer T, et al. Impact of depressed mood on relapse in patients with inflammatory bowel disease: a prospective 18-month follow-up study. *Psychosomatic Medicine* 2004;66:79–84.

3 Wilhelm K, Kotze B, Waterhouse M, et al. Screening for depression in the medically ill: a comparison of self-report measures, clinical judgment, and DSM-IV diagnoses. *Psychosomatics* 2004;45:461–469.

4 Severijnen R, Bayat N, Bakker H, et al. Enteral drug absorption in patients with short small bowel. *Clin Pharmacokinet* 2004;43:951–962.

5 de Wet C, Reed L, Glasper A, et al. Benzodiazepine codependence exacergates the opioid withdrawal syndrome. *Drug Alcohol Depend* 2004;76:31–35.

6 Richards DM and Irving MH. Assessing the quality of life of patients with intestinal failure on home parenteral nutrition. *Gut* 1997;40:218–222.

7 Richards DM, Scott NA, Shaffer JL, Irving M. Opiate and sedative dependence predicts poor outcome for patients receiving home parenteral nutrition. *JPEN J Parenter Enteral Nutr* 1997;21:336–338.

8 Daniell HW. Narcotic induced hypogonadism during therapy for heroin addiction. *J Addict Dis* 2002;21:42–53.

9 Engstrom I, Bjornestam B, Finkel Y. Psychological distress associated with home parenteral nutrition in Swedish children, adolescents, and their parents. *J Pediatr Gastroenterol Nutr* 2003;37:246–250.

10 Wamboldt MZ, Wamboldt FS. Role of the family in the onset and outcome of childhood disorders: selected research findings. *J Am Acad Child Adol Psychiatry* 2000;39:1212–1219.

11 Goble LA. The impact of a child's chronic illness on Fathers. *Issues in Comprehensive Pediatric Nursing* 2004;27:153–162.

12 Sudan D. Quality of life after intestinal transplantation. *Prog Transplant* 2004;14:284–288.

13 Rovera GM, DiMartini A, Schoen RE, et al. Quality of life of patients after intestinal transplantation. *Transplantation* 1998;66:1141–1145.

14 Jowsey SG, Talyor ML, Schneekloth TD, Clark MM. Psychosocial challenges in transplantation. *J Psychiatr Pract* 2001;7:404–414.

23 Munchausen Syndrome by Proxy

Paul E. Hyman and Brenda Bursch

Key points

- Munchausen syndrome by proxy is a form of child abuse characterized by a caretaker secretly causing illness with the inadvertent collusion of medical professionals.

- Muchausen syndrome by proxy commonly involves gastrointestinal symptoms, and may mimic chronic intestinal pseudo-obstruction, a cause of intestinal failure.

- Absence of bowel dilation, normal intestinal manometry, accelerating disease trajectory, daily pain, and absence of urinary bladder involvement characterize Muchausen by proxy, simulating chronic intestinal pseudo-obstruction.

- Centers of excellence caring for children with chronic intestinal pseudo-obstruction and intestinal failure must be prepared to identify and report Munchausen by proxy.

Over 20 years, more than 200 children with intestinal failure and a diagnosis of chronic intestinal pseudo-obstruction have been referred for confirmatory intestinal manometry (Hyman, unpublished data). Just over half the children had severe abnormalities in contraction patterns, explaining their symptoms. About 25% of the children, nearly all preteens and teens with pain or nausea as the chief complaint, met criteria for functional bowel disorders. These patients had normal or nearly normal motility studies. Sixteen percent of children referred for intestinal failure had normal motility and features suggesting that the illness was fal-

Intestinal Failure: Diagnosis, Management and Transplantation.
Edited by Alan N. Langnas, Olivier Goulet, Eamonn M.M. Quigley and Kelly A. Tappenden. © 2008 Blackwell Publishing. ISBN 978-1-4051-4637-1.

sified [1]. A few of these children died unexpectedly. One underwent intestinal transplantation [2].

It is important for professionals working with children diagnosed with pediatric gastrointestinal diseases to be aware of the frequency, warning signs, and ways of falsifying vomiting, diarrhea, feeding problems, abdominal distension, and pain. Because chronic intestinal pseudo-obstruction with intestinal failure is exceedingly rare, it is essential that intestinal transplant teams routinely place illness falsification on the differential diagnosis and are adept at assessing for this potentially lethal form of child abuse. The purpose of this chapter is to educate clinicians how to approach the assessment of illness falsification.

Definition

Munchausen by proxy is a form of child maltreatment in which an adult falsifies signs or symptoms in a victim, causing that victim to be regarded as ill or impaired [3]. There are two components to this term: victimization of the child and psychopathology of the abuser. The term *pediatric condition/illness falsification* describes the abusive behavior, regardless of motivation. *Factitious disorder by proxy* is the psychiatric diagnostic term for the abuser whenever the motivation for abuse is to satisfy personal psychological needs.

There are multiple methods of illness falsification, including exaggeration, fabrication, simulation, and induction. Exaggeration is embellishment of a genuine problem. Fabrication refers to completely false statements made by the abuser about the child's medical history or symptoms. Abusers simulate problems by falsifying records, medical tests, or symptoms. Examples include moving a pH probe during an evaluation, adding nail polish remover to a urine sample, or contaminating a diaper with one's own blood. Induction is the direct triggering of a problem or aggravating a genuine problem. Examples include poisoning, injecting air into a gastrostomy, or manipulation of insulin or asthma medications. All these methods take place under the unwitting collusion of unsuspecting medical professionals. The evaluation of illness falsification must take into account these potential forms of falsification.

Any gastrointestinal illness can be falsified, including: appendicitis, bacterial overgrowth, celiac disease, chronic intestinal pseudo-obstruction, cystic fibrosis, gastroesophageal reflux, functional GI disorders, infections, inflammatory bowel disease, intestinal obstructions, malnutrition, secretory diarrhea, and pancreatitis [2,4–8]. The most frequent complaints reported by caregivers who falsify illness in their children included the GI-related symptoms of anorexia/feeding problems (24.6%), diarrhea (20.0%), and pain (8.0%) [9]. Apnea, cyanosis, and vomiting were the most frequently reported symptoms among 6% of victims who had died. A previous review also found high rates of reports of vomiting (10%) among suspected abusers [10].

Diarrhea can be simulated by adding fluid to feces or by presenting someone else's diarrhea in place of the child's stool sample. Unexpectedly low electrolyte and osmolar concentrations may indicate water was added to the sample. Diarrhea can be induced by altering the diet or medications of an ill child or by poisoning with osmotic agents, stimulants, or bacteria (i.e., feces); with suppositories or by repeated enemas. Fasting is can be used to distinguish between osmotic and secretory diarrhea [8,11,12]. Persistent osmotic diarrhea during fasting suggests laxative abuse. Vomiting, hematemesis, and rectal bleeding can also be simulated by presenting someone else's emesis, feces, or blood in place of the child's sample. Induction of vomiting can involve gagging the child or poisoning. Rectal bleeding can be simulated by mixing the child's or someone else's blood or feces with that of the child [13–15]. Induction of hematemesis or rectal bleeding can be caused by corrosives or direct injury.

Warning signs

While insufficient for diagnosis, warning signs *related to the illness* include that the illness (or test result) does not make medical sense, is oddly difficult to effectively treat, is exceedingly rare, or does not follow a normal illness or recovery trajectory. Preliminary research [1] suggests that warning signs in cases of falsified chronic intestinal pseudo-obstruction include: (a) daily abdominal pain, (b) illness involving three or more organ systems, (c) an accelerating disease trajectory, (d) a reported history of preterm birth, (e) absence of dilated bowel on X-ray, (f) normal antroduodenal manometry, and (g) no urinary neuromuscular disease. Although these findings are not presented as diagnostic criteria, the index of illness falsification suspicion should rise with the number of warning signs. General warning signs *of a suspected abuser* include symptoms only occur in the caregiver's presence or after the caregiver has been present; the caregiver is unusually attentive to medical issues; the caregiver appears less or more worried about child's illness than medical staff (doesn't take cues related to level of alarm from clinicians); the caregiver is medically knowledgeable or attempts to appear so; the caregiver requests unnecessary or dangerous medical procedures; or the caregiver has a pattern of lying. *Family history warning signs* include: caregiver reports medical interests or experience; or the caregiver or the family has an extensive history of illness.

Clinical assessment

General recommendations and planning

Because abusers are often well liked and consequently team members typically do not agree about the likelihood of pediatric illness falsification, we recommend a team approach to assessment with the assistance of a written protocol. The goal is to conduct a scientific, systematic, safe, thorough, and objective assessment without unnecessarily alarming the family or creating undo conflict among team members. Team members might include attending physicians and residents, nursing, the hospital child protection team, social work, psychiatry/psychology, child life, security, and other consultants involved (such as nutrition services, medical consultants, physical therapy, experts on the topic of pediatric illness falsification).

The written protocol delineates task responsibility and outlines procedures, including frequent communication with the family and among team members; obtaining and reviewing past records; collateral contacts with past clinicians and other caregivers; guidelines for documentation and for the collection of physical specimens that could be evidence; planning for family, child and team emotional support; developing an assessment and treatment plan; discussing and arranging safety parameters for the child and family members; and deciding when/if contact with outside authorities is required. Safety issues to consider for inpatients include location of the child (intensive care unit, private room, near nurses station, etc.); level of monitoring (telemetry, sitter, visitation, hours, covert videotape, etc.); and emergency response plans (in case of acute medical event or attempted discharge against medical advice). It is also useful for the protocol to include guidance related to how decisions will be made and how to proceed in the event of disagreement among team members.

Medical record review

A careful medical record review and summary is the cornerstone to assessment of illness falsification. Diagnoses based solely on reports of the suspected caregiver should be questioned, and the records should be assessed for inconsistencies, exaggerations, potential induction, and other patterns of illness falsification.

Most parents will sign consent forms for all past medical and insurance records, as well as other records that might be useful (school nurse records). It is important to acquire records from all outpatient appointments, hospitalizations, home visits, and emergency department visits. If there has been a sibling death, it is important to obtain those records.

Chronologically summarizing the medical contacts into a table will reveal patterns of health care utilization, illness and medical treatment trajectories, and the behaviors of family members. For each health care contact, the table should include: date, location, reported symptoms as stated by caregiver, objective observations of health care provider, lab/test results, conclusions/diagnoses, treatment provided, efficacy of treatment, and other comments or observations. Be sure to identify the source of information, examine primary data (test results rather than the interpretation), evaluate if clinician conclusions match objective data, consider if objective findings could have been simulated or induced, and assess if the record makes sense. If the

Table 23.1 Specific examples of signs of pediatric illness falsification.

Sign	Examples
Recurrent illness that appears unusual	Persistent and severe vomiting with no other signs or symptoms of illness, unexplained weight loss while on TPN, or multiple episodes of poly-microbial sepsis in a child without dilated bowel.
Unexpected symptom occurrence	Symptoms occurring on particular days or during particularly stressful times for the parent, or unexpected similar symptoms in multiple family members.
Lack of continuity of care	False representation of health care contacts or parental refusal to release records.
Inconsistencies	Reported symptoms do not match objective findings (a caretaker reports severe diarrhea and vomiting for six days, however the child appears well hydrated); reported medical history does not match previous medical records (false report of a premature birth); a pattern of frequent diagnoses that do not match objective findings; behavior of parent does not match expressed distress or reports of symptoms; other false or concerning history provided by parent; medical record names and numbers do not match.

abuser is lying but not inducing symptoms, the veracity of claims can be determined by inconsistencies [16]. If the caregiver is actively inducing illness, the medical record summary can be used to evaluate the logic and likelihood of the medical presentation, and to search for signs of induction. Collateral records or interviews with others are helpful to determine the truth of inconsistencies. See Table 23.1 for examples of potential signs of this form of abuse.

Observation and documentation

If a child is admitted for evaluation, it is important to initially observe the child and family without altering factors that one would expect might impact symptoms, such as medical care or diet. This allows objective assessment of symptoms directly observed by the team compared to the reports of symptoms by the patient and family members.

Conduct in-depth individual interviews with the suspected caregiver and others to document the entire history as well as delineate the complete list of current symptoms, concerns, and limitations. Audio record these interviews for accuracy or have two professionals taking notes. Likewise, carefully interview and observe the child to document the status of the child medically, cognitively, developmentally, socially, and emotionally. This facilitates comparison with information that others report. Although it is rare that the child will report abuse, this may occur. It is more likely that you will hear different accounts of symptoms, abilities, and history. Medical record documentation is improved when team members document who said what to whom; if a symptom was directly observed by a clinician, already present when the clinician arrived (such as vomit) or simply reported by caregiver to clinician; unusual verbatim comments by caregiver; discrepancies between verbal reports made by caregivers and objective data/observations; no shows to appointments; episodes of noncompliance; and if a diagnosis is based solely on caregiver report.

Two legal concerns related to covert videotape are potential violation of the 4th amendment right to privacy and lack of court admissibility if evidence is obtained in violation. The clinical issues focus on safety and financial concerns such as who will monitor the video, if it will be continuously monitored, and deciding when intervention is indicated. Video surveillance has been found to be effective at identifying episodes of illness induction [17], but it is unpredictable how helpful the evidence will be in court. Based on the current laws in the United States, video surveillance in a child's hospital room may be permissible for protection of the child patient, assistance in diagnoses and treatment, or protection of the facility and employees from allegations of negligence. Legal protections to consider include: a video clause in the admission consent forms, warning signs posted in the hospital, specific consent, overt video monitoring, or a specific warrant. Development of a protocol is recommended for the use of video surveillance, with the inclusion of guidelines regarding monitoring and emergency intervention. Finally, videotaping without audio may be equally effective and less intrusive.

Clinical evaluation

In order to conduct an objective evaluation, one must discount the parental report of symptoms and rely on direct observations and on closely monitored medical tests. It is important to think about how one could simulate or induce a particular symptom and then assess for evidence of such behavior. For example, abnormal results of a pH probe might be discounted if a suspicious parent was alone with the child during the procedure, especially if someone tampered with the tape. Tap water can be added to stools to simulate diarrhea. The history provided by the parent will enable the clinician to challenge claims. For example, claims of lactose intolerance can be tested under observation. A bedside commode and a sitter can reveal or stop false claims of diarrhea. Medications can be systematically removed if it is suspected that they are not needed. Physical therapy or other interventions can be recommended to optimize functioning. Because it is not the normal process for determining a differential diagnosis, and because it can be highly stressful, it is helpful to discuss the assessment plan with an experienced consultant.

At admission and during increases in observed symptoms, obtain lab specimens for toxicology. An emetine screen may be indicated for persistent vomiting. The chain of evidence must be preserved to establish that specimens were not contaminated.

There is no consistent psychological profile of someone who has engaged in illness falsification [18]. Many abusers appear "normal" as parents. Therefore, a psychiatric interview and/or psychological testing of the suspected caretaker may not indicate any psychopathology. However, children are adversely impacted by this form of abuse and may become distressed during the hospitalization [19,20]. Psychiatric and developmental evaluations of the child are indicated as part of the initial evaluation. Additionally, ongoing support to the child, family, and team, and assistance with rehabilitation treatment planning can be helpful contributions by mental health professionals.

Separation test

Separation of the child from the suspected abuser can be a powerful way to determine if illness falsification has occurred. However, persistent symptoms do not rule out past illness falsification. Continued symptoms suggest that some or all of the symptoms are legitimate, that the child has been permanently injured, or that the child is not being sufficiently protected. Additionally, if medical treatment is altered at the time that separation occurs, it can be difficult to discern the cause for a change in health.

Conclusion

Given the risks associated with transplantation, it is imperative for both child and professional protection that intestinal transplant teams are skilled at routinely assessing for illness falsification in patients with unexpected, unexplained or rare symptoms. See Bursch and Hyman [21] for a more detailed review of this topic, along with recommendations regarding next steps and family feedback, recommendations to child protection authorities, risk assessment, placement, and treatment.

References

1 Hyman PE, Bursch B, Beck D, et al. Discriminating Munchausen syndrome by proxy from chronic digestive disease in toddlers. *Child Maltreatment* 2002;7:132–137.

2 Kosmach B, Tarbell S, Reyes J, Todo S. "Munchausen by proxy" syndrome in a small bowel transplant recipient. *Transplant Proc* 1996;28:2790–2791.

3 Ayoub CC, Alexander R, Beck D, et al. Position paper: definitional issues in Munchausen by proxy. *Child Maltreat* 2002;7:105–111.

4 Croft PR, Racz MI, Bloch JD, Palmer CH. Autopsy confirmation of severe pulmonary interstitial fibrosis secondary to Munchausen syndrome presenting as cystic fibrosis. *J Forensic Sci* 2005;50:1194–1198.

5 de Ridder L, Hoekstra JH. Manifestations of Munchausen syndrome by proxy in pediatric gastroenterology. *J Pediatr Gastroenterol Nutr* 2000;31:208–211.

6 Keswani RN, Sauk J, Kane SV. Factitious diarrhea masquerading as refractory celiac disease. *South Med J* 2006;99:293–295.

7 Lasher LJ, Feldman MD. Celiac disease as a manifestation of Munchausen by proxy. *South Med J* 2004;97:67–69.

8 Chuang E, Piccoli DA. Gastrointestinal manifestations. In: Levin AV, Sheridan MS, eds. *Munchausen Syndrome by Proxy*. New York: Lexington Books, 1995:121–128.

9 Sheridan MS. The deceit continues: an updated literature review of Munchausen Syndrome by Proxy. *Child Abuse Negl* 2003;27:431–451.

10 Rosenberg DA. Web of deceit: a literature review of Munchausen syndrome by proxy. *Child Abuse Neglect* 1987;11:547–563.

11 Ladefoged K, Schaffalitzky de Muckadell OB, Jarrum S. Faecal osmolality and electrolyte concentrations in chronic diarrhoea: Do they provide diagnostic clues? *Scand J Gastroenterol* 1987;22:813–820.

12 Phillips S, Donaldson L, Geisler K, et al. Stool composition in factitial diarrhea: A 6-year experience with stool analysis. *Ann Intern Med* 1995;123:97–100.

13 Kurlandsky L, Lukoff JY, Zinkham WH, et al. Munchausen syndrome by proxy: Definition of factitious bleeding in an infant by 51Cr labeling of erythrocytes. *Pediatrics* 1979;63:228–231.

14 Malatack JJ, Wiener ES, Gartner JC, et al. Munchausen by proxy: A new complication of central venous catheterization. *Pediatrics* 1985;75:523–525.

15 Mengarda G, Pittschieler K, Platzgummer S. A case of Munchausen syndrome by proxy with digestive symptoms and severe growth retardation. *Pediatr Med Chir* 1995;17:107–110.

16 Sanders MJ, Bursch B. Forensic assessment of illness falsification, Munchausen by proxy, and Factitious Disorder, NOS. *Child Maltreat* 2002;7:112–124.

17 Hall DE, Eubanks L, Meyyazhagan S, Kenney RD, Johnson, SC. Evaluation of covert video surveillance in the diagnosis of Munchausen syndrome by proxy: lessons from 41 cases. *Pediatrics* 2000;105:1305–1312.

18 Parnell TF, Day DO, eds. *Munchausen by Proxy Syndrome: Misunderstood Child Abuse*. Thousand Oaks, CA: Sage Publications, Inc, 1998.

19 Ayoub CC. Emotional impact of Munchausen by proxy on the child victims: A five-year follow-up study. In Schreier H. (Chair), Munchausen by proxy: Psychiatric presentations, treatment findings, what to do when a new child is born. Symposium meeting of the Ameri-

can Academy of Child & Adolescent Psychiatry, Chicago. October 1999.

20 Bools CN, Neale BA, Meadow SR. Follow-up of victims of fabricated illness (Munchausen syndrome by proxy). *Arch Dis Child* 1993;69:625–630.

21 Bursch B, Hyman PE. Gastrointestinal Features of Pediatric Illness Falsification. In: Kleinman RE, Goulet OJ, Mieli-Vergani G, et al., ets. *Walker's Pediatric Gastrointestinal Disease: Pathophysiology, Diagnosis, Management*, 5th ed. B C Decker Publisher, in press.

5 Pharmacological Approaches to Intestinal Failure

24 Luminal Nutrient Factors in Intestinal Adaptation and Their Use in Therapy

Jon A. Vanderhoof and Rosemary J. Young

Key points

- The success of intestinal adaptation is highly dependent on the appropriate use of luminal nutrients.
- Age and reason for intestinal resection impact on the initial selection of nutrients to enhance adaptation.
- Carbohydrates, proteins, and fats all play unique and specific roles in the adaptation process.
- Micronutrient, humoral, and other intestinotrophic substances are also significant factors that can be utilized to maximize overall bowel adaptation.
- Ongoing reassessment and manipulation of specific nutrients at different stages in the postresection period are necessary to achieve and maintain full enteral tolerance.

Introduction

Weaning a patient with short bowel syndrome (SBS) from parenteral to enteral nutrition usually necessitates numerous adaptive changes in order to permit long-term survival without parenteral nutrition (PN). These adaptive changes are very heavily dependent upon luminal nutrition. Most attention has been paid to changes in absorptive surface area as a result of intestinal dilatation, and especially in small infants, significant lengthening of the remaining small bowel. Numerous functional changes at the level of the absorptive surface area also occur, including lengthen-

Intestinal Failure: Diagnosis, Management and Transplantation.
Edited by Alan N. Langnas, Olivier Goulet, Eamonn M.M. Quigley and Kelly A. Tappenden. © 2008 Blackwell Publishing.
ISBN 978-1-4051-4637-1.

ing of the villi and changes in the microvillus structure. Other adaptive changes are related to functional modifications in the absorptive process itself, which may result in more efficient absorption or metabolism of micro- and macronutrients at the absorptive surface. Finally, in order to accommodate the reduced availability of energy substrate, there is significant downregulation of systemic metabolic activity at multiple levels, permitting the individual to survive on fewer calories.

Many adaptive responses occur solely as a response to a reduction in surface area and the need for more energy and enhanced absorptive surface. Others are probably stimulated by higher concentrations of micro- and macronutrients in the lumen relative to what was present prior to the resection. Additionally, individual nutrients supplied in higher levels than normal appear to have some unique abilities to stimulate the adaptive response. It is these nutrients, or luminal factors, that will be primarily discussed in this chapter. An understanding of these data and concepts are important in order to design an appropriate dietary and enteral feeding program for the rehabilitating patient with SBS.

Our full understanding of these nutrients and their effects is inhibited by a lack of controlled human trials. This is, of course, because of the limited number of patients available, the impact of patient age on the adaptive response, the differences in underlying disease processes, and the anatomic differences between patients with SBS. Consequently, we are forced to rely on the number of animal studies that compare the adaptive response to various dietary changes. It is always difficult to relate changes in an animal model directly to the human situation, especially in view of the anatomic and functional differences between species, including differences in their normal diets, how that species responds to changes in nutrition, and overall differences in their digestive processes. The rat, for example, utilizes extensive fecal fermentation, coprophagia, and other processes to enhance its digestive function; these are not normal processes in the human. Nonetheless, these animal studies have often provided us with useful information for directing human investigations into the effect of micro- and macronutrients on the adaptive response.

General processes

Traditionally, enteral nutrients have been thought to impact the adaptation response at a number of different levels. These include a direct stimulation of the workload of the enterocyte with subsequent enhancement of digestive and absorptive function at the local level. In the non-resected bowel the jejunal villi are greater in length than the ileum; however, after a resection, the adaptive capacity of the ileum has been shown to be greater than the jejunum [1] demonstrating structural adaptation occurring partially due to the direct nutrient stimulatory effect. In other instances, enhanced production of trophic hormones or growth factors in response to the enhanced presence of enteral nutrients may occur [2]. Some, but less, attention has been paid to the impact of intraluminal effects of the products of digestion, or intraluminal fermentation, which also may play an important role in stimulating the adaptive response [3].

Recently, technology has permitted us to study how nutrients may impact the upregulation of certain genes which may be involved in the adaptation response. The specific functions of these genes are also being better defined, allowing us to understand exactly how intraluminal nutrients regulate intestinal adaptation. In addition, we know that nutrients are capable of stimulating the production of normal intestinal secretions, including pancreatic or biliary secretions, which may themselves assist in the adaptation process. It is well known that both a fasting state and provision of nutrients parenterally does impair intestinal function and structure, thus emphasising the necessity for aggressive enteral nutrition.

In general, the adaptive response is thought to be more of one of hyperplasia than hypertrophy, meaning an actual increase in number rather than size of cells. Increasing the replication rate of these cells in the crypt certainly plays a role; additionally; changes in maturation and cell survival may also be factors. Conflicting data has been observed on whether apoptosis may increase or decrease cell survival or overall lifespan [4,5]. Nonetheless, the overall effect of these adaptive responses is an increase in the epithelial cell population within a given length of intestine. Finally, the importance of the adaptive response of the colon is often overlooked. Here, nutrients can play a significant role in enhancing absorptive function, in some instances through fluid, electrolyte, and micronutrient absorption, and, in some instances, through uptake of the fermentation products of macronutrient malabsorption, such as short chain fatty acids [6].

Macronutrients involved in adaptation

Carbohydrates

Carbohydrates exist in the diet as monosaccharides, disaccharides, starches (usually as amylose and amylopectin), and complex non-digestible or poorly digestible carbohydrates which may be partially utilized through fermentation. Digestible carbohydrates are broken down through the action of amylase enzymes from the salivary glands and, more importantly, from the pancreas, as well as through the brush border enzymes, sucrase, isomaltase, maltase, and lactase. The form through which carbohydrates are presented in the diet may significantly influence rates of digestion. For example, wheat starch in the form of pasta is digested much more slowly than rice flour [7,8]. This is quite important in patients with short bowel syndrome since it influences the percentage of carbohydrates which may be rapidly digested in the small bowel and absorbed, or conversely which may be malabsorbed and fermented more slowly in the colon, providing short chain fatty acids but also influencing intestinal gas and bloating. The presentation of large volumes of carbohydrates in the form of bolus feedings or large meals, and especially rapidly digested carbohydrates, may produce major fluid and electrolyte imbalance in the short bowel patient [9].

An enhancement in carbohydrate uptake has been clearly observed in children with short bowel syndrome. Both glucose absorption and sucrose hydrolysis have been found to significantly increase following bowel resection [10]. Most nutrients produce some enhancement of intestinal adaptation and carbohydrates are certainly no exception. Carbohydrates, because they are important stimulators of insulin secretion, are likely to provide significant benefit. Insulin has been shown to play an important role in small intestinal growth and development in animal studies [11,12]. Here, the more rapidly digested and absorbed carbohydrates, such as highly available amylopectin or small oligosaccharides or maltose would clearly be important in eliciting this effect.

In the small bowel, carbohydrates are broken down to monosaccharides which are normally important facilitators of sodium and water absorption. Consequently, the continuous provision of adequate glucose to the small intestine without overloading the transport mechanisms can facilitate continuous water and sodium absorption without osmotic diarrhea. The same is true for the colon, but as a result of the less porous colonic epithelium, the potential for marked fluid losses from the colon is significantly less.

Nonabsorbable carbohydrates are perhaps nutritionally much more important in the short bowel patient than in the normal individual as they are broken down into short chain fatty acids through the metabolism of endogenous bacterial flora. They consist primarily of acetate, propionate and butyrate and can be rapidly absorbed by both passive and active transport in small quantities in the ileum and to larger degree in the colon. Acetate is present in the greatest proportions with lesser amounts of propionate. Butyrate accounts for the least amount of short chain fatty acids in the bowel and, at a cellular level, is the one most preferred for oxidation by epithelial cells. Short chain fats also may be a significant source of energy via colonic salvage, contributing 4.4 kcal per gram. The absence of luminal SCFAs have been noted to be associated with diversion colitis and therefore when present an important anti-inflammatory role [13]. Specifically, butyrate, has been shown to reduce paracellular permeability [14], modulate immune responses [15,16] and has shown some clinical benefit in inflammatory bowel disease [17].

Short chain fatty acids themselves may have some direct effect on the adaptation response [18]. Their presence has been shown to enhance fluid and electrolyte transport in animal studies through the promotion of sodium absorption in the intestine [19–21]. Tappenden et al. have demonstrated that resected rats given short chain fatty acid supplemented TPN have an increase in a specific sodium/glucose transporter in the enterocyte brush border [22]. Additionally, Tappenden et al. have demonstrated an increase in the intestinal adaptive factors of proglucagon and ornithine decarboxylase in rodents fed SCFA supplemented TPN [23].

SCFAs may have more specific influences on the adaptation process including the ability to modulate expression of genes important to the processes maintaining colonic tissue homoeostasis [24]. Another benefit of short chain fatty acids and some enteric bacteria is their ability to promote cytoprotective heat shock proteins, which help prevent mucosal injury [25,26]. Additionally, by reducing intraluminal pH, short chain fats may stimulate cell turnover and stimulate pancreatic secretions, which may be important trophic factors. Short chain fatty acid supplementation of intravenous solutions has also been shown to reduce mucosal atrophy in TPN dependent animals [22,27,28].

Nondigestible carbohydrates also may have trophic benefits independent of short chain fatty acid production, which may influence the adaptation process. For example, pectin and guar gums appear to slow gastric emptying and, consequently, reduce levels of postprandial glucose elevation [29]. This reduction in gastric emptying allows more continuous provision of nutrients to the small bowel for constant saturation and stimulation of the enterocytes. Many animal studies have directly demonstrated the trophic effects of these fibers on the gastrointestinal tract [30]. A decrease in mucosal inflammatory responses has also been demonstrated when pectin is administered enterally [31]. Supplementing diets with pectin and guar gum also have been shown to produce a stimulatory effect on jejunal and ileal crypt cell proliferation and migration, suggesting enhancement of the intracelluar regeneration process [32,33].

Lipids

Lipids are very important stimulators of the adaptation process. Lipids are involved in the stimulation of a number of potentially trophic substances including GLP-2 and neurotensin (discussed in Chapter 25). The effect of malabsorbed lipids on the ileal brake, resulting in reduced intestinal transit time and, perhaps, delayed gastric emptying, may be a significant advantage in enhancing nutrient contract with the mucosal epithelium and, thereby, stimulating intestinal adaptation. These effects may be partially mediated through peptide YY (PYY) [34,35]. It has been shown that high levels of PYY are present in SBS patients with a colon in continuity [36]; however, the extent to which massive ileal resection impairs this mechanism merits further investigation.

In rat models, low-fat diets significantly impair postresectional adaptation [37]. Long chain fats appear to be significantly better at stimulating intestinal adaptation in rat models than medium chain fats [38]. This may be partially, but not totally, a result of deficiencies in linoleic acid, an important substrate for synthesis of N-6 prostaglandins [39]. Eicosapentaenoic acid, an N-3 highly unsaturated, long chain, polyunsaturated fatty acid, and an important substrate for N-3 prostaglandin synthesis, appears to be an even more potent stimulator of intestinal adaptation [40]. Reducing prostaglandin synthesis through aspirin administration reduces, at least to some degree, the stimulatory benefits of N-6 fatty acids, suggesting that prostaglandin synthesis may be an important part of the adaptation process [41].

Protein

Most protein in the diet is present in the form of complex proteins, large molecules with complex secondary and tertiary structures. In early work with animal models, high protein diets have been shown to enhance jejunal amino acid transport [42] and, more recently, colostrum protein concentrate has been shown to enhance intestinal adaptation [43]. It has been found that dipeptide absorption may, in some cases, proceed more rapidly than amino acid absorption [44]. Proteins may also be important regulators of the secretion of numerous trophic hormones and regulatory peptides, such as ghrelin and insulin-like growth factor-1 (IGF-1) [45].

There has been extensive work on the role of certain amino acids in influencing the adaptation process. Certain amino acids, such as glutamine and arginine, and branched chain amino acids (leucine, valine, isoleucine) appear to be utilized differentially. Specifically, glutamine appears to be an important fuel for enterocyte function and also is the major mechanism of circulatory transport for amine groups. Numerous studies in animals have shown the important role of glutamine in maintaining intestinal mass [46–48]. A recent study utilizing Caco-2 cells has demonstrated that glutamine may have a gene-specific effect on

intestinal cells by altering the expression of certain proteins [49]. Even provision of parenteral glutamine may prevent mucosal atrophy in certain situations, in animal models [48].

The effect of glutamine on influencing intestinal adaptation after massive bowel resection has been controversial. Studies comparing glutamine with other amino acids and carbohydrates in the rat model of resection have shown no specific benefit [50,51]. In combination with growth hormone, glutamine has been shown, in some human clinical studies, to enhance intestinal adaptation [52,53]. Not all studies show benefit to the same degree nor did all demonstrate a prolonged effect on overall nutritional status [54]. Pediatric studies of glutamine supplementation also have demonstrated conflicting results, with some benefit in improving intestinal barrier function being noted in malnourished children [55]; however, improvement in intestinal absorption or barrier function was not seen in a group of children with surgical gastrointestinal disease [56].

Arginine deficiency has been demonstrated to be associated with poor weight gain in animals who have undergone bowel resection [57] and parenteral arginine may enhance the intestinal mucosal barrier in a similar group of animals undergoing resection [58]. It functions not only as a precursor to polyamines but is broken down to nitric oxide, which may play a role in maintaining the intestinal mucosal barrier [59], although studies are also controversial in this area [60].

Polyamine activity is important in fueling tissues undergoing rapid replication and has been shown to be increased after small bowel resection [61]. The endogenous polyamines include putrescine, spermidine, and spermine. They are regulated by ornithine decarboxylase, an enzyme which, when deficient, leads to and inhibition of adaptation in rats who have undergone jejunal resection [62]. However, human clinical trials in short bowel syndrome have not been reported. Epidermal growth factor (EGF) discussed in Chapter 25 is important in the maintenance and repair of the intestinal mucosa and has been studied in relationship to polyamines [63]. Additionally, trefoil peptides, have recently been identified as important factors in the maintenance of mucosal integrity through cytoprotective effects [64]; however, human studies are lacking.

Micronutrients

Micronutrients, composed of vitamins and minerals, may also be important in the adaptation process. Many poorly absorbed micronutrients are frequently complexed with other luminal contents, making absorption difficult. For example, maintaining adequate calcium and magnesium intake in short bowel syndrome is often problematic and certain luminal factors may result in excessive binding of these ions [65]. Phytate is a well known inhibitor of calcium, iron, and zinc absorption. However, various forms of carbohydrate are actually capable of enhancing absorption of certain minerals [66,67]. Magnesium absorption, particularly difficult in short bowel syndrome, may be enhanced by some fibers [68].

Luminal bacteria often receive too little attention, yet they are important constituents that may affect the adaptation process. The dilated small bowel with its poor motility, a frequent finding in patients with short bowel syndrome, often contains much larger numbers of luminal bacteria than is present in the anatomically normal small intestine. Short chain fatty acids and other metabolites are often produced in these dilated loops. A byproduct of bacterial metabolism, D-lactate, may have significant untoward effects on the host, especially in small infants and children [69]. A large percentage of the luminal contents contain both live and dead bacteria and bacterial fragments which alters gastrointestinal function in a number of ways. The presence of inflammation related to gut flora reduces effective absorptive surface area, creates an immature epithelium, and ultimately impaired absorption. However, anti-inflammatory short chain fatty acids produced via bacterial fermentation provide a significant benefit.

We know that a number of genes can be influenced by bacteria or bacterial metabolites [70,71], especially in the immune cells in the gut [72]. For example, in a rabbit model, the combination of *Bacteroides fragilis* and *Bacillus subtilis* was found to promote gut associated lymph tissue development and the early phases of antibody development, whereas clostridium subterminale, *Escherichia coli* and *Staphylococcus epidermidis* did not [73]. It is also likely that genes involved in the adaptation response may be sensitive to certain, as yet unidentified, gut bacteria. The numbers of these bacteria present will likely be influenced by different dietary factors and macronutrients. Much more data is needed to create a reasonable understanding of how this process may be manipulated. Eventually, probiotic therapy may even play a role in intestinal adaptation; however, the selection of the appropriate probiotic organism must be preceded by careful work to elucidate exactly what genes are involved in the adaptation process and how various gut bacteria may influence the activity of these genes.

Summary

What does this all mean from the standpoint of the patient? The dietary management of the short bowel patient is a difficult process and the complexity of the various interactions of dietary nutrients within the lumen and at the level of the brush border is often not given sufficient consideration. The relative rates of absorption and fermentation, the influence of the by products of fermentation and the provision of nutrients in the right quantity, quality, and frequency in order to optimize absorption are each factors that require careful consideration. Provision of adequate micro- and macronutrients for optimal stimulation of adaptation, must be balanced with avoidance of overtaxing the workload capacity of the intestine. Careful interaction between gastrointestinal physiologists, nutritionists, gastroenterologists, and surgeons, and a comprehensive intestinal rehabilitation program, is needed to optimize all this information for the benefit of the rehabilitating patient with SBS.

References

1 Dowling RH, Booth CC. Structural and functional changes following small intestinal resection in the rat. *Clin Sci* 1967;32:139–149.

2 Ziegler TR, Estivariz CF, Jonas CR, et al. Interactions between nutrients and peptide growth factors in intestinal growth, repair, and function. *JPEN J Parenter Enteral Nutr* 1999;23(suppl):S174–S183.

3 Olesen M, Gudmand-Hoyer E, Holst JJ, et al. Importance of colonic bacterial fermentation in short bowel patients: small intestinal malabsorption of easily digestible carbohydrate. *Dig Dis Sci* 1999;44:1914–1923.

4 Sukhotnik I, Bernshteyn A, Mogilner JG. The basic biology of apoptosis and its implications for pediatric surgery. *Eur J Pediatr Surg* 2005;15:229–235.

5 Juno RJ, Knott AW, Profitt SA, et al. Preventing enterocyte apoptosis after massive small bowel resection does not enhance adaptation of the intestinal mucosa. *J Pediatr Surg* 2004;39: 907–911.

6 Nordgaard I, Hansen BS, Mortensen PB. Importance of colonic support for energy absorption as small-bowel failure proceeds. *Am J Clin Nutr* 1996;64:222–231.

7 Jarvi AE, Karlstrom BE, Granfeldt YE, et al. The influence of food structure on postprandial metabolism in patients with non-insulin-dependent diabetes mellitus. *Am J Clin Nutr* 1995;61:837–842.

8 Foster-Powell K, Holt SH, Brand-Miller JC. International table of glycemic index and glycemic load values: 2002. *Am J Clin Nutr* 2002;76:5–56.

9 Ameen VZ, Powell GK, Jones LA. Quantitation of fecal carbohydrate excretion in patients with short bowel syndrome. *Gastroenterology* 1987;92:493–500.

10 Schmitz J, Rey F, Bresson JL, et al. [Perfusion study of intestinal sugar absorption after extensive intestinal resection (author's transl)]. *Arch Fr Pediatr* 1980;37:491–495.

11 Sukhotnik I, Shehadeh N, Shamir R, et al. Oral insulin enhances intestinal regrowth following massive small bowel resection in rat. *Dig Dis Sci* 2005;50:2379–2385.

12 Huo YJ, Wang T, Xu RJ, et al. Dietary insulin affects leucine aminopeptidase, growth hormone, Insulin-like growth factor I and insulin receptors in the intestinal mucosa of neonatal pigs. *Biol Neonate* 2006;89:265–273.

13 Lim AG, Langmead FL, Feakins RM, et al. Diversion colitis: a trigger for ulcerative colitis in the in-stream colon? *Gut* 1999;44:279–282.

14 Kinoshita M, Suzuki Y, Saito Y. Butyrate reduces colonic paracellular permeability by enhancing PPARgamma activation. *Biochem Biophys Res Commun* 2002;293:827–831.

15 Bocker U, Nebe T, Herweck F, et al. Butyrate modulates intestinal epithelial cell-mediated neutrophil migration. *Clin Exp Immunol* 2003;131:53–60.

16 Inan MS, Rasoulpour RJ, Yin L, et al. The luminal short-chain fatty acid butyrate modulates NF-kappaB activity in a human colonic epithelial cell line. *Gastroenterology* 2000;118:724–734.

17 Hallert C, Bjorck I, Nyman M, et al. Increasing fecal butyrate in ulcerative colitis patients by diet: controlled pilot study. *Inflamm Bowel Dis* 2003;9:116–121.

18 Cavaglieri CR, Nishiyama A, Fernandes LC, et al. Differential effects of short-chain fatty acids on proliferation and production of pro- and anti-inflammatory cytokines by cultured lymphocytes. *Life Sci* 2003;73:1683–1690.

19 Binder HJ, Mehta P. Short-chain fatty acids stimulate active sodium and chloride absorption in vitro in the rat distal colon. *Gastroenterology* 1989;96:989–996.

20 Ramakrishna BS, Venkataraman S, Srinivasan P, et al. Amylase-resistant starch plus oral rehydration solution for cholera. *N Engl J Med* 2000;342:308–313.

21 Musch MW, Bookstein C, Rocha F, et al. Region-specific adaptation of apical Na/H exchangers after extensive proximal small bowel resection. *Am J Physiol Gastrointest Liver Physiol* 2002;283:G975–G985.

22 Tappenden KA, Thomson AB, Wild GE, et al. Short-chain fatty acid-supplemented total parenteral nutrition enhances functional adaptation to intestinal resection in rats. *Gastroenterology* 1997;12:792–802.

23 Tappenden KA, Thomson AB, Wild GE, et al. Short-chain fatty acids increase proglucagon and ornithine decarboxylase messenger RNAs after intestinal resection in rats. *JPEN J Parenter Enteral Nutr* 1996;20:357–362.

24 Cuff MA, Shirazi-Beechey SP. The importance of butyrate transport to the regulation of gene expression in the colonic epithelium. *Biochem Soc Trans* 2004;32:1100–1102.

25 Kojima K, Musch MW, Ren H, et al. Enteric flora and lymphocyte-derived cytokines determine expression of heat shock proteins in mouse colonic epithelial cells. *Gastroenterology* 2003;124:1395–1407.

26 Ren H, Musch MW, Kojima K, et al. Short-chain fatty acids induce intestinal epithelial heat shock protein 25 expression in rats and IEC 18 cells. *Gastroenterology* 2001;121:631–639.

27 Tappenden KA, Drozdowski LA, Thomson AB, et al. Short-chain fatty acid-supplemented total parenteral nutrition alters intestinal structure, glucose transporter 2 (GLUT2) mRNA and protein, and proglucagon mRNA abundance in normal rats. *Am J Clin Nutr* 1998;68:118–125.

28 Thompson JS, Quigley EM, Palmer JM, et al. Luminal short-chain fatty acids and postresection intestinal adaptation. *JPEN J Parenter Enteral Nutr* 1996;20:338–343.

29 Jenkins DJ, Jenkins AL. Dietary fiber and the glycemic response. *Proc Soc Exp Biol Med* 1985;180:422–431.

30 Brunsgaard G, Bach Knudsen KE, Eggum BO. The influence of the period of adaptation on the digestibility of diets containing different types of indigestible polysaccharides in rats. *Br J Nutr* 1995;74:833–848.

31 Rolandelli RH, Saul SH, Settle RG, et al. Comparison of parenteral nutrition and enteral feeding with pectin in experimental colitis in the rat. *Am J Clin Nutr* 1988;47:715–721.

32 Pell JD, Gee JM, Wortley GM, et al. Dietary corn oil and guar gum stimulate intestinal crypt cell proliferation in

rats by independent but potentially synergistic mechanisms. *J Nutr* 1992;122:2447–2456.

33 Tamura M, Suzuki H. Effects of pectin on jejunal and ileal morphology and ultrastructure in adult mice. *Ann Nutr Metab* 1997;41:255–259.

34 Lin HC, Zhao XT, Wang L, et al. Fat-induced ileal brake in the dog depends on peptide YY. *Gastroenterology* 1996;110:1491–1495.

35 Cuche G, Cuber JC, Malbert CH. Ileal short-chain fatty acids inhibit gastric motility by a humoral pathway. *Am J Physiol Gastrointest Liver Physiol* 2000;279:G925–G930.

36 Nightingale JM, Kamm MA, van der Sijp JR, et al. Gastrointestinal hormones in short bowel syndrome. Peptide YY may be the "colonic brake" to gastric emptying. *Gut* 1996;39:267–272.

37 Sukhotnik I, Mor-Vaknin N, Drongowski RA, et al. Effect of dietary fat on early morphological intestinal adaptation in a rat with short bowel syndrome. *Pediatr Surg Int* 2004;20:419–424.

38 Vanderhoof JA, Park JH, Mohammadpour H, et al. Effects of dietary lipids on recovery from mucosal injury. *Gastroenterology* 1990;98:1226–1231.

39 Hart MH, Grandjean CJ, Park JH, et al. Essential fatty acid deficiency and postresection mucosal adaptation in the rat. *Gastroenterology* 1988;94:682–687.

40 Kollman-Bauerly KA, Thomas DL, Adrian TE, et al. The role of eicosanoids in the process of adaptation following massive bowel resection in the rat. *JPEN J Parenter Enteral Nutr* 2001;25:275–281.

41 Vanderhoof JA, Park JH, Grandjean CJ. Reduced mucosal prostaglandin synthesis after massive small bowel resection. *Am J Physiol* 1988;254:G373–G377.

42 Lis MT, Crampton RF, Matthews DM. Effect of dietary changes on intestinal absorption of L-methionine and L-methionyl-L-methionine in the rat. *Br J Nutr* 1972;27:159–167.

43 Nagy ES, Paris MC, Taylor RG, et al. Colostrum protein concentrate enhances intestinal adaptation after massive small bowel resection in juvenile pigs. *J Pediatr Gastroenterol Nutr* 2004;39:487–492.

44 Minami H, Morse EL, Adibi SA. Characteristics and mechanism of glutamine-dipeptide absorption in human intestine. *Gastroenterology* 1992;103:3–11.

45 Teresa Vallejo-Cremades M, Gomez de Segura IA, Gomez-Garcia L, et al. A high-protein dietary treatment to intestinally hypotrophic rats induces ghrelin mRNA content and serum peptide level changes. *Clin Nutr* 2005;24:904–912.

46 Zhou X, Li YX, Li N, et al. Effect of bowel rehabilitative therapy on structural adaptation of remnant small intestine: animal experiment. *World J Gastroenterol* 2001;7:66–73.

47 Tamada H, Nezu R, Matsuo Y, et al. Alanyl glutamine-enriched total parenteral nutrition restores intestinal adaptation after either proximal or distal massive resection in rats. *JPEN J Parenter Enteral Nutr* 1993;17:236–242.

48 Chen K, Nezu R, Sando K, et al. Influence of glutamine-supplemented parenteral nutrition on intestinal amino acid metabolism in rats after small bowel resection. *Surg Today* 1996;26:618–623.

49 Lenaerts K, Mariman E, Bouwman F, et al. Glutamine regulates the expression of proteins with a potential health-promoting effect in human intestinal Caco-2 cells. *Proteomics* 2006.

50 Vanderhoof JA, Blackwood DJ, Mohammadpour H, et al. Effects of oral supplementation of glutamine on small intestinal mucosal mass following resection. *J Am Coll Nutr* 1992;11:223–237.

51 Michail S, Mohammadpour H, Park JH, et al. Effect of glutamine-supplemented elemental diet on mucosal adaptation following bowel resection in rats. *J Pediatr Gastroenterol Nutr* 1995;21:394–398.

52 Byrne TA, Morrissey TB, Nattakom TV, et al. Growth hormone, glutamine, and a modified diet enhance nutrient absorption in patients with severe short bowel syndrome. *JPEN J Parenter Enteral Nutr* 1995;19:296–302.

53 Byrne TA, Wilmore DW, Iyer K, et al. Growth hormone, glutamine, and an optimal diet reduces parenteral nutrition in patients with short bowel syndrome: a prospective, randomized, placebo-controlled, double-blind clinical trial. *Ann Surg* 2005;242:655–661.

54 Scolapio JS, Camilleri M, Fleming CR, et al. Effect of growth hormone, glutamine, and diet on adaptation in short-bowel syndrome: a randomized, controlled study. *Gastroenterology* 1997;113:1074–1081.

55 Lima AA, Brito LF, Ribeiro HB, et al. Intestinal barrier function and weight gain in malnourished children taking glutamine supplemented enteral formula. *J Pediatr Gastroenterol Nutr* 2005;40:28–35.

56 Duggan C, Stark AR, Auestad N, et al. Glutamine supplementation in infants with gastrointestinal disease: a randomized, placebo-controlled pilot trial. *Nutrition* 2004;20:752–756.

57 Wakabayashi Y, Yamada E, Yoshida T, et al. Effect of intestinal resection and arginine-free diet on rat physiology. *Am J Physiol* 1995;269:G313–G318.

58 Welters CF, Dejong CH, Deutz NE, et al. Effects of parenteral arginine supplementation on the intestinal adaptive response after massive small bowel resection in the rat. *J Surg Res* 1999;85:259–266.

59 Sun Y, Fihn BM, Jodal M, et al. Inhibition of nitric oxide synthesis potentiates the colonic permeability

increase triggered by luminal bile acids. *Acta Physiol Scand* 2004;180:167–175.

60 Tuncyurek P, Sari M, Firat O, et al. Does pharmaconutrition with L-arginine and/or alpha-tocopherol improve the gut barrier in bile duct ligated rats? *Eur Surg Res* 2006;38:4–10.

61 Tsujikawa T, Fukunaga T, Itoh A, et al. Alteration in expression of polyamine and glucose-related enzyme mRNA after small bowel resection in the rat residual ileum. *Int J Mol Med* 2002;10:489–492.

62 Bamba T, Vaja S, Murphy GM, et al. Role of polyamines in the early adaptive response to jejunectomy in the rat: effect of DFMO on the ileal villus:crypt axis. *Digestion* 1990;46(suppl):410–423.

63 Tsujikawa T, Bamba T, Hosoda S. The trophic effect of epidermal growth factor on morphological changes and polyamine metabolism in the small intestine of rats. *Gastroenterol Jpn* 1990;25:328–334.

64 Playford RJ, Marchbank T, Calnan DP, et al. Epidermal growth factor is digested to smaller, less active forms in acidic gastric juice. *Gastroenterology* 1995;108:92–101.

65 Greger JL. Nondigestible carbohydrates and mineral bioavailability. *J Nutr* 1999;129(suppl):1434S–1435S.

66 Scholz-Ahrens KE, Schaafsma G, van den Heuvel EG, et al. Effects of prebiotics on mineral metabolism. *Am J Clin Nutr* 2001;73(suppl):459S–464S.

67 Vermorel M, Coudray C, Wils D, et al. Energy value of a low-digestible carbohydrate, NUTRIOSE FB, and its impact on magnesium, calcium and zinc apparent absorption and retention in healthy young men. *Eur J Nutr* 2004;43:344–352.

68 Coudray C, Demigne C, Rayssiguier Y. Effects of dietary fibers on magnesium absorption in animals and humans. *J Nutr* 2003;133:1–4.

69 Mack DR. D(-)-lactic acid-producing probiotics, D(-)-lactic acidosis and infants. *Can J Gastroenterol* 2004;18:671–675.

70 Di Caro S, Tao H, Grillo A, et al. Bacillus clausii effect on gene expression pattern in small bowel mucosa using DNA microarray analysis. *Eur J Gastroenterol Hepatol* 2005;17:951–960.

71 Di Caro S, Tao H, Grillo A, et al. Effects of Lactobacillus GG on genes expression pattern in small bowel mucosa. *Dig Liver Dis* 2005;37:320–329.

72 Mutch DM, Simmering R, Donnicola D, et al. Impact of commensal microbiota on murine gastrointestinal tract gene ontologies. *Physiol Genomics* 2004;19:22–31.

73 Rhee KJ, Sethupathi P, Driks A, et al. Role of commensal bacteria in development of gut-associated lymphoid tissues and preimmune antibody repertoire. *J Immunol* 2004;172:1118–1124.

25 The Role of Humoral Factors in Intestinal Adaptation

Jennifer N. Woodard and Kelly A. Tappenden

Key points

- Numerous endogenous signals are likely important in intestinal adaptation.
- Intestinal adaptation involves both structural and functional responses that do not occur in parallel and are likely provoked by different stimuli.
- Exogenous administration of putative adaptive stimuli may augment intestinal adaptation and provide potential therapies for individuals with intestinal failure.
- Long-term effects of these factors are unknown.

Introduction

Following injury or resection, the residual intestine has the capability to adapt. Basic adaptive mechanisms include: dilation and elongation of the residual bowel; epithelial hyperplasia resulting in expansion of the mucosal architecture; enhanced digestion and absorption secondary to increased expression of functional proteins; and increased transit time allowing for increased contact between nutrients and the mucosa. The residual intestine will adapt in response to a variety of stimuli including enteral nutrients, pancreaticobiliary secretions, and humoral factors (reviewed in [1]). The purpose of this chapter is to discuss humoral stimuli, particularly glucagon-like peptide-2 (GLP-2), growth hormone (GH), epidermal growth factor (EGF), insulin-like growth factor-1

Intestinal Failure: Diagnosis, Management and Transplantation.
Edited by Alan N. Langnas, Olivier Goulet, Eamonn M.M. Quigley and Kelly A. Tappenden. © 2008 Blackwell Publishing.
ISBN 978-1-4051-4637-1.

(IGF-I), keratinocyte growth factor (KGF), and transforming growth factor-α (TGF-α), as potential mediators of intestinal adaptation.

Glucagon-like peptide 2

Glucagon-like peptide 2 (GLP-2) is a 33-amino acid intestinotrophic factor released from the L cells located in the ileum and colon upon nutrient ingestion [2]. GLP-2 is one of five main peptides encoded by the proglucagon gene [3]. In the intestine, proglucagon is post-translationally cleaved by prohormone convertase 1/3 (PC 1/3) to release GLP-2, as well as GLP-1, glicentin, and oxyntomodulin [4].

Interest in the intestinotrophic action of GLP-2, distinct from its inclusion as a proglucagon-derived-peptide, intensified in 1996 with a report from Drucker and associates [5] that nude mice bearing three different proglucagon-derived peptide producing tumors exhibited a doubling in small intestinal weight that was associated with increased crypt-villous length and epithelial proliferation. Exogenous administration of the various proglucagon-derived peptides revealed that GLP-2 was the intestinotrophic mediator.

As it relates to intestinal failure, GLP-2 has received much attention as a newly established stimulator of small intestinal growth [6,7] and function [6,8,9]. In adult rats, exogenous administration of GLP-2 prevents parenteral nutrition-induced intestinal atrophy [10] and following a 90% intestinal resection, prevents postsurgical compromise in barrier function as well as increases length, villous height, and abundance of the sodium-glucose transporter, SGLT-1, in the residual ileum [11].

The impact of GLP-2 appears to be broad in scope, with redundancies in underlying mechanisms. The structural and functional adaptations induced by GLP-2 are not limited to the adult intestine, but have also been reported in the developing intestine of neonatal piglets [12–14]. Furthermore, GLP-2 effects extend beyond the post-surgical period and appear to have utility during the refeeding period following chronic parenteral nutrition support. GLP-2 administration increases the expression of numerous enterocyte-associated nutrient transporters in both rodents [15] and piglets, thereby improving the transport capacity for hexoses [16]. In addition, GLP-2 has been shown to reduce gastric acid secretion [17] and slow gastric emptying [18]. Finally, GLP-2 administration increases blood flow in the superior mesenteric artery in a nitric oxide-dependent mechanism mediated via intrinsic, noncholinergic enteric neurons [19,20].

Given these promising results in animal studies, it should not be surprising that human clinical trials are underway. Jeppesen and colleagues [21] reported improvements in intestinal absorption and nutritional status following the treatment with native GLP-2 given to subjects for 35 days in an open label study and found improvements in intestinal absorption of energy (3.5%), wet weight (11%), and nitrogen (4.7%) and associated with increases in body weight (1.2 kg), lean body mass (2.9 kg), and 24-hour urine creatinine excretion. However, GLP-2 itself has a very short half-life of approximately 7 minutes because of cleavage of two amino acids at the N-terminus by the enzyme dipeptidyl peptidase IV (DPP-IV). Therefore, the therapeutic strategy currently employed in human trials involves a DPP-IV resistant GLP-2 analog called teduglutide. Reports from Phase II clinical trials in human subjects with short bowel syndrome given teduglutide reveal heightened, albeit reversible, improvements in relative wet weight absorption (22%), urine weight (555 g/day) and urine sodium excretion (53 mmol/day), decreases in fecal wet weight (711 g/day), and fecal energy excretion (347 kcal/day; [22]) and with parallel changes in crypt-villous architecture. Little is currently known about long-term effects, optimal dosing regime, or the most efficacious window of administration following surgery. However, initial results indicate that GLP-2 administration, particularly in the form of a degradation resistant analog, may become an important medical therapy for individuals with intestinal failure.

Epidermal growth factor

Epidermal growth factor (EGF) is a 53-amino acid peptide that is involved in the proliferation and differentiation of a wide variety of cell types. Sources of EGF include saliva, pancreaticobiliary secretions, Brunner's glands of the duodenum, and Paneth cells. EGF receptors are found throughout the gastrointestinal tract and are thought to be critically important in the mechanism whereby EGF mediates adaptation of the intestinal epithelium.

Similar to other humoral factors involved in intestinal adaptation, exogenous EGF induces both structural and functional enhancements in the absorptive epithelium. Following a 50% intestinal resection in mice, EGF treatment increases ileal villous height and crypt depth by the concomitant cytokinetic upregulation of proliferation and reduction in apoptosis [23]. Additionally, in a rat intestinal transport model, EGF administration improved functional aspects of the intestine, including induction of SGLT-1 and PepT1 transporters, as well as maltase and sucrase activities [24].

Manipulation of endogenous plasma EGF concentration and receptor abundance suggests that both are important for intestinal adaptation. When mice received a 50% intestinal resection and had the submandibular salivary glands removed, the typical morphological adaptations induced by EGF were not observed [25]. Furthermore, studies involving mutations in the EGF receptor revealed impaired structural adaptations as assessed by epithelial cell proliferation, mucosal DNA and protein concentration, and villous length [26]. Moreover, when EGF-overexpressing transgenic mice were subjected to partial enterectomy, mucosal protein and DNA concentration, villous length, and crypt depth were elevated over those measured in wild type resection controls [27].

Human trials with exogenous EGF administration are also underway. In one such study, pediatric patients with intestinal failure given daily doses of EGF for 6 weeks, demonstrated improved carbohydrate absorption and tolerance of enteral feedings; however, these effects reversed on treatment cessation [28]. Further studies are needed to determine the optimal timing, duration, and administration methods to validate the feasibility of EGF as a treatment option in humans with intestinal failure.

Transforming growth factor-α

Transforming growth factor-α (TGF-α) is a 50-amino acid peptide that is similar in structure to EGF and also binds EGF receptors. TGF-α is constitutively produced in the enterocytes of the intestine. When administered following a 75% resection in rats, TGF-α augmented morphological aspects of intestinal adaptation, including increases in villous height, epithelial proliferation, and mucosal DNA and protein content [29]. However, studies using Waved-1 mice, which lack TGF-α expression, showed that intestinal adaptation induced by resection occurs to the same extent as that observed in wild type mice [30]. Thus, although exogenous TGF-α appears to stimulate adaptation, TGF-α does not appear to be an essential ligand for intestinal adaptation and may reveal redundancies with EGF receptor signaling following intestinal resection.

Keratinocyte growth factor

Keratinocyte growth factor (KGF) is a 163-amino acid peptide that is produced in the dermis, lungs, heart, liver, pancreas, and GI tract and functions as a potent epithelial cell specific growth factor. When exogenous KGF is administered, KGF receptor mRNA abundance increases, suggesting that the beneficial effects of KGF are partially a result of receptor up-regulation [31]. Exogenous KGF administration prevents total parenteral nutrition-induced intestinal atrophy by increasing proliferation and decreasing apoptosis within the intestinal epithelium [32]. Following an 85% intestinal resection in rats, KGF administration increases mucosal thickness, crypt-villous architecture, and mucosal DNA and protein content [33]. Functional adaptations following intestinal resection include enhanced barrier function, active ion transport, and glucose and amino acid transport [31,32]. The utility of KGF therapy for intestinal failure is largely unexplored beyond rodent models of total parenteral nutrition and short bowel syndrome.

Insulin-like growth factor-I

Insulin-like growth factor-I (IGF-I) is a 70-amino acid peptide similar to insulin in structure. It is produced primarily by the liver, although local production occurs in the mesenchymal cells of the intestine as well. IGF mediates GH action, stimulates insulin activity, and assists in growth and development. IGF-I has numerous effects that augment intestinal adaptation. In a parenteral nutrition mouse model, administration of IGF-I reversed the associated atrophy by increasing jejunal mass, protein, and DNA concentration [34]. Following a 70% intestinal resection in rats, exogenous IGF treatment increases jejunal mucosal mass (20%), mucosal DNA (33%) and protein (36%) content, and enterocyte proliferation and crypt depth [35]. During cirrhosis-induced intestinal atrophy in the rat, IGF-I treatment also reversed the intestinal atrophy and improved epithelial glucose and amino acid transport [36]. In transgenic mice that overexpress IGF-I within the muscularis layer of the intestine, partial enterectomy increased the length of the remnant intestine and was associated with an early decline and subsequent increase in the relative mucosal surface area, revealing the IGF-I signaling within the muscle wall may play an important role in intestinal adaptation [37]. Despite these effects, IGF-I appears less promising than other potential therapies for intestinal failure with negligible effects reported in many studies of key variables of adaptation, including mucosal architecture and epithelial cytokinetics [35,37,38].

Growth hormone

Growth hormone (GH) is a 191 amino acid anabolic protein. It is responsible for stimulating growth via initiation of cell division, and provides regulatory effects on macronutrient metabolism by stimulating protein synthesis, gluconeogenesis, and lipolysis. After release of GH from the anterior pituitary, there are numerous locations within the GI tract in which it can bind its receptor, including the stomach, small intestine, and colon.

Several studies have shown structural adaptations following GH administration. Following an 80%

resection in piglets, GH increased the adaptive process through increases in the length of the small bowel remnant [39]. Growth hormone also increased mucosal thickness and crypt-villous length in rats following resection [40].

Exogenous GH administration in humans has produced conflicting results. On the positive side, GH given to pediatric patients dramatically improved growth status, both in terms of height and weight, while aiding weaning from parenteral nutrients [41]. GH treatment of parenteral-nutrient dependent adults with intestinal failure increased intestinal absorption of energy (15%), nitrogen (14%), carbohydrates (10%), and lipid (12%; [42]). Effects such as these, demonstrated by other investigators [42–45], prompted the Food and Drug Administration (FDA) in the United States to approve the use of GH in the treatment of patients with SBS (recently reviewed in [46]).

By contrast, evidence of GH stimulation of intestinal adaptation has been less consistent; indeed, little to no effects of GH administration have been reported either in animals or human clinical trials [47–49]. For instance, Vanderhoof and associates reported that the administration of GH in rats had no effect on intestinal adaptation as mucosal mass, protein, and sucrase activity were actually higher in the control animals than those receiving treatment following intestinal resection [50]. A randomized, double-blind, crossover placebo-controlled trial in humans with SBS reported no change in intestinal absorption of a variety of nutrients including carbohydrates, fat, and nitrogen, as well as macrominerals such as sodium, potassium, calcium, and magnesium [51]. With such mixed results, it is difficult to ascertain the true effects of GH on intestinal adaptation and the therapeutic specificity of GH on the intestine, versus widespread, systemic effects. Many differences exist in these studies, not only in the effects described but also in the dose administered, treatment time, and the patients' disease or animal model used. Further exploration of GH, as it is now used in the clinic, will surely determine its efficacy as a viable treatment option for patients with intestinal failure.

Conclusions

Numerous studies reveal that humoral factors do promote intestinal adaptation and may provide therapeutic options for humans with intestinal failure. Although the majority of studies have appropriately studied each candidate stimulus in isolation, it is important to note that these factors exist simultaneously in the body and it is certainly their synchronized interactions that are important in regulating intestinal adaptation. While these factors are studied and optimal doses, administration methods, and timing and duration of therapy are determined, complimentary therapies aimed at coupling synergistic humoral stimuli, interactions with oral nutrient consumption, and sustainable alleviation of parenteral nutrient requirements should be key considerations.

References

1 Tappenden KA. Mechanisms of enteral nutrient-enhanced intestinal adaptation. *Gastroenterology* 2006; 130(suppl):S93–S9.

2 Lovshin J, Drucker DJ. Synthesis, secretion and biological actions of the glucagon-like peptides. *Pediatr Diabetes* 2000;1:49–57.

3 White JW, Saunders GF. Structure of the human glucagon gene. *Nucleic Acids Res* 1986;14:4719–4730.

4 Dhanvantari S, Seidah NG, Brubaker PL. Role of prohormone convertases in the tissue-specific processing of proglucagon. *Mol Endocrinol* 1996;10:342–355.

5 Drucker DJ, Erlich P, Asa SL, Brubaker PL. Induction of intestinal epithelial proliferation by glucagon-like peptide 2. *Proc Natl Acad Sci USA* 1996;93:7911–7916.

6 Kato Y, Yu D, Schwartz MZ. Glucagonlike peptide-2 enhances small intestinal absorptive function and mucosal mass in vivo. *J Pediatr Surg* 1999;34:18–20; discussion 20–1.

7 Tsai CH, Hill M, Asa SL, et al. Intestinal growth-promoting properties of glucagon-like peptide-2 in mice. *Am J Physiol* 1997;273:E77–E84.

8 Brubaker PL, Izzo A, Hill M, Drucker DJ. Intestinal function in mice with small bowel growth induced by glucagon-like peptide-2. *Am J Physiol* 1997;272:E1050–E1058.

9 Cheeseman CI. Upregulation of SGLT-1 transport activity in rat jejunum induced by GLP-2 infusion in vivo. *Am J Physiol* 1997;273:R1965–7R191.

10 Chance WT, Foley-Nelson T, Thomas I, Balasubramaniam A. Prevention of parenteral nutrition-induced gut hypoplasia by coinfusion of glucagon-like peptide-2. *Am J Physiol* 1997;273:G559–G563.

11 Martin GR, Wallace LE, Sigalet DL. Glucagon-like peptide-2 induces intestinal adaptation in parenterally fed rats with short bowel syndrome. *Am J Physiol Gastrointest Liver Physiol* 2004;286:G964–G972.

12 Petersen YM, Burrin DG, Sangild PT. GLP-2 has differential effects on small intestine growth and function in fetal and neonatal pigs. *Am J Physiol Regul Integr Comp Physiol* 2001;281:R1986–R1993.

13 Burrin DG, Stoll B, Guan X, et al. Glucagon-like peptide 2 dose-dependently activates intestinal cell survival and proliferation in neonatal piglets. *Endocrinology* 2005;146:22–32.

14 Burrin DG, Stoll B, Jiang R, et al. GLP-2 stimulates intestinal growth in premature TPN-fed pigs by suppressing proteolysis and apoptosis. *Am J Physiol Gastrointest Liver Physiol* 2000;279:G1249–G1256.

15 Au A, Gupta A, Schembri P, Cheeseman CI. Rapid insertion of GLUT2 into the rat jejunal brush-border membrane promoted by glucagon-like peptide 2. *Biochem J* 2002;367:247–54.

16 Cottrell JJ, Stoll B, Buddington RK, et al. Glucagon-like peptide-2 protects against TPN-induced intestinal hexose malabsorption in enterally refed piglets. *Am J Physiol Gastrointest Liver Physiol* 2006;290:G293–G300.

17 Meier JJ, Nauck MA, Pott A, et al. Glucagon-like peptide 2 stimulates glucagon secretion, enhances lipid absorption, and inhibits gastric acid secretion in humans. *Gastroenterology* 2006;130:44–54.

18 Wojdemann M, Wettergren A, Hartmann B, Holst JJ. Glucagon-like peptide-2 inhibits centrally induced antral motility in pigs. *Scand J Gastroenterol* 1998;33:828–832.

19 Deniz M, Bozkurt A, Kurtel H. Mediators of glucagon-like peptide 2-induced blood flow: Responses in different vascular sites. *Regul Pept* 2007;7–15.

20 Stephens J, Stoll B, Cottrell J, et al. Glucagon-like peptide-2 acutely increases proximal small intestinal blood flow in TPN-fed neonatal piglets. *Am J Physiol Regul Integr Comp Physiol* 2006;290:R283–R289.

21 Jeppesen PB, Hartmann B, Thulesen J, et al. Glucagon-like peptide 2 improves nutrient absorption and nutritional status in short-bowel patients with no colon. *Gastroenterology* 2001;120:806–815.

22 Jeppesen PB, Sanguinetti EL, Buchman A, et al. Teduglutide (ALX-0600), a dipeptidyl peptidase IV resistant glucagon-like peptide 2 analogue, improves intestinal function in short bowel syndrome patients. *Gut* 2005;54:1224–1231.

23 Helmrath MA, Shin CE, Erwin CR, Warner BW. The EGF\EGF-receptor axis modulates enterocyte apoptosis during intestinal adaptation. *J Surg Res* 1998;77:17–22.

24 Nakai K, Hamada Y, Kato Y, et al. Further evidence that epidermal growth factor enhances the intestinal adaptation following small bowel transplantation. *Life Sci* 2004;75:2091–2102.

25 Helmrath MA, Shin CE, Fox JW, et al. Adaptation after small bowel resection is attenuated by sialoadenectomy: the role for endogenous epidermal growth factor. *Surgery* 1998;124:848–854.

26 Helmrath MA, Erwin CR, Warner BW. A defective EGF-receptor in waved-2 mice attenuates intestinal adaptation. *J Surg Res* 1997;69:76–80.

27 Erwin CR, Helmrath MA, Shin CE, et al. Intestinal overexpression of EGF in transgenic mice enhances adaptation after small bowel resection. *Am J Physiol* 1999;277:G533–G540.

28 Sigalet DL, Martin GR, Butzner JD, et al. A pilot study of the use of epidermal growth factor in pediatric short bowel syndrome. *J Pediatr Surg* 2005;40:763–768.

29 Sukhotnik I, Yakirevich E, Coran AG, et al. Effect of transforming growth factor-alpha on intestinal adaptation in a rat model of short bowel syndrome. *J Surg Res* 2002;108:235–242.

30 Falcone RA, Jr., Stern LE, Kemp CJ, et al. Intestinal adaptation occurs independent of transforming growth factor-alpha. *J Pediatr Surg* 2000;35:365–370.

31 Yang H, Wildhaber BE, Teitelbaum DH. 2003 Harry M. Vars Research Award. Keratinocyte growth factor improves epithelial function after massive small bowel resection. *JPEN J Parenter Enteral Nutr* 2003;27:198–206; discussion 206–207.

32 Yang H, Wildhaber B, Tazuke Y, Teitelbaum DH. 2002 Harry M. Vars Research Award. Keratinocyte growth factor stimulates the recovery of epithelial structure and function in a mouse model of total parenteral nutrition. *JPEN J Parenter Enteral Nutr* 2002;26:333–340; discussion 340–341.

33 Johnson WF, DiPalma CR, Ziegler TR, et al. Keratinocyte growth factor enhances early gut adaptation in a rat model of short bowel syndrome. *Vet Surg* 2000;29:17–27.

34 Murali SG, Nelson DW, Draxler AK, et al. Insulin-like growth factor-I (IGF-I) attenuates jejunal atrophy in association with increased expression of IGF-I binding protein-5 in parenterally fed mice. *J Nutr* 2005;135:2553–2559.

35 Dahly EM, Guo Z, Ney DM. IGF-I augments resection-induced mucosal hyperplasia by altering enterocyte kinetics. *Am J Physiol Regul Integr Comp Physiol* 2003;285:R800–R808.

36 Castilla-Cortazar I, Pascual M, Urdaneta E, et al. Jejunal microvilli atrophy and reduced nutrient transport in rats with advanced liver cirrhosis: improvement by

Insulin-like Growth Factor I. *BMC Gastroenterol* 2004;4:12.

37 Knott AW, Juno RJ, Jarboe MD, et al. Smooth muscle overexpression of IGF-I induces a novel adaptive response to small bowel resection. *Am J Physiol Gastrointest Liver Physiol* 2004;287:G562–G570.

38 Gillingham MB, Dahly EM, Murali SG, Ney DM. IGF-I treatment facilitates transition from parenteral to enteral nutrition in rats with short bowel syndrome. *Am J Physiol Regul Integr Comp Physiol* 2003;284:R363–R371.

39 Benhamou PH, Canarelli JP, Richard S, et al. Human recombinant growth hormone increases small bowel lengthening after massive small bowel resection in piglets. *J Pediatr Surg* 1997;32:1332–1336.

40 Gu Y, Wu ZH, Xie JX, et al. Effects of growth hormone (rhGH) and glutamine supplemented parenteral nutrition on intestinal adaptation in short bowel rats. *Clin Nutr* 2001;20:159–166.

41 Ladd AP, Grosfeld JL, Pescovitz OH, Johnson NB. The effect of growth hormone supplementation on late nutritional independence in pediatric patients with short bowel syndrome. *J Pediatr Surg* 2005;40:442–445.

42 Seguy D, Vahedi K, Kapel N, et al. Low-dose growth hormone in adult home parenteral nutrition-dependent short bowel syndrome patients: a positive study. *Gastroenterology* 2003;124:293–302.

43 Byrne TA, Persinger RL, Young LS, et al. A new treatment for patients with short-bowel syndrome. Growth hormone, glutamine, and a modified diet. *Ann Surg* 1995;222:243–254; discussion 254–255.

44 Byrne TA, Morrissey TB, Nattakom TV, et al. Growth hormone, glutamine, and a modified diet enhance nutrient absorption in patients with severe short bowel syndrome. *JPEN J Parenter Enteral Nutr* 1995;19:296–302.

45 Byrne TA, Wilmore DW, Iyer K, et al. Growth hormone, glutamine, and an optimal diet reduces parenteral nutrition in patients with short bowel syndrome: a prospective, randomized, placebo-controlled, double-blind clinical trial. *Ann Surg* 2005;242:655–661.

46 Messing B, Blethen S, DiBaise JK, et al. Treatment of adult short bowel syndrome with recombinant human growth hormone: a review of clinical studies. *J Clin Gastroenterol* 2006;40(suppl):S75–S84.

47 Scolapio JS. Effect of growth hormone, glutamine, and diet on body composition in short bowel syndrome: a randomized, controlled study. *JPEN J Parenter Enteral Nutr* 1999;23:309–312; discussion 312–313.

48 Scolapio JS, Camilleri M, Fleming CR, et al. Effect of growth hormone, glutamine, and diet on adaptation in short-bowel syndrome: a randomized, controlled study. *Gastroenterology* 1997;113:1074–1081.

49 Scolapio JS. Short bowel syndrome: recent clinical outcomes with growth hormone. *Gastroenterology* 2006;130(suppl):S122–S126.

50 Vanderhoof JA, Kollman KA, Griffin S, Adrian TE. Growth hormone and glutamine do not stimulate intestinal adaptation following massive small bowel resection in the rat. *J Pediatr Gastroenterol Nutr* 1997;25:327–331.

51 Szkudlarek J, Jeppesen PB, Mortensen PB. Effect of high dose growth hormone with glutamine and no change in diet on intestinal absorption in short bowel patients: a randomised, double blind, crossover, placebo controlled study. *Gut* 2000;47:199–205.

6 Autologous Reconstruction of the GI Tract

26 Autologous Reconstruction of the GI Tract

Debra Sudan

Key points

- Patients with short bowel syndrome may benefit from nontransplant surgery to improve intestinal function.

- Standard general surgical interventions include recruitment of unused intestine by closing fistulas or ostomies.

- Novel surgical techniques for the treatment of short bowel syndrome that appear to be beneficial in improving function include tapering and lengthening procedures, that is, Bianchi or serial transverse enteroplasty (STEP).

- Bianchi tapering and lengthening is technically demanding, but has excellent long-term results with 80% of patients weaning from TPN and the majority have sustained improvement.

- STEP tapering and lengthening has been only recently introduced and long-term results have not been established. The short-term results suggest that the overall ability to wean TPN may not be as good as Bianchi tapering; however, a direct comparison in a randomized trial has not been performed.

- Repeated lengthening can be performed by applying the STEP after the Bianchi procedure. In patients with the shortest remnant bowel lengths, the Bianchi procedure should therefore be applied as the first tapering and lengthening procedure, whenever feasible.

Before the introduction of parenteral nutrition (PN), short bowel syndrome was often fatal. The introduc-

Intestinal Failure: Diagnosis, Management and Transplantation.
Edited by Alan N. Langnas, Olivier Goulet, Eamonn M.M. Quigley and Kelly A. Tappenden. © 2008 Blackwell Publishing.
ISBN 978-1-4051-4637-1.

tion of parenteral nutrition in the 1970s provided an opportunity for survival in many patients. Despite long-term survival in many, overall life expectancy of patients permanently dependent on PN is less than that of the age matched general population due to life-threatening complications such as line sepsis, loss of venous access and parenteral nutrition-associated liver disease [1,2]. Intestinal transplantation has achieved clinical success in a few centers, but because of the requirement of long-term immunosuppression with its attendant risks, nontransplant surgical procedures continue to have a place in the treatment of permanent intestinal failure [3]. In this chapter, we will review these surgical procedures as a treatment for short bowel syndrome.

Recruitment of unused intestine

In TPN-dependent patients, the best way to increase enteral function is to recruit any bypassed or unused remnant bowel that is functional. This can be done by closing enterocutaneous fistulas or surgical ostomies. In patients that had intestinal atresia, one must maintain a high index of suspicion for other sites of stricture in the remnant small bowel or colon when restoring continuity. Passage of a balloon catheter through the remnant bowel intra-operatively can identify strictures that may not be visualized with radiographic studies. In patients with jaundice, provided that the hepatic synthetic function is intact, restoration of intestinal continuity appears worth the risk if there is reasonable expectation of weaning the TPN and avoiding transplantation afterward. In contrast, patients with advanced liver disease or who have remnant lengths or small bowel function that suggest little chance of weaning TPN are better served by transplantation.

Reversed segments, colonic interposition, nipple valve construction

Several novel surgical procedures have been suggested to enhance intestinal adaptation. The most commonly performed of these rare procedures is a reversed segment, which is formed at the junction of remnant small bowel and colon by isolating 3 to 10 cm of jejunum (or ileum if present) and rotating it 180 degrees [4–6]. This segment of small intestine is then sutured back into place and acts as a break to the rapid transit of succus entericus allowing for longer contact with the intestinal mucosa and theoretically better absorption. Only 38 cases have been reported in the world literature and this technique is rarely used today although 50–70% of reports suggested some benefit. Unfortunately, as many as one-third developed obstruction at the site of reversed segment requiring further surgical intervention and often resection. Less commonly, interposition of a segment of colon in the central portion of the remnant small bowel has been reported to slow motility. Fewer than 20 cases are identified in the world literature and several of these patients developed severe lactic acidosis or eosinophilic colitis requiring reversal [7]. There have been ten reported cases of construction of a nipple valve, which has been suggested to recreate the effects of the ileocecal valve [8,9] The partially obstructing nature appears to lead to proximal bowel dilation and has been combined with later longitudinal lengthening in six patients in one center [9]. Although there are theoretical advantages with each of these procedures, there has not been widespread adoption of any into clinical practice.

Intestinal lengthening procedures

Longitudinal lengthening (Bianchi)

In 1980, Bianchi published the first manuscript describing a longitudinal intestinal lengthening procedure (depicted in Figure 26.1) in a pig model [10]. This technique was performed with linear stapling of the bowel longitudinally after creation of a tunnel in the avascular plane between vessels in each leaf of the mesentery. He described lengthening of segments varying from 10 to 30 cm. Although two of the pigs died from perioperative complications, seven survived, thus verifying that the technique was reproducible. In 1984, Bianchi reviewed four clinical cases and the earlier experimental results in the pig model and suggested an alternative hand-sewn technique, as depicted in Figure 26.2 [11]. The modification was recommended as a result of the finding of inter-loop fistulas in two of the experimental cases in which stapling had been performed. A simplification of the stapled technique of longitudinal lengthening was described by Chahine et al. in 1998 (see Figure 26.3), which required only one anastomosis while maintaining the proximal and distal bowel in continuity [12].

Experimental results

Buie and colleagues in 1993 demonstrated the superiority of Bianchi lengthening over simple adaptation in a 75% resection model [13]. He demonstrated uniformly poor weight gain in three experimental short bowel groups compared to sham operated controls. He then demonstrated significantly more catch-up growth in two experimental groups randomized to either proximal or distal Bianchi lengthening compared to the adaptation-only control short bowel pigs (see Figure 26.4).

Clinical results of Bianchi procedure

Table 26.1 is a summary of the clinical results of all published cases identified through a PubMed search for the terms intestinal lengthening, short bowel syndrome, and Bianchi. Careful examination of manuscripts was performed to prevent duplication and references to patients in follow-up articles were pooled leading to the identification of 113 unique patients from at least 11 institutions [3,9,14–22]. The first published report in 1981 by Boeckman and Traylor described a 4-year-old child with gastroschisis, who had 50 cm of remnant small intestine [14]. This patient was weaned from TPN 10 weeks after the procedure. It appears from the published reports that, in most cases, the Bianchi procedure was applied to patients that were less than 1 year of age and had complications of TPN administration with up to 50% of patients being jaundiced in some series. The procedure was applied more often in patients that had undergone weeks or months of adaptation after their initial bowel resection and no reports

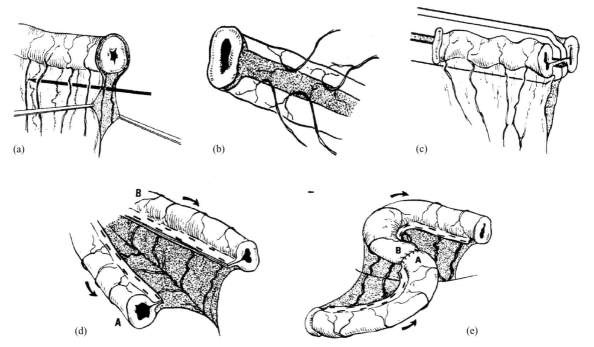

Figure 26.1 Longitudinal intestinal lengthening. (a) The small bowel is divided at either end of a dilated loop. The mesentery is dissected to create a plane along the axis of the intestine between branches of mesenteric blood vessels. (b) The mesentery has two leaves. Arterial and venous branches of mesenteric vessels alternate from one leaf of the mesentery to the other. (c) A gastrointestinal stapling device can be passed between the leaves of the mesentery. (d) When the stapler is fired, the single loop of dilated intestine is divided into two parallel loops. (e) The parallel loops can then be turned in a "lazy S" fashion to approximate the distal end of one loop to the proximal end of the second loop. In this way, the parallel loops are anastomosed end-to-end to reestablish continuity and double the length of small bowel. In addition, the lengthened segment is then reanastomosed to the normal small bowel or colon proximally and distally (not shown). (Reproduced from Bianchi [11], with permission from Elsevier.)

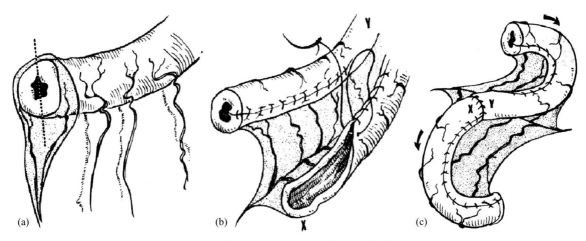

Figure 26.2 Hand-sewn technique for longitudinal intestinal lengthening. After the initial description of the stapled technique shown in Figure 26.1, this alternate technique of a hand-sewn closure was described. This was suggested to decrease the risk for fistula formation between adjacent staple lines. (Reproduced from JRSM supplement No. 3, Volume 77, 1984 pages 35–41, with permission from Royal Society of Medicine Press, London.)

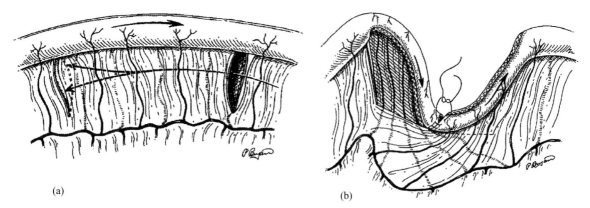

(a)   (b)

Figure 26.3 Modification of intestinal lengthening technique. The most recent modification of the technique utilizes the stapled technique described in Figure 26.1, however the bowel lumen is not completely transected proximally and distally in order to gain access to the mesentery. A small window is made in the side of the mesentery, as shown in Figure 26.3a. This allows continuity of the intestine to be maintained proximally and distally as shown in Figure 26.3b, rather than requiring 3 anastomoses. (Reproduced from Chahine and Ricketts [12], with permission from Elsevier.)

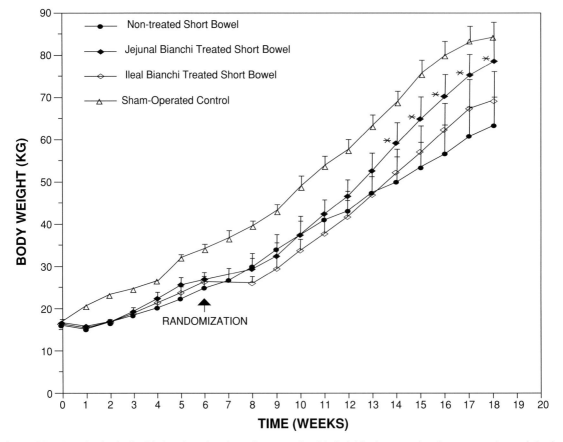

Figure 26.4 Growth of animals with short bowel syndrome (-•-,-◇- and -◇-) is diminished compared to sham operated controls (-△-). In the three groups with short bowel lengths, both Bianchi treated groups had improved growth compared to the group that was untreated. (Reproduced from Buie et al. [13], with permission from Elsevier.)

Table 26.1 Summary of all published reports of Bianchi-type longitudinal intestinal lengthening procedures identified through PubMed search including number of patients (N), year of publication, length of residual small intestine before and after lengthening (pre/post), length of follow-up (F/U) in weeks (wks), months (mos) or years (yrs), number of patients weaned off of TPN (off) or improved in degree of enteral tolerance, complications reported, summary of metabolic studies performed, deaths and cause of death.

	N	Year	SB length, cm (Pre/post)	F/U	TPN	Complications	Metabolic findings	Deaths	Causes of death
Boekman	1	1981		10 wks	1 off		↑ fat absorption	0	
Aigrain	1	1985	25/?	6 mos	1 off		↑ fat absorption and d-xylose	0	
Pokorny	2	1991	50,47/?	4,6 mos	2 off		↑ transit time	0	
Georgeson	9	1994	49 ± 28/ 98 ± 46	5–49 mos	2 off/ 5 improved	Duodenal stenosis, bowel obstruction, Jejunal perforation, fistula	Catch-up growth observed	2/9 (22%)	
Thompson	14	1995			7 off/ 5 improved	16% not sustained benefit, reoperation		1/14 (7%)	
Bianchi	20	1997	A: 45 (38–110) D: 35 (25–90)	6.4 yrs	7 off/ 2 part			11/20 (55%)	Liver failure (10), Sepsis (1)
Weber	16	1999	42–50/ 58–90		14 off/ 2 improved	Obstruction (5), fistula (1)	↑ fat absorption and d-xylose ↑ transit time	0	
Waag	25	1999	28 (6–48)/ 46 (11–73)	6 yrs	17 off/ 1 improved	Poor linear growth		7/25 (28%)	Liver failure (3) Sepsis (2) Aspiration (1) Venous thrombosis (1)
Sudan	20	2005	33 (16–91) 61 (29–130)/	2 yrs	13 off/ 5 improved			2/20 (10%)	Line sepsis (1), Influenza pneumonia (1)

Table 26.2 A summary of functional results of Bianchi-type lengthening in a clinical series of patients. The number of stools decreased (from 8 to 3 per 24 hour period) correlating with the prolonged transit time of contrast through the intestine as measured by small bowel contrast study (52 minutes prior to lengthening vs. 205 minutes 6 months after lengthening). In addition, there was less stasis due to contrast remaining in dilated small bowel loops after lengthening (i.e. clearance). There is also a measured improvement in absorption of carbohydrates (D-xylose absorption) and fat (Fecal fat) after intestinal lengthening.

Results of functional and absorptive studies performed pre- and post-operatively			
		Post-operatively	
	Pre-operatively	1 mo	6 mo
Stool count	8 ± 2	4 ± 1	3 ± 1
Transit time (min)	52 ± 14	135 ± 31	205 ± 28
Clearance (h)	4.5 ± 0.6	2.4 ± 0.8	2.6 ± 1.1
D-xylose absorption (1 h, g/dL)	5.0 ± 2.0	18.6 ± 5.1	22.4 ± 5.8
Fecal fat (% diet)	40 ± 8.2	20 ± 6.5	18 ± 7.8

Note. Data are expressed as mean ±SEM.
(Reproduced from Weber et al. [23], with permission from Elsevier.)

of lengthening at the time of initial resection or anastomosis of atretic segments were identified. Most of the experience in Bianchi lengthening and tapering is in children (109 patients), although reports from the University of Nebraska include 4 adults [3,17]. The median age for the pediatric patients at the time of Bianchi lengthening was 1 year (range = 3 weeks to 16 years) and the median remnant length of bowel (measured in most series from the ligament of Treitz to the small bowel colonic junction) was 45 (range 14–110) cm. The overall median additional length achieved by the procedure was 25 cm yielding a median total bowel length of 70.5 (20–160 cm). Overall patient survival was 81%, but varied widely in the different series from 48% to 100%. In most series, the majority of patients demonstrated an improvement in enteral tolerance with 84 % of survivors achieving independence from parenteral nutrition (mean follow-up time of 2 years).

Weber et al. demonstrated excellent clinical improvement in his series with complete enteral dependence in 4 out of 5 patients within 6 months of lengthening [23]. In addition, he carefully described measurements reflecting improved bowel function and increased nutrient absorption [23]. The narrower luminal diameter and additional longitudinal length produced by the Bianchi procedure improves intestinal motility, as demonstrated by prolonged transit time for charcoal. Prolonging transit time leads to longer mucosal contact with nutrients and, in the Weber series, a decrease in stool number and volume. In addition, Weber and others have shown improved carbohydrate and fat absorption with specific metabolic studies including D-xylose absorption and measurements of fecal fat, which were all improved at 6 and 12 months compared to measurements performed 1 week before lengthening (see Table 26.2) [14,15,23]. Finally, improved clearance of barium after Bianchi tapering and lengthening suggests the elimination of stasis, which likely allows for improved function of the mucosa by decreasing bacterial overgrowth and mucosal inflammation [16,20].

The variability in survival after the Bianchi procedure is likely related to wide variations in the degree of liver disease present in patients at the time of the procedure, experience of the team in the care of patients with short bowel syndrome, and the availability of transplantation for salvage in patients who failed to wean from TPN, or developed other significant complications after lengthening.

Complications of Bianchi tapering and lengthening

The most frequent complication overall was progression of the underlying liver disease (n = 13; 12%),

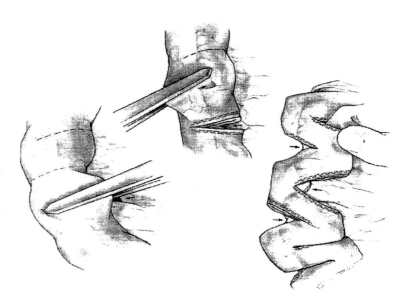

Figure 26.5 Serial transverse enteroplasty (STEP). The dilated segment of small bowel is narrowed by alternate firings of the gastrointestinal stapling device from the mesenteric and anti-mesenteric border of the intestine. The final luminal diameter reflects the distance between firings as well as the distance across the bowel diameter that is left undivided. The goal is to decrease the bowel diameter to normal, which ranges from 1 cm to 2.5 cm in small children and adults, respectively. Narrowing the lumen too much can lead to the development of a stricture and obstructive symptoms. (Reproduced from Kim et al. [24], with permission from Elsevier.)

which was uniformly fatal in the published cases. In more recent years, intestinal transplantation has become an option that could salvage such patients. Other complications reported include intestinal obstruction, (n = 10), intestinal leak (n = 2), inter-loop fistula (n = 5), loss of venous access (n = 2) and bacterial sepsis (n = 5). Although the procedure was described 26 years ago, the world experience appears to be limited. The complexity of the procedure, the severity of complications in selected patients, the difficulty in predicting which patients are likely to achieve enteral independence through adaptation alone and the introduction of intestinal transplantation have all contributed to the infrequency of the application of Bianchi tapering and lengthening to patients with short bowel syndrome.

STEP (serial transverse enteroplasty)

A novel alternative technique of bowel lengthening was described by Kim et al. in a pig model in 2003 [24]. The operative technique is depicted in Figure 26.5. STEP lengthening is performed by firing linear staplers alternatively from the mesenteric and anti-mesenteric edge of the dilated small bowel. The distance between subsequent firings of the stapler is guided by the normal diameter of the small bowel in the patient and ranges between 1 and 2.5 cm.

Experimental results

After the initial description of feasibility, a series of experiments in 10 pigs was reported by Chang et al. [25]. The pigs were randomized to 90% resection with or without STEP lengthening and then observed for a 6-week period. During the 6 weeks of follow-up, the control pigs with 10% retained native intestine demonstrated a 17% weight loss, whereas the STEP animals maintained their initial weight at the time of resection. In addition, the STEP pigs demonstrated improved D-xylose absorption, had higher levels of triglyceride and fat-soluble vitamins, and had higher plasma citrulline levels than the control animals [25].

Clinical results of STEP procedure

Because of the recent description of the technique, clinical experience is limited to 15 patients in the published literature from four centers [3,22,26,27]. The clinical information from these cases is summarized in Table 26.3. In contrast to the Bianchi procedure, one-third of the experience in published cases of STEP lengthening is in adults (5/15). The median remnant lengths of small bowel in children and adults undergoing lengthening by the STEP were 57 (22–135) and 55 (22–84) cm, respectively. The median total bowel lengths after STEP were 105 (38–200) and 67 (38–140) cm, in children and adults respectively. Patient survival was 97% with median follow-up of 10.5 (3–24) months. Two patients failed to improve their enteral tolerance after

Table 26.3 A summary of the published reports of STEP lengthening procedures including the number of patients (N), the year of publication, the length of remnant small bowel before and after the procedure and complications reported.

Author	Year of Publication	Number of Patients	Age, yrs.	Jaundice (Y/N)	Small bowel length, cm (pre/post)	Length of follow-up, months	Alive (Y/N)	TPN (off or % of total calories)
Kim	2003	1	1.9	N	135/200	6	Y	50%
Wales	2005	1	0.01	N	90/112	7	Y	Off
Ismail	2005	1	0.01	N	50/75	6	Y	Off
Sudan	2005	8	5	N	80/110	10	Y	40%
			3	Y*	23/38	8	Y	Off
			14	N	65/105	24	Y	Off[b]
			18	N	55/67	15	Y	100%
			25	Y*	80/140	12	Y	Off
			38	N	64/76	21	Y	Off[b]
			40	N	52/65	19	Y	Off
			54	Y	25/38	3	N	100%
Javid	2005	5	1.9[a]					
			0.7	Y*	27/59	8	Y	?
			1.2	Y	84/113	15	Y	20%
			1.2	N	39/69	11	Y	Off
			0.01	N	22/51		Y	?

Yrs. = years, Y = yes, N = no, cm = centimeters, pre = prior to lengthening, post = after lengthening, TPN = total parenteral nutrition, a = same patient as reported above in Kim, * = patients with jaundice in past and biopsy-proven cirrhosis, but not jaundiced at time of procedure, [b] = patient restarted TPN after initial weaning due to weight loss, ? = not reported in the manuscript.

STEP and had progression of their liver disease resulting in death in one patient and combined liver/small bowel transplantation in the other. Complete weaning from TPN was achieved in 50% of patients undergoing the technique.

Complications of STEP

The STEP appears quite safe and very few complications have been described in the initial cohort of 15 patients. There was one reported death in this group of patients (7%). The death occurred 2 months after the procedure and was related to the development of line sepsis in a patient with severe liver disease and in the absence of any surgical complications. The other major complication was intestinal obstruction, most likely a result of adhesions, requiring 3 months of full TPN support before spontaneous resolution [3]. Other minor complications, primarily line sepsis, occurred in several patients. Failure to wean from TPN was more common after STEP (50%) than after Bianchi lengthening

(16%) and resulted in the need for transplantation in 1 patient undergoing STEP [28].

Comparison of results—Bianchi vs. STEP

The initial reported case and two other patients underwent STEP lengthening after previous Bianchi lengthening as a result of recurrent bowel dilatation [3,22]. In these patients, the STEP was able to augment the prior lengthening achieved and appears an ideal application of both techniques in the patient with extremely short remnant bowel lengths. In addition, the STEP procedure has been applied to several patients where the Bianchi procedure was not feasible technically because of a foreshortened mesentery or prior injury to the vasculature in one leaf of the mesentery. In large part, both procedures have been applied as primary definitive therapy with the expectation that either lengthening procedure alone may provide enough improvement in enteral function to avoid TPN related complications and the need for intestinal transplantation. Although the Bianchi has generally been applied only after significant adaptation has occurred, the STEP has been performed in several patients on the first day of life for intestinal atresia [26–28].

Although published clinical results of the Bianchi procedure suggest potentially greater risk for perioperative complications compared to the STEP procedure, the benefit, in terms of successful weaning from parenteral nutrition, may also be greater in patients who have undergone the Bianchi procedure compared to STEP. In light of this, the Bianchi procedure appears indicated as a primary procedure for patients at highest risk for poor outcome, that is, shortest remnant bowel length/or jaundice. The additional benefit of primary Bianchi lengthening is that this leaves the potential for further lengthening with later application of the STEP. The STEP procedure is therefore reserved for primary application in circumstances where a foreshortened mesentery or vascular injury of one leaf of the mesentery prevents the application of Bianchi lengthening and as an alternative to simple tapering where long lengths of dilated remnant small bowel exist.

Indications and patient selection

Based on the review of the experience with both intestinal lengthening surgeries and intestinal transplantation, the following recommendations are suggested. In patients with complications of their short bowel syndrome (including recurrent bacteremia, loss of venous access, PN-related liver disease) a tapering and lengthening procedure (when feasible) or transplantation is indicated. The decision on which procedure is performed is based on the balance of risk and potential benefit as well as the technical feasibility of the appropriate procedure. Those patients that have advanced liver disease as demonstrated by hepatic synthetic dysfunction, thrombocytopenia, and jaundice should be placed on the transplant waiting list. The patient with advanced liver disease is medically fragile and should undergo the procedure that is most likely to provide them with the best possibility of long-term survival, which usually is a combined liver/small

bowel transplant. Lengthening procedures are not indicated because a severe complication may preclude transplantation.

Lengthening procedures and recruitment of unused bowel segments (i.e. closure of an ostomy or enteric fistula and repair of strictures) are the treatment of choice in patients that are not jaundiced, but have dilated or discontinuous bowel segments leading to bacterial overgrowth, diarrhea, malabsorption, or recurrent bacteremia. Provided that venous access is not an issue, these patients have the longest period of time to allow slow and gradual adaptation and can usually avoid the need for transplantation with careful management in an experienced center. The candidate for lengthening is typically a patient that has markedly dilated small bowel (usually >10 cm in length) and this dilation is thought to be leading to bacterial overgrowth and diarrhea or recurrent bacteremia, which then interferes with the ability to wean TPN. The expectation is that return to normal caliber of this segment of bowel and the additional length achieved with either Bianchi or STEP will be sufficient to discontinue TPN.

Lengthening procedures may also be performed in patients with jaundice, who have preserved albumin levels, prothrombin time, and normal platelet count. Although these patients require very close follow-up to avoid missing the window of opportunity for transplantation, more than two-thirds of jaundiced patients with preserved synthetic function are able to wean from TPN and clear the jaundice and thereby avoid transplantation. Although there is not an absolute length of remnant small bowel required to perform lengthening, it is unlikely to be of benefit in patients with less than 15 cm of residual small intestine, especially beyond the first few months of life. Lengthening procedures in the jaundiced patient appears to be riskier than in the nonjaundiced patient and should be performed only after careful consideration. Complications are not well tolerated and progression of the liver disease is generally rapid if severe complications arise. Many of the patients with severe complications may be salvageable with transplantation, but this must be performed without prolonged delay. The jaundiced patient is the most difficult to manage and must be followed very closely while attempting to wean the TPN.

These surgical procedures are an important part of the successful treatment of intestinal failure, but are not sufficient to "cure" the patient. A multidisciplinary team including a dedicated gastroenterologist, surgeon, dietician, and nursing staff experienced in the care of patients with short bowel syndrome will maximize the benefits of the procedure. Intestinal transplantation is a good alternative to lengthening in patients who have loss of venous access and are unable to continue PN longterm during the period of intestinal adaptation and when liver disease is advanced. Recent survival rates after intestinal transplantation are similar to published reports of survival on TPN. Transplantation, however, requires the administration of immunosuppressive medications with their attendant risks and therefore when TPN weaning is likely, nontransplant surgeries are very effective and preferable alternatives.

(There is a registry available for the STEP procedure that can be accessed through the website http://www.childrenshospital.org/cfapps/step/index.cfm.)

References

1 Howard L, Heaphey L, Fleming CR, et al. Four years of North American registry home parenteral nutrition outcome data and their implications for patient management. *JPEN J Parenter Enteral Nutr* 1991;15:384–393.

2 Vantini I, Benini L, Bonfante F, et al. Survival rate and prognostic factors in patients with intestinal failure. *Dig Liver Dis* 2004;36:46–55.

3 Sudan D, DiBaise J, Torres C, et al. A multidisciplinary approach to the treatment of intestinal failure. *J Gastrointest Surg* 2005;9:165–176; discussion 176–177.

4 Panis Y, Messing B, Rivet P, et al. Segmental reversal of the small bowel as an alternative to intestinal transplantation in patients with short bowel syndrome. *Ann Surgery* 1997;225:401–407.

5 Pigot F, Messing B, Chaussade S, et al. Severe short bowel syndrome with a surgically reversed small bowel segment. *Dig Dis Sci* 1990;35:137–144.

6 Thomas JF, Jordan GL, Jr. Massive Resection of Small Bowel and Total Colectomy: Use of Reversed Segment. *Arch Surg* 1965;90:781–786.

7 Garcia VF, Templeton JM, Eichelberger MR, et al. Colon interposition for the short bowel syndrome. *J Pediatr Surg* 1981;16:994–995.

8 Vernon A, Georgeson K. Surgical options for short bowel syndrome. *Semin Pediatr Surg* 2001;10:91–98.

9 Georgeson K, Figueroa H, Vencente Y, Hardin WJ. Sequential intestinal lengthening procedures for refractory short bowel syndrome. *J Pediatr Surg* 1994;29:316–321.

10 Bianchi A. Intestinal loop lengthening—a technique for increasing small intestinal length. *J Pediatr Surg* 1980;15:145–151.

11 Bianchi A. Intestinal lengthening: an experimental and clinical review. *J R Soc Med* 1984;77(suppl):35–41.

12 Chahine AA, Ricketts RR. A modification of the Bianchi intestinal lengthening procedure with a single anastomosis. *J Pediatr Surg* 1998;33:1292–1293.

13 Buie WD, Thurston OG, vanAerde JE, et al. Jejunum is preferable for construction of a Bianchi bowellengthening procedure in swine short bowel. *J Pediatr Surg* 1993;28:102–109.

14 Boeckman CR, Traylor R. Bowel lengthening for short gut syndrome. *J Pediatr Surg* 1981;16:996–997.

15 Aigrain Y, Cornet D, Cezard JP, Boureau M. Longitudinal division of small intestine: a surgical possibility for children with the very short bowel syndrome. *Z Kinderchir* 1985;40:233–236.

16 Pokorny W, Fowler C. Isoperistaltic intestinal lengthening for short bowel syndrome. *Surg Gynecol Obstetr* 1991;172.

17 Thompson J, Langnas A, Pinch L, et al. Surgical approach to short-bowel syndrome. *Ann Surg* 1995;222:600–607.

18 Flageole H, Adolph VR, Sigalet DL, et al. The Bianchi procedure in a patient with jejunal atresia. *Eur J Pediatr Surg* 1997;7:361–363.

19 Bianchi A. Longitudinal intestinal lengthening and tailoring: results in 20 children. *J R Soc Med* 1997;90:429–432.

20 Weber T. Isoperistaltic bowel lengthening for short bowel syndrome in children. *Am J Surg* 1999;178:600–604.

21 Waag KL, Hosie S, Wessel L. What do children look like after longitudinal intestinal lengthening. *Eur J Pediatr Surg* 1999;9:260–262.

22 Kim HB, Lee PW, Garza J, et al. Serial transverse enteroplasty for short bowel syndrome: a case report. *J Pediatr Surg* 2003;38:881–885.

23 Weber T, Powell M. Early improvement in intestinal function after isoperistaltic bowel lengthening. *J Pediatr Surg* 1996;31:61–64.

24 Kim H, Fauza D, Garza J, et al. Serial transverse enteroplasty (STEP): A novel bowel lengthening procedure. *J Pediatr Surg* 2003;38:425–429.

25 Chang RW, Javid PJ, Oh JT, et al. Serial transverse enteroplasty enhances intestinal function in a model of short bowel syndrome. *Ann Surg* 2006;243:223–228.

26 Wales PW, Dutta S. Serial transverse enteroplasty as primary therapy for neonates with proximal jejunal atresia. *J Pediatr Surg* 2005;40:E31–E34.

27 Ismail A, Alkadhi A, Alnagaar O, Khirate A. Serial transverse enteroplasty in intestinal atresia management. *J Pediatr Surg* 2005;40:E5–E6.

28 Javid PJ, Kim HB, Duggan CP, Jaksic T. Serial transverse enteroplasty is associated with successful short-term outcomes in infants with short bowel syndrome. *J Pediatr Surg* 2005;40:1019–1023; discussion 1023–1024.

7 Organ Replacement Therapy for Intestinal Failure

27 Intestinal Transplantation: Indications and Patient Selection

Kareem M. Abu-Elmagd

Key points

- Intestinal transplantation is used more frequently for irreversible gastrointestinal failure patients who no longer can be maintained on TPN or effectively treated for complex abdominal pathology.

- Short bowel syndrome, gut dysmotility, gastrointestinal neoplastic syndromes, and enterocyte dysfunction are the leading causes of gut failure and indications for transplantation.

- The anatomic and functional status of each of the solid abdominal and visceral organs dictate the type of intestinal allograft needed for each patient.

- The therapeutic role of isolated liver replacement in SBS patients with TPN induced liver failure and the medical necessity for composite visceral replacement in patients with hollow visceral myopathy or neuropathy have yet to be fully defined.

- The recent achievement of patient survival rates similar to, or better than, those achieved on home parenteral nutrition justify the early consideration of intestinal transplantation and before the development of TPN failure.

For nearly three decades, the small bowel was considered a forbidden organ for clinical transplantation because of the associated massive lymphoid tissue, high antigenicity, and microbial colonization [1]. With the clinical introduction of effective immunosuppressive agents, the formidable risks of allograft rejection and subsequent lethal host infection were ameliorated and

Intestinal Failure: Diagnosis, Management and Transplantation.
Edited by Alan N. Langnas, Olivier Goulet, Eamonn M.M. Quigley and Kelly A. Tappenden. © 2008 Blackwell Publishing. ISBN 978-1-4051-4637-1.

the procedure has become a clinical reality for the last 16 years [2,3]. Furthermore, the survival advantages of the procedure have significantly improved over the last 5 years because of novel immunosuppressive protocols, better postoperative management, and new surgical innovations [4]. With better survival outcome and recent recognition by the Center for Medicare and Medicaid Services (CMS), intestinal and multivisceral transplantation have been used more frequently for patients with irreversible gastrointestinal failure who can be no longer maintained on total parenteral nutrition (TPN) therapy or effectively treated for complex abdominal pathology. Nonetheless, this chapter focuses on current practical guidelines, disease indications, pre-transplant evaluation, and proper patient selection, with special reference to each of the three main types of intestinal transplantation.

Indications

Current practical guidelines

Irreversible intestinal failure and complex abdominal visceral pathology with failure of the currently available conventional therapeutic modalities including TPN are essential prerequisites for intestinal and multivisceral transplantation [5–7]. Accordingly, the procedure is currently utilized and recognized by most health care providers as a rescue therapy for patients with irreversible gastrointestinal failure. However, the recently published data of the Pittsburgh intestinal transplant experience with patient survival rates similar to, or better than, those achieved on home parenteral nutrition may justify a modification of the current practical guidelines with a lifting of such restricted criteria [8]. To provide a definitive conclusion, a well-designed prospective study that compares isolated intestinal transplantation with TPN therapy may be required, particularly among patients who meet an agreed-on definition of low and high risk for TPN failure.

The definition of TPN failure was fully addressed in our formal request for national coverage [1]. Significant biochemical or histological evidence of liver injury, loss of central venous access with thrombosis of at least two central veins, frequent line sepsis or a single episode of fungal infection, and recurrent episodes of severe dehydration despite intravenous fluid supplement are TPN-associated complications that declare therapy failure.

Disease etiology and type of intestinal allograft

Short bowel syndrome (SBS), defective gastrointestinal motility, gastrointestinal neoplastic syndromes, impaired enterocyte function, and other gastrointestinal pathologic disorders are the main etiologic categories of gut failure and indications for transplantation. Patients with chronic gastrointestinal failure are candidates for intestinal transplant either alone (Figure 27.1a), combined with liver (Figure 27.1b) or as part of a multivisceral graft that includes stomach, duodenum, pancreas, and small bowel with, or without, the liver (Figure 27.1c). The type of intestinal allograft required for each patient is dictated by the anatomic and functional status of each solid and visceral abdominal organ. The entire length or a segment of the large bowel may be included in the allograft particularly in those patients who could benefit from a pull-through operation, or any other reconstructive surgical procedures.

Isolated intestine

SBS is the most common indication for intestine-only transplantation. Congenital disorders such as gastroschisis, volvulus, and atresia are the leading causes in children. In adults, the main causes are visceral ischemia, Crohn's disease, trauma, mesenteric desmoid tumor, and surgical adhesions. Splanchnic ischemia is commonly precipitated by hypercoagulable states, such as protein C, S or antithrombin III deficiencies, factor V/II mutations or the presence of lupus anticoagulant or anticardiolipin antibodies [9].

Hereditary neoplastic and congenital motility disorders such as familial polyposis, Gardner syndrome, total intestinal aganglionosis, and hollow visceral myopathy/neuropathy (Figure 27.2) are not uncommon indications among both adults and children. The extent of the disease, however, may dictate whether or not spontaneous en-bloc replacement of more than one of the abdominal visceral organs will be necessary. A deficiency of enterocyte absorptive capacity with the development of intestinal failure is commonly seen in children with microvillus inclusion disease and in adults with radiation enteritis, autoimmune enteropathy, lymphangectasia, and inflammatory bowel disease.

An accurate assessment of the extent of TPN-associated liver injury is very crucial for successful outcome after transplantation. The decision to perform simultaneous hepatic replacement is very challenging, particularly in patients with asymptomatic porto-mesenteric venous thrombosis and significant liver damage. The decision, however, should be guided by the presence or absence of portal hypertension, as well as the extent of liver disease [2]. For example, SBS patients with isolated splenic vein thrombosis should undergo isolated intestinal transplantation accompanied by splenectomy or, preferably, a splenorenal shunt, particularly in cases with a recannalized distal splenic segment. However, those with extensive thrombosis of the portomesenteric and splenic venous systems may be considered for composite visceral grafts with combined liver-intestinal or multivisceral transplantation.

The diagnosis of portal hypertension is based upon standard criteria including low blood cell counts, a low platelet count, an enlarged spleen, the detection of gastroesophageal varices or portal hypertensive gastropathy, and the presence of ascites. Some of these overt manifestations are less pronounced in patients with SBS because of reduced or absent mesenteric arterial flow. In general, patients with modest portal hypertension (mild splenic enlargement, platelet count >50,000, no gastroesophageal varices, and portal fibrosis without significant hepatic cholestasis) should be cautiously considered for intestinal transplantation alone. Under these circumstances, the venous outflow of the intestinal allograft may be preferably drained to the recipient systemic circulation via the inferior vena cava.

Combined liver and intestine

The operation is commonly indicated for SBS patients with TPN-associated hepatic failure. The en bloc

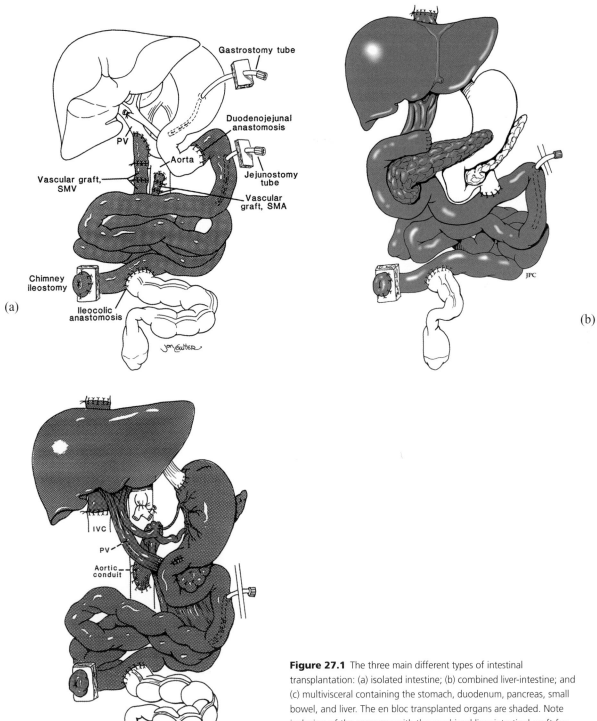

Figure 27.1 The three main different types of intestinal transplantation: (a) isolated intestine; (b) combined liver-intestine; and (c) multivisceral containing the stomach, duodenum, pancreas, small bowel, and liver. The en bloc transplanted organs are shaded. Note inclusion of the pancreas with the combined liver-intestinal graft for technical and logistic reasons. A jejunostomy tube was placed for early feeding and chimney ileostomy for surveillance ileoscopy and guided mucosal biopsy.

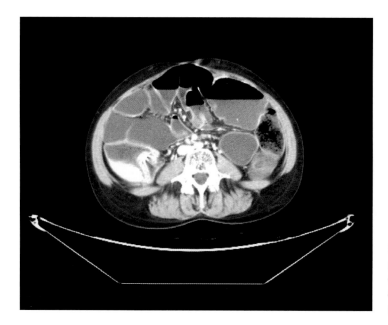

Figure 27.2 Abdominal CT in a patient with pseudo-obstruction syndrome. Note diffuse dilation of the intestinal loops. Patient received a modified multivisceral transplantation with preservation of the native liver three years ago.

replacement of both organs is also the only technically feasible and safe procedure that can be offered to the liver failure patient with concomitant portomesenteric venous thrombosis. It is our common observation that most SBS patients with TPN-induced severe hepatic cholestasis develop accelerated liver failure without histologically documented cirrhosis (Figure 27.3). As stated earlier, gastroesophageal varices and ascites are less likely to develop in some of these patients because of the reduced splanchnic vascular bed.

Multivisceral

Full or modified multivisceral transplantation is indicated for patients with complex abdominal pathology including massive gastrointestinal polyposis, traumatic loss of the abdominal viscera, extensive abdominal desmoid tumors, locally aggressive non-metastasizing neoplasms, generalized hollow visceral myopathy/neuropathy, and complete thrombosis of the splanchnic arterial (Figure 27.4A) or portal venous system(s) (Figure 27.4B) with vascular or hepatic decompensation. In our clinical practice, the number of organs to be replaced is limited to those affected by the abdominal pathology.

According to the data of the Intestinal Transplant Registry (ITR), the need for the intestine alone was more frequent in adults (55%) compared to children (37%) with more simultaneous hepatic replacement in children (50%) versus adults (21%). Multivisceral grafts were given to more adults (24%) than children (13%). Such a disparity in the number of transplanted organs between children and adults could be related to differences in the nature of the primary intestinal

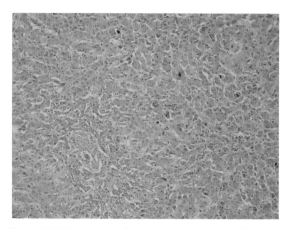

Figure 27.3 Liver biopsy of a patient with TPN-induced liver failure with a total serum bilirubin level of 21.0 mg/dl. Note the histopathologic absence of classic cirrhosis despite the clinical and biochemical evidence of cholestatic liver failure.

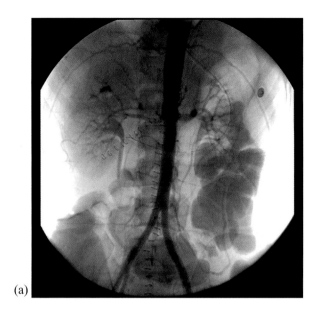
(a)

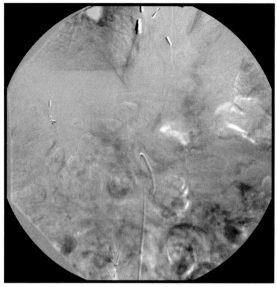
(b)

Figure 27.4 (a) A flush aortogram with complete occlusion of the celiac and superior mesenteric artery. The patient underwent total enterectomy for mesenteric infarction and was referred to the Pittsburgh Medical Center for visceral transplantation. (b) The venous phase of a visceral angiogram in a patient with extensive symptomatic gastrointestinal varices. Note complete thrombosis of the portomesenteric and splenic venous systems that dictated the need for en bloc multivisceral transplantation.

disease and the higher susceptibility of the pediatric liver to the metabolic injury of both TPN and SBS.

Gut failure and survival outcome

Similar to other abdominal and thoracic organ transplantations, the survival of the intestinal and multivisceral transplant recipient is influenced by the disease etiology and indication for transplantation. Because of disease heterogenicity and differences between adults and children, Kaplan Meier calculations of patient survival were focused on those with common disorders among both age groups. According to the Pittsburgh experience, patients with microvillus inclusion disease and pseudo-obstruction syndromes had better survival in both the pediatric and adult population (Figure 27.5).

Controversies

The cumulative improvement in long-term survival outcome with en bloc liver-intestinal and multivisceral

transplantation has questioned the therapeutic role of isolated liver replacement in SBS patients with TPN-induced liver failure. This controversial issue is further fueled by the previously reported unsatisfactory outcomes with liver transplantation alone [10], the improved outcome, reported by others, in highly selected cases [11] and the current high mortality rate among children awaiting composite visceral grafts [12]. Nonetheless, the procedure is justifiable in children with a sufficient length of small bowel, increasing tolerance of enteral feeding, and high expectation of achieving full nutritional autonomy [11]. However, it remains to be seen if these patients will sustain long-term successful outcome without further need for TPN therapy and avoidance of its potential deleterious effects on the liver allograft [1].

The recently defined syndromes of hollow visceral myopathy or neuropathy are not uncommon indications for visceral transplantation. The criteria of medical necessity to replace other visceral organs en bloc with the intestine have yet to be fully defined. It is our

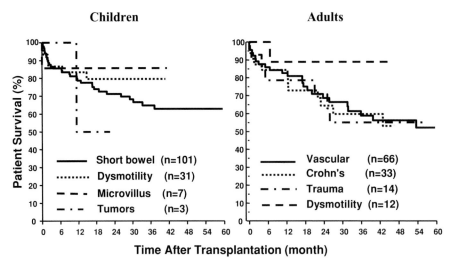

Figure 27.5 Kaplan Meier intestinal and multivisceral recipient survival according to the etiology of the gastrointestinal disease and leading indications for transplantation. Note better survival with microvillus disease in children and with dysmotility syndromes in both adults and children. Vascular occlusion, Crohn's disease and trauma had similar survival outcomes (unpublished Pittsburgh data).

current practice to simultaneously replace the stomach, duodenum, and pancreas en bloc with the intestine to eliminate the inevitable morbidities and mortalities associated with disease progression. Other transplant centers, however, have advocated a less extensive operation by limiting the visceral replacement to the small bowel alone with surgical drainage of the atonic native stomach to the proximal jejunal allograft. With both techniques, hepatic replacement is limited to patients with irreversible damage of the native liver.

Patient selection

Early referral

Patients with gut failure are commonly referred for transplantation after the development of life-threatening TPN complications, particularly liver failure. Universal adherence to this practice has been associated with significant morbidity and mortality among candidates awaiting composite visceral transplantation [12,13]. Furthermore, recent data from the ITR has shown a significantly higher survival rate for patients who were transplanted while waiting at home (Figure 27.6). In addition, the Pittsburgh pilot study of early transplantation has shown better therapeutic indices including survival, quality of life and cost effectiveness [14].

Early referral followed by successful transplantation of the intestine alone undoubtedly broadens the therapeutic benefits of the procedure. In addition to salvaging the native liver, the rehabilitation of most patients and their primary caregivers could be easily achieved with early restoration of their socioeconomic status. Equally important, is the technical feasibility of removing the isolated intestinal allograft as a rescue therapy for graft failure or life-threatening opportunistic infections of the recipient without the need for simultaneous retransplantation. With discontinuation of immunosuppression and reinstitution of TPN therapy, most patients could be saved and, at a later time, considered for retransplantation.

The evaluation process

The algorithm of the initial evaluation is guided by etiology and extent of the underlying disorder, associated extra-gastrointestinal pathology, and coexistence of systemic morbidity(s) that could contraindicate candidacy or increase the risk of transplantation. As a simple practical guideline, failure to maintain patients at their calculated ideal body weight without TPN therapy or during a weaning process is usually a surrogate marker of poor enteric functional reserve and indicative of irreversible gastrointestinal failure. Nonetheless, initial comprehensive assessment of the patient nutritional status including thorough medical and surgical history,

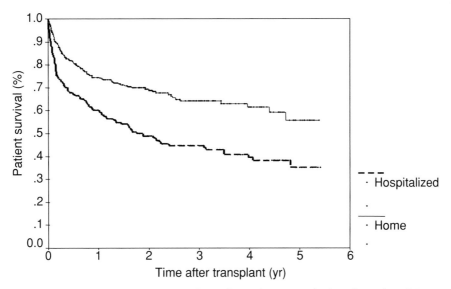

Figure 27.6 The intestinal transplant registry patient survival according to the status at the time of transplantation. Note a significantly higher survival rate for patients who were transplanted while waiting at home. (Reproduced from Grant et al. [3] with permission from Lippincott, Williams & Wilkins.)

full clinical examination and pertinent biochemical nutritional indices is the Achilles heel of the targeted and cost effective evaluation process.

The anatomic and functional assessment of the gastrointestinal tract, as well as the other abdominal organs, is usually the first step in the investigation process. The methods utilized include radiologic imaging, endoscopic instrumentation, and histologic examination of the remaining components of the gastrointestinal tract. Candidates with pseudo-obstruction syndromes often require gut motility studies to define the type of the defect, as well as the extent of organ involvement. The prior documentation of visceral or systemic vascular thromboses dictates the need for full hypercoagulable studies with the aim to identify one or more of the precipitating factors, including specific protein deficiencies, genetic mutations of the coagulation cascade factors and the development of prothrombotic antibodies. In addition, complete abdominal visceral angiography is mandatory to assess the extent of splanchnic thrombosis and guide the type of visceral allograft needed. In these and other high-risk patients with a history of central vein thrombosis, radiologic mapping of the major upper and lower torso central venous channels is essential for prompt and safe establishment of the required venous access at the time of transplantation. Without the local availability of other innovative venous access techniques [15,16], patients who are undergoing simultaneous liver replacement must have reliable wide-bore venous access above the diaphragm for volume resuscitation and delivery of blood products during the anhepatic phase.

Defining the degree of hepatic dysfunction, evidence of portal hypertension, and extent of liver pathology is essential in order to determine the need for the en bloc replacement of the native liver with the intestine. Accordingly, the biochemical profiling of liver injury, a full hematologic panel, the endoscopic evaluation of the gastrointestinal tract, and liver biopsy, preferably transjugular, are required for the decision-making process. The extent of assessment of the cardiopulmonary and other body systems is guided by patient age, past medical history, the nature of the primary gastrointestinal disorder and the detection of other coexistent pathologic abnormalities. Full details of the routine evaluation process are described elsewhere [17].

Contraindications

The contraindications for intestinal, liver-intestinal, and multivisceral transplantation were primarily established based upon historical experience with other abdominal organ transplantation procedures [18].

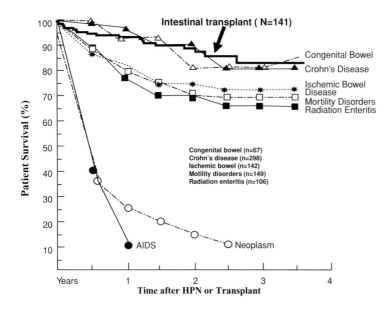

Figure 27.7 Survival curves of 762 HPN patients with benign intestinal diseases and 141 intestinal recipients (thick solid curve) who were transplanted at the University of Pittsburgh Medical Center since July 2001 under the new immunosuppressive protocol. The survival data of the HPN patients were extrapolated from the Oley A.S.P.E.N. Information System (OASIS) as previously reported. (Reproduced from Abu-Elmagd *Gastroenterology* 2006;S132–S137, with permission from the American Gastroenterological Association.)

These contraindications are either relative or absolute and include, but are not limited to, significant cardiopulmonary insufficiency, incurable malignancy, persistent life-threatening intra-abdominal or systemic infections, and severe immune deficiency syndromes. A remote history of gastrointestinal malignancy, the presence of resectable desmoid or stromal tumors, and active abdominal infection at the time of referral, should not be considered as absolute contraindications for transplantation [8,19,20]. In addition, loss of central venous access should not preclude transplantation and age should not be considered as a contraindication, unless it is associated with one or more of the above prohibitive risk factors [1,15,16].

Summary

The optimal management of patients with SBS and other gastrointestinal disorders can only be delivered through a multidisciplinary team with expertise in the medical and surgical management of these complex patients. In these highly complex patients possessing a wide variety of pathologic disorders, a thorough and systematic evaluation is essential in order to establish a proper management strategy. With clearly defined selection criteria, a treatment algorithm which incorporates medical management, autologous

surgical reconstruction, or transplantation will undoubtedly achieve the best outcome for each individual patient. When indicated, intestinal transplantation should be considered early and before the development of TPN-related complications. Such a statement is supported by the recent achievement of patient survival similar to, or better than, that achieved by patients on home parenteral nutrition despite the use of the procedure to rescue patients with TPN failure (Figure 27.7). In addition, transplantation achieves full nutritional autonomy in most patients and eliminates the need for TPN early after surger.

Acknowledgments

With thanks to Guilherme Costa MD, Geoffrey Bond MD, Kyle Soltys MD, Rakesh Sindhi MD, Robert Squires MD, Stephen O'Keefe MD, and George Mazariegos MD.

References

1 Abu-Elmagd KM, Bond G, Reyes J, Fung J. Intestinal transplantation: a coming of age. *Adv Surg* 2002;6:65–101.

2 Abu-Elmagd K, Reyes J, Bond G, et al. Clinical intestinal transplantation: a decade of a single center experience. *Ann Surg* 2001;234:404–417.

3 Grant D, Abu-Elmagd K, Reyes J, et al. 2003 Report of the intestine transplant registry: a new era has dawned. *Ann Surg* 2005;241:607–613.

4 Abu-Elmagd K. Intestinal transplantation for short gut syndrome and gut failure: Rewarding outcomes and current consensus. *Gastro* 2006;130:132–137.

5 Sudan D, DiBaise J, Torres C, et al. A multidisciplinary approach to the treatment of intestinal failure. *J Gastrol Surg* 2005;9:165–177.

6 Bond G, Costa G, Mazariegos G, et al. Intestinal failure and visceral transplantation: a new era of colossal achievement. In: Matarese L, Steiger E, D L Seidner, eds. *Intestinal Failure and Rehabilitation: A Clinical Guide*. New York: CRC Press, Boca Raton, 2004;295–319.

7 Abu-Elmagd K, Bond G, Matarese L, et al. Gut rehabilitation and intestinal transplantation. *Therapy* 2005;2:853–864.

8 Abu-Elmagd KM Mazariegos G, Bond G, et al. Intestinal transplantation: current status and future considerations. *Am J Gastroenterol* 2006;101:307.

9 Giraldo M, Martin D, Colangelo J, et al. Intestinal transplantation for patients with short gut syndrome and hypercoagulable states. *Transplant Proc* 2000;32:1223–1224.

10 Lawrence JP, Dunn SP, Billmire DE, et al. Isolated liver transplantation for liver failure in patients with short bowel syndrome. *J Pediatr Surg* 1994;29:751–753.

11 Botha JF, Grant WJ, Torres C, et al. Isolated liver transplantation in infants with end-stage liver disease due to short bowel syndrome. *Liver Trans* 2006;12:1062–1066.

12 Bueno J, Ohwada S, Kocoshis S, et al. Factors impacting on the survival of children with intestinal failure referred for intestinal transplantation. *J Pediatr Surg* 1999;34:27–33.

13 Fryer J, Pellar S, Ormond D, et al. Mortality in candidates waiting for combined liver-intestine transplants exceeds that for other candidates waiting for liver transplants. *Liver Trans* 2003;9:748–753.

14 Schuster B, Bond G, Koritsky D, et al. Early intestinal transplantation for patients with acute irreversible intestinal failure. *Transplanation* 2006;2:279.

15 Lang E, Reyes J, Faintuch S, et al. Central venous recannalization and restoration of candidacy for intestinal and multivisceral transplantation: an innovative radiologic approach. *J Vasc Interv Radiol* 2005;16:1203–1213.

16 Boucek CD, Abu-Elmagd KM. Alternative route transfusion for transplantation surgery in patients lacking accessible veins. *Anesth Analg* 2006;102:1591–1592.

17 Abu-Elmagd K, Reyes J, Fung JJ. Clinical intestinal transplantation: recent advances and future considerations. *AST Primer on Transplantation*, 2001.

18 Fung JJ, Abu-Elmagd K, Todo S. Intestinal and multivisceral transplantation. In: Bell RH Jr., ed. Digestive Tract Surgery: A Text and Atlas. JB Lippincott Company, 1996;1229–1261.

19 Stamos J, Martin L, Colangelo J, et al. Intestinal and multivisceral transplantation in patients with abdominal malignancy: disease recurrent and survival outcomes. *Transplantation* 2004;78(suppl):057.

20 Chatzipetrou MA, Tzakis AG, Pinna AD, et al. Intestinal transplantation for the treatment of desmoid tumors associated with familial adenomatous polyposis. *Surgery* 2001;129:277–281.

28 Isolated Small Bowel Transplantation and Combined Liver-Small Bowel Transplantation

Douglas G. Farmer

Key points

- The technical aspects of both the donor and recipient operation are well established.

- There are four general types of intestinal grafts commonly transplanted including isolated intestinal graft, combined liver intestinal graft, modified multivisceral graft, and multivisceral graft.

- The surgical techniques used for transplantation of an isolated intestinal graft, combined liver intestinal graft, modified multivisceral graft and multivisceral graft are reviewed in a step-by-step fashion.

- Inclusion of the pancreaticoduodenal complex in liver intestinal grafts is now common and alleviates the need for biliary reconstruction.

- The liberal use of both arterial and venous conduits is strongly recommended and facilitates allograft implantation.

- The use of enteral feeding tubes such as gastrostomy tubes and jejunostomy tubes are common and allow access for enteral administration of medications and nutrition.

- Abdominal wall closure/reconstruction can be challenging and there are now many prosthetic options available to assist with this procedure.

Intestinal Failure: Diagnosis, Management and Transplantation.
Edited by Alan N. Langnas, Olivier Goulet, Eamonn M.M. Quigley and Kelly A. Tappenden. © 2008 Blackwell Publishing.
ISBN 978-1-4051-4637-1.

Introduction

The techniques for intestinal transplantation have evolved with experience and may differ somewhat between transplant centers. The techniques also differ depending on the organ(s) to be transplanted. The purpose of this chapter is to review the surgical techniques used to perform the most common transplant procedures involving the intestine. For clarity, the following terminology will be applied: *intestinal transplantation* (ITx; general term for transplantation of any graft inclusive of the intestine), *isolated intestinal transplantation* (I-ITx; graft that includes all or part of the donor jejunoileum only), *liver-intestinal transplantation* (L-ITx; graft that includes all or part of the liver and jejunoileum), *multivisceral transplantation* (MVTx; graft that includes an en bloc set of organs based on the liver, duodenum, pancreas, and jejunoileum with or without part or all of the stomach), *modified multivisceral transplantation* (mMVTx; same as MVT except liver is not included). This chapter will review the landmark developments in these techniques followed by a step-by-step outline of the procedures.

Background/history

Richard Lillehei is largely acknowledged to have established the early techniques used for I-ITx when he performed canine experiments in the 1950s designed to determine the susceptibility of the intestine to ischemia [1]. Likewise, Thomas Starzl introduced the techniques of MVTx with his canine experiments reported in the

1960's [2]. Although there were several case reports of unsuccessful human attempts in the 1960–70s, the modern era of ITx was not ushered until successful cases of human MVTx [3,4], I-ITx [5], and L-ITx [6] were reported in the 1990s. Together, these landmark reports established the foundations for the techniques used in many centers throughout the world.

Donor selection

In general, the intestinal grafts are procured from a highly selected subset of cadaveric organ donors. Because of the exquisite sensitivity of the intestine to ischemic injury, many of the event surrounding brain death and trauma reduce the number of potential intestinal donors dramatically. Most centers, select hemodynamically stable, brain-dead donor who do not have a significant history of down-time/cardiac arrest and do not require significant doses of pressor medications. In addition, to to size constraints from the recipient standpoint, most centers attempt to obtain donors that are of equal or lesser size when compared to the recipient. This further constrains the donor availability. Attempts to overcome these constraints have led to the development of surgical techniques such as split or reduced cadaveric grafts as well as live donor grafts. Both of these are beyond the scope of this chapter.

Donor/graft techniques

The surgical approach to the cadaveric intestinal donor is the same as that described for multiorgan procurements [7–11]. Abdominal midline and median sternotomy incisions are used for exposure. Careful co-ordination between the various procurement teams is essential. Initially, preparation for rapid cross-clamp is performed with cannulation of the inferior mesenteric vein, encircling the distal abdominal aorta and proximal supraceliac aorta. After these steps, all visceral organs including the liver, pancreas, and small intestine can be procured either separately or in any combination depending on recipient needs (Figure 28.1) [10].

For I-ITx, the entire jejunoileum is mobilized and an intra-abdominal colectomy performed. The jejunum is stapled just past the ligament of Treitz and the small

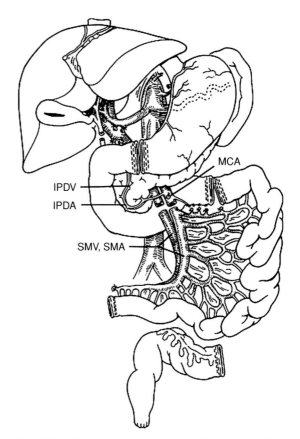

Figure 28.1 Diagram demonstrating the graft options resulting from a multiorgan procurement. Divisions at duodenum and jejunum indicate potential levels of transection, both vascular and gastrointestinal. Thus all organs can be procured either separately or in any combination. (Reproduced from Abu-Elmagd et al. [10], with permission from Lippincott, Williams and Wilkins.)

mesenteric vessels connecting the proximal mesentery are ligated. The superior mesenteric artery (SMA) and vein (SMV) can be used at the level of the root of the mesentery thus preserving the pancreas for whole organ transplantation. Alternatively, if the pancreas is not allocated, the SMA can be dissected down to the aorta and the SMV dissected up to the portal vein (PV) (Figure 28.2a) [12].

For L-ITx, there are basically 2 procurement techniques—the traditional and "Omaha technique." In the traditional technique, the donor head of the pancreas and duodenum are removed during the procurement (FIgure 28.2b) or during back-table preparation. As this technique is no longer commonly used,

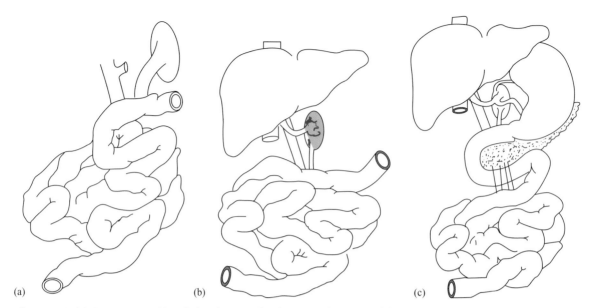

Figure 28.2 (a) demonstrates a jejunoileal graft procured with its vascular pedicle consisting of the SMA and SMV. (b) demonstrates a liver-intestine (L-ITx) graft procured using the traditional technique; the entire liver and jejunoileal segment is present. The vascular inflow is shown off a cuff of donor aorta. (c) demonstrates a multivisceral graft (MVTx) including the whole liver, stomach, pancreas, duodenum, and jejunoileum. The vascular inflow is shown off a cuff of donor aorta. (Reproduced from Moon and Tzakis [12], with permission from Yonsei Medical Journal.)

procurement of the L-ITx graft using the Omaha technique will be described [13,14]. Briefly, the liver is mobilized using standard techniques. The duodenum is stapled distal to the pylorus. The bile duct is left intact and the head of the pancreas is mobilized off the retroperitoneum. A distal subtotal pancreatectomy is performed removing the body and tail of the pancreas beyond the PV. Note, this latter step is optional as the entire pancreas can be left intact as originally described in the reference. A total abdominal colectomy is performed and the entire jejunoileum is mobilized. When complete, the composite graft consists of the liver, duodenum and head of the pancreas, and entire jejunoileum with the arterial inflow off the aorta/celiac trunk/SMA and leaving the donor PV intact (Figure 28.3a) [15]. The popularity of this technique rests in the elimination of the need for a donor pancreaticoduodenectomy and for biliary reconstruction in the recipient as the donor bile duct remains intact.

Procurement of the MVTx graft is really quite similar to that described earlier for the L-ITx graft. The major difference lies in the pancreatic portion of the operation. Rather than perform a subtotal pancreatectomy, the entire pancreaticoduodenal-splenic complex is mobilized and contained within the graft. Additionally, the stomach can be included in this graft simply by moving the proximal gastrointestinal transection up to the distal esophagus. Thus, the organ complex consists of the liver, stomach, duodenum, pancreas, spleen and jejunoileum. The vascular inflow is similar to that described above and the entire celiac trunk, including the left gastric and splenic arteries, is preserved (Figure 28.2c) [12].

An important modification of the above procedures is the reduced/split procurement techniques [15,16]. These techniques were driven by the long waiting times and high wait-list mortality rates for small children in need of a liver-inclusive MVTx or L-ITx. They were derived from split/reduced liver techniques developed to address liver allograft shortages in children waiting for isolated liver transplantation. In general, the procedure proceeds as outlined earlier except that the liver portion of the graft is split or reduced as described elsewhere [17]. This procedure results in a more

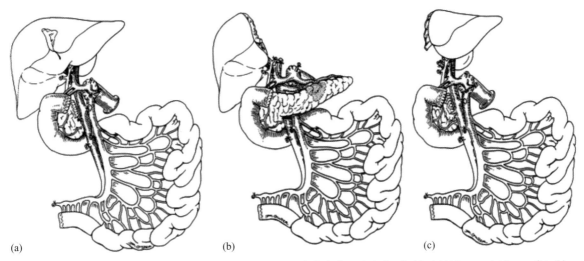

(a)   (b)   (c)

Figure 28.3 Diagram indicating several options for liver-intestine grafts including whole liver in (a), right trisegmental liver graft in (b), and left lateral segment liver graft in (c). Note, the duodenum, together with the head of the pancreas, is retained a and c (Omaha Technique) while the entire pancreas is retained in (b)). (Reproduced from Reyes et al. [15], with permission from Blackwell Publishing.)

size-appropriate en bloc graft (Figures 28.3a and b) [15].

Once all warm dissection is complete, and once all procuring teams are prepared, cannulation and cross-clamping proceed in a coordinated fashion. First, the donor is administered heparin intravenously. Then the distal aorta is ligated and cannulated. Although the optimal preservation solution for the intestine has not been established, the University of Wisconsin Solution (ViaSpan®, Barr Laboratories) is currently the gold standard. All organs are then flushed and topically cooled with ice. Removal of the organs proceeds with the thoracic organs first, followed by the liver (and any associated en bloc organs), intestine, pancreas, and kidneys. Back-table preparation is usually required and consists of establishing vascular cuffs, suturing conduits onto vascular orifices, and removing excess tissue. This preparation usually occurs at the recipient hospital.

Recipient operative steps

The recipient operation can essentially be divided into ten key parts. The first portion is always the *establishment of vascular access*. As many ITx candidates

have a long history of central venous catheters and access site limitations, preoperative mapping of potential vascular access sites is strongly recommended to facilitate this step. An MR venogram performed during transplant evaluation is usually sufficient. Central venous access, both above and below the diaphragm, is recommended using large bore catheters. Furthermore, approximately two to four ports are recommended. For adults, right heart monitoring using a Swan-Ganz Catheter should be considered.

The second portion of the procedure is the *abdominal incision* and *adhesion lysis*. For liver-inclusive grafts, a bilateral subcostal incision with an upper midline extension is mandatory. To achieve optimal lower abdominal exposure, extending the midline portion of the incision below the umbilicus is frequently needed, although this can complicate abdominal wall closure. For recipients of I-ITx or mMVTx without the liver, a midline incision, with or without a transverse/subcostal component, is standard. This provides optimal exposure to achieve venous outflow into the portomesenteric circulation when needed, as well as to establish gastrointestinal continuity. Once the appropriate incision is created, most ITx recipients require an extensive adhesion lysis to obtain abdominal cavity exposure.

The third portion of the operation is the appropriate *"organectomy"*. This, of course varies, based on the

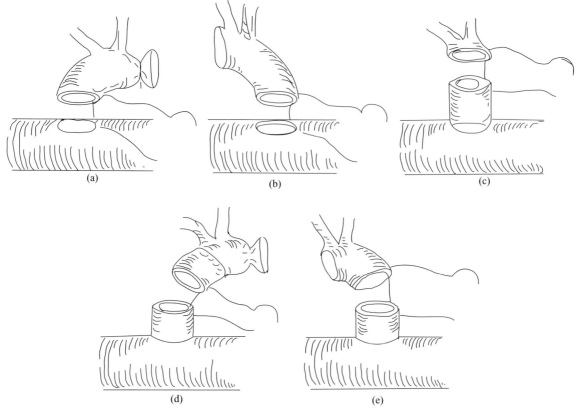

Figure 28.4 Diagram demonstrating various arterial conduit options. (a) Direct anastomosis between the donor and recipient infrarenal aorta. (b) Direct anastomosis between the donor and recipient supraceliac aorta. (c) Placement of an interposition conduit on the recipient aorta. (d) Placement of an interposition conduit on both the donor and recipient aorta. (e) Placement of an interposition conduit on the aorta with the use of a donor aortic segment in which the distal end is oversewn with a patch technique. (Reproduced from Nishida et al. [18], with permission from John Wiley & Sons Ltd on behalf of the British Journal of Surgery Society Ltd.)

organ(s) to be transplanted. For the I-ITx recipient, the remnant jejunoileum is mobilized and resected leaving a suitable portion of proximal jejunum and preserving as much distal colon as possible for later anastomosis. For L-ITx recipients, a total hepatectomy is performed with or without excision of the retrohepatic inferior vena cava (IVC). Additionally, the remnant small bowel resection should also take place as outlined above. Finally, for MVTx recipients, a total abdominal resection of the appropriate viscera is undertaken. For stomach-inclusive grafts, the proximal GI transection is at the level of the distal esophagus/proximal stomach while for stomach-exclusive MVTx grafts, either a subtotal or partial gastrectomy is performed. Additionally, an en bloc total hepatectomy, pancre-

aticoduodenectomy, and splenectomy are performed including the stomach and remnant small bowel, as described earlier. The fourth portion of the recipient operation is the *establishment of vascular inflow and outflow*. The liberal use of both arterial and venous conduits is strongly recommended to optimize graft implantation (Figure 28.4) [18]. Again, this step depends on the organ(s) to be transplanted and the donor vascular situation. For the I-ITx recipient, the graft usually has at least a segment of donor SMA and SMV. The infrarenal aorta is usually appropriate for suturing an arterial inflow conduit. The outflow can vary depending on recipient anatomy with options including the recipient PV, splenic vein, SMV, or IVC. The use of a venous outflow conduit is helpful. For L-ITx recipients, arterial inflow can be obtained off either the supraceliac or infrarenal aorta using a donor conduit. When en bloc organs are procured, a segment of donor abdominal and/or thoracic aortic is generally included to simplify this portion of the surgery. Outflow is via the suprahepatic IVC of the donor graft and recipient. Lastly, for recipients of MVTx grafts, the inflow and outflow are the same as described for L-ITx recipients.

The next step of the transplant procedure is performing the *vascular anastomoses*. In general, the venous anastomosis/outflow anastomosis is performed first and this should be done without redundancy to prevent kinking and twisting. For recipients of I-ITx, this is an end-to-end anastomosis between the donor SMV/PV and the venous outflow conduit using a fine monofilament suture. The venous outflow for the ITx can be either the native splanchnic venous system or the inferior vena cava. The vena cava is used for technical ease or if there is underlying liver disease. For recipients of L-ITx and MVTx, this anastomosis is between the supraceliac IVC of the donor and that of the recipient. Leaving the recipient vena cava intact simplifies the procedure at this stage, as there is no need to perform an anastomosis between the infrahepatic IVC of the donor and recipient. Once the venous anastomoses are completed, arterial inflow is obtained. For the I-ITx recipient, the donor SMA is sutured to the aortic conduit. For L-ITx and MVTx, the donor aorta is sutured to the aortic conduit. After flushes are completed, the organ(s) are reperfused simultaneously.

The native PV in the recipient of L-ITx grafts must also be addressed. Most commonly, an end-to-side native *portocaval shunt* is performed. The optimal time for this is after the hepatectomy and prior to implantation of the graft. Alternatively, this can occur after reperfusion although this is less ideal due to the position of the transplanted graft. Another option for the native PV is an anastomosis to the donor PV. Again, this is less than ideal due to positioning/orientation and the portocaval shunt is highly recommended.

The next operative step is the *biliary surgical step*. Obviously, this step is not applicable to I-ITx recipients and only to those with liver-inclusive grafts. The donor gallbladder should always be removed. In some instances, this is performed during the donor operation but can be safely done after reperfusion. If the L-ITx was procured using the standard technique, then biliary reconstruction is required usually with a Roux-en-Y defunctionalized limb of transplanted jejunum. If the L-ITx graft was procured using the Omaha Technique, or in the case of MVTx graft recipients, the biliary anastomosis is not needed.

After completion of the above steps, *restoration of intestinal continuity* is addressed. The general steps include proximal and distal gastrointestinal targets and the creation of an ileostomy. For I-ITx recipients, the proximal gastrointestinal targets are either the native jejunum or stomach—the former is preferred as it is more physiologic. Anastomoses should be performed according to surgeon preference/experience. The same applies for L-ITx recipients. For MVTx recipients, there are several options. If the stomach was included then a gastrogastrostomy or esophagogastrostomy is performed. A pyloroplasty must also be performed to prevent gastric outlet obstruction after vagal denervation. If the stomach was not included in the graft, then the proximal gastrointestinal connection can vary. A defunctionalized Roux-en-Y limb of transplanted jejunum anastomosed to the native stomach or esophagus probably results in the best long-term function. Alternatively, a loop gastrojejunostomy can be performed but may be associated with chronic bile reflux. The distal gastrointestinal hookup also has variability depending on the patient's underlying gastrointestinal disease and motility issues, as well as the length of remnant colon and the method of ileostomy creation. As there are many options, only principles will be discussed. First, an ileostomy is usually created to allow graft monitoring in the perioperative period. This can be an end ileostomy, a loop ileostomy, or diverting proximal ileostomy. Second, the transplanted ileum should be anastomosed to the remnant colon and this can occur at the initial operation or at a later date. Third, in patients with functional colonic remnants, internalizing gastrointestinal secretions is preferred for optimal long-term function which translates into ileostomy takedown some months after the ITx. In patients in which distal gastrointestinal continuity has been established at ITx, this takedown procedure is greatly simplified. Otherwise, takedown requires a concomitant surgical distal ileocolostomy.

The *placement of enteral feeding tubes* is the next surgical step. Again, several options exist. For patient's who do not receive grafts containing the stomach, a

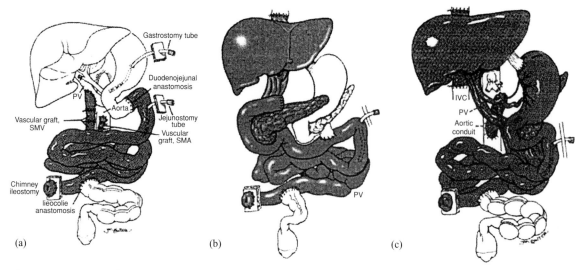

Figure 28.5 Diagrams demonstrating an isolated intestinal graft after implantation (a), and liver-intestinal graft with inclusion of the whole pancreas (b), and a Multivisceral graft (c). The vascular anastomoses are indicated. Abbreviations used in figure: SMV: superior mesenteric vein; PV: portal vein; SMA: superior mesenteric artery; IVC: inferior vena cava. (Reproduced from Abu-Elmagd et al. [23], with permission from Elsevier.)

gastrostomy tube is usually placed using the Stamm technique. Alternatively, this can be a "2-in-1" tube or gastrojejunostomy tube with the gastric portion in the stomach and the jejunal portion in the transplanted intestine. Some centers prefer separate jejunal feeding tubes in the transplanted intestine. The latter is optimal in patients who receive grafts that include the stomach or have an esophagojejunostomy performed. Nasoenteric feeding tubes are usually discouraged due to the potential need for long-term GI access in many of these patients.

The last and perhaps one of the most complex/ challenging portions of the transplant operation is *abdominal wall closure*. The presence of a complex incision, prior abdominal scars, feeding tubes, ostomies, and potentially lost abdominal domain complicate closure. Primary fascial closure is of course the goal in all patients. This goal is not achieved, at least initially, in many cases. There are multiple methods to handle this situation [19]. The first and foremost principle is to avoid a closure under tension. The liberal use of prosthetic patches/mesh allows temporary coverage and flexibility while the recipient recovers from the operation and the edema of the organs reduces. A second-look operation is then required to

achieve closure. In some instances, a skin-only closure is obtained leaving the patient with an abdominal hernia that may require future surgical correction. Fascial coverage using a prosthetic mesh, Gore-Tex® (WL. Gore & Assoc), or AlloDerm® (LifeCell Inc) is increasingly used [20,21]. Abdominal wall transplantation has been performed for extreme abdominal wall defect situations [22]. In general, the safest and most expeditious method to achieve closure is prudent.

Diagrams demonstrating the completed transplant procedures are shown for an I-SBT (Figure 28.5a), L-ITx (Figure 28.5b), and MVTx (Figure 28.5c) [23].

Summary

In conclusion, ITx is a complex procedure with many surgical variances depending on the organ(s) transplanted. Recipient anatomy and disease dictate the organ(s) required. The techniques described here provide a brief but detailed description of multiorgan procurement and transplantation. Of course, variations do exist and are commonly and successfully used.

References

1 Lillehei R, Goott B, Miller F. The physiologic response of the small bowel of the dog to ischemia including prolonged in vitro preservation of the bowel with successful replacement and survival. *Ann Surg* 1959;150:543–561.

2 Starzl T, Kaupp H. Mass homotransplantations of abdominal organs in dogs. *Surg Forum* 1960;11:28–30.

3 Starzl T, Rowe M Todo S, et al. Transplantation of multiple abdominal viscera. *JAMA* 1989;261:1449–1458.

4 Williams, JW, Sankary, H, Foster, P, et al. Splanchnic transplantation: an approach to the infant dependent on parenteral nutrition who develops irreversible liver disease. *JAMA* 1985;261:1458–1462.

5 Deltz E, Schroeder P, Gebhard H, et al. Successful clinical small bowel transplantation: a report of a case. *Clin Transpl* 1989;21:89–91.

6 Grant D, Wall W, Mineuualt R, et al. Successful small bowel/liver transplantation. *Lancet* 1990;335:181–184.

7 Starzl T, Hakala T, Shaw B, et al. A flexible procedure for multiple cadaveric organ procurement. *Surg Gynecol Obstet* 1984;158:228–03.

8 Starzl T, Miller C, Bronznick B, et al. An improved technique for multiple organ harvesting. *Surg Gynecol Obstet* 1987;165:343–348.

9 Starzl T, Todo S, Tzakis A. et al. The many faces of multivisceral transplantation. *Surg Gynecol Obstet* 1991; 172:335–344.

10 Abu-Elmagd K, Fung J, Bueno J, et al. Logistics and technique for procurement of intestinal, pancreatic, and hepatic grafts from the same donor. *Ann Surg* 2000; 232:680–687.

11 Yersiz H, Renz J, Hisatake G, et al. Multivisceral and isolated intestinal procurement techniques. *Liver Transpl* 2003;9:881–886.

12 Moon JI, Tzakis AG. Intestinal and multivisceral transplantation. *Yonsei Med J* 2004;31:1101–1106.

13 Sudan D, Iyer K, Deroover A, et al. A new technique for combined liver-intestinal transplantation. *Transplantation* 2001;72:1846–1849.

14 Bueno J, Abu-Elmagd K, Mazariegos G, et al. Composite liver-small bowel allografts with preservation of donor duodenum and hepatic biliary system in children. *J Pediatr Surg* 2000;35:291–299.

15 Reyes J, Mazariegos GV, Bond GM, et al. Pediatric intestinal transplantation: historical notes, principles and controversies. *Pediatr Transplant* 2002;6:193–207.

16 de Ville de Goyet J, Mitchell A, et al. En block combined reduced-liver and small bowel transplants: from large donors to small children. *Transplantation* 2000; 27:555–559.

17 Renz JF, Yersiz H, Reichert PR, et al. Split-liver transplantation: a review. *Am J Transplant* 2003;3:1323–1335.

18 Nishida S, Vaidya A, Kato T, et al. Use of donor aorta for arterial reconstruction in paediatric liver and multivisceral transplantation. *Br J Surg* 2004;91: 705–708.

19 Carlsen, BT, Farmer, DG, Busuttil, RW, et al. Incidence and Management of Abdominal Wall Defects after Intestinal and Multivisceral Transplantation, *Plastics and Reconstructive Surgery* 2007;119:1247–1255.

20 Di Benedetto F, Lauro A, Masetti M, et al. Use of prosthetic mesh in difficult abdominal wall closure after small bowel transplantation in adults. *Transplant Proc* 2005;37:2272–2274.

21 Drosou A, Kirsner RS, Kato T, et al. Use of a bioengineered skin equivalent for the management of difficult skin defects after pediatric multivisceral transplantation. *J Am Acad Dermatol* 2005;52:854–858.

22 Levi DM, Tzakis AG, Kato T, et al. Transplantation of the abdominal wall. *Lancet* 2003;361:2173–2176.

23 Abu-Elmagd KM. Intestinal transplantation for short bowel syndrome and gastrointestinal failure: current consensus, rewarding outcomes, and practical guidelines. *Gastroenterology* 2006;130(suppl 1):S132–S137.

29 Living Donor Intestinal Transplantation

Enrico Benedetti, Fabrizio Panaro and Giuliano Testa

Key points

- Living donor bowel transplantation may be beneficial in selected candidates.
- The risk for donors is the main concern in considering living donor bowel transplantation.
- To date, no significant morbidity or mortality has been reported in living donors.
- The results of living donor bowel transplant are similar to those obtained with standard cadaver donor.
- Pediatric candidates with intestinal and hepatic failure may be treated with combined transplants from a living donor.

Introduction

Living donors have been extensively used in kidney and liver transplantation with excellent results in terms of outcomes. In fact, kidney transplantation from living donors has been associated with superior patient and graft survival compared to cadaveric donors in all age groups [1]. This strategy is currently the most efficacious, although partial, solution to the cadaveric donor shortage.

The role of living donors in intestinal transplantation (ITx) is not as well defined, mostly because the limited experience with the procedure. To date, according to

Intestinal Failure: Diagnosis, Management and Transplantation.
Edited by Alan N. Langnas, Olivier Goulet, Eamonn M.M. Quigley and Kelly A. Tappenden. © 2008 Blackwell Publishing. ISBN 978-1-4051-4637-1.

registry data, only 41 living donor segmental intestinal transplants (LDITx) have been performed worldwide [2]. The potential advantages of LDITx, in analogy to other living donor transplant procedures, include elimination of waiting time, better matching, the opportunity for preoperative donor and recipient optimization, elective surgery, minimal cold ischemia, and expansion of the donor pool (Table 29.1).

The experience with LDITx is still limited to a few centres around the world. However, the recent standardization of the surgical technique has improved the results in both adult and pediatric patients with results now comparable to those obtained with cadaver intestinal transplantation according to the international registry [2]. The purpose of this chapter is to review the current status of LDITx, with particular reference to the specific indications of the procedure in comparison to cadaver intestinal transplantation.

Brief history

The first reported human ITx was performed by Lillihei in 1967 [3]. Unfortunately, this attempt and several others that followed were uniformly unsuccessful. In 1988, under Cyclosporine immunosuppression, Deltz et al. performed, in Kiel, Germany, the first successful LDITx [4]. The recipient of this living related allograft remained TPN-free for 4 years before the graft was lost to chronic rejection.

Attempts in the mid-1990s before the standardization of the surgical technique failed either because too short segments of intestine (only 60 cm, not adequate to free the recipient from total parental nutrition), or because segments of jejunum prone to vascular complications, were used [5]. It is significant, however, that success in LDITx was achieved by various groups when identical twins were utilized [6–8].

In 1997 Gruessner described a standardized technique based on procurement of a segment of distal ileum of appropriate length and vascularized by a single pedicle [9]. The technique was later perfected and initial data on donor safety published by the University of Illinois group [10]. Recently, the same group has presented a technique for combined living donor liver/intestinal transplantation, extending the potential of the strategy to children affected by short bowel syndrome complicated by liver failure [11].

Indications for living donor intestinal transplantation

The indications and contraindications for LDITx are the same as for cadaver intestinal transplantation and are discussed in detail in other chapters of the book. Briefly, ITx is indicated in patients with irreversible intestinal failure suffering from life-threatening TPN-related complications. Any patient who is a candidate for ITx is potentially a candidate to LDITx.

Table 29.1 summarizes the potential advantages and disadvantages of LDITx versus standard cadaver intestinal transplant. Clearly, the main concern in using LDITx is the potential risk to the donor. Therefore, the

Table 29.1 Living versus cadaver bowel transplant.

Living related bowel transplant	Cadaver bowel transplant
Advantages	**Disadvantages**
Elimination of waiting time	Long waiting time
Optimal HLA matching	Inferior HLA matching
Short cold ischemia time	Long ischemia time
Optimal bowel graft decontamination	Inferior bowel graft decontamination
Elective surgery	Emergency surgery
Disadvantages	**Advantages**
Risk for donor	Donor risk not applicable
Shorter bowel graft	Whole bowel graft
Small vascular pedicle	Optimal vascular pedicle

benefits for the recipient should be carefully balanced with concern for donor safety.

The issue of the elimination of waiting time may be of particular importance in pediatric candidates for ITx. As of July 2003, 173 patients were listed for ITx in the United States, of whom 131 (76%) were of pediatric age, of which about 65% were in need of combined liver/intestinal transplant. The mortality on the waiting list for ITx is particularly elevated in children waiting for combined liver/bowel transplant (25–30%), according to UNOS data. The University of Pittsburgh has reported that out of 257 children evaluated for ITx 120 died while awaiting surgery [12]. Interestingly, the University of Nebraska reported that in a group of 47 children listed for cadaver isolated intestinal transplant, 13 also had to be listed for liver transplant while waiting. Therefore, in children, the elimination of waiting time may be particularly advantageous in decreasing mortality and avoiding progression to liver failure. It is hard to understand the reason for the relatively long waiting time on the transplant list, despite the striking discrepancy between the numbers of potentially available donors (12,227 in the United States in 2001) versus the number of bowel transplants performed (111 in the same year). One possible explanation is the objective difficulty in obtaining a "perfect" cadaveric donor. The majority of transplant centers are willing to consider only young, hemodynamically stable, size-matched donors, preferably CMV negative. Therefore, the waiting time is prolonged and associated with high mortality, especially for pediatric patients waiting for combined liver/bowel transplant.

The recent development of the technique of combined living donor intestinal and liver transplantation may help even those children affected by established failure of both organs, the most likely to die on the waiting list. LDITx may prove life-saving for patients referred for lack of central venous access after multiple thromboses, allowing an immediate solution to this challenging problem.

Most experts would agree that, in the presence of an identical twin as a potential donor, LDITx can be performed with an extremely high rate of success and without immunosuppression, as reported by Morel et al and others [6–8]. Of course, caution must be exercised to avoid using an identical twin in the setting of diseases that are hereditary. The effect of HLA matching on the outcomes of intestinal transplantation is not known. However, the specific case of an HLA identical sibling as a donor can confer some immunological advantages, according to the limited experience currently available. It is important to stress that with modern immunosuppression, excellent patient and graft survival, and a low rate of rejection have been achieved in leading centers with poorly HLA-matched cadaver donors [13,14].

Finally, LDITx may have a role in highly sensitized patients waiting for ITx. It has been recently shown that transplanting intestinal grafts against a positive cross-match can be quite harmful [15]. In an analogy to the current practice in living donor kidney transplantation, highly sensitized candidates to ITx can be treated with plasmapheresis and intravenous immune globulin to electively obtain a negative cross-match to the intended living related donors. Our group has performed a successful LDITx in a highly sensitized young adult converting the cross-match from positive to negative by plasmapheresis before transplantation of a fraternal intestinal graft.

The living donor for intestinal transplantation

The pre-requisite for using living donors for ITX is the safety of the donor operation. The transplant community has accepted and considered ethically appropriate the use of living donors in kidney, liver, pancreas and lung transplantation. The donor's risk is quite significant in the setting of adult-to-adult liver transplantation and still present, although reduced, for all of the other organs mentioned. The operative risk of a healthy adult undergoing elective segmental bowel resection is quite low, surely comparable to the risks taken by a living kidney donor for elective nephrectomy and inferior to the risk of right hepatectomy.

To date, no major morbidity or mortality has been reported among donors of segmental bowel grafts. The University of Illinois group has published the largest single center experience with ileal resection from donors for LDITx [10]. In a series of nine consecutive donors, no significant technical complications were reported. Moreover, the donors did not suffer from persistent diarrhea, weight loss or Vitamin B_{12} deficiency. To date, our center has performed 20 LDITx with no complications, except for one superficial wound infec-

tion which was successfully treated conservatively. Of course, the risk of postoperative bowel obstruction is present and should be included in the pre-operative information session with the donor.

Although further data will be needed to assess more precisely the donor's morbidity in this setting, the information currently available suggest that segmental bowel donation performed according a standardized technique is quite safe.

Donor evaluation

Potential living donor small bowel donor selection starts with the preliminary determination of ABO blood type and Human Leukocyte Antigen (HLA) type. The donor and the recipient ABO blood types must be compatible; in the presence of multiple potential donors, the candidate with the best HLA match is selected. A careful evaluation of possible cardiopulmonary risk factors must follow; Table 29.2 summarizes the step-wise evaluation of potential donors for LDITx proposed by University of Illinois team.

Historically, in order to evaluate the relevant arterial anatomy of the distal ileum, conventional selective mesenteric angiography has been performed (Figure 29.1). More recently, in an analogy to the experience with living donor kidney and liver evaluation,

---

Table 29.2 Donor evaluation protocol.

- History and physical examination
  - No history of intestinal surgery
- ABO-compatibility
- Lymphocytotoxic cross-match
- Anatomical assessment: abdominal CT scan, selective superior mesenteric angiogram or 3D-angio-CT-scan
- Laboratory tests: glucose, BUN, electrolytes, creatinine, bilirubin, alkaline phosphotase, AST, ALT, GGT, albumin, ammonia, alpha-fetoprotein, prothrombin time, partial thromboplastin time, triglycerides, Vitamin A-D-E-K-B_{12}
- Infectious diseases assessment: hepatitis screen, HIV, CMV (IgG, IgM), EBV (IgG, IgM), Herpes zoster (IgA, EIA), stool culture, urine culture
- Chest X-Ray
- ECG
- Anesthesiology assessment: consultation, anesthesia and surgical history, drug allergies
- Psychosocial assessment: psychiatry and psychological consultation, social worker consultation

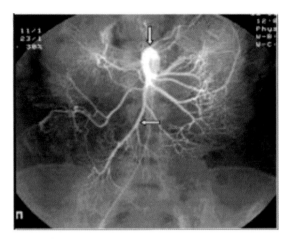

Figure 29.1 Selective angiography of mesenteric vessels.

the technique of angio-CT with 3D reconstruction of the vasculature has been proposed and applied to the intestinal living donor candidate. In our experience, the latter provides images that are comparable to those obtained with conventional angiography, but minimizes donor discomfort and potential risks [16].

Table 29.3 provides the most important characteristics in determining the best potential donor.

Donor operation

The elective nature of LDITx allows standard bowel preparation for the donor, which is given the night before surgery. No specific intraoperative monitoring is usually necessary and therefore neither central venous nor arterial lines are used in our center. The operation is performed with a standardized technique, slightly modified from the original description of Gruessner [9].

The donor is explored through a lower midline incision; the length of the small bowel is measured using an umbilical tape from the ligament of Treitz to the

Table 29.3 Conditions to be a good donor.

- Age less than 65 years
- Low operative risk—body mass index (BMI) < 30
- ABO-compatibility and negative cross-match—best HLA match available
- Preferably CMV/EBV negative
- No GI-tract pathology
- No psycho-social contraindications

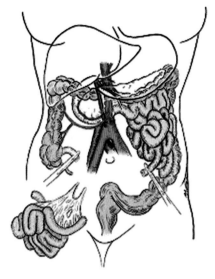

Figure 29.2 Schematic representation of the donor operation.

ileocecal valve (ICV). Then, after controlling the position of the vascular arcades for the terminal ileum, 150 cm (for pediatric patients) to 200 cm (for adults) of ileum are marked as the intended graft, preserving 20 cm of bowel proximal to the ICV (Figure 29.2). Finally, the remainder of the small bowel is measured again to ensure that at least 60% is left for the donor.

The distal portion of the mesenteric artery and vein are dissected free. The mesentery is divided in a "V"-shaped fashion with the tip of the V at the level of the dissected vessels and extending toward the two stitches marking the selected ileal graft. Finally, the small bowel is divided using a GIA stapler. After heparinization, the graft is removed and the vascular stumps over sewn. On the back table, the graft is perfused though the artery with University of Wisconsin solution until the perfusate is clear.

Intestinal continuity is reestablished with a side-to-side stapled anastomosis and the incision is closed with subcutaneous and intradermic suture in a cosmetic fashion. No drains are used. The donor is recovered in the regular ward. A nasogastric suction tube is left in place for 24 hours, after which the donor is started on a clear liquid diet and rapidly advanced to solid food. The epidural catheter is removed 2 days after the surgery. Antibiotic prophylaxis is given for only 3 doses after the surgery.

Our average length of stay in the hospital is 4 days. All donors operated at the University of Illinois at Chicago have resumed their work an average of 3 weeks after the surgery.

The recipient for living donor intestinal transplantation

The pre-transplant work-up for LDITx is not different from the standard preparation used for cadaver ITx candidates and described in other chapters of this book. Once a suitable living donor is identified, the transplant can be immediately scheduled avoiding any further risk of developing complications on the waiting list. The elective nature of LDITx allows easy rescheduling of the transplant in case of the interval development of any complication in the recipient, such as a sudden line sepsis.

For those cases of children referred for intestinal failure complicated by decompensated liver failure, we perform the living donor liver transplant as an emergency and the LDITx as soon as the patient's condition stabilizes. LDITx is also scheduled as an emergency for patients referred for lack of central venous access due to multiple venous thromboses. After standard bowel preparation, the timing of the recipient operation is set in synchrony with the donor with the goal of minimizing ischemia time.

Recipient operation

A midline incision is routinely used to explore the abdomen; meticulous dissection of all adhesions is performed. The proximal and distal ends of the residual small bowel are exposed for the intestinal reconstruction with the donor ileal graft. The arterial and venous anastomoses are completed in an end-to-side fashion between the mesenteric vessels and the infrarenal aorta and vena cava.

Once the vascular anastomoses have been completed and the graft is properly reperfused, the operation continues with the re-establishment of the intestinal tract continuity.

We routinely perform the proximal and distal enteric anastomoses in a double layer, hand-sewn and side-to-side fashion.

Finally, a loop ileostomy is performed about 10–15 cm proximally to the distal enteric anastomosis in

order to permit access for post-transplant surveillance graft biopsies. We routinely insert a gastro-jejunal tube to allow gastric decompression and early enteral feeding. The tip of the jejunal tube is manually placed past the proximal enteric anastomosis.

The closure of the abdomen can be quite challenging in ITx because of the loss of domain caused by the extensive enterectomy. In the setting of LDITx, the limited size of the segmental graft almost invariably allows for easy primary closure. However, in pediatric patients less than 5 years of age it is impossible to attempt primary closure even with only 150 cm adult ileal segment.

Our technique, in this setting, consists in closing without tension the resulting abdominal defect with Vycril mesh secured to the edges of the fascia. In our experience, the resulting open wound granulates and contracts quite rapidly allowing closure with an autologous skin graft 6 weeks after transplant.

Post-transplant management and complications

The post-transplant issues in LDITx are similar to those encountered in cadaver intestinal transplant and are described in detail elsewhere in this book. We will briefly review only specific details pertinent to LDITx.

Immunosuppression

The immunosuppression currently used for LDITx is not different from the highly refined protocols currently used in leading intestinal transplant centers for cadaver ITx; these are extensively treated in other section of the book. We originally used a standard 5 dose induction with Thymoglobulin followed by maintenance with Tacrolimus and steroids. Recently, we have adopted a protocol consisting of short high-dose thymoglobulin induction with rapid steroid elimination, as suggested by the Pittsburgh group [13]. Our maintenance consists of Tacrolimus and either Mycophenolate Mofetil or Rapamycin.

Infectious complications

Infectious complications are the leading cause of death after ITx [2]. Any insult to the allograft, whether ischemic or immunologic, can lead to bacteremia and potential sepsis. We have reported a low incidence of infectious complications in recipients of LDITx [17]. Prolonged cold ischemia time has been linked with an increased rate of bacterial translocation in cadaver ITx [18]. It is possible that the extremely short cold ischemia time (about 5–10 minutes in our experience) may contribute to a decreased rate of infections in LDITx.

Surgical complications

Surgical complications are relatively common in cadaver ITx [2]. Despite the greater challenge in vascular reconstruction for LDITx because of the small size of the vessels, registry data do not demonstrate a higher rate of vascular complications in LDITx. In our series, we did not observe any technical complications either from the intestinal anastomosis or from the vascular anastomosis. Although it is not appropriate to generalize these findings due to the small sample size, the elective nature of LDITx, the short ischemia time and the optimal quality of the graft may, theoretically, contribute to the technical success.

Results of living donor intestinal transplant

Registry data clearly document that patient and graft survival are comparable between cadaver and living donor intestinal transplant recipients [2]. Twelve of the 32 LDITx reported in the latest version of the ITR database were performed in a standardized fashion at the University of Illinois at Chicago. The overall 1- and 3-year patient survival rate was 82% and graft survival 75%. In the last eight patients, transplanted after January 2000, the 1-year patient and graft survival rates have been 100% and 88%, respectively. The median hospital stay was 36 days [13–290]. During the first year after transplantation only the single patient who received a totally mismatched graft experienced one episode of rejection [8%]. All the surviving patients are currently supported by enteral diet without fluid requirements.

Conclusions

LDITx is a promising strategy that may complement cadaver ITx in the treatment of irreversible intestinal failure in patients unable to tolerate long-term TPN.

Although very limited information is currently available, the procedure seems to be safe for the donor and reasonably successful for the recipient. In patients with an available identical twin as the donor, who highly sensitized, or who at high risk of dying because total lack of central venous access, LDITx may be the preferred approach. Probably the most promising application of LDITx is in children with established or impending liver failure secondary to short bowel syndrome. Early LDITx may prevent the progression to irreversible liver failure in some children waiting in the cadaver list, whereas combined living donor liver/intestinal transplant may prove life-saving for children with decompensated liver failure.

Further studies will be needed to fully evaluate the role of LDITx in the treatment of these complex patients.

References

1 United Network for Organ Sharing. Available at http://www.unos.org. Accessed February 2006.

2 Intestinal Transplant Registry. Available at http://www.intestinaltransplant.org. Accessed February 2006.

3 Lillehei RC, Idezuki Y, Feemster JA, et al. Transplantation of stomach, intestine, and pancreas: experimental and clinical observation. *Surgery* 1967;62:721–741.

4 Deltz E, Schroeder P, Gebhardt H, et al. Successful clinical small bowel transplantation: report of a case. *Clin Transplant* 1989;3:89.

5 Tesi R, Beck R, Lambiase L, et al. Living related small bowel transplantation; donor evaluation and outcome. *Transplant Proc* 1997;29:686–687.

6 Morris JA, Johnson DL, Rimmer JA, et al. Identical twin small bowel transplant for desmoid tumor. *Lancet* 1995;345:1577–1578.

7 Calne RY, Friend PJ, Middleton S, et al. Intestinal transplant between two of identical triplets. *Lancet* 1997;350:1077–1078.

8 Morel P, Kadry Z, Charbonnet P, et al. Paediatric living related intestinal transplantation between two monozygotic twins: a 1-year follow-up. *Lancet* 2000;355:723–724.

9 Gruessner RW, Sharp HL. Living-related intestinal transplantation: first report of a standardized surgical technique. *Transplantation* 1997;11:1605–1607.

10 Testa G, Panaro F, Schena S, et al. Living Related Small Bowel Transplantation—Donor Surgical Technique. *Ann Surg* 2004;240:779–784.

11 Testa G, Holterman M, John E. Combined living donor liver/bowel transplantation. *Transplantation* 2005;79:1401–1404.

12 Bueno J, Ohwada S, Kocoshis S, et al. Factors impacting the survival of children with intestinal failure referred for intestinal transplantation. *J Pediatr Surg* 1999;34:27–32.

13 Reyes J, Mazariegos GV, Abu-Elmagd K, et al. Intestinal transplantation under tacrolimus monotherapy after perioperative lymphoid depletion with rabbit antithymocyte globulin (thymoglobulin). *Am J Transplant* 2005;5:1430–1436.

14 Langnas AN. Advances in small-intestine transplantation. *Transplantation* 2004;77(suppl):S75–S78.

15 Wu T, Abu-Elmagd K, Bond G, et al. A clinicpathologic study of isolated intestinal allografts with preformed IgG lymphocytotoxic antibodies. *Hum Pathol* 2004;35:1332–1339.

16 Panaro F, Testa G, Balakrishnan N, et al. Living related small bowel transplantation in children: 3-dimensional computed tomography donor evaluation. *Pediatr Transplant* 2004;8:65–70.

17 Cicalese L, Sileri P, Asolati M, et al. Low infectious complications in segmental living related small bowel transplantation in adults. *Clin Transplant* 2000;14:567–571.

18 Cicalese L, Sileri P, Green M, et al. Bacterial translocation in clinical intestinal transplantation. *Transplantation* 2001;71:1414–1417.

19 Benedetti E, Holterman M, Asolati M, et al. Living related segmental bowel transplantation: From experimental to standardized procedure. *Ann Surg* 2006;244:694–699.

20 Porubsky M, Testa G, John E. Pattern of growth after pediatric living donor small bowel transplantation. *Pediatr Transplant* 2006;10:701–706.

21 Nightingale J. The short bowel syndrome. *Eur J Gastroenterol Hepatol* 1995;7:514–520.

22 Howard L, Ament M, Fleming R, et al. Current use and clinical outcomes of home parenteral and enteral nutrition therapies in the United States. *Gastroenterology* 1995;109:355.

23 Kaufman S, Tzakis AG, et al. Indications for pediatric intestinal transplantation: A position paper of the American Society of transplantation. *Pediatr Transplant* 2001;5:80–87.

24 Grant DR. Intestinal transplantation: 1997 report of the international registry. *Transplantation* 1999;67:1061.

25 Kusne S, Manez R, Frye B, et al. Use of DNA amplification for diagnosis of cytomegalovirus enteritis after intestinal transplantation. *Gastroenterology* 1997;112:1121–1128.

26 Kato T, Nishida S, Levi D, et al. Multivisceral transplantation without the liver. *Transplant Proc* 2002;34:910.

27 de Ville de Goyet J. Surgical aspects. Presented at the VII International Small Bowel Transplantation Symposium. Sept 2001;12–15; Stockholm, Sweden.

28 Spada M, Alessiani M, Fabbi M, et al. Bacterial translocation is enhanced in pig intestinal transplantation when the colon is included in the graft. *Transplant Proc* 1996;28:2658.

29 Goulet O, Michel JL, Jobert A, et al. Small bowel transplantation alone or with the liver in children: changes by using FK506. *Transplant Proc* 1998;30:1569–1570.

30 Todo S, Tzakis AG, Abu-Elmagd K, et al. Intestinal transplantation in composite visceral grafts or alone. *Ann Surg* 1992;216:223–233.

31 Reyes J, Bueno J, Kocoshis S, et al. Current status of intestinal transplantation in children. *J Pediatr Surg* 1998;33:243–254.

32 Langnas AN, Sudan DL, Kaufman S, et al. Intestinal transplantation: a single-center experience. *Transplant Proc* 2000;32:1228.

33 Pinna AD, Weppler D, Nery J, et al. Intestinal transplantation at the University of Miami-five years of experience. *Transplant Proc* 2000;32:1226–1227.

34 Jan D, Michel JL, Goulet O, et al. Up-to-date evolution of small bowel transplantation in children with intestinal failure. *J Pediatr Surg* 1999;34:841–844.

35 Beath SV, Protheroe SP, Brook GA, et al. Early experience of paediatric intestinal transplantation in the United Kingdom, 1993 to 1999. *Transplant Proc* 2000;32:1225.

36 Farmer DG, McDiarmid SV, Yersiz H, et al. Improved outcome after intestinal transplantation: an 8-year, single-center experience. *Transplant Proc* 2000;32:1233–1234.

37 Kato T. New techniques for prevention and treatment of rejection in intestinal transplantation. *Current Opinion in Organ Transplantation* 2000;5:284–289.

38 Abu-Elmagd K, Fung J, McGhee W, et al. The efficacy of daclizumab for intestinal transplantation: preliminary report. *Transplant Proc* 2000;32:1195–1196.

39 Demetris AJ, Nalesnik MA. Transplant Pathology Internet Services. Available at: http://tpis.upmc.edu.

40 Sigurdsson L, Kocoshis S, Todo S, Putnam P, Reyes J. Severe exfoliative rejection after intestinal transplantation in children. *Transplant Proc* 1996;28:2783–2784.

41 Langnas AN, Shaw BW, Antonson DL, et al. Preliminary experiencewith intestinal transplantation in infants and children. *Pediatrics* 1996;97:443–448.

42 Jan D, Michel JL, Goulet O, et al. Up-to-date evolution of small bowel transplantation in children with intestinal failure. *J Pediatr Surg* 1999;34:841–844.

43 Langrehr JM, Hoffman RA, et al. Induction of graft versus host disease and rejection by sensitized small bowel allograft. *Transplantation* 1991;52:399–405.

44 Pirenne J, Benedetti E, et al. Graft versus host response: clinical and biological relevance after transplantation of solid organs. *Transplantation Review* 1996;10:46–48.

45 Allen U, Hebert D, Moore D, et al. Epstein-Barr virus-related post-transplant lymphoproliferative disease in solid organ transplant recipients, 1988–97: a Canadian multi-centre experience. *Pediatr Transplant* 2001;5:198–203.

46 Bates WD, Gray DW, Dada MA, et al. Lymphoproliferative disorders in Oxford renal transplant recipients *J Clin Pathol* 2003;56:439–446.

47 Smets F, Vajro P, Cornu G, et al. Indications and results of chemotherapy in children with posttransplant lymphoproliferative disease after liver transplantation. *Transplantation.* 2000;69:982–984.

48 Sudan DL, Kaufman SS, Shaw BW Jr, et al. Isolated intestinal transplantation for intestinal failure. *Am J Gastroenterol* 2000;95:1506–1515.

49 Green M, Michaels MG, Webber SA, et al. The management of Epstein-Barr virus associated post-transplant lymphoproliferative disorders in pediatric solid organ transplant recipients. *Pediatr Transplant* 1999;3:271–281.

50 Talisetti A, Testa G, Holterman M, et al. Successful Treatment of Post-Transplant Lymphoproliferative Disorder with Removal of Small Bowel Graft and Subsequent Second Bowel Transplant. *J Pediatr Gastrenterol Nutr* 2005;41:354–356.

51 Kim J, Fryer J, Craig RM. Absorptive function following intestinal transplantation. *Dig Dis Sci* 1998;43:1925–1930.

52 Abu-Elmagd, Todo S, Tzakis A, et al. Three years clinical experience with intestinal transplantation. *J Am Coll Surg* 1994;179:385–400.

30 Isolated Liver Transplantation for Intestinal Failure-Associated Liver Disease

Jean F. Botha and Alan N. Langnas

Key points

- The development of intestinal failure-associated end stage liver disease in children showing evidence of gut adaptation poses significant challenges in terms of therapeutic options.

- Wait-list mortality for combined liver and intestinal transplantation exceeds that for all other organs.

- In selected patients, isolated liver transplant may allow time and optimal circumstances for full enteral adaptation to take place and independence from parenteral nutrition to be achieved.

Introduction

Children and infants with short bowel syndrome (SBS) are at risk of developing serious intestinal failure-related complications before full intestinal adaptation has taken place. Catheter related sepsis; loss of intravenous access and intestinal failure (IF)-associated liver disease may be life threatening complications that result in treatment failure and the need for intestinal transplantation. Parenteral nutrition (PN) is the major supportive therapy for children with short bowel syndrome until intestinal adaptation occurs and enteral autonomy is achieved. Once liver disease develops survival at 5 years is 0% with most children dying within 2 years of the onset of liver disease.

Intestinal Failure: Diagnosis, Management and Transplantation.
Edited by Alan N. Langnas, Olivier Goulet, Eamonn M.M. Quigley and Kelly A. Tappenden. © 2008 Blackwell Publishing.
ISBN 978-1-4051-4637-1.

When liver failure develops before weaning from PN has occurred, a vicious cycle of intolerance to feeding and progressive liver disease ensues. Ascites, bowel wall edema, and recurrent gastrointestinal bleeding as a result of impaired synthetic function of the liver and portal hypertension suppresses bowel adaptation and intestinal function. Other factors such as bacterial overgrowth, bowel dysmotility, bile salt depletion, and recurrent central line infections delay further weaning from PN.

In some patients referred for liver and small bowel transplantation, end-stage liver disease (ESLD) occurs despite a seemingly adequate length and function of the small intestinal remnant, and, were it not for the presence of liver disease, may in time achieve enteral autonomy. Advanced liver disease and portal hypertension have been shown to negatively impact the process of intestinal adaptation [3]. Portal hypertension results in malabsorption of sugar, fluid and electrolytes [4]. Furthermore, children with extrahepatic portal vein obstruction have shown improvement of nutrient absorption as well as improved growth after portal decompressive procedures [5]. Transplantation of the liver alone in these patients with SBS and intestinal failure-associated liver disease (IFALD) will remove factors such as ascites, bowel wall edema, gastrointestinal bleeding, and luminal bile salt deficiency, thus allowing time and optimal conditions for complete enteral adaptation to occur.

There are advantages to isolated liver transplantation over combined liver and small bowel transplantation. Lower levels of immunosuppression are required and steroids can more easily be weaned, organ availability is greater because of standardized reduction techniques, and the availability of living donor transplantation. A recent study by Fryer and colleagues highlighted the disproportionately high waiting-list mortality between liver transplant only candidates and liver intestine candidates [2]. Analysis of the OPTN/SRTR database for 2003 revealed substantial waiting times for intestinal transplant candidates which translate into a waiting list death rate of 635 per 1000 patient years at risk [10]. In the United States, the national median wait list time is longer than 9 months with a wait list mortality of 35% (http://www.ustransplant.org).

Intestinal failure-associated liver disease (IFALD)

Parenteral nutrition has improved the outcome for infants with intestinal failure. Particularly following neonatal small bowel resection, PN provides time for the process of intestinal adaptation to take place. Intestinal failure associated liver dysfunction, however, remains a life-threatening complication. Premature babies appear to be to be most at risk suggesting that liver dysfunction is related to the immaturity of the neonatal liver. Lack of enteral intake and recurrent episodes of sepsis, whether from central lines or bacterial overgrowth, are the other major factors associated with the development of IFALD. Components of the PN formula may also be related to the development of IFALD. Deficiencies of the amino acids taurine and cysteine have been cited and the toxic effects of manganese have recently been highlighted. Jaundice is the most obvious sign of IFALD, however portal fibrosis and splenomegaly may develop in the absence of jaundice and despite extensive fibrosis esophageal varices are an infrequent finding. This is discussed in greater detail in Chapter 21.

Suitability for isolated liver transplant

Predicting which patients are likely to achieve enteral tolerance after liver transplantation is difficult to define. The criteria that we use to determine successful weaning of PN after liver transplant involve careful clinical assessment of bowel function past and present. The key functional parameter that we use is maximum enteral tolerance, which is defined as that portion of total caloric requirement that has been tolerated by the

Table 30.1 Predictors of enteral autonomy after isolated liver transplant for IFALD.

Predictor	
Maximal enteral tolerance	>50% of calories by the enteral route
	• Stool frequency and consistency
	• Maintain hydration
	• Maintain growth
Bowel length	>25 cm from ligament of Treitz
Patient age	<2 years

enteral route at any time in the patient's history. This also takes into account the fact that caloric requirements in children with SBS are greater than that of normal children. An enteral tolerance of 50% of required calories is the benchmark that we have used in considering children for isolated liver transplant. This includes assessment of stool output and consistency as well as patient hydration and growth. Bowel length has always been a key predictor of weaning from PN in children with SBS. The lower limit of small bowel length measured from the ligament of Treitz, which we consider likely to result in weaning from PN is 25 cm. Children less than 2 years of age have a greater capacity for intestinal adaptation (Table 30.1).

Nebraska experience

The largest experience with liver transplantation in children with SBS and IFALD has recently been reported by the group from the University of Nebraska. This series builds on their previous experience and now represents 23 children who had been referred to their center for evaluation for combined liver and small bowel transplantation that, after thorough evaluation, were deemed to be suitable candidates for isolated liver transplantation, based on their criteria [11,12]. The etiology of SBS represented the usual spectrum of diseases causing SBS in infants. All 23 children had SBS and ESLD. Median serum bilirubin was 19 mg/dl (range 2.9–40), median prothrombin time was 17 seconds (range 13.3–37), median serum albumin was 2.5 mg/dl (range 2.1–3.0) and median pediatric end-stage liver disease (PELD) score was 30 (range 18–44). All patients were severely growth retarded as manifested by median z-score for height of −2.29 (range −4.6–0.06) and median z-score for weight of −1.68 (range −3.17–0.6). At the time of transplantation, the median age was 11 months (range 6.5–48) and median weight of 7.5 kg (range 5.2–15). As a group, the median enteral tolerance was 50% (range 30–100%). The median small bowel length was 50 cm (range 20–100 cm) and 13 patients had retained their ileocecal valves. Twenty-three patients underwent 28 liver transplants, of which 14 were whole organs and 14 partial livers (12 left lateral segments and 2 full left lobes). Five transplants were from living donors. The method of biliary reconstruction was by Roux-en-Y choledochojejunostomy in 12 cases and duct-to-duct anastomosis in 16.

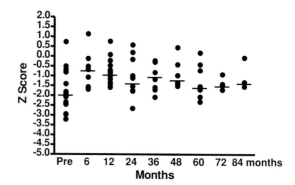

Figure 30.1 Standardized weight Z-score by time of follow-up (median ± range)

Survival and nutritional outcome after liver transplant

Patient and graft survival is 82% and 75% at 1 year and 72% and 60% at 5 years. Fourteen patients (82%) have been completely weaned from PN at a median of 3 months (range 1–72 months) after transplantation. Six of these patients meet all their nutritional requirements from oral intake; the remaining eight still require supplemental or full tube feeds. When examining differences between the successes and the failures there appeared to be no differences in median bowel length (56 cm vs. 45 cm, p = 0.17) and percentage enteral tolerance (55% vs. 45%, p = 0.06). A similar number of patients had retained ileocecal valves (p = 1.0). Changes in the anthropometric parameters were assessed in the surviving children with at least 1 year of follow-up. There were modest improvements in the individual height-for-age and weight for age z-scores over time. The median change in height-for-age z-score was 0.57 (range) over a 4-year period. Similarly, the median change in weight-for-age z-score was 0.42 (range) over the same period indicating maintenance of linear growth with some catch up growth occurring in the first year post transplant (Figures 30.1 and 30.2). In the patients that are alive, the current median albumin concentration is 3.9 mg/dl (range 2.7–4.8), indicating adequate visceral protein stores. Four children in this series required autologous gut reconstruction. One child underwent a Bianchi procedure 2 years after transplant followed by a serial transverse

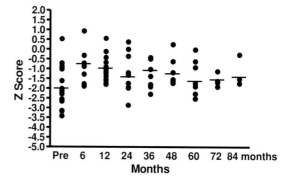

Figure 30.2 Standardized height Z-score by time of follow-up (median ± range)

enteroplasty (STEP) 3 years later, after which he was successfully weaned from PN. The first patient in the series who is now over 10 years post-transplant underwent a Bianchi procedure 8 years after transplant and is currently off PN. Gastric outlet obstruction occurred in a child who had previously had duodenal atresia repaired as a neonate and required reconstruction of his gastric outlet. A patient with NEC and a long transverse colon stricture underwent takedown of her end jejunostomy and resection of the colon stricture and jejunocolostomy 6 months after liver transplant was successfully weaned from PN.

World experience

Small series and a few case reports have suggested that isolated liver transplantation for SBS and IF related

Table 30.2 World experience with isolated liver transplant in children with short bowel syndrome.

Series	Number of patients	Alive	Off PN
Hassan [7]	1	1	1
Gottrand [8]	1	1	1
Lawrence [6]	5	4	3
Muiesan [10]	5	3	3
Diamond [9]	3	2	0
Botha [13]	23	17	14

liver failure is a feasible treatment option in selected patients with features suggestive of eventual enteral autonomy. Lawrence reported on five patients with SBS and ESLD who underwent six liver transplants. Of the four long-term survivors, two remain on PN [6]. Case reports from Hassan and colleagues and Gottrand and colleagues confirm that long-term success can be achieved and that autologous gut reconstruction after isolated liver transplant is also feasible [7,8]. Diamond and colleagues recently reported on three children who underwent liver transplantation alone for IFALD; one child died 7 months after transplantation from recurrent IFALD. The remaining children, despite tolerating enteral feeds, remain on PN for poor weight gain [9]. Muiesan and colleagues reported a series of five children with SBS and ESLD, three of which underwent isolated liver transplantation with the expectation of full enteral adaptation and eventual weaning from PN and two patients in whom combined liver and intestinal transplantation were indicated but, because of life-threatening liver failure, underwent liver transplantation with a sequential isolated intestinal transplant planned in the future. All three children transplanted with the expectation of eventual enteral adaptation were successfully weaned from PN. The two children who were "bridged" to intestinal transplant both died, one while waiting and the other after sequential isolated intestinal transplantation [10] (Table 30.2).

Conclusion

Children with SBS are dependent on parenteral nutrition in order to survive while the remnant gut undergoes adaptation. Complications related to IF include loss of venous access, central line related infections and progressive liver failure, which results in failure of PN [1]. Patients who have failed PN support as a result of the development of liver disease are considered for combined liver and intestinal transplantation. The youngest patients with ultra-short gut are the most susceptible to the development of PN associated liver disease, which may develop in up to 50% of these patients. The etiology of liver disease in children on long-term PN is multifactorial; however, the role of intra-abdominal infections and sepsis is increasingly being recognized. Whatever the pathogenesis, once ESLD develops the survival at 5 years is 0% [2].

In carefully selected patients with SBS and ESLD with favorable prognostic features for eventual enteral autonomy, liver transplantation alone can provide the time and the optimal circumstances required for full intestinal adaptation to take place. Survival is acceptable and independence from PN is durable. Liver transplants in patients with SBS should not performed with the intent of bridging patients to sequential small bowel transplantation as suggested by some, but, rather, with the expectation that these children could be weaned from PN in the presence of normal liver function and the absence of portal hypertension. To do otherwise would lead to unacceptable graft and patient loss. It is important to emphasize that these are challenging patients that require an intense level of postoperative care and should be managed in a multidisciplinary setting at centers with experience in pediatric liver and intestinal transplantation.

References

1 Buchman AL, Scolapio J, Fryer J. AGA technical review on short bowel syndrome and intestinal transplantation. *Gastroenterology* 2003;124:1111–1134.

2 Fryer J, Pellar S, Ormond D, et al. Mortality in candidates waiting for combined liver-intestine transplants exceeds that for other candidates waiting for liver transplants. *Liver Transplantation* 2003;9:748–753.

3 Weber TR, Keller MS. Adverse effects of liver dysfunction and portal hypertension on intestinal adaptation in short bowel syndrome in children. *Am J Surg* 2002;184:582–586.

4 Jacobs DL, Lof J, Quigley EM, et al. The effect of mesenteric venous hypertension on gut motility and absorption. *J Surg Res* 1990;48:562.

5 Kato T, Romero R, Koutouby R, et al. Portosystemic shunting in children during the Era of endoscopic therapy: improved postoperative growth parameters. *J Pediatr Gastroenterol Nutr* 2000;30:419–424.

6 Lawrence JP, Dunn SP, Billmire DF, et al. Isolated liver transplantation for liver failure in patients with short bowel syndrome. *J Pediatr Surg* 1994;29:751–753.

7 Hassan KO, Beath SV, McKiernan PJ, et al. Difficult management choices for infants with short bowel syndrome and liver failure. *J Pediatr Gastroenterol Nutr* 2002;35:216–219.

8 Gottrand F, Michaud L, Bonnevalle M, et al. Favorable nutritional outcome after isolated liver transplantation for liver failure in a child with short bowel syndrome. *Transplantation* 1999;67:632–634.

9 Diamond IR, Wales PW, Grant DR, Fecteau A. Isolated liver transplantation in pediatric short bowel syndrome: is there a role? *J Pediatr Surg* 2006;41:955–959.

10 Muiesan P, Dhawan A, Novelli M, et al. Isolated liver transplant and sequential small bowel transplantation for intestinal failure and related liver disease in children. *Transplantation* 2000;69:2323–2326.

11 Harmon WE, McDonald RA, Reyes JD, et al. Pediatric Transplantation. *Am J Transplant* 2005;4:887–903.

12 Horslen SP, Sudan DL, Iyer KR, et al. Isolated liver transplantation in infants with end-stage liver disease associated with short bowel syndrome. *Ann Surg* 2002;235:435–439.

13 Botha JF, Grant WJ, Torres C, et al. Isolated liver transplantation in infants with end-stage liver disease due to short bowel syndrome. *Liver Transpl* 2006;12:1062–1066.

31 Preservation of the Intestine

**Vincent B. Nieuwenhuijs, Mihai Oltean,
Henri G. Leuvenink and Rutger J. Ploeg**

Key points

- Small bowel preservation starts with donor selection and management.
- Non-heart-beating donors are currently not considered.
- Cold storage after vascular perfusion with University of Wisconsin solution (UW) is most commonly used.
- Luminal preservation strategies may offer further improvement of graft quality.
- The maximum cold ischemia time is 9 hours.

Introduction

Intestinal transplantation (ITx) has become an effective treatment option for intestinal failure with graft survival gradually improving over time [1]. The outcome of solid organ transplantation in general is greatly dependent of the organ quality at the time of implantation [2]. The quality of the organs starts to deteriorate promptly after, or even before, the diagnosis of braindeath [3]. Therefore, optimal donor management, correct surgical technique during the multi-organ retrieval procedure and effective preservation strategies are key issues in achieving favorable outcomes after transplantation (Figure 31.1).

The intestine has functional and morphologic characteristics that raise special concerns and obstacles in the choice of preservation solution and the storage technique. An effective preservation strategy for an

Intestinal Failure: Diagnosis, Management and Transplantation.
Edited by Alan N. Langnas, Olivier Goulet, Eamonn M.M. Quigley and Kelly A. Tappenden. © 2008 Blackwell Publishing.
ISBN 978-1-4051-4637-1.

intestinal graft should allow for a reasonable period of cold storage, preserve mucosal integrity and limit ischemia- and reperfusion (IR) injury. This chapter discusses the current issues related to the preservation of the intestinal graft.

Donor selection and management

The shorter waiting lists and the relative underutilization of the intestine allow a more selective policy on donor and graft selection than with other organs. Because the recipients often have contracted abdominal cavities as a result of the loss of the native intestine, smaller, ABO identical donors are typically preferred. Selective gut decontamination with an antibiotic mixture (amphotericin B/mycostatin, tobramycin/gentamycin, and polymyxin E) administered through a nasogastric tube, early after acceptance for donorship and at the time of organ procurement, is advocated by many U.S. centers [4]. Because the intestine is extremely vulnerable to ischemia and hypoperfusion, donors with prolonged hemodynamic instability, episodes of cardiac arrest as well as non-heart-beating donors are deemed unsuitable. Because of the concern that older grafts would have impaired repair mechanisms, younger, less than 50-year-old, donors are usually selected.

Inotropes should be used judiciously to maintain an acceptable mean arterial blood pressure since they may compromise splanchnic perfusion and the intestinal microcirculation, particularly that of the capillary loops in the villus. Experimental evidence suggests that several donor preconditioning strategies may be effective in reducing IR injury, yet clinical data are missing [5]. Table 31.1 provides an overview of the

Table 31.1 Donor variables to consider in donor selection.

Variable	Favorable	Unfavorable
Age[1]	<50 years	>50 years
Donor weight[1]	<recipient weight	>recipient weight
ABO matching	identical	compatible
Hemodynamic instability	none, minor inotropic support	significant inotropic support, cardiac arrest
Donor type	heart-beating or living-(un)related	non-heart beating
Cold ischemia time	<9 hours	>9 hours
Multivisceral Tx	Good liver and/or kidney function	Impairment of hepatic and/or renal function

[1]Different criteria apply for pediatric recipients which need to be age and size matched

donor variables that need to be considered for donor selection.

Donor surgery of the intestine

The first important steps toward maintaining organ viability and allowing effective preservation of the intestine relate to intestinal procurement. Effective organ preservation is based on three principles: (1) temperature effect (rapid cooling to 0–4°C); (2) an effective wash-out; and (3) a solution effect depending on the physical and biochemical environment created by the compounds included in the preservation solution.

The surgical procedure of multi-organ procurement is complex, often involving several surgical teams. A dedicated intestinal procurement team should be present at the time of retrieval to ensure optimal graft preparation and to check whether the retrieved graft meets the recipient requirements, in terms of graft length and inclusion of required additional organs (liver, pancreas, stomach). An experienced surgical team can also avoid excessive manipulation of the viscera. This may be deleterious for the intestine and triggers the development of a complex pro-inflammatory milieu that, together with brain death and IR injury, could worsen the transplant outcome [6]. Several techniques allowing the simultaneous retrieval of the abdominal organs and their transplantation as separate or composite grafts have been developed [4]. Most approaches aim for a careful, yet not excessive, dissection of the main vascular trunks with an intact donor circulation.

After dissection, the organs are cooled in-situ through infradiaphragmatic aortic retrograde perfusion. The most commonly used method for vascular perfusion is that of isolated infradiaphragmatic aortic low-pressure perfusion performed with a cold preservative solution by gravitation. It has been demonstrated for rat liver grafts that high-pressure perfusion and rapid washout may shorten the warm-ischemia time and improve organ function, yet no such studies

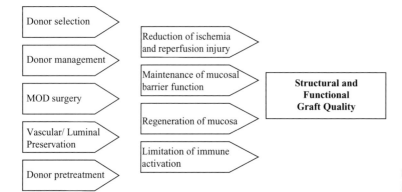

Figure 31.1 Factors determining small bowel graft quality.

exist regarding the intestine [7]. A high volume of the aortic perfusate ensures rapid cooling, but the ideal core temperature of the organs (0–4 degrees) is not reached until after packaging and storage on ice. Despite complete bleaching after perfusion, the intestine may still feel warm, due to its hollow structure and contents. Therefore, it should be left immersed in the cold solution for at least 30 minutes to achieve adequate cooling before attempting any organ separation or graft reduction techniques [4].

The various organs are then separated on the backtable, according to the need of transplanting centers and after consultation with the implantation teams. Besides transplanting the entire gastrointestinal and liver complex as a multivisceral graft, individual grafts may be fashioned from the cluster of the splanchnic viscera. To facilitate the transplant procedure vascular grafts should be included as a "toolkit" (iliac vessels, thoracic aorta, and neck vessels).

Donor type and the effect of brain death

Currently, non-heart-beating donors are not considered because the intestine is very sensitive to IR- and preservation injury. Heart-beating, brain-dead donors are used most in ITx, but the experience with living-(un)related intestinal transplantation (LR-ITx) is growing.

Although the experience with LR-ITx is still limited, the results both in adults and children are promising [8]. Less than half of the donor intestine (the ileum), vascularized by the terminal ileocolic artery is resected. LR-ITx enables optimal donor and recipient preparation, shortens the waiting time, helps overcome size-matching incongruence and enables very short cold and warm ischemic periods [9]. The advantages and disadvantages of the method are discussed elsewhere. There could be a potential advantage of transplanting grafts from living donors because, after brain death, the quality of the organs progressively deteriorates; several studies have shown a negative impact on the immunological and inflammatory status of both liver and kidney [3,10]. Despite the lack of evidence in humans, a study in rodents shows alterations in intestinal morphology after one and four hours of brain death, with mucosal changes and increased inflammatory activity [11].

Recently, the progressive pro-inflammatory and pro-coagulatory response induced during brain death and aggravated by warm or cold ischemia was confirmed in clinical kidney donation and transplantation [3,10].

Although this stress-induced response is followed by an attempt of the body to upregulate protective mechanisms such as hemoxygenase-1 (HO-1), the systemic inflammatory activation could be too overwhelming to prevent primary nonfunction or delayed graft function, especially in organs retrieved from older and more marginal donors. As in living donation, stress-induced responses are minimal compared to those in deceased donors, the actual preservation solution used is probably not crucial, provided that the washout achieves rapid cooling and an effective rinse of blood components. Most centers will use the same solution as in deceased donors, for the intestine this would be UW solution.

Key pathophysiological events during intestinal ischemia and reperfusion

The epithelial cells covering the intestinal villi are held together by tight junctions, whose proper functioning is maintained by several energy-dependent processes including tyrosine kinase and GTP kinase signaling [12]. During ischemia, the alteration in the functioning of intercellular junctions will result in increased permeability and fluid shifts between the lumen and the intestinal wall within minutes from the start of oxygen deprivation.

Even in normal, physiologic, conditions, a certain oxygen gradient occurs in the villi, due to oxygen shunting at the base of the villus [13]. This phenomenon becomes more evident in low flow states such as hypotension and shock, leading to a pronounced oxygen deficit toward the tip of the villus. The subsequent breakdown of the epithelial lining favors bacterial translocation. The intestine has, accordingly, been called "the motor of multi-organ dysfunction syndrome (MODS)" [14].

In normal circumstances, oncotic and osmotic pressures are tightly regulated at the epithelial/luminal and epithelial/lamina propria interfaces. During ischemia, physiologic homeostasis is disrupted and fluid shifts between these compartments are further promoted.

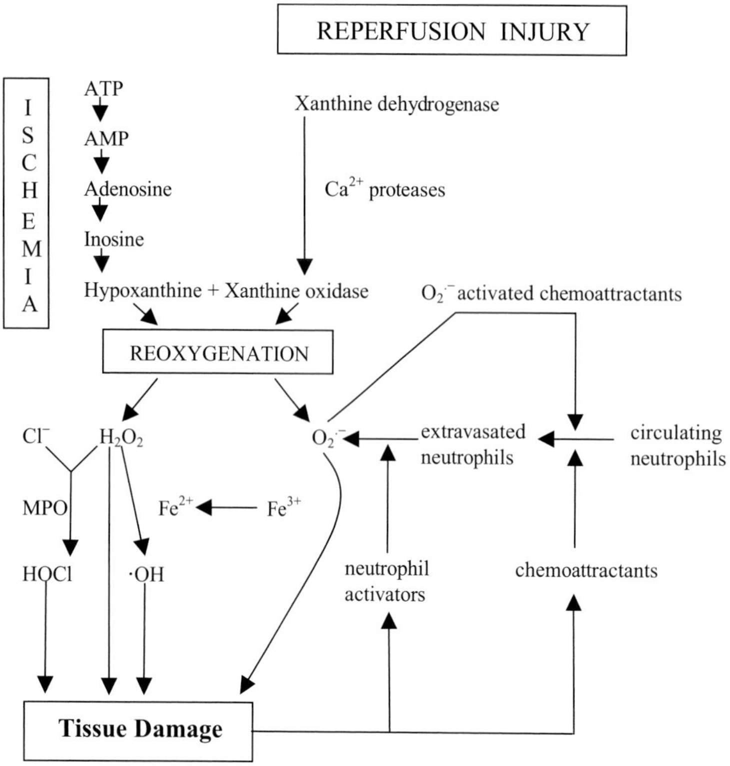

REPERFUSION INJURY

Figure 31.2 Pathways of generation of reactive oxygen species and tissue damage during ischemia and reperfusion.

The metabolic alterations secondary to anoxia lead to changes in intracellular pH with resultant mitochondrial injury and lysosomal activation. On the luminal side, the aggression of protease-containing intestinal contents inflicts further damage on a mucosa which is temporarily devoid of its repair and defense mechanisms. Although these phenomena have originally been described in the setting of warm ischemia, these changes may also occur during the cold preservation of the intestine, albeit at a lower rate and extent.

Upon reperfusion, an intense oxidative stress mediated by the abundantly present enzyme xanthine-oxidase as well as mitochondrial dysfunction will occur. The generation of reactive oxygen and nitrogen species will lead to lipid peroxidation and cellular injury together with the activation of various transcription factors with the up-regulation or de-novo synthesis of numerous biomolecules [15]. Figure 31.2 gives an overview of the pathways involved in the generation of reactive oxygen species during ischemia and reperfusion.

Vascular flush and cold storage

Until recently, virtually all intestinal graft were preserved in University of Wisconsin solution (UW) because this was the preservation solution used by most transplant centers [4]. Recently, centers around the world have manifested a renewed interest in HTK solution (Histidine-Triptophane-Ketoglutarate, Custodiol) and, thus, HTK also started to be used for preserving intestinal grafts. HTK proved as effective as UW in kidney and liver transplantation, at least for average cold ischemia times. In-situ cooling of the intestine is achieved through retrograde, slow, aortic perfusion with UW or HTK, taking care not to overperfuse the bowel, a precaution particularly important when using HTK. Many centers with intestinal transplant programs recommend stopping intestinal perfusion after 1–1.5 L and removing the intestinal graft at that time. Cold perfusion is followed by static storage in a UW or HTK bath, in a manner similar to other abdominal organs. The high content of potassium in the UW will require a wash-out prior graft reperfusion [2].

Because of its high potassium content, grafts preserved in UW display an increased vascular resistance and a partly constricted capillary bed. The microvasculature may suffer further endothelial injury after the period of cold preservation [16]. Any additional perfusate may further augment microvascular injury. Moreover, in contrast to organs with a firm capsule and a parenchymatous structure such as the liver and the kidneys, passing an additional volume of fluid through a cavitary organ such as the intestine may cause an expansion of the already damaged, partly denuded lamina propria.

Recently, a nonrandomized study was conducted at the University of Pittsburgh Medical Center, which compared the efficacy of HTK (52 transplants) and UW (79 transplants) in grafts containing intestinal segments. The study concluded that, although similarly effective and safe in preserving the intestine, the frequency of postreperfusion syndrome and the occurrence of pancreatic complications in composite grafts (containing the intestine and the pancreas) were increased when using HTK, because of as yet unidentified reasons [17]. This finding could reopen a discussion of the importance of a colloid in the preservation solution. As a matter of fact, for most organs with shorter cold ischemia times the addition of hydroxy-ethyl starch (HES) is not necessary. Previously, it has been shown, however, that, especially in preservation of the pancreas, omitting HES leads to a higher rate of graft failure and pancreatitis [18]. HES (250 kD), on the one hand, has beneficial properties on matrix metalloproteases (e.g. protecting cell membranes in the liver); it will, on the other hand, aggregate with erythrocytes in microcapillaries when not properly perfused. In this respect, the replacement of HES by polyethylene glycol (PEG), as in the newer preservation solution IGL-1, could be an advantage. PEG is a potent oncotic agent counteracting cellular edema, is non-toxic and a prominent scavenger in lipid peroxidation.

Rationale for luminal preservation, the third compartment

The classical principles of solid, parenchymatous organ preservation are only partly applicable to the intestine because of the cavitary structure of the intestine. In addition to the classical intravascular (or extracellular) and extravascular (or intracellular) compartments, as present in parenchymatous organs, the presence of the intestinal lumen creates a third compartment that is not reached by vascular flush. The luminal compartment is critical if one considers its highly variable osmolarity and osmolality, its surface and volume as well as the "leaky" epithelium covering the intestinal mucosa.

The intestine further differs from the other organs in its absorptive capacity, designed to cope with rapid shifts of fluids and osmotic changes. Moreover, the intestinal epithelial membrane differs from the membranes of other organs in various ion transport channels (Na/H, Na/glucose, Na/HCO3, Cl). Likewise, the basolateral membrane, which is in contact with the subepithelial space is structurally, chemically and functionally different from the apical membrane, bordering on the intestinal lumen.

The tight junctions seal the intercellular space but allow and regulate the passive paracellular transport of ions. The function of the tight junctions, having extracellular, transmembrane and intracellular domains, is ATP-dependent. An altered, increased paracellular transport is to be expected during and after reperfusion.

In the past, several studies have explored the efficacy of UW delivered to the luminal side. Intestinal segments preserved with luminal UW flush compared to intestinal segments undergoing vascular flush alone showed improved morphology [19,20]. It is unclear how luminal UW flush attenuates preservation injury, maybe due to partial control of the osmolarity and reduction of the mucosal injury by diluting the protease-rich, cytotoxic intraluminal content.

Another approach that attempts to reduce preservation injury involved the intraluminal instillation of various tailored solutions. Their composition included a mixture of amino acids in addition various impermeants [20,21]. Besides gaining a partial control over the above-mentioned factors (the cytotoxic content, highly variable osmolarity) the improved results could have been because the amino acids did not readily pass through the tight junctions and the ion channels and remained in the lumen, thus maintaining its osmotic parameters. Few, if any, of these preservation studies were followed by transplantation of the intestinal graft.

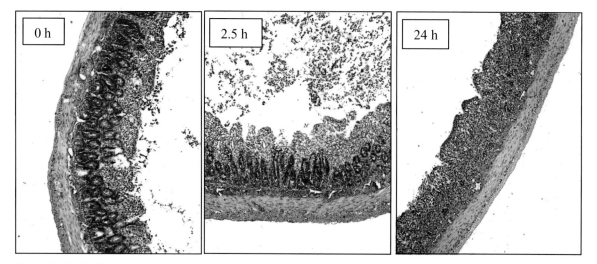

Figure 31.3 Histology of reperfused small bowel graft after cold preservation in UW solution followed in WagRy Rats. HE staining, magnification 100×. Immediate reperfusion after procurement (0 hours) shows villous atrophy with intact crypts. After 2.5 hours of preservation: sloughing of the villi with intact crypts. After 14 hours of preservation, no villi are seen and injury to the crypts is noted.

This leaves the relevance and clinical application of these methods to be established.

The introduction of perfluorocarbon as a small molecule capable of retaining and slowly releasing oxygen into the intestinal lumen, allowed an extended preservation of up to 24 hours in canine intestinal transplantation [22].

Despite issues related to practical application and a lack of clarity on mechanism of action, these approaches indicate that adequately addressing the intraluminal compartment could further improve intestinal graft quality and may provide superior transplant results when compared with the current approaches using vascular perfusion alone. In clinical practice, however, intraluminal flush is not (yet) used, the intestines are perfused through the vasculature while the gut lumen is stapled off. The fear of structural damage to the mucosa is mainly based on rodent models. Olson et al. have, however, shown that the human small bowel is more resistant to mechanical damage and that a luminal flush offers structural and functional advantages compared to vascular flush alone [20].

Development of intestinal ischemic injury

Intestinal ischemic injury presents as a gradual detachment of the epithelial layer from the underlying lamina propria. The subepithelial cleft (the space of Gruenhagen) initially occurs at the villus tip and gradually extends toward the base of the villus. The advanced stages are characterized by epithelial breakdown and disintegration of the lamina propria, then the subsequent disappearance of the other mucosal compartments [23].

The more moderate, typical, preservation injury occurring after about four to six hours of cold storage consists in epithelial detachment down the length of the villi but not reaching the crypts. Longer preservation periods above 9–10 hours are associated with more advanced injury, that presents with denuded or even partly destroyed villi [20,24]. On graft reperfusion, advanced injuries will turn to diffuse, bleeding ulcerations. Prolonged cold ischemic time for more than 9 hours is also associated with a high rate of bacterial translocation as a result of the breakdown of the mucosal barrier [25]. The degree of intestinal ischemic injury can easily be assessed by the Park scoring system [23]. A histological example of the structural change to bowel after preservation and IR injury is given in Figure 31.3.

Conclusions

The goal of intestinal preservation is to maintain the morphological and functional integrity of the epithelial barrier and thus to reduce bacterial translocation and the potential for septic complications after transplantation.

To date, there has been overall agreement that the intestine adheres only partly to the classical principles of organ preservation. This may be because the intestine has its luminal compartment as a third entity besides the intracellular and the extracellular compartments. Although existing preservation solutions address the composition of the latter two compartments, the former has previously been disregarded. Several studies, which have intuitively addressed the control of its composition, showed that attempts to control the composition of the luminal compartment improve the results of preservation. However, a solid theoretical basis and clinical application are still lacking. Until such studies provide more effective strategies for intestinal preservation, transplant teams using the available preservation fluids should strive to maintain the intestinal cold ischemia time below 9 hours.

As in other organs, the basic principles of organ preservation remain important: to rapidly cool the intestine with a flush-out of blood components; to equilibrate the tissue with the preservation solution; to use hypothermia (0–4°C) as a critical factor in reducing metabolic activity; to use effective preservation solutions that maintain membrane and intracellular integrity, prevent cellular edema, and buffer for acidosis. Furthermore, preservation solutions should include biochemical agents to support energy metabolism and counteract reactive oxygen species during cold ischemia and at the time of reperfusion.

References

1 Grant D, Abu-Elmagd K, Reyes J, et al. 2003 report of the intestine transplant registry: a new era has dawned. *Ann Surg* 2005;241:607–613.

2 Southard JH, Belzer FO. Organ preservation. *Annu Rev Med* 1995;46:235–247.

3 Nijboer WN, Schuurs TA, van der Hoeven JA, et al. Effect of brain death on gene expression and tissue activation in human donor kidneys. *Transplantation* 2004;15:978–986.

4 Abu-Elmagd K, Fung J, Bueno J, et al. Logistics and technique for procurement of intestinal, pancreatic, and hepatic grafts from the same donor. *Ann Surg* 2000;232:680–687.

5 Oltean M, Pullerits R, Zhu C, et al. Donor pretreatment with FK506 reduces reperfusion injury and accelerates intestinal graft recovery in rats. *Surgery* 2007;667–676.

6 Turler A, Kalff JC, Heeckt P, et al. Molecular and functional observations on the donor intestinal muscularis during human small bowel transplantation. *Gastroenterology* 2002;122:1886–1897.

7 't Hart NA, van der Plaats A, Leuvenink HGD, et al. Initial blood washout during organ procurement determines liver injury and function after preservation and reperfusion. *Am J Transplant* 2004;4:1836–1844.

8 Cicalese L, Rastellini C, Sileri P, et al. Segmental living related small bowel transplantation in adults. *J Gastrointest Surg* 2001;5:168–172.

9 Testa G, Panaro F, Schena S, et al. Living related small bowel transplantation—Donor surgical technique. *Ann Surg* 2004;240:779–784.

10 Schuurs TA, Morariu AM, Ottens PJ, et al. Time-dependent changes in donor brain death related processes. *Am J Transplant* 2006;25:2903–2911.

11 Koudstaal LG, 't Hart NA, Ploeg RJ, et al. Inflammation and structural changes in donor intestine and liver after brain death induction. *Eur J Gastroenterol Hepatol* 2005;17:A44–A45.

12 Bush KT, Keller SH, Nigam SK. Genesis and reversal of the ischemic phenotype in epithelial cells. *J Clin Invest* 2000;106:621–626.

13 Lundgren O. Studies on blood flow distribution and countercurrent exchange in the small intestine. *Acta Physiol Scand Suppl* 1967;303:1–42.

14 Deitch EA. The role of intestinal barrier failure and bacterial translocation in the development of systemic infection and multiple organ failure. *Arch Surg* 1990;125:403–404.

15 Yeh KY, Yeh M, Glass J, Granger DN. Rapid activation of NF-kappaB and AP-1 and target gene expression in postischemic rat intestine. *Gastroenterology* 2000;118:525–534.

16 Clavien PA, Harvey PR, Strasberg SM. Preservation and reperfusion injuries in liver allografts. An overview and synthesis of current studies. *Transplantation* 1992;53:957–978.

17 Bond G, Aggarwal S, Schuster B, et al. Is Histadine-Tryptophan-Ketoglutarate (HTK) a better cold preservative solution for intestinal and multivisceral allografts? *Am J Transplant* WTC Abstract book, Abstract 65 p88. 2006.

18 Ploeg RJ, Boudjema K, Marsh D, et al. The importance of a colloid in canine pancreas preservation. *Transplantation* 1992;53:735–741.

19 DeRoover A, de Leval L, Gilmaire J, et al. Luminal contact with University of Wisconsin solution improves human small bowel preservation. *Transplant Proc* 2004;36:273–275.

20 Olson DW, Jijon H, Madsen KL, et al. Human small bowel storage: The role for luminal preservation solutions. *Transplantation* 2003;27:709–714.

21 Salehi P, Zhu JZJ, Castillo EG, et al. Preserving the mucosal barrier during small bowel storage. *Transplantation* 2003;27:911–917.

22 Fujino Y, Kakinoki K, Suzuki Y, et al. Successful 24-hour preservation of ischemically damaged canine small intestine by the cavitary two-layer method. *Transplantation* 2003;15:777–780.

23 Park PO, Haglund U, Bulkley GB, Falt K. The sequence of development of intestinal tissue injury after strangulation ischemia and reperfusion. *Surgery* 1990;107:574–580.

24 Tesi RJ, Jaffe BM, McBride V, Haque S. Histopathologic changes in human small intestine during storage in viaspan organ preservation solution. *Arch Pathol Lab Med* 1997;121:714–718.

25 Cicalese L, Sileri P, Green M, et al. Bacterial translocation in clinical intestinal transplantation. *Transplantation* 2001;27:1414–1417.

32 Immediate Postoperative Care of the Intestinal Transplant Recipient

Gabriel J. Hauser, Jeffrey S. Plotkin and Thomas Fishbein

Key points

- Optimizing hemodynamics is critical to allograft viability.
- Many patients have intrinsic respiratory problems before transplant that can have an impact on postoperative care.
- Postoperative renal dysfunction is common and is often related to administered medications.
- Postoperative infections are frequent despite prophylactic strategies.
- Allograft function and the development of rejection can have a profound impact on the postoperative care of the patient.

Introduction

Care of the patient immediately after intestinal transplantation can be considered in terms of recipient organ system management, and monitoring of, and response to, the function of the allograft organs. These may include the intestine alone, or the intestine along with the stomach, liver, pancreas, kidney, or colon. Early support required will be determined by aspects of the surgical procedure as well as early graft function.

Cardiovascular

The primary challenge of the early post-operative management of patients after intestinal transplantation is

Intestinal Failure: Diagnosis, Management and Transplantation.
Edited by Alan N. Langnas, Olivier Goulet, Eamonn M.M. Quigley and Kelly A. Tappenden. © 2008 Blackwell Publishing.
ISBN 978-1-4051-4637-1.

maintenance of adequate graft perfusion. This may be monitored with bedside Doppler examination of the stoma and can be used to help manipulate hemodynamic and fluid management (Figure 32.1). Assurance of oxygen delivery to the newly grafted organ is of paramount importance. Oxygen delivery (DO_2) is defined by the following equation: $DO_2 = [(Hgb \times 1.3 \times SaO_2) + (PaO_2 \times .003)] \times$ cardiac output. As such, the hematocrit should be maintained between 27% and 30%, as this has been shown to provide the optimal balance between oxygen carrying capacity and increased viscosity leading to decreased cardiac output (Table 32.1) [3]. Another means of manipulating blood viscosity is the maintenance of a relatively hypocoagulable state. As such, an INR of 3–4 and platelet counts as low as 20×10^{-6}/L are usually tolerated without bleeding, and plasma and platelet transfusions should be avoided, unless there is a clinical indication. Furthermore, the PaO_2 should be maintained to yield a hemoglobin oxygen saturation >95%. Cardiac output should be normal to high; adequate volume status and avoidance of high afterload should be ensured.

The maintenance of hemodynamic stability is critical in promoting graft viability and function. Ideally, maintaining adequate hematocrit, oxygenation, and fluid balance will lead to adequate cardiac output and perfusion pressure; however, if vasopressor or inotropic support are necessary, it is best to avoid agents with a predominance of alpha receptor activity (i.e. neosynephrine). The rationale for this is to achieve adequate perfusion pressure with flow (cardiac output) rather than resistance (vasoconstriction), which may yield an acceptable blood pressure at the expense of tissue perfusion.

After the acute postoperative phase, some patients develop hypertension as a result of hypervolemia, renal

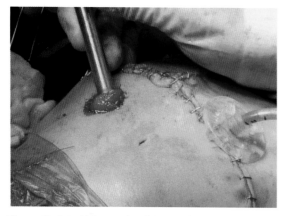

Figure 32.1 Bedside stomal perfusion can be assessed frequently using Doppler flow assessment as shown intraoperatively here.

insufficiency, calcineurin nephrotoxicity, and steroid use. Calcium channel blockade is usually preferred for

control. If the patient requires frequent doses, long-acting agents may help, although this may be determined by absorption and intestinal graft function. Beta-blockers are commonly employed in patients with liver failure who have left ventricular hypertrophy. Many medications prolong the QT interval. These include tacrolimus, pentamidine, octreotide, macrolides (azithromycin, erythromycin), methadone, and chloral hydrate. It is recommended to obtain a preoperative baseline QTc measurement when such agents are used as a result of the risk of torsade de pointes.

Respiratory

Many recipients have compromised respiratory function either because of prematurity or chronic lung disease (bronchopulmonary dysplasia) in pediatric patients, or hepatopulmonary syndrome, recurrent

Table 32.1 Main points in management by organ system.

Organ system	Parameters	Optimal	Acceptable	Possible complication
Cardiovascular	1. Hgb/Hct* 2. PaO₂/SaO₂ 3. Perfusion	Hct 27–30% O₂ Sat > 95% Normal MAP for age range	Above 22% 95% Increase C.O., avoid alpha vasoconstrictors	Graft ischemia and dysfunction Poor graft perfusion
Respiratory	Avoid high pressures and high FiO₂; prior lung injury common among these patients	1. Target TV 6–8 cc/kg 2. Plateau Pressures <30 cm H₂0	Permissive hypercarbia	1. Barotrauma 2. Watch for transient diaphragmatic paralysis—usually resolves
Renal	Good perfusion; avoid oliguric state	Maintain 0.5 cc/k/h output	low dose Dopamine (2.5–5.0 µg/kg/min) or Fenoldopam (0.03–0.1 µg/kg/min)	1. Need for CVVH 2. Be aware of possible abdominal compartment syndrome when poor renal function
Infectious disease	1. Should be afebrile early 2. INR should begin to correct within 48 hours 3. Should clear serum lactate within 48 hours	1. Afebrile 2. Decreasing INR from first postoperative value 3. Falling lactate immediately postoperatively	1. Increased WBC often due to reperfusion injury to graft 2. Well perfused stoma 3. Lactate slower to fall if aortic clamping required	1. Line sepsis from TPN catheter if not removed 2. Perforation or anastomotic leak 3. Spontaneous peritonitis 4. Liver graft dysfunction

*Oxygen delivery (DO₂) is defined by the following equation: $DO_2 = [(Hgb \times 1.3 \times SaO_2) + (PaO_2 \times .003)] \times$ cardiac output

pulmonary infections, and sepsis-related acute respiratory distress syndrome, in both adults and children. The trachea of most patients with isolated small intestinal transplants can be extubated within the first 24–48 hours. Patients with multivisceral transplants usually remain intubated for several days. This is particularly the case when a large graft size mandates delayed abdominal closure. Reoperations for partial closure may be required several times in the first week.

Generous fluid administration to maintain graft capillary blood flow may result in pulmonary edema, which may lead to significant intrapulmonary shunts, especially in the presence of bronchopulmonary dysplasia. Decreased chest wall and abdominal wall compliance secondary to edema, large graft size, ascites, and pleural effusions may further compromise pulmonary function. The high inspired oxygen concentrations or distending airway pressures needed to maintain the target hemoglobin oxygen saturations of >95% may lead to further pulmonary injury. In patients with severe lung disease, permissive hypercarbia may minimize such injury, with target tidal volumes of 6–8 cc/Kg body weight and plateau pressures <30 cmH$_2$O, as per the ARDSnet protocol. Patients after multivisceral transplants are at an increased risk for transient diaphragmatic dysfunction. This can be assessed with ultrasonography or fluoroscopy. Although this complication may lead to prolonged ventilation, it is almost always reversible with conservative management.

Renal

Renal dysfunction is common in transplant recipients. Factors such as preoperative renal dysfunction, episodic hypotension, calcineurin use, and nephrotoxic antibiotics conspire to cause renal dysfunction in up to 25% of patients with temporary dialysis required in up to 10% [10]. In addition, liver allograft dysfunction may lead to impairment in renal function. In general, the hemodynamic parameters discussed above to yield maximal oxygen delivery to the new intestine also insure renal perfusion (Table 32.1). In addition, the use of low-dose Dopamine (2.5–5.0 ug/kg/min) or Fenoldopam (0.03–0.1 ug/kg/min) may be of some benefit, despite the lack of clear proof in the literature. While in the intensive care unit, should dialysis be necessary, we prefer the use of continuous venovenous hemodialysis or hemofiltration to avoid rapid volume shifts which may adversely affect organ perfusion. In the presence of compromised renal function, leaky capillaries and hypoalbuminemia, high venous pressures may lead to generalized edema and worsening third space losses. Increased abdominal wall edema may also delay abdominal closure in patients with a prosthetic mesh covering the abdominal wound, In these cases, planned sequential abdominal lavage and staged closure after diuresis removes interstitial edema may be required. Albumin and loop diuretic administration are usually effective in achieving diuresis while maintaining intravascular volume.

Electrolyte

Imbalances must be corrected aggressively with intravenous delivery. The transplanted bowel will often exhibit calcium and magnesium malabsorption with high ileostomy outputs. Water, sodium, and bicarbonate are often lost in large quantities with high ileostomy outputs. This is more common after the first few days, and may lead to metabolic acidosis requiring sodium bicarbonate replacement. Hypomagnesemia will potentiate tacrolimus neurotoxicity and serum levels should therefore be maintained. Postoperative hyperglycemia is common in these patients. When the pancreas is transplanted with the allograft, close blood glucose monitoring is required. Hypoglycemia is a rare complication, even in small infants with compromised liver function, but may occur in patients receiving a pancreas transplant in whom the native pancreas is maintained. Based on recent evidence linking tight glycemic control with improved outcomes in critically ill surgical patients, insulin infusions are frequently used to maintain serum glucose levels between 80 and 150. This may be particularly relevant to the transplant population, as the reported survival advantage with this strategy was attributable to reduced septic complications.

Hematologic

Abnormalities including anemia, thrombocytopenia, prolonged prothrombin time, and increased INR are common in the postoperative period, especially in patients with preoperative liver dysfunction or when a hepatic graft is included, and are monitored closely. Packed red blood cells are administered to reach the target hematocrit levels. As mentioned above, plasma and platelet transfusions are used sparingly.

Infections

A major cause of morbidity and mortality in organ transplant recipients is infection (Table 32.1). Two of the easiest and most effective methods for preventing infections are strict adherence to aseptic technique when performing invasive procedures and dressing changes and hand washing before and after each patient contact. Furthermore, indwelling lines should be changed to a new site whenever there is external evidence of infection or positive blood cultures, keeping in mind the challenges imposed in finding venous access sites in these patients. The usual signs of infection such as fever and leukocytosis may be masked or absent in these patients. Furthermore, bacterial, viral, fungal, and protozoal infections are common in these patients and may be missed by general infection surveillance procedures [5]. It has been shown that conditions such as diabetes mellitus, hepatitis and uremia may predispose patients to infections following solid organ transplantation, as does the treatment of rejection episodes [5]. Intestinal transplant recipients are frequently colonized with multiple nosocomial organisms, some resistant to multiple antibiotics. Fungal colonization is also common, particularly in those with disorders of motility. Postoperatively, these patients are susceptible to bacterial translocation across the fragile intestinal graft. Sepsis in the first day or so may prompt reexploration. Positive cultures obtained later from abdominal drain fluid may come from graft lymphatic leakage and translocation of bacteria. These cultures usually grow gram-negative organisms and require antibiotic treatment. If there is no adequate response to antibiotic treatment, the patient will require exploration and washout.

Intravenous broad-spectrum antibiotics should be provided for several days after transplantation or until the first biopsy confirming mucosal integrity of the transplanted bowel has been obtained. The choice of antibiotics depends on results of cultures and sensitivities in the late pre-transplant period in the case of patients with recurrent bouts of line-related sepsis. After this time, antibiotic choice should be guided by culture results. The intestinal graft is very fragile and prone to perforations. High-dose steroids frequently mask the typical signs of peritonitis. Careful attention must be paid to subtle signs such as feeding intolerance, abdominal distention, low grade fever, persistent leukocytosis, falling hemoglobin, or rising or falling ileostomy output. A low threshold for reexploration has proved life-saving. Serum lactate levels may rise in the first 12–24 hours after intestinal transplantation, depending on pre-transplant graft ischemia time. A continuing rise of lactate levels after that time may indicate ongoing gut ischemia and may require surgical exploration.

Rejection

The diagnosis of allograft rejection is based on multiple parameters, the three most important of which are the clinical course, the endoscopic appearance of the allograft (Figure 32.2), and the histology of biopsy specimens. There is currently no reliable serum marker for intestinal rejection. Clinical changes that may indicate the onset of a rejection episode are various and nonspecific, so that clinical acumen and close observation are critical. The ileostomy output should be assessed for volume, color and consistency. Stomal output in the first week after transplantation is usually 1–2 liters/day for adults and 40–60 cc/kg/day for children, and this is usually clear or blood-tinged in the first few days. Effluent that becomes increasingly bloody and that is associated with a cyanotic or congested stoma is indicative of possible rejection or allograft ischemia. Increased stomal output is also a typical sign of rejection, and this may involve a secretory component of diarrhea. This will result in very high outputs and require cc/cc fluid replacement to avoid severe dehydration. Rejection may also be associated with any, or all, of the following symptoms and signs: abdominal pain, cramping, decreased stomal output, and an obstructive picture. These complaints should prompt radiologic evaluation to rule out mechanical obstruction and endoscopic biopsy of the allograft, not necessarily immediate operative intervention. Internal herniation of the intestine can occur; obstruction should be dealt with operatively if this situation is confirmed. If the graft includes other organs, appropriate serum markers for injury of those organs can be followed, but the majority

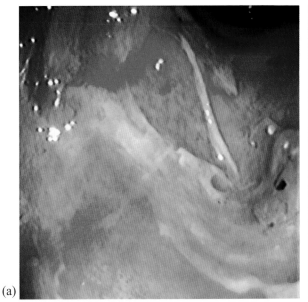

(a)

(b)

Figure 32.2 Graft investigation by ileoscopy is often performed at the bedside in the ICU early after transplantation in. (a) demonstrates severe rejection occurring early after transplantation (1 week) with sloughing of the mucosal lining from the submucosa. Although rarely encountered, this may be accompanied by a septic state during a period of heightened immunosuppression. (b) by contrast, demonstrates the normal appearance of transplanted intestinal mucosa, sometimes associated with mild increased lymphatic congestion as shown here. (Courtesy of Stuart S. Kaufman, MD.)

of intestinal rejection episodes occur in isolation, even when the bowel is transplanted with other organs. Serum amylase and lipase levels should be followed daily for multi-visceral allografts. Liver chemistries are followed with liver-containing allografts.

The stomach is never the site of severe rejection and should not be used as the basis for judging allograft integrity. Furthermore, when the colon is included in the allograft, the small intestine must be examined as well, as the colon is much less likely to be the site of rejection and therefore unreliable, if normal in appearance.

Nutritional management

Patients who are critically ill have significantly increased caloric and protein needs due to their hypermetabolic state leading to negative nitrogen balance and protein loss [7]. Furthermore, transplant patients may be malnourished preoperatively, and require nutritional support to enhance wound healing and leukocyte function. General guidelines for nutritional support include 1.75–2 grams protein/kilogram/day and 30–35 kilocalories/kilogram/day during the immediate postoperative period and at times of significant physiologic stress. Patients are continued on total parenteral nutrition in the early postoperative period. The function of the intestinal allograft is assessed daily, beginning in the operating room at the time of transplantation. Preservation injury or a positive lymphocytotoxic cross-match may result in edema and congestion of the allograft mucosa in the first few days after transplantation. Furthermore, the migrating motor complex and ordered motility are disrupted as a result of dennervation of the graft; these functions return at variable times after transplantation. Even when the allograft appears grossly normal, the histology taken at the time of transplantation may reveal severe mucosal disruption that would cause malabsorption. These factors conspire to produce a state of malabsorption in the early postoperative period.

Tube feedings are initially begun as an electrolyte solution followed by dipeptide-based isotonic or hypotonic formula in small volumes. Full strength feeds are not typically started until several weeks after transplantation, when the gut lymphatics adjust to absorb the fats. Intravenous fluids may still be required until free water can be given via an enteral tube to compensate for losses. These elemental feedings can later be modified, as tolerated, to provide increased caloric or protein needs, as guided by nutritional support recommendations.

High stomal output

The management of high stomal output in the absence of rejection will depend on studies of absorption, fecal fat content, motility and transit time. Watery diarrhea may respond initially to loperamide. Paragoric and pectin can be added to the enteral intake, but pectin should not be placed through a jejunostomy tube. Tincture of opium is effective if there is rapid transit. Furthermore, the addition of an alpha-adrenergic agent may improve intestinal motility because of an effect of the efferent reflex arc. Fat malabsorption and steatorrhea may be improved by the administration of pancreatic enzymes in patients who have had parenteral nutrition-related pancreatitis and who did not receive a pancreas with the allograft. Finally, cholestyramine may decrease choleretic diarrhea in patients with no ileocecal valve and bile salt malabsorption. These problems are at times difficult to delineate, and the evaluation for such etiologies of diarrhea, in the absence of evidence of rejection, should be thorough.

Summary

In summary, the immediate care of the intestinal transplant patient requires a knowledge of the organs transplanted and the early outcome of surgery, as well as the application of general principles of intensive care management of the transplant patient. The quality of early graft function of the intestine, liver, or pancreas components of the allograft will guide the delivery of metabolic, nutritional and cardiovascular support. The integration of the efforts and knowledge of the intensivist, transplant surgeon, and gastroenterologist assure

competent decision making in this critical phase of care of the transplant recipient.

References

1 United Network for Organ Sharing Web site (http:www.unos.org), 10/99.

2 Plotkin JS, Njoku MJ, Howell CD, et al. The evolution of a successful liver transplant program in 1996; The clinical and administrative role of the anesthesiologist. *Liver Transpl Surg* 1997;3:468–470.

3 Valeri CR, Crowley JP, Loscalzo J. The red cell transfusion trigger: has a sin of commission become a sin of omission? *Transfusion* 1998;38:602–610.

4 Flye MW. Immunosuppressive therapy. In: Flye MW, ed. *Principles of Organ Transplantation.* Philadelphia: WB Saunders, 1989.

5 Dunn DL, Najarian JS. Infectious complications in transplant surgery. In: Shires GT, Davis J, eds. *Principles and Management of Surgical Infection.* Philadelphia: JB Lippincott, 1990;425–464.

6 Brayman KL, Stephanian E, Matas AJ, et al. Analysis of infectious complications occurring after solid-organ transplantation. *Arch Surg* 1992;127:38–48.

7 Jeejeebhoy KN. Nutrition in critical illness. In: Ayres SM, Grenvik A, Holbrook PR, Shoemaker WC, eds: *Textbook of Critical Care, Third Edition.* Philadelphia: W.B. Saunders, 1995;1106–1115.

8 Parsa MH, Shoemaker WC. Enteral feeding. In: Ayres SM, Grenvik A, Holbrook PR, Shoemaker WC, eds: *Textbook of Critical Care, Third Edition.* Philadelphia: W.B. Saunders, 1995;1126–1134.

9 Aggarwal S, Kang Y, Freeman JA, et al. Postreperfusion syndrome: Cardiovascular collapse following hepatic reperfusion during liver transplantation. *Transplant Proc* 1987;19:54–55.

10 McCauley J, Van Thiel D, Starzl TE, et al. Acute and chronic renal failure after liver transplantation. *Nephron* 1990;55:121–128.

11 Marquez JM. Citrate intoxication during hepatic transplantation. In: Winter PM, Kang Y, eds. *Hepatic Transplantation: Anesthetic and Perioperative Management.* New York: Praeger, 1986;110–119.

12 Scott VL, De Wolf AM, Kang Y, et al. Ionized hypomagnesemia in patients undergoing orthotopic liver transplantation: A complication of citrate intoxication. *Liver Transpl Surg* 1996;2:343–347.

13 Carmichael FJ, Crawford MW, Khayyam N, et al. Effect of propofol infusion on splanchnic hemodynamics and

liver oxygen consumption in the rat: A dose response study. *Anesthesiology* 1993;79:1051–1060.

14 de Groen PC, Aksamit AJ, Rakela J, et al. Central nervous system toxicity after liver transplantation. *N Engl J Med* 1987;317:861–866.

15 Lee YJ, Lee SG, Kwon TW, et al. Neurologic complications after orthotopic liver transplantation including central pontine myelinolysis. *Transplant Proc* 1996;28:1674–1675.

16 Bernuau J, Rueff B, Benhamou JP. Fulminant and subfulminant liver failure: Definitions and causes. *Semin Liver Dis* 1986;6:97–106.

17 Schiodt FV, Atilasoy E, Shakil AO, et al. Etiology and outcome for 295 patients with acute liver failure in the United States. *Liver Transpl Surg* 1999;5:29–34.

18 Hoofnagle JH, Carithers RL, Shapiro C, Ascher N. Fulminant hepatic failure: Summary of a workshop. *Hepatology* 1995;21:240–252.

19 Williams R, Gimson AES. Intensive care and management of acute hepatic failure. *Dig Dis Sci* 1991;36:820–826.

20 Inagaki M, Shaw B, Schafer D, et al. Advantages of intracranial pressure monitoring in patients with fulminant hepatic failure. *Gastroenterology* 1992;102:A826.

21 Rolando N, Harvey F, Brahm J, et al. Prospective study of bacterial infection in acute liver failure: An analysis of fifty patients. *Hepatology* 1990;11:49–53.

33 Surgical Complications of Intestinal Transplantation

Wendy J. Grant

> **Key points**
>
> - Intestinal transplantation is a technically challenging operation.
> - Complications can be broken down into three categories—postoperative, vascular access, and endoscopic.
> - Reoperations are common.
> - Despite the challenges and complications, intestinal transplantation remains the standard therapy for patients with life-threatening complications of intestinal failure.

Intestinal transplantation is now accepted as life-saving therapy for patients with severe complications of intestinal failure. As with all transplants, the operative procedure is just one stage in the life-long commitment to transplantation. Although the transplant procedure is a small part of the whole process, the operation is technically challenging and therefore is fraught with potential complications. The spectrum of operations is addressed elsewhere in this text, and can be divided into those in which just the intestine (with or without the pancreas) is transplanted versus operations in which the liver is included (with stomach, duodenum, pancreas, intestine, or colon). The choice of organs to be transplanted is dependent on the needs of the patient and the experience of the transplant center. Essentially all patients that are candidates for

intestinal transplantation or undergo intestinal transplantation will have had previous abdominal operations and central line placements. One can break down the categories of complications into those involving the transplant operation itself and those resulting from other related procedures, such as procedures to achieve vascular access and endoscopy.

Operative complications

The history of intestinal transplantation is relatively short, and technical advances in performing the operation have made an impact on graft and patient survival. Two groups have described modifications to the combined liver and small bowel operation that have led to a decrease in biliary and vascular complications [1,2]. The original operation as described by Grant et al. [3] called for a complete hilar dissection and creation of a hepaticojejunostomy using the transplanted bowel. Biliary complication rates as high as 12% were reported. These complications, which included leaks and stenosis of the bile duct, were a result of the need for a donor hepaticojejunostomy to the donor bile duct [1]. The modification of leaving the hilum intact has essentially eliminated biliary complications from the liver-small bowel transplant operation. Clinically significant pancreatitis has been reported [2], but our experience with over 100 of these grafts has not revealed any instance of or life-threatening pancreatitis in the graft.

Intra-operative complications begin with the challenges of reoperative surgery, including inadvertent enterotomies, bleeding, and unexpected anatomical findings. Enterotomies in the bowel to be removed are not a problem, but injury to the native duodenum in

Intestinal Failure: Diagnosis, Management and Transplantation.
Edited by Alan N. Langnas, Olivier Goulet, Eamonn M.M. Quigley and Kelly A. Tappenden. © 2008 Blackwell Publishing.
ISBN 978-1-4051-4637-1.

patients undergoing isolated small bowel transplant, or those in whom the foregut is preserved, can pose long-term problems as the duodenum can be slow to heal and is prone to reperforation. Bleeding can be related to hepatic dysfunction in patients undergoing combined liver and small bowel transplants, but as anesthesia teams have become more adept at managing these patients intra-operatively, these problems occur less frequently.

Closure of the abdominal wall is a potential problem in patients who have had multiple prior operations and in whom loss of peritoneal domain may mean that the organs being transplanted necessitate tension on the abdominal wall at the time of closure. Use of prosthetic material is occasionally necessary, but is avoided, if at all possible. This being said, undue tension on the abdominal wall closure puts the patient at risk for dehiscence of the abdominal wall closure. The Miami group has reported transplantation of the abdominal wall in several patients undergoing intestinal transplantation. The vascular pedicle was based on the donor inferior epigastric vessels and the iliac vessels which were implanted separately onto the recipient iliacs. They reported that five of nine patients transplanted have long-term survival with an intact abdominal wall [4].

In the United Kingdom, pediatric donors are rare, so the group in Birmingham have routinely used adult donors as a source for their pediatric patients in need of liver and small bowel transplants. They use reduced size grafts—splitting the liver and removing a part of the intestine in order to have the organs fit into their patients [5].

Postoperatively, surgical complications can result from injury to the native or transplanted organs at the time of the initial operation or from preservation injury or immunologic insult which make the intestine prone to perforation. Intra-abdominal abscesses develop even without intestinal perforation, most likely from contamination of the peritoneal cavity at the time of removal of the native bowel. Fluid or blood that accumulates in the abdomen postoperatively may become secondarily infected and the most effective way to alleviate this problem is by reexploration with irrigation of the abdominal cavity. Hemostasis at the end of the transplant operation is essential to minimize the development of hematomas that may become secondarily infected.

Chylous ascites is not a well-reported complication, but might be expected given the extensive dissection performed in removing the remaining intestine and the implantation of the transplanted bowel without attention being paid to establishing lymphatic drainage. Reyes et al. reported in 1998 their experience to date with intestinal transplantation in children and reported that 4 of the 55 patients developed chylous ascites [6]. In the recent experience at the University of Nebraska, this complication had not been clinically significant. Many centers approach early feeding of the patients with low fat elemental formulas, which may decrease the lymphatic stimulation of the graft and allow the divided lymphatics to heal.

Complications of ostomies are uncommon, but prolapse and incarceration are possible. Long-term complications such as bowel obstruction are possible and would require operative intervention, as with obstruction of the native small bowel.

Rarely, surgical complications will result in the need to remove the graft. According to the Intestine Transplant Registry, 20.6% of grafts that were removed were due to thrombosis/ischemia or bleeding. An additional 13.1% do not specify the reasons for graft removal and could represent technical failures of the operation. Other reasons from graft removal are infectious and immunologic [7]. In a review of late causes of graft loss, Iyer et al. found that none were due to technical causes [8]. The updated experience at the University of Nebraska reveals that 63% of grafts lost in the first 90 days were a result of complications, such as thrombosis or perforation, and these primarily were isolated small bowel grafts.

Kato et al. reviewed the Miami experience with 141 intestinal transplants in 123 children. They found that 74 of the 123 children required reexploration following intestinal transplantation for bleeding, dehiscence, intraabdominal sepsis, obstruction, anastomotic leak, and a few other reasons. Their reoperative rate was 0.87 per patient [9]. Ruemele et al reviewed their experience in patients with microvillous inclusion disease undergoing intestinal transplantation. In the seven patients, six patients experienced technical complications following transplantation which included the need for colectomy, cholecystectomy, the creation of an ileostomy, as well as the development of a biliary leak, stoma prolapse and an abdominal wall abscess [10]. The Paris group described their experience

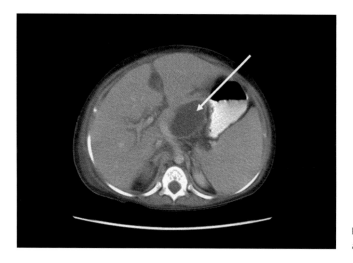

Figure 33.1 Contrast-enhanced CT showing abscess adjacent to aortic conduit.

with 52 children undergoing intestinal transplantation. Thirty-five of the 52 children had surgical complications that required return to the operating room. These complications included bleeding, thrombosis, biliary leak, perforation, obstruction, graft volvulus, and prolapse of the stoma. They also experienced problems with the abdominal wall in 12 of their patients. On average, their patients underwent 1.3 additional surgical procedures following the original intestinal transplant operation [11].

On review of 182 patients undergoing intestinal transplantation over a 15-year period at the University of Nebraska, only 41 patients did not require return to the operating room for exploration of the abdomen. The procedures performed included repair of perforation (n = 202), exploration without findings of perforation (n = 148), evacuation of hematoma (n = 36), relief of bowel obstruction (n = 23) and revision of intestinal anastomosis (n = 17). Other procedures included splenectomy (n = 34), placement of surgical feeding tubes (n = 18) and tracheostomy (n = 18). In addition, 42 procedures were performed for dehiscence and 5 for evisceration. To look specifically at the operations for bowel perforation, these 202 operations were performed in only 66 patients. Of these 66 patients, 40 of them underwent only 1 or 2 explorations for perforation, representing 47 of the 202 operations. The remaining 26 patients accounted for the bulk of the operations for perforation and underwent an average of 5.9 operations for perforation per patient.

Imaging of the abdomen plays an important role in diagnosing intra-abdominal pathology. Because of the degree of immunosuppression, physical exam and laboratory markers of infection (white cell count, acidosis) may also be unreliable.

In a review of radiographic findings after intestinal transplantation, Unsinn and his group demonstrated their experience with contrast-enhanced CT scans to diagnose intra-abdominal abscesses and vascular complications [12]. Contrast-enhanced CT scans are relatively easy to obtain and can be done in a timely fashion. Enhancement of a fluid collection indicates likely infection and often vascular structures can be delineated (Figure 33.1). Because of renal dysfunction that can be seen following transplant, the use of IV contrast is often undesirable. We have extensive experience with the use of non-contrast enhanced CT scans in patients in the early postoperative period and although there are limitations to these exams, they are often useful as screening tools when deciding about a patient's clinical status (Figure 33.2).

Vascular access

A lack of, or loss of, vascular access is a relatively common indication for small bowel transplantation. All

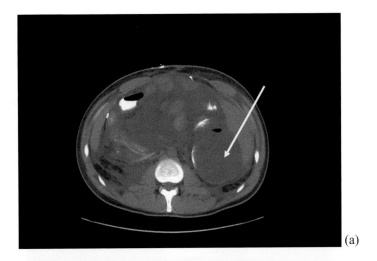

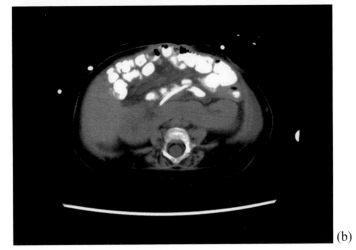

Figure 33.2 (a) Non-contrast-enhanced CT showing abscess—arrow indicates the fluid collection with air-fluid level. (b) Non-contrast-enhanced CT showing loops of transplanted bowel without abscess of perforation. Abdominal wall defect from open wound.

patients require central venous access for the transplant procedure and for management during the immediate post-operative period for TPN and other medications.

This patient population is unique in that thrombosis of the central veins is commonplace. There is a classification for degree of loss of vascular access [13]. A forum from the VIIIth International Small Bowel Transplant Symposium proposes that patients be classified according to number of thrombosed central veins as diagnosed by Doppler ultrasound. Although the group from Miami does not specifically address complications from line placement, they indicate that the degree of

vascular access lost does not have an impact on operative time for line placement. They examined 91 patients undergoing intestinal transplantation. The challenge of line placement in these patients is represented by "anesthesia time," which ranged from 15 to 240 minutes. Most of this time was consumed by line placements. Patients have an ongoing need for central venous access in the immediate postoperative period until they are weaned from TPN and this analysis predicts the challenge that could be faced. The Miami group again reported that 15% of the cases that they examined required balloon angioplasty of a central vein to maintain access following transplantation [13].

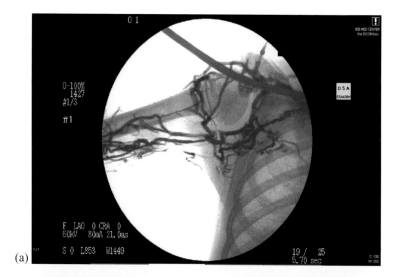

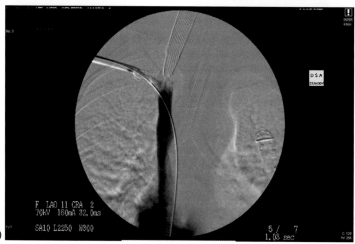

Figure 33.3 (a) Angiogram showing collateral flow around subclavian occlusion. (b) Angiographic image following stent placement in the internal jugular vein for treatment of SVC syndrome.

Braun et al. described their challenges with two patients with very limited vascular access, one of them requiring access following intestinal transplant. In this patient, the need for central venous access and anticoagulation led to complications with the stoma and the abdominal wall. Fortunately, once the patient was able to be sustained with enteral nutrition, the line was removed and by their report, the patient did well [14]. At the University of Nebraska, all patients undergo Doppler ultrasound of their central veins at the time of evaluation in order to document the degree of central venous thrombosis. The vast majority of central lines are placed by surgeons with occasional assistance from the interventional radiologists

in the few cases in which stent placement or angioplasty has been required (Figure 33.3). In reviewing 182 patients (159 children and 23 adults) undergoing intestinal transplantation, we found that 598 lines had been placed either at the time of transplantation or in the postoperative period. There were no deaths associated with these line placements. The most common indication for line placement was bacteremia. Patients with blood cultures positive for gram-positive bacteria and any hemodymanic instability have their lines removed as do patients with blood cultures positive for yeast or gram-negative rods. Lines are left out if possible for at least 24 hours before replacement.

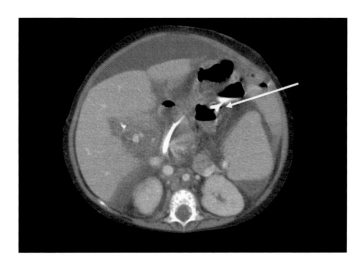

Figure 33.4 CT scan showing tip of the feeding tube outside of the lumen of the bowel—free fluid and air result from perforation.

Endoscopic complications

For patients undergoing intestinal transplantation, to date the only reliable method for detection of rejection is mucosal biopsy. Noninvasive methods for detection of rejection are being explored, but, as of yet, have not been validated. Biopsy surveillance requires endoscopy, most commonly through a stoma created partly for this purpose during the early post-transplant course. Complications of endoscopy include bleeding, hematoma causing obstruction of the lumen of the bowel, perforation and disruption of the stoma. All of these complications have been seen in intestinal transplant recipients; fortunately, no grafts have been lost or patients have died as a result of an endoscopic complication, but these do add to the morbidity of the intestinal transplant procedure. In addition, once patients have undergone take-down of the ileostomy, most patients require general anesthesia for endoscopic evaluation of the graft which poses additional risk. Intestinal transplant patients may be at increased risk of bleeding complications following endoscopic biopsy if they are on platelet inhibiting drugs, such as aspirin. In addition, many of these patients have hypersplenism as a result of their history of liver disease and may be thrombocytopenic.

Another aspect of patient care that is unique to intestinal transplantation is the need for feeding tube access to the graft. Most patients, especially children,

have oral aversion and require tube feedings until they relearn to eat. Perforations from feeding tube placement were common in our early experience (Figure 33.4) and we, therefore, avoid placement of feeding tubes into the graft at the time of transplant. Feeding jejunostomies present unique management issues and, in general, gastro-jejunostomies or nasal jejunal tubes are used for those patients that do not tolerate gastric feedings, or have had a partial gastrectomy. Placement of these tubes into the jejunum endoscopically presents another unique challenge for the endoscopist and remains a big part of management of the patient following intestinal transplantation.

Conclusions

Surgical complications following intestinal transplantation are universal and are to be expected. A need for reexploration is common. Complications of endoscopy, which is necessary for surveillance of rejection, are uncommon, but do represent a source of morbidity associated with intestinal transplantation. Placement of central venous catheters is a very common procedure that is necessary for the care of the intestinal transplant patient. It is made more challenging by the fact that all of these patients have had previous central lines placed, but it can be done safely without a significantly high complication rate. This review is limited by the lack of published data, but provides an overview of the surgical challenges faced when operating on patients with intestinal failure that require life-saving intestinal transplantation.

References

1 Sudan D, Iyer KR, Deroover A, et al. A new technique for combined liver/small intestinal transplantation. *Transplantation* 2001;72:1846–1848.

2 Bueno J, Abu-Elmagd K, Mazariegos G, et al. Composite liver-small bowel allografts with preservation of donor duodenum and hepatic biliary system in children. *J Pediatr Surg* 2000;35:291–296.

3 Grant D, Wall W, Mimeault R, et al. Successful small-bowel/liver transplantation. *Lancet* 1990;335:181–184.

4 Levi DM, Tzakis AG, Kato T, et al. Transplantation of the abdominal wall. *Lancet* 2003;361:2173–2176.

5 De Ville DG, Mitchell A, Mayer AD, et al. En block combined reduced-liver and small bowel transplants: from large donors to small children. *Transplantation* 2000;69:555–559.

6 Reyes J, Bueno J, Kocoshis S, et al. Current status of intestinal transplantation in children. *J Pediatr Surg* 1998;33:243–254.

7 Intestinal Transplant Registry, http://www. intestinaltransplant.org.

8 Iyer K, Kaufman S, Sudan D, et al. Long-term results of intestinal transplantation for pseudo-obstruction in children. *J Pediatr Surg* 2001;36:174–177.

9 Kato T, Tzakis A, Selvaggi G, et al. Intestinal and Multivisceral Transplantation in Children. *Ann Surg* 2006;243:756–766.

10 Ruemmele FM, Jan D, Lacaille F, et al. New perspectives for children with microvillous inclusion disease: rarly small bowel transplantation. *Transplantation* 2004;77:1024–1028.

11 Goulet O, Sauvat F, Ruemmele F, et al. Results of the paris program: ten years of pediatric intestinal transplantation. *Transplant Proc* 2005;37:1667–1670.

12 Unsinn KM, Koenigsrainer A, Rieger M, et al. Spectrum of imaging findings after intestinal, liver-intestinal, or multivisceral transplantation: part 2, posttransplantation complications. *Am J Roentgenol* 2004;183:1285–1291.

13 Selvaggi G, Gyamfi A, Kato T, et al. Analysis of vascular access in intestinal transplant recipients using the miami classification from the VIIIth international small bowel transplant symposium. *Transplantation* 2005;79:1639–1643.

14 Braun F, Platz KP, Faendrich F, et al. Management of venous access problems before and after intestinal transplantation: case reports. *Transplant Proc* 2004;36:392–393.

34 Infections in Small Bowel Transplant Recipients

Alison Freifeld and Andre Kalil

Key points

- Infections are the major cause of morbidity and mortality among small bowel transplant recipients, with over 90% developing an infection, primarily as a result of bacteria.

- Bacterial translocation across the intestinal wall, as a consequence of preservation injury, allows bacteria to enter normally sterile spaces.

- Early infections are acquired postoperatively in the hospital and may be caused by drug-resistant nosocomial pathogens.

- Increased immunosuppression, such as that used for managing rejection episodes, is associated with increased risk for infection.

- CMV is a common viral infection after small bowel transplantation but it is now often successfully prevented by antiviral prophylaxis and blood viral load testing with preemptive therapy.

Introduction: infection incidence

Infectious complications are a common cause of medical morbidity, graft loss and mortality in recipients of small bowel transplants [1–5]. Although surgical complications, acute rejection, multi-organ failure syndrome, and post-transplant lymphoproliferative disease (PTLD) may be anticipated in a minority of patients, infections occur in nearly every recipient of a small bowel graft and account for most of the poor

Intestinal Failure: Diagnosis, Management and Transplantation.
Edited by Alan N. Langnas, Olivier Goulet, Eamonn M.M. Quigley and Kelly A. Tappenden. © 2008 Blackwell Publishing.
ISBN 978-1-4051-4637-1.

outcomes following this procedure [6]. In a review of 117 intestinal transplants from the University of Nebraska in 2002, 93% of recipients experienced a bacterial infection, 25% had a fungal infection and 14% developed cytomegalovirus (CMV) infection [1]. Similarly, a series from the University of Pittsburgh in 2001 found that among 50 pediatric small bowel transplant recipients all had at least one infectious episode, with bacterial infections being observed in over 90% of patients [7]. In another series, from the Paris intestinal transplant program, viral infections such as adenovirus, rotavirus, CMV and Epstein-Barr (EBV) have been the predominant infections [8].

Infectious complications appear to be most frequent following multi-visceral organ transplants that include small intestine as well as in liver-small bowel transplants. By comparison, among isolated liver transplant recipients, rates of infection are in the range of 60–75% [9–11].

Pathogenesis: bacterial translocation

Under normal conditions, the bowel lumen acts a vessel for endogenous flora that aid in digestion and drug detoxification, whereas the bowel mucosa acts as a barrier to prevent those resident bacteria from gaining access to the bloodstream and other sites. It is hypothesized that trauma associated with transplantation compromises the barrier function of the bowel mucosa, allowing for translocation of endogenous intraluminal bacteria across a damaged mucosal surface and into otherwise sterile spaces such as the bloodstream or abdominal cavity [7]. Bacterial translocation has been associated with a variety of situations, including antibiotic therapy, total parenteral nutrition (TPN), ischemia/reperfusion injury, bacterial overgrowth, intestinal motility disorders, hepatic insufficiency, and an immunosuppressed state, all of which may occur in the setting of intestinal transplantation. In a study that measured bacterial translocation by the simultaneous identification of microorganisms in the blood or liver biopsy and in the stool, Cicalese and colleagues found that bacterial translocation episodes occurred in 44% of all small bowel transplant recipients [7]. Acute rejection was linked to nearly 40% of all episodes. A cold ischemia preservation time of less than 7 hours was associated with a 14% incidence of bacterial translocation whereas prolongation to 9 hours or longer was associated with bacterial translocation in 76% of patients. Efforts to limit cold ischemia times and decrease rejection episodes by employing more effective immunosuppressive regimens, such as tacrolimus, are associated with a lower risk of infection [12].

Early studies showed a trend toward higher rates of early bacterial infections in patients with small bowel grafts that included a colonic segment versus those that did not [13–15]. Higher graft and fecal bacterial counts found in these patients were thought to result in increased rates of bacterial translocation from the colonic portion of the graft, with consequent high rates of sepsis. The exclusion of the colonic segment has subsequently become standard in many centers that perform mall bowel transplantation, with significant improvements in survival [15,16]. However, others have successfully transplanted the right colonic segment on a routine basis, without any adverse effect on outcome [5].

Major risk factors for infection

Infection risk in intestinal transplantation is largely related to the surgical procedure itself and to the fact that the transplanted organ represents a reservoir of pathogens, as well as to associated peri-transplant medical conditions such as malnutrition, immunosuppression, and, especially, the impact of episodes of acute rejection [4,12]. Age at small bowel transplant of less than 1 year was associated with significantly higher death rates related to infections, in recent studies [17,18].

Although no studies have systematically assessed the many other potential risk factors for infection in this population, it is clear that many such factors exist. Renal insufficiency and increased blood product transfusion requirements peri-operatively have been associated with increased risk for bacterial infections after liver transplantation, and are likely to play a role in small bowel transplant recipients [10,19]. CMV and EBV reactivations and other serious viral infections are generally related to increased immunosuppression in organ transplant patients. Risk factors for candidemia in seriously ill patients include the presence of indwelling venous catheters, acute renal failure, recent abdominal surgery, broad spectrum antibiotics, and use of TPN, all of which are common among small bowel recipients postoperatively [20].

Bacterial infections

Bacterial infections are reported to occur in a majority of recipients after small bowel transplantation, generally in the first few weeks after surgery [21–23]. Common sites of infection, as identified in a recent prospective Italian study of 19 small bowel recipients, are bloodstream infections (including those related to catheters) 18%, urinary tract infections 15%, intra-abdominal infections, and peritonitis 14%, and pneumonias 14% [21]. Loinaz et al. from Miami found that catheter-related infections accounted for 30% of all infections, whereas wound infections and peritonitis were also very common [23]. These bacterial infections are largely related to the physical alterations in the abdomen that are consequent on surgery itself (e.g. anastomotic leak, vascular compromise, wound infection), as well as to the ubiquitous presence of indwelling plastic catheters and to the postoperative stresses of mechanical ventilation, malnutrition and exposure to nosocomial pathogens [14]. Skin and gut flora predominate as the most common pathogens, including Staphylococcal spp., enterococci, and enteric gram-negative rods such as *E. coli, Klebsiella*, and *Enterobacter*. Enteric gram-negative bacteremias especially tend to occur in association with rejection or gastrointestinal post-transplant lymphoproliferative disease and should prompt an evaluation for these possibilities [24]. Most postoperative pneumonias in SBT recipients are caused by gram-negative bacteria, predominantly *Pseudomonas aeruginosa* [21–23]. It is notable that ileoscopy with biopsy is an essential tool in the postoperative assessment of intestinal transplant recipients, particularly in cases of fever, diarrhea, or bleeding, where rejection or infection must be defined [25]. Complications of this procedure, including bacterial sepsis, are rare.

Gram-negative infections are often readily treated with agents such as piperacillin-tazobactam or a later generation cephalosporin (e.g. cefepime) that have good activity against nosocomially acquired resistant organisms. Piperacillin-tazobactam or a carbapenem (i.e. meropenem, imipenem) are also good choices for many strains of *Pseudomonas aeruginosa* (usually used in conjunction with a second active agent such as an aminoglycoside) as well as for intra-abdominal infections that are often due to a mixture of aerobic and anaerobic bacteria of gut origin. In hospitals where extended-spectrum beta-lactamases (ESBLs) are an intrinsic problem among *E. coli or Klebsiella* species, a carbapenem (i.e. imipenem or meropenem) may be required since they are the only drugs consistently reliable against these multiresistant pathogens. The restricted use of certain antibiotics is associated with significant reductions in these drug-resistant pathogens, so care should be taken to use antibiotics as specifically and appropriately as possible, for the bacteria isolated [26].

Staphylococcus epidermidis (coagulase negative staphylococcus) is the most common Gram positive bloodstream isolate in SBT patients [21]. Because coagulase negative staphylococci are common blood culture contaminants, a true bloodstream infection is diagnosed only if multiple blood cultures grow the organism. It tends to be a very weak pathogen, often associated with catheter infections. In most instances, coagulase negative staphylococcal catheter infections are readily cured with intravenous vancomycin. If vancomycin or another gram-positive active agent is started empirically (i.e. linezolid, daptomycin), it should be stopped as soon as cultures are deemed negative so as to avoid overuse of these antibiotics.

S. aureus bacteremias must be dealt with swiftly and effectively, as mortality is at least 20% [27]. Ideally, this should entail using a semisynthetic penicillin (oxacillin, nafcillin) for rapid killing of methicillin-susceptible organisms (MSSA), removal of the catheter in most cases, and a transesophageal echocardiogram to evaluate for endocarditis, which occurs in about 13% of individuals with *S. aureus* bacteremia [27,28].

Vancomycin should only be used for MRSA or in penicillin-allergic patients who have MSSA, as it has slower bacterial killing than penicillins. A minimum of 2 weeks of intravenous antibiotic therapy is regarded as the standard for uncomplicated *S. aureus* bacteremia, with 4–6 weeks for endocarditis, or other deep, or complicated, infections [28]. Daptomycin is an effective alternative for *S. aureus* bacteremia, but linezolid (a bacteristatic agent) has not been as rigorously studied [29,30].

Vancomycin-resistant enterococcus (VRE) is an increasingly problematic among hospitalized patients, especially following abdominal surgery. In liver transplantation, VRE infections have been associated with prior antibiotic use, multiple abdominal surgeries, biliary complications, and decreased survival compared to non-VRE control patients. Linezolid is a useful therapy for VRE and may improve survival [31].

Empirical antibiotic regimens for presumptive infections should be selected based upon clinical presentation and hospital flora susceptibility patterns. Every effort should be made, however, to obtain a specific microbiological diagnosis through procedures such as blood, urine or stool cultures, broncho-alveolar lavage (BAL) or percutaneous needle drainage or biopsy of collections or masses. Ultimately, the choice of a specific antibiotic regimen depends on the susceptibility of the isolate causing the infection. Surgical interventions such as drainage of abdominal collections or debridement of infected wounds are required for cure, along with adjunctive antibiotic therapy.

Viral infections

Primary or reactivated infections due to CMV and EBV are the most frequent causes of serious viral infection after small bowel transplant. These herpes viruses are typically acquired early in life and subsequently establish lifelong latency, with intermittent reactivations that are usually asymptomatic in the normal host. These viruses may be transmitted via the graft, so transfer of an organ from a CMV or EBV sero-positive donor to a sero-negative recipient confers the highest risk for developing invasive viral disease. Higher levels of immunosuppression and the use of anti-lymphocyte antibodies are also associated with increased risk for reactivations of these viruses [32].

Serious CMV infections and EBV-related PTLD are typically seen in seronegative recipients during the intermediate postoperative phase, usually between 1 and 6 months after small bowel transplantation when levels of immunosuppression are still relatively high, and both may be associated with significant graft loss and death [2,22].

EBV viremia is common following small bowel transplantation, occurring in as many as 60% of patients [33,34]. However, EBV-related PTLD has been reported to occur in about 11 to 30% of small bowel transplant recipients, occurring most often in the first 18 months but being reported as late as 4 years later [33,35,36] (see Chapter 39). Ganciclovir prophylaxis of high-risk patients (EBV seronegative recipients from seropositive donors) may reduce the incidence of PTLD [37]. Monitoring of EBV viral load by PCR may be a useful screening tool; however, prospective studies are still needed to evaluate the frequency and utility of this test for EBV-related diseases. Rising EBV viral load should prompt a careful examination searching for lymphadenopathy, and CT scans of chest and sinuses to look for signs of lymphoma. Biopsy of any abnormal lymph nodes should be pursued aggressively in an effort to make a diagnosis of PTLD. The negative predictive value of a low or undetectable EBV viral load is excellent [33]. In patients with a rising EBV viral load, the reduction of immunosuppression is a critical intervention, in an effort to allow natural immune defenses to control EBV replication. Intravenous ganciclovir may have some utility, although studies are not definitive [37,38]. In the event that PTLD is pathologically proven, an oncologist should become involved as therapy may involve cytotoxic chemotherapy and/or rituximab (anti-CD20 antibody). There is no evidence to suggest that rituximab should be given in the absence of a PTLD diagnosis.

CMV accounted for the majority of viral infections noted in a recent study of post-intestinal transplant infections, and most of these were asymptomatic reactivations in CMV seropositive (R+) recipients [21]. Invasive CMV infection can present with a wide range of symptoms and severity. Enteritis is the most common manifestation of severe disease in small bowel transplant recipients, with pneumonitis or hepatitis being much less frequent. Biopsy confirms the diagnosis of deep tissue CMV infection. "CMV syndrome" characterized by fever, leukopenia, thrombocytopenia, and atypical lymphocytosis may also occur in SBT recipients. The development of any of these symptoms or signs should prompt testing for peripheral blood CMV viral load by PCR or pp65 antigenemia test, to evaluate for CMV as the possible etiology. Because CMV PCR is not standardized (as most PCRs) among different transplant centers, the frequency of testing and cutoff number of copies/ml is based on each institution's assay validation and clinical experience. For example, at University of Nebraska, most of patients who develop CMV disease have greater than 10,000 copies/ml at initial PCR evaluation. Intravenous ganciclovir is the therapy of choice for invasive CMV disease; intravenous gamma globulin may provide additional benefit but more studies are needed. For "CMV syndrome" or asymptomatic reactivation, oral valganciclovir is an effective therapy. It is important to recognize that the "indirect effects" of primary or reactivation CMV infection (even asymptomatic reactivations) include immune dysregulation and white blood cell dysfunction with increased susceptibility to invasive bacterial and fungal infections [39,40].

The incidence of adenovirus infection ranged from 4% to 100% in one outbreak among SBT recipients, with the majority of invasive enteric infections occurring in the first month post-transplant; disease may also occur sporadically at >1 year after transplant [41,42]. Adenovirus enteritis appears to be most frequent in pediatric patients receiving composite liver and intestinal allografts. It often causes ulcerations in the bowel and may be clinically indistinguishable from graft rejection, CMV infection, or other causes of enteritis. Biopsy with immunohistochemical stains specific for adenovirus will aid accurate diagnosis. Nosocomial transmission can occur, although it has been hypothesized that the graft is the viral source due to the persistence of adenovirus in an infected host for months to years. Dissemination is uncommon but if it occurs, is associated with a mortality rate of at least 50% in immunosuppressed patients. No association between intensity of immunosuppression, incidence of acute rejection and risk for adenovirus invasive disease could be found in a recent study of intestinal transplant recipients, making it difficult to predict which patients might develop disease [42]. There is no current standard therapy for adenovirus disease, although a reduction in immunosuppression is an important measure [32,41]

Recently described calicivirus infections, caused by noroviruses, are a common cause of mild gastroenteritis in normal children but may cause a prolonged diarrheal illness and graft dysfunction in pediatric small bowel transplant recipients [43]. Molecular testing of emesis or stools makes the diagnosis; there is no specific treatment for norovirus diarrhea.

Fungal infections

Fungal infections are reported to occur in 10–70% of small bowel recipients, usually in the first postoperative month [14,21]. *Candida* spp. account for nearly all fungal infections in the small bowel transplant setting and are usually associated with intra-abdominal or indwelling venous catheter infections. Candidemia is generally associated with attributable mortality rates as high as 40% in some series, and is a risk for death and graft loss specifically in SBT recipients [5]. Early initiation of therapy for presumed candidemia in high risk patients such as those who are postoperative or in the intensive care unit, decreases hospital mortality [44].

The management of candidemia requires catheter removal and replacement at a different site as well as, and an ophthalmologic exam to rule out candida endophthalmitis. A minimum of 2 weeks antifungal therapy from the first documented negative blood culture. In most cases, *C. albicans* is the culprit and is generally susceptible to fluconazole. Species such as *C. krusei* or *C. glabrata* should be treated with a newer azole or echinocandin as they are often less susceptible to fluconazole.

Infectious diarrhea

Diarrhea is a common occurrence following SBT and is often multifactorial in origin. Standard evaluation for infectious causes should include stool assays for *Clostridium difficile*, adenovirus, rotavirus and norovirus. Enteric pathogen cultures can be sent for Salmonella, Shigella and *E. coli* 0157:H7 if the patient has been living outside of the hospital environment. Post-transplant lymphoproliferative disorder, bacterial overgrowth, cryptosporidiosis or cytomegalovirus may be identified by endoscopy and biopsy, which should be performed in all cases of unexplained post-transplant diarrhea [5,45,46].

Preventive strategies for infection

Some transplant programs provide prophylactic intravenous broad spectrum systemic antibiotics and oral bowel decontaminating antibiotics until recovery of intestinal transit while others do not continue antibiotics past surgery [1,8]. General recommendations for antimicrobial prophylaxis for colorectal operations include a preoperative parenteral antimicrobial, such as cefotetan or cefoxitin, given for no more than 24 hours after surgery. There is no clear evidence of benefit for longer antibiotic coverage in the SBT recipient. However, high-dose immunosuppression, the presence of wounds, drains and catheters, intubation, and potential anastamotic leaks are risk factors that require physicians to maintain vigilance for detecting infections in the immediate postoperative period. Daily examination of the patient, with special attention to changes in the abdominal examination, catheter and wound sites, temperature and white blood count trends, and stool outputs are essential. A recent retrospective study of surveillance stool cultures after pediatric small bowel transplantation revealed no predictive value for such cultures [47]. There are no data to support protective isolation of SBT recipients but, again, this practice varies by program.

The prevention of CMV reactivation and symptomatic infection can be effectively accomplished by either universal antiviral prophylaxis of all recipients, or by preemptive strategies to selectively treat only those with an increased CMV viral load detected by PCR or pp65 antigen assay. Current data from a large meta-analysis of trials in other solid organ transplant types suggest that universal prophylaxis reduces several indirect effects from CMV, such as bacterial and fungal infections, allograft rejection, and death [48].

High-dose acyclovir, valacyclovir, ganciclovir, valganciclovir, and CMVIG have all been used to prevent CMV infections among other SOT patients. No comparative trial data are specifically available for small bowel transplant patients. However, valganciclovir prophylaxis did not receive the FDA indication for liver recipients because of a significantly higher rate of CMV invasive disease than prophylaxis with ganciclovir. No drugs have been proved to fully prevent EBV-induced PTLD. However, one observational study [49] and one cohort (with historical controls) study [50] suggest that EBV viral load monitoring (monthly or bimonthly) followed by preemptive reduction of immunosuppression may prevent PTLD in pediatric liver transplant recipients. This data is promising, but it needs to be tested in prospective studies with concurrent controls in order to change standard of care.

A recent meta-analysis of fluconazole prophylaxis in critically ill patients with significant risk factors for invasive candidiasis showed that the intervention reduces invasive fungal infections by one-half and total mortality by one-quarter [51]. Risk factors for invasive candidiasis include immunosuppression, indwelling catheters, broad-spectrum antibiotics, hyperalimentation, acute renal failure, and Candida colonization. Extending this data to SBT recipients, we recommend that patients found to be colonized at any site with *Candida* spp. in the early postoperative period should start prophylaxis with fluconazole or an echinocandin, until their risk for invasive candidiasis is diminished [51,52].

References

1 Langnas A, Chinnakotla S, Sudan D, et al. Intestinal transplantation at the University of Nebraska Medical Center: 1990 to 2001. *Transplant Proc* 2002;34:958–960.

2 Todo S, Reyes J, Furukawa H, et al. Outcome analysis of 71 clinical intestinal transplantations. *Ann Surg* 1995;222:270–280; discussion 280–2.

3 Cicalese L, Sileri P, Coady N, et al. Proposed protocol to reduce bacterial infectious complications in living related small bowel transplant recipients. *Transplant Proc* 2002;34:950.

4 Nishida S, Levi D, Kato T, et al. Ninety-five cases of intestinal transplantation at the University of Miami. *J Gastrointest Surg* 2002;6:233–239.

5 Sauvat F, Dupic L, Caldari D, et al. Factors influencing outcome after intestinal transplantation in children. *Transplant Proc* 2006;38:1689–1691.

6 Farmer DG, McDiarmid SV, Yersiz H, et al. Outcome after intestinal transplantation: results from one center's 9-year experience; discussion 1031–2. *Arch Surg* 2001;136:1027–1031.

7 Cicalese L, Sileri P, Green M, et al. Bacterial translocation in clinical intestinal transplantation. *Transplantation* 2001;71:1414–1417.

8 Goulet O, Sauvat F, Ruemmele F, et al. Results of the Paris program: ten years of pediatric intestinal transplantation. *Transplant Proc* 2005;37:1667–1670.

9 Garcia S, Roque J, Ruza F, et al. Infection and associated risk factors in the immediate postoperative period of pediatric liver transplantation: a study of 176 transplants. *Clin Transplant* 1998;12:190–197.

10 Hadley S, Samore MH, Lewis WD, et al. Major infectious complications after orthotopic liver transplantation and comparison of outcomes in patients receiving cyclosporine or FK506 as primary immunosuppression. *Transplantation* 1995;59:851–859.

11 Singh N, Gayowski T, Wagener M, Yu VL. Infectious complications in liver transplant recipients on tacrolimus. Prospective analysis of 88 consecutive liver transplants. *Transplantation* 1994;58:774–778.

12 Di Benedetto F, Lauro A, Masetti M, et al. Outcomes after adult isolated small bowel transplantation: experience from a single European centre. *Dig Liver Dis* 2005;37:240–246.

13 Cicalese L, Sileri P, Green M, et al. Bacterial translocation in clinical intestinal transplantation. *Transplant Proc* 2000;32:1210.

14 Kusne S, Furukawa H, Abu-Elmagd K, et al. Infectious complications after small bowel transplantation in adults: an update. *Transplant Proc* 1996;28:2761–2762.

15 Furukawa H, Reyes J, Abu-Elmagd K, et al. Intestinal transplantation at the University of Pittsburgh: six-year experience. *Transplant Proc* 1997;29:688–689.

16 Abu-Elmagd K, Reyes J, Todo S, et al. Clinical intestinal transplantation: new perspectives and immunologic considerations. *J Am Coll Surg* 1998;186:512–25; discussion 525–7.

17 Gaynor JJ, Kato T, Selvaggi G, et al. The importance of analyzing graft and patient survival by cause of failure: an example using pediatric small intestine transplant data. *Transplantation* 2006;81:1133–1140.

18 Kato T, Tzakis AG, Selvaggi G, et al. Intestinal and multivisceral transplantation in children. *Ann Surg* 2006;243:756–64; discussion 764–6.

19 Husain S, Tollemar J, Dominguez EA, et al. Changes in the spectrum and risk factors for invasive candidiasis in liver transplant recipients: prospective, multicenter, case-controlled study. *Transplantation* 2003;75:2023–2029.

20 McKinnon PS, Goff DA, Kern JW, et al. Temporal assessment of Candida risk factors in the surgical intensive care unit. *Arch Surg* 2001;136:1401–1408; discussion 1409.

21 Guaraldi G, Cocchi S, Codeluppi M, et al. Outcome, incidence, and timing of infectious complications in small

bowel and multivisceral organ transplantation patients. *Transplantation* 2005;80:1742–1748.

22 Lauro A, Di Benedetto F, Masetti M, et al. Twenty-seven consecutive intestinal and multivisceral transplants in adult patients: a 4-year clinical experience. *Transplant Proc* 2005;37:2679–2681.

23 Loinaz C, Kato T, Nishida S, et al. Bacterial infections after intestine and multivisceral transplantation. *Transplant Proc* 2003;35:1929–1930.

24 Sigurdsson L, Reyes J, Kocoshis SA, et al. Bacteremia after intestinal transplantation in children correlates temporally with rejection or gastrointestinal lymphoproliferative disease. *Transplantation* 2000;70:302–305.

25 Sigurdsson L, Reyes J, Putnam PE, et al. Endoscopies in pediatric small intestinal transplant recipients: five years experience. *Am J Gastroenterol* 1998;93:207–211.

26 Owens RC, Jr., Rice L. Hospital-based strategies for combating resistance. *Clin Infect Dis* 2006;42(Suppl 4):S173–S181.

27 Chang FY, MacDonald BB, Peacock JE, et al. A prospective multicenter study of Staphylococcus aureus bacteremia: incidence of endocarditis, risk factors for mortality, and clinical impact of methicillin resistance. *Medicine (Baltimore)* 2003;82:322–332.

28 Mitchell DH, Howden BP. Diagnosis and management of Staphylococcus aureus bacteraemia. *Intern Med J* 2005;35 (Suppl 2):S17–S24.

29 Fowler VG, Jr., Boucher HW, Corey GR, et al. Daptomycin versus standard therapy for bacteremia and endocarditis caused by Staphylococcus aureus. *N Engl J Med* 2006;355:653–665.

30 Shorr AF, Kunkel MJ, Kollef M. Linezolid versus vancomycin for Staphylococcus aureus bacteraemia: pooled analysis of randomized studies. *J Antimicrob Chemother* 2005;56:923–929.

31 Gearhart M, Martin J, Rudich S, et al. Consequences of vancomycin-resistant Enterococcus in liver transplant recipients: a matched control study. *Clin Transplant* 2005;19:711–716.

32 Manez R, Kusne S, Abu-Elmagd K, et al. Factors associated with recurrent cytomegalovirus disease after small bowel transplantation. *Transplant Proc* 1994;26:1422–1423.

33 Green M, Bueno J, Rowe D, et al. Predictive negative value of persistent low Epstein-Barr virus viral load after intestinal transplantation in children. *Transplantation* 2000;70:593–596.

34 Pascher A, Klupp J, Schulz RJ, et al. CMV, EBV, HHV6, and HHV7 infections after intestinal transplantation without specific antiviral prophylaxis. *Transplant Proc* 2004;36:381–382.

35 Quintini C, Kato T, Gaynor JJ, et al. Analysis of risk factors for the development of posttransplant lymphoprolipherative disorder among 119 children who received primary intestinal transplants at a single center. *Transplant Proc* 2006;38:1755–1758.

36 Finn L, Reyes J, Bueno J, Yunis E. Epstein-Barr virus infections in children after transplantation of the small intestine. *Am J Surg Pathol* 1998;22:299–309.

37 McDiarmid SV, Jordan S, Kim GS, et al. Prevention and preemptive therapy of postransplant lymphoproliferative disease in pediatric liver recipients. *Transplantation* 1998;66:1604–1611.

38 Holmes RD, Orban-Eller K, Karrer FR, et al. Response of elevated Epstein-Barr virus DNA levels to therapeutic changes in pediatric liver transplant patients: 56-month follow up and outcome. *Transplantation* 2002;74:367–372.

39 Paya CV. Indirect effects of CMV in the solid organ transplant patient. *Transpl Infect Dis* 1999;1(suppl 1):8–12.

40 Preiksaitis JK, Brennan DC, Fishman J, Allen U. Canadian society of transplantation consensus workshop on cytomegalovirus management in solid organ transplantation final report. *Am J Transplant* 2005;5:218–227.

41 Parizhskaya M, Walpusk J, Mazariegos G, Jaffe R. Enteric adenovirus infection in pediatric small bowel transplant recipients. *Pediatr Dev Pathol* 2001;4:122–128.

42 Pinchoff RJ, Kaufman SS, Magid MS, et al. Adenovirus infection in pediatric small bowel transplantation recipients. *Transplantation* 2003;76:183–189.

43 Morotti RA, Kaufman SS, Fishbein TM, et al. Calicivirus infection in pediatric small intestine transplant recipients: pathological considerations. *Hum Pathol* 2004;35:1236–1240.

44 Morrell M, Fraser VJ, Kollef MH. Delaying the empiric treatment of candida bloodstream infection until positive blood culture results are obtained: a potential risk factor for hospital mortality. *Antimicrob Agents Chemother* 2005;49:3640–3645.

45 Gerber DA, Green M, Jaffe R, et al. Cryptosporidial infections after solid organ transplantation in children. *Pediatr Transplant* 2000;4:50–55.

46 Mack DR, Dhawan A, Kaufman SS, Langnas AN, Seemayer TA. Small bowel bacterial overgrowth as a cause of chronic diarrhea after liver transplantation in children. *Liver Transpl Surg* 1998;4:166–169.

47 John M, Gondolesi G, Herold BC, et al. Impact of surveillance stool culture guided selection of antibiotics in the

management of pediatric small bowel transplant recipients. *Pediatr Transplant* 2006;10:198–204.

48 Kalil AC, Levitsky J, Lyden E, et al. Meta-analysis: the efficacy of strategies to prevent organ disease by cytomegalovirus in solid organ transplant recipients. *Ann Intern Med* 2005;143:870–880.

49 Kogan-Liberman D, Burroughs M, Emre S, et al. The role of quantitative Epstein-Barr virus polymerase chain reaction and preemptive immunosuppression reduction in pediatric liver transplantation: a preliminary experience. *J Pediatr Gastroenterol Nutr* 2001;33:445–449.

50 Lee TC, Savoldo B, Rooney CM, et al. Quantitative EBV viral loads and immunosuppression alterations can decrease PTLD incidence in pediatric liver transplant recipients. *Am J Transplant* 2005;5:2222–2228.

51 Playford EG, Webster AC, Sorrell TC, Craig JC. Antifungal agents for preventing fungal infections in non-neutropenic critically ill and surgical patients: systematic review and meta-analysis of randomized clinical trials. *J Antimicrob Chemother* 2006;57:628–638.

52 Sobel JD, Rex JH. Invasive candidiasis: turning risk into a practical prevention policy? *Clin Infect Dis* 2001;33:187–190.

35 Immunosuppression after Intestinal Transplantation

Raquel Garcia-Roca and Rainer Gruessner

Key points

- The general principles of immunosuppressive therapy for intestinal transplant recipients are the same as for other solid-organ recipients.

- For induction therapy, the use of antibodies has resulted in favorable outcomes, although the appropriate amount of antibody induction therapy remains controversial.

- Maintenance immunosuppressive therapy after intestinal transplants should be tacrolimus-based. The use of other maintenance agents has been much less consistent over time, but sirolimus appears to be more frequently used than others.

- In contrast to other solid-organ transplants, severe rejection after intestinal transplants has been associated not only with graft loss but also with a relatively high rate of recipient death.

- Most rejection episodes, particularly those associated with sloughing of mucosa, ulcers, and exfoliation, are treated with a 5- to 7-day course of antibody therapy.

Introduction

The intestine is the most immunogenic of all transplanted solid organs. Its high immunogenicity is one of the main reasons that the results of intestinal transplants trail those of all other solid-organ transplants. To improve outcome in this field, the quest for optimal immunosuppressive therapy is crucial. According to the

Intestinal Failure: Diagnosis, Management and Transplantation.
Edited by Alan N. Langnas, Olivier Goulet, Eamonn M.M. Quigley and Kelly A. Tappenden. © 2008 Blackwell Publishing. ISBN 978-1-4051-4637-1.

Intestinal Transplant Registry (ITR), 1-year graft survival rates in all three intestinal recipient categories—intestinal transplant alone (ITA), simultaneous intestinal and liver transplant (SILT), and multivisceral transplant (MVT)—are very similar, ranging from 59% to 65% [1]. In contrast, 1-year patient survival rates differ by category: higher for ITA recipients (77%) than for SILT (60%), and MVT (66%) recipients [2].

The first intestinal transplant was performed in 1967 by Richard Lillehei at the University of Minnesota [2], yet a breakthrough in this field was not achieved until the immunosuppressant tacrolimus became available in the early 1990s [3]. Just as cyclosporine 10 years earlier had propelled kidney, liver, and heart transplantation into a new era, the introduction of tacrolimus marked the beginning of a new era in intestinal transplantation.

The general principles of immunosuppressive therapy for intestinal transplant recipients are the same as for other solid-organ recipients. But, because of the high immunogenic load and the strong expression of histocompatibility antigens by intestinal grafts, it was initially believed that the amount of immunosuppression required had to be more than that for kidney, liver, or heart transplant recipients [4,5]. This dictum is certainly true for preventing frequent and refractory rejection episodes (and concurrent infections, given the intestinal graft's mucosal breakdown and resulting bacterial translocation). Nonetheless, it was realized in the mid-1990s that "overimmunosuppression" could cause posttransplant lymphoproliferative disease (PTLD) and, less frequently, graft-vs-host-disease (GVHD). Over the last decade, it has become apparent that immunosuppressive therapy after intestinal transplants must be finessed, such that rejection, PTLD, and GVHD are all prevented.

The appropriate amount of antibody induction therapy for achieving this goal remains controversial and has included options ranging from a full 5- to 7-day course of polyclonal antibodies to no antibody treatment at all. The need for concurrent immunomodulatory strategies is also unclear (e.g., donor-specific cell augmentation, donor or graft pretreatment). What is certain at this time is that maintenance immunosuppressive therapy after intestinal transplants must be based on tacrolimus (not cyclosporine [CSA]). A second drug, such as sirolimus (rapamycin) or mycophenolate mofetil (MMF), might be added as a potential adjunct. Steroid withdrawal or avoidance is as much a goal after intestinal transplants as after other solid-organ transplants, but most intestinal transplant recipients remain on steroids for maintenance therapy [1,6].

Other unresolved issues include the following:

1 Should the amount of immunosuppression be based on the recipient category, with more immunosuppression given to ITA (vs. SILT and MVT) recipients? Intestinal grafts are believed to be protected immunologically by a simultaneously transplanted liver [5,7].

2 Should the amount of immunosuppression be the same for recipients of living donor (LD) and deceased donor (DD) grafts? ITR data currently do not show an impact of HLA-matching on outcome; however, intestinal transplants between HLA-identical twins do not require posttransplant immunosuppression at all and, in our own experience, transplants between HLA-identical nontwin siblings require significantly less immunosuppressive therapy [8–11].

3 Should the amount of immunosuppression be different for pediatric and adult intestinal recipients, based on age-related differences in the pharmacokinetics of immunosuppressive drugs?

All available drugs for induction and maintenance therapy have been used in intestinal transplant recipients. To the best of our knowledge, no prospective or randomized study comparing immunosuppressive regimens after intestinal transplants has been reported, because of the overall small number of recipients. The quest for more specific, yet less toxic immunosuppression is also crucial for improving long-term outcomes after intestinal transplants. To achieve this goal, two approaches are possible. First, immunosuppressive trials should focus less on short-term (i.e., 1 year posttransplant) outcome and more on long-term graft function, reducing drug toxicity, and long-term economic and quality of life issues. Second, genotype and molecular or immune monitoring should be used to individualize immunosuppressive therapy. Currently in its infancy, genotype and molecular monitoring may allow identification of low, intermediate, and high (recipient and donor) responder groups. Such individualized immunosuppressive therapy may ultimately result in improved patient and graft outcome, reduced comorbidities (e.g. bone loss, hypertension, nephrotoxicity), reduced metabolic complications (e.g. hyperlipidemia, diabetes mellitus), and improved compliance—thanks to simpler dosing and fewer drug-related side effects.

Induction therapy

The term "induction therapy" is used to describe the administration of mono- or polyclonal antilymphocyte antibody therapy for a short course, immediately pre- or posttransplant. The rationale for potent immunosuppressive antibody therapy is to diminish the host immune response to the graft. It also provides a therapeutic window during which the administration of calcineurin inhibitors can be delayed, reduced in terms of dose, or avoided altogether. Induction therapy has also been associated with "conditioning" effects in the recipient that may induce immunologic hyporesponsiveness by eliciting peripheral and central depletion of all lymphocyte subsets.

Over time, all types of available polyclonal antibodies (e.g. equine and rabbit antithymocyte or antilymphocyte preparations) and monoclonal antibodies (e.g. muromonab-CD3, interleukin-2 receptor blockers, alemtuzumab) have been used after intestinal transplants without one agent establishing clinical predominance. However, the most recent ITR report indicates that, in a log-logistical model, factors associated with improved graft and patient survival rates include the use of induction antibody therapy, either with interleukin-2 receptor blockers or with antithymocyte or antilymphocyte preparations [1]. In contrast, the monoclonal antibody muromonab-CD3 (Orthoclone OKT3, Orthobiotec, Raritan, NJ) is rarely used anymore for induction therapy. Cyclophosphamide is no longer used for induction therapy, because it was shown that it did not prolong survival [12,13] but, rather, increased the risk of bacterial infections [14].

Recent single-center publications have reported favorable outcome with the following antibodies: (1) interleukin-2 receptor (IL2R) blockers; (2) antilymphocyte antibodies; and (3) alemtuzumab (Table 35.1). Favorable results with the use of interleukin-2 receptor blockers were first noted by the Pittsburgh group [15,16]. The Miami group reported that the use of daclizumab (a humanized, genetically engineered, IgG 1 monoclonal antibody specific for CD25) resulted in a significant reduction in the incidence and severity of acute rejection episodes [17]. Because daclizumab blocks the binding of interleukin-2 to its receptor on T cells undergoing activation, its specific, targeted mechanism of action eliminates many of the unwarranted side effects of polyclonal antibodies.

In the Miami protocol, daclizumab (2 mg/kg) was given intravenously intraoperatively and once every 14 days thereafter for a total of 6 doses, followed by a dose of 1 mg/kg once every 14 days for an additional 6 doses (12 in all) [17]. Likewise, the Nebraska group reported that the use of basiliximab led to a significant decrease in the incidence and in the median number of acute rejection episodes after intestinal transplants. At 1 year posttransplant, 68% of patients receiving basiliximab remained free from rejection versus only 18% of controls [4]. According to the Nebraska protocol, basiliiximab was given immediately after reperfusion of the intestinal graft in the operating room; a second dose was administered on posttransplant day 4. The Miami and the Nebraska studies included ITA, SILT, and MVT recipients. The incidence of infectious complications did not increase with daclizumab or basiliximab; in fact, in the Nebraska experience, it even decreased. According to the ITR, the use of induction antibody therapy directed against interleukin-2 receptors resulted in significantly higher graft and patient survival rates in recipients who did (vs. did not) receive such antibodies (p > 0.002) [1]. However, despite these encouraging results, interleukin-2 receptor blockers have not eliminated the occurrence of exfoliative rejection.

The Miami group recently reported their preliminary experience with the humanized monoclonal CD52 antibody alemtuzumab in all three intestinal recipient categories (n = 24). Alemtuzumab was administered in four doses: preoperatively, at the completion of the transplant procedure, and on posttransplant days 3 and 7. With alemtuzumab, the Miami group observed a trend toward a reduced incidence and a reduced severity of rejection episodes; it also enabled most recipients to avoid maintenance adjuvant steroid treatment and to halving their usual dose of tacrolimus. Of note, the incidence of opportunistic infections did not increase (follow-up, 2 to 16 months) [18]. However, a subsequent study on the use of alemtuzumab in pediatric recipients showed unfavorable results, so its use was then limited to patients at least 4 years of age [19,20]. Another study revealed increased intraoperative bleeding in liver transplant recipients when a preoperative dose of alemtuzumab was used, so the initial four doses were changed to two doses (on posttransplant days 1 and 4) [21].

The Pittsburgh group has reported favorable outcome with pretransplant administration of 5 mg/kg of rabbit antilymphocyte globulin and with posttransplant tacrolimus monotherapy, with subsequent dose spacing [22,23]. In pediatric recipients, it was technically difficult to infuse the whole dose before graft reperfusion, so the dose was divided and given pre- and postreperfusion [13]. This protocol produced higher 1-year graft (100%) and patient survival rates (100%), as compared with earlier protocols that used cyclophosphomide or daclizumab for induction therapy (75%, graft; 77%, patient) or as compared with maintenance tacrolimus and steroid therapy without induction therapy (76%, graft; 81%, patient). The use of antilymphocyte conditioning for induction and steroid-free posttransplant tacrolimus monotherapy resulted in less immunosuppression and in a lower rate of infectious diseases, such as cytomegalovirus and Epstein-Barr virus [13]. The strategy to raise the intervals between doses rather than to reduce daily amounts of tacrolimus is novel; the ultimate objective is to find the lowest maintenance drug dose consistent with stable graft function [22]. According to ITR data, graft and patient survival rates were significantly higher when induction antibody therapy directed against T or B lymphocytes was (vs. was not) used (p > 0.008) [1].

Thus, antibody-based induction therapy of any kind has been one of the main reasons for improved outcome after intestinal transplants. Not surprisingly, a United Network for Organ Sharing (UNOS) analysis noted a 43% increase in the use of antibody induction therapy over the last decade [6]. Yet, the optimal type of induction therapy remains to be defined, given the overall low number of intestinal transplants and the

Table 35.1 Review of current immusuppressive protocols at leading intestinal transplant centers worldwide.

Transplant program	Donor pre treatment	Induction	Calcineurin inhibitor	Mycophenolate	Sirolimus
University of Nebraska	Thymoglobulin	Anti-IL2R agent or thymoglobulin (6 mg/kg divided doses)	Tacrolimus 12 h trough 15 ng/dl for 3 months	Only for renal sparing	Refractory rejection or renal sparing
University of Pittsburgh	None	Thymoglobulin 5 mg/kg single dose or Campath 30 mg	Tacrolimus 12 h trough 8–10 ng/dl for 3 months	None	
University of Miami	None	Campath 30 mg day 0 and day 3	Tacrolimus 12 h trough of 10 ng/dl	None	
University of Paris Hospital Necker	None	Anti-IL2R agent	Tacrolimus trough or 25 ng/dl for isolated bowel transplants and 20 for combined liver and small bowel first 4 weeks	None	Severe or chronic rejection
Birmingham Children's Hospital	None	Anti IL-2R agent	Tacrolimus 12 h trough of 15 to 20 for first 3 weeks	Only for rejection	

(Source: personal communications with individual programs.)

lack of prospective or randomized single- or multicenter studies.

The use of antibody therapy for induction has been associated with a higher PTLD rate in intestinal (vs. other solid-organ) transplant recipients [24,25]. According to ITR data, the incidence of PTLD in children <18 years of age and in adults was 11% and 3% for ITA, 10% and 3% for SILT, and 19% and 6% for MVT recipients [1]. In one study, however, of all the various antibodies used after intestinal transplants, OKT3 was the only significant risk factor for the development of PTLD [26].

Maintenance therapy

The introduction of tacrolimus in the early 1990s led to a renewed interest in intestinal transplants [3,27]. Previous CSA-based immunosuppressive protocols had been disappointing. According to the 1996 ITR report of 180 transplants, 1-year graft survival rates for recipients on CSA improved from 17% (ITA), 44% (SILT), and 41% (MVT) to 65% (ITA), 64% (SILT), and 51% (MVT) for recipients on tacrolimus [28]. These clinical results were consistent with earlier small and large animal studies showing that tacrolimus was much more effective than CSA in preventing intestinal graft rejection [29,30].

Despite the significant improvement in outcome after the introduction of tacrolimus, the most recent ITR report compiling the worldwide experience since 1998, published about a decade after the previously quoted ITR report, demonstrated very similar 1-year graft survival rates: 65%, ITA; 59%, SILT; and 61%, MVT recipients. Although the 1-year survival rates have changed little, long-term results (3- and 5-year survival rates) have improved since then, possibly indicating better long-term management of posttransplant immunosuppression [1].

Tacrolimus in the immediate posttransplant period can be administered either intravenously or orally [31]. Because most transplant centers use some type of induction therapy, tacrolimus is usually started orally; therapeutic levels are reached by the time antibody therapy is discontinued (Table 35.1). If no induction antibody therapy is given, initial (3 to 7 days) intravenous tacrolimus therapy is preferable to achieve therapeutic levels immediately posttransplant. Most centers aim for blood levels between 15 and 20 ng/ml within the first 3 months posttransplant and then for levels between 8 and 15 ng/ml thereafter [16,32,33]. According to UNOS data, tacrolimus is now used in all recipient categories to the absolute exclusion of CSA [6,33,34]. However, side effects of tacrolimus therapy have not been uncommon, including deteriorating kidney function, hemolytic uremic syndrome, and diabetes mellitus [20,35–37]. Sirolimus has been used in patients with tacrolimus-related side effects, in particular, nephrotoxicity. The Nebraska group reported the use sirolimus in 15 pediatric intestinal transplant recipients with elevated creatinine levels and hypertension. With sirolimus plasma levels between 8 and 10 ng/ml, the tacrolimus dose was reduced by about 50% [32]. Kidney function improved in 11 of the 15 recipients, but two recipients lost their grafts to rejection while on sirolimus, and four died (sepsis, ruptured aneurysm). Other complications such as hypertriglyceremia, neutropenia, and wound healing and infectious complications increased.

Tacrolimus remains the gold standard agent for all intestinal transplant regimens, but centers have not reached consensus regarding the most efficacious adjunctive agents [38] (Table 35.1). Most intestinal transplant centers use tacrolimus in combination with steroids for maintenance therapy. According to ITR and UNOS data, 90% of intestinal transplant recipients are being maintained on tacrolimus and steroids. This pattern has remained constant for almost a decade [1,6,34].

The use of other maintenance agents has been much less consistent over time, but sirolimus appears to be more frequently used now. Fishbein et al. recommended the use of sirolimus after showing that 1-year graft survival rates were 92% with (n = 12) vs 50% without (n = 19) sirolimus in ITA and SILT recipients; the incidence of biopsy-proven rejection in the first 30 days posttransplant was 70% for recipients with, versus 74% without, sirolimus (likewise, the severity of rejection was significantly lower with sirolimus) [38]. In their experience, the combined use of sirolimus, tacrolimus, and steroids for maintenance, and basiliximab for induction, significantly decreased the incidence of early rejection and eliminated early graft loss caused by fulminant rejection; these favorable results were observed in both adult and pediatric recipients [38,39]. However, sirolimus had to be temporarily withheld or discontinued in 60% of the recipients because of neutropenia, viral infections, and PTLD; of note, the rate of wound-related complications did not increase. The relatively high incidence, in the Fishbein study, of sirolimus-related complications was similar to the studyreported by the Nebraska group [32]. In addition, Fishbein et al. [38] noted that in recipients with liver disease who were on sirolimus, the recovery of peripheral blood counts posttransplant was delayed; the rate of discontinuing sirolimus was high. Therefore, they concluded that sirolimus was most useful as a short-term adjunct to tacrolimus, rather than as a regular maintenance drug.

According to UNOS data, the use of MMF peaked at 57% in 1996, and has since fallen out of favor and is not as common anymore [34]. Earlier studies by the Miami group had suggested that the oral route can be effectively used early after intestinal transplants, not only for tacrolimus but also for MMF. However, a subsequent study by that same group, and by others showed oral-specific differences in MPA pharmacology and bioavailability: intestinal transplant recipients displayed the lowest MPA levels of any solid-organ transplant group, suggesting the need for separate dosing by type of transplant. Because of poor absorption, which may be compounded during rejection episodes, and the gastrointestinal side effects associated with MMF, its long-term benefit still needs to be demonstrated in intestinal transplant recipients [40,41].

with sloughing of mucosa, ulcers, and exfoliation, are treated with a 5- to 7-day course of antibody therapy (OKT3, alemtuzumab, polyclonal antilymphocyte preparations) [43]. Sloughing of the intestinal mucosa with resultant sepsis has frequently been fatal [42,43]. Attempts to control severe rejection are often futile, and graft enterectomy is the only hope to save the recipeint's life [38,44]. Recipients with sepsis as a result of a severe rejection episode should be treated with antibody therapy, under broad-spectrum antibiotic coverage. Conversion to sirolimus or MMF has been reported in recipients with refractory rejection [32,43]. Of note, Fishbein et al. reported successful treatment of recipients with late ulcerating rejection (refractory to standard antibody treatment) with infliximab, the monoclonal antibody to tumor necrosis factor-α [46]. Interestingly, the mucosal ulcerations were similar to those seen in ulcerating inflammatory bowel disease. Mild rejection (as judged by biopsy) can be successfully treated with steroid boluses or with increased doses of the standard maintenance drugs [17,18].

According to the Pittsburgh group, 8% of intestinal transplant recipients develop chronic rejection [47]. Although the etiology of chronic intestinal rejection appears to be multifactorial, better control of acute rejection episodes may decrease its incidence. If obliterative arteriopathy is suspected, conversion to sirolimus should be considered, to prevent the progression of intimal hyperplasia and subsequent luminal occlusion.

Graf rejection

According to ITR data, rejection remains a formidible problem: of 919 intestinal recipients, 49 (11%) died of graft rejection—and another 213 (49%) of sepsis and multiorgan failure (some of those deaths were the result of underlying rejection) [1]. Graft rejection rates reported by the ITR were 57% for ITA, 39% for SILT, and 48% for MVT recipients [1]. Single centers have reported rejection rates of up to 95% [4,18,44], requiring additional bolus corticosteroid or antibody therapy, and graft removal rates of up to 20% because of uncontrolled rejection [4].

Graft biopsy remains the gold standard for diagnosing rejection. The introduction of zoom endoscopy for surveillance [45] has further improved timely diagnosis. Most rejection episodes, particularly those

Immune monitoring

To monitor the level of immune function after intestinal transplants, the Pittsburgh group reported that the Cylex(R) immune cell function assay can be used as an objective tool. It measures global immune responses (ATP in ng/ml) of CD4-positive cells from whole blood samples. In a blinded retrospective study, Zeei et al. compared immune function to the clinical course and histologic biopsy results of 20 intestinal transplant recipients. Eight recipients with no major adverse events or changes in immunosuppressive therapy had only moderate to low immune function and were categorized as immunologically and clinically stable. Twelve patients displayed strong immune responses and required addition of steroids, OKT3, or both [48]. Further studies are needed to validate the reliability of such monitoring and to determine if it does, in fact, allow safe minimization, or weaning off, of immunosuppressive therapy.

The Pittsburgh group also showed that the presence of donor-specific T-suppressor cells (CD8$^+$, CD28$^-$) in the circulation may characterize transplant recipients whose graft function can be maintained with minimal or no immunosuppression [49]. If validated in larger studies, such immune monitoring may allow indidivual minimization of immunosuppressive therapy.

Immunomodulatory strategies

In the CSA era, immunomodulatory strategies in the form of graft or donor pretreatment were already used in intestinal transplant recipeints, in an attempt to prolong graft survival. Williams et al. used a cobalt-60 source that delivered 1,750 RAD to the ex vivo intestinal graft [50]. Despite CSA and prednisone treatment, biopsies showed acute rejection already on the third posttransplant day. Also in the 1980s, two teams— led by Starzl et al. [51] and by Williams et al. [52]— attempted to deplete the donor lymphocytes from SILT and MVT grafts. Starzl et al. gave 10 mg of OKT3 intravenously 90 minutes before graft removal. Williams et al. irradiated both grafts and gave one donor 5 mg of OKT3. However, two recipients died of perioperative bleeding; another two died of lymphomas. Thus, early attempts at graft and donor pretreatment failed.

Immunolomodulatory strategies shifted from graft or donor pretreatment to recipient conditioning in the 1990s. The Pittsburgh group attempted to augment (micro)chimerism and to induce tolerance by infusing of unmodified donor bone marrow cells (most commonly, a single infusion of 3 to 5×10^8 donor cells/kg given over 20 minutes within the first 12 hours after revascularization) [5,16]. The Pittsburgh group and, later, the Miami group continued to give unmodified donor bone marrow infusions for about a decade but this strategy failed to significantly improve outcome. Specifically, clinical results failed to show that bone marrow augmentation reduced the incidence of acute or chronic rejection; the question of whether chimerism plays a role in the development and maintenance of tolerance has not been conclusively answered [53–55].

Future considerations

Intestinal transplantation will be more broadly applied only if immunosuppressive or immunodulatory strategies are developed that diminish or eliminate the rate of severe, exfoliative rejection with its associated risks of graft loss and recipient death. Currently, most patients with intestinal failure who do not have TPN-associated complications are not routinely considered for intestinal transplants. As with the introduction of tacrolimus in the 1990s, the advent of new immunosuppressive agents and of more potent, yet less toxic, regimens may further improve the results after intestinal transplants.

References

1 Grant D, Abu-Elmagd K, Reyes J, et al. 2003 report of the intestine transplant registry: a new era has dawned. *Ann Surg* 2005;241:607–613.

2 Lillehei RC, Idezuki Y, Feemster JA, et al. Transplantation of stomach, intestine, and pancreas: experimental and clinical observations. *Surgery* 1967;62:721–741.

3 Hoffman AL, Makowka L, Banner B, et al. The use of FK-506 for small intestine allotransplantation. *Transplantation* 1990;49:483–490.

4 Sudan DL, Chinnakotta S, Horslen S, et al. Basiliximab decreases the incidence of acute rejection after intestinal transplantation. *Transplant Proc* 2002;34:940–941.

5 Abu-Elmagd K, Reyes J, Todo S, et al. Clinical intestinal transplantation: new perspectives and immunologic considerations. *J Am Coll Surg* 1998;186:512–527.

6 Shiffman ML, Saab S, Feng S, et al. Liver and intestine transplantation in the United States, 1995–2004. *Am J Transpl* 2006;6:1170–1187.

7 Goulet O, Damotte D, Sarnacki S. Liver-induced immune tolerance in recipients of combined liver-intestine transplants. *Transplant Proc* 2005;37:1689–1690.

8 Gruessner RWG, Sharp HL. Living related intestinal transplantation—first report of a standardized surgical technique. *Transplantation* 1997;64:1605–1607.

9 Calne RY, Friend PK, Middleton S, et al. Intestinal transplant between two of identical triplets. *Lancet* 1997;350:1077–1078.

10 Morel P, Kadry Z, Charbonnet P, et al. Paediatric living related intestinal-transplantation between two monozygotic twins: a 1-year follow-up. *Lancet* 2000; 355:723–724.

11 Benedetti E, Holterman M, Asolati M, et al. Living related segmental bowel transplantation: from experimental to standardized procedure. *Ann Surg* 2006;244: 694–699.

12 Todo S, Reyes J, Furukawa H, et al. Outcome analysis of 71 clinical intestinal transplantations. *Ann Surg* 1995;222:270–282.

13 Bond GJ, Mazariegos GV, Sindhi R, et al. Evolutionary experience with immunosuppression in pediatric intestinal transplantation. *J Pediatr Surg* 2005;40:274–280.

14 Pinna AD, Weppler D, Nery JR, et al. Induction therapy for clinical intestinal transplantation: comparison of four different regimens. *Transplant Proc* 2000;32:1193–1194.

15 Abu-Elmagd K, Fung J, McGhee W, et al. The efficacy of daclizumab for intestinal transplantation: preliminary report. *Transplant Proc* 2000;32:1195–11964.

16 Abu-Elmagd K, Reyes J, Bond G, et al. Clinical intestinal transplantation: a decade of experience at a single center. *Ann Surg* 2001;234:404–417.

17 Carreño MR, Kato T, Weppler D, et al. Induction therapy with daclizumab as part of the immunosuppressive regimen in human small bowel and multiorgan transplants. *Transplant Proc* 2001;33:1015–1017.

18 Tzakis AG, Kato T, Nishida S, et al. Preliminary experience with Campath 1H (C1H) in intestinal and liver transplantation. *Transplantation* 2003;75:1227–1231.

19 Kata T, Tzakis AG, Selvaggi G, et al. Intestinal and multivisceral transplantation in children. *Ann Surg* 2006;243:756–766.

20 Kato T, Gaynor JJ, Selvaggi G, et al. Intestinal transplantation in children: a summary of clinical outcomes and prognostic factors in 108 patients from a single center. *J Gastrointest Surg* 2005;9:75–89.

21 Tzakis AG, Kata T, Levi DM, et al. 100 multivisceral transplants at a single center. *Ann Surg* 2005;242:480–493.

22 Starzl TE, Murase N, Abu-Elmagd K, et al. Tolerogenic immunosuppression for organ transplantation. *Lancet* 2003;361:1502–1510.

23 Reyes J, Mazariegos GV, Abu-Elmagd K, et al. Intestinal transplantation under tacrolimus monotherapy after perioperative lympoid depletion with rabbit antithymocyte globulin (Thymoglobulin(R)). *Am J Transplant* 2005;5:1430–1436.

24 Nalesnik MA. Clinicopathologic features of posttransplant lymphoproliferative disorders. *Ann Transplant* 1997;2:33–40.

25 Shpilberg O, Wilson J, Whiteside TL, et al. Pre-transplant immunological profile and risk factor analysis of post-transplant lymphoproliferative disease development: the results of a nested matched case-control study. *Leukemia and Lymphoma* 1999;36:109–121.

26 Quintini C, Kata T, Gaynor JJ, et al. Analysis of risk factors for the development of posttransplant lymphoproliferative disorder among 119 children who received primary intestinal transplants at a single center. *Transplant Proc* 2006;38:1755–1758.

27 Todo S, Tzakis AG, Abu-Elmgadt K, et al. Cadaveric small bowel and small bowel-liver transplantation in humans. *Transplantation* 1992;53:369–376.

28 Grant D. Current results of intestinal transplantation: early report. *Lancet* 1996;347:1801–1803.

29 Gruessner RWG, Fryer JP, Fasola C, et al. A prospective study of FK506 versus CsA and pig ATG in a porcine model of small bowel transplantation. *Transplantation* 1995;59:164–171.

30 Hoffman AL, Makowka L, Cai X, et al. The effect of FK 506 on small intestine allotransplantation in the rat. *Transplant Proc* 1990;22:76–77.

31 Allers C, Eichhom J, Leckel K, et al. Tacrolimus, daclizumab, sirolimus, and budesonide after small bowel transplantation in order to reduce nephrotoxicity. *Transplant Proc* 2002;34:942.

32 Horslen S, Torres C, Collier D, et al. Initial experience using rapamycin immunosuppression in pediatric intestinal transplant recipients. *Transplant Proc* 2002;34:934–935.

33 Langnas AN Advances in small-intestine transplantation. *Transplantation* 2004;77:S75–S78.

34 Kaufman DB, Shapiro R, Lucey MR, et al. Immunosuppression: practice and trends. *Am J Transplant* 2004; 4(Suppl 9):38–53.

35 Ueno T, Kato T, Gaynor J, et al. Renal dysfunction following adult intestinal transplant under tacrolimus-based immunosuppression. *Transplant Proc* 2006;38:1762–1764.

36 Ueno T, Kato T, Gaynor J, et al. Renal function after pediatric intestinal transplant. *Transplant Proc* 2006;38:1759–1761.

37 Humar A, Jessurun J, Sharp HL, et al. Thrombotic microangiopathy after liver-small bowel transplant—a case report. *Clin Transplant* 1998;12:600–601.

38 Fishbein TM, Florman S, Gondolesi G, et al. Intestinal transplantation before and after the introduction of sirolimus. *Transplantation* 2002;73:1538–1542.

39 Fishbein TM, Kaufman SS, Florman SS, et al. Isolated intestinal transplantation: proof of clinical efficacy. *Transplantation* 2003;76:636–640.

40 Tsaroucha AK, Zuker K, Esqunazi V, et al. Levels of mycohphenolic acid and its glucuronide derivative in the plasma of liver, small bowel, and kidney transplant

patients receiving tacrolimus and CellCept combination therapy. *Transpl Immunol* 2000;8:143–146.

41 Al-Hussaini A, Tredger M, Dhawan A. Immunosuppression in pediatric liver and intestinal transplantation: a closer look at the arsenal. *J Pediatr Gastroenterol Nutr* 2005;41:152–165.

42 Lee RG, Nakamura K, Tsamandas AC, et al. Pathology of human intestinal transplantation. *Gastroenterology* 1966;110:1820–1834.

43 Selvaggi G, Kato T, Gaynor JJ, et al. Analysis of rejection episodes in over 100 pediatric intestinal transplant recipients. *Transpl Proc* 2006;38:1711–1712.

44 Sudan DL, Kaufman SS, Shaw BW Jr, et al. Isolated intestinal transplantation for intestinal failure. *Am J Gastroenterol* 2000;95:1506–1515.

45 Kato T, O'Brien CB, Nishida S, et al. The first case report of the use of a zoom videoendoscope for the evaluation of small bowel graft mucosa in a human after intestinal transplantation. *Gastrointest Endosc* 1999;50:257–261.

46 Fishbein TM. The current state of intestinal transplantation. *Transplantation* 2004;78:175–178.

47 Parizhskaya M, Redondo C, Demetris A, et al. Chronic rejection of small bowel grafts: pediatric and adult study of risk factors and morphologic progression. *Pediatr Dev Pathol* 2006;6:240–250.

48 Zeevi A, Britz JA, Bentlejewski CA, et al. Monitoring immune function during tacrolimus tapering in small bowel transplant recipients. *Transplant Immunol* 2005;15:17–24.

49 Sindhi R, Manavalan JS, Magill A, et al. Reduced immunosuppression in pediatric liver-intestine transplant recipients with CD8+CD28-T-suppressor cells. *Hum Immunol* 2005;66:252–257.

50 Tattersal C, Gebel H, Haklin M, et al. Lymphocyte responsiveness after irradiation in canine and human intestinal allogafts. *Curr Surg* 1989;46:16–19.

51 Starzl TE. Personal communication. 1991 (unpublished).

52 Williams JW, Sankary HN, Foster PF, et al. Splanchnic transplantation: an approach to the infant dependent on parenteral nutrition who develops irreversible liver disease. *JAMA* 1989;261:1458–1462.

53 Abu-Elmagd K, Reyes J, Todo S, et al. Clinical intestinal transplantation: new perspectives and immunologic considerations. *J Am Coll Surg* 1998;186:512–525.

54 Gruessner RWG, Uckun FM, Pirenne J, et al. Recipient preconditioning and donor-specific bone marrow infusion in a pig model of total bowel transplantation. *Transplantation* 1997;63:12–20.

55 Pirenne J, Gruessner AC, Benedetti E, et al. Donor specific unmodified bone marrow transfusion does not facilitate intestinal engraftment after bowel transplantation in a porcine model. *Surgery* 1997;121:79–88.

36 Immunology of Intestinal Allograft Rejection

Kenneth A. Newell and Jonathan P. Fryer

Key points

- Intestines elicit a more vigorous recipient immune response than do other commonly transplanted organs.

- The presence of specialized lymphoid organs and the vast number of hematopoietic cells contained within the transplanted intestine likely contribute to the enhanced immunogenicity of transplanted intestines.

- The immunologic microenvironment of the intestine is predisposed toward inflammatory responses that may favor harmful heterologous immune responses (cross-reactive immune responses between pathologic bacteria or viruses and alloantigens) and consequent graft damage.

- Migration of immune cells to transplanted intestines may be regulated by chemokines and integrins that confer some degree of tissue specificity suggesting potential therapeutic targets.

Overview of basic aspects of alloimmunity

Although many components of the alloimmune response to transplanted intestines are shared with other transplanted organs, the unique vigor of the rejection response following intestinal transplantation suggests the involvement of unique immune mechanisms. Before discussing these unique mechanisms, the basic elements of alloimmune rejection responses will be reviewed.

Intestinal Failure: Diagnosis, Management and Transplantation.
Edited by Alan N. Langnas, Olivier Goulet, Eamonn M.M. Quigley and Kelly A. Tappenden. © 2008 Blackwell Publishing.
ISBN 978-1-4051-4637-1.

Components of the basic immune response

Cellular components

Alloimmunity is comprised of both cellular and soluble elements. Cellular responses can be subdivided into innate, or antigen nonspecific, and adaptive, or antigen-specific, responses. Lymphocytes are the main components of the adaptive immune system with T and B lymphocytes playing a critical role in the process of rejection. Mice lacking T and B cells accept fully mismatched skin grafts indefinitely, whereas the transfer of T cells into these mice causes allograft rejection. Similarly, mice that lack T cells expressing the $\alpha\beta$ T cell receptor (TCR) (the vast majority of peripheral T cells) fail to reject intestinal allografts, whereas those lacking T cells that express the $\gamma\delta$ TCR (relatively overexpressed in the intestine and skin) promptly reject intestinal allografts [1]. In humans, depletion of T cells or lymphocytes using antibodies such as muromonab-CD3 (OKT3) or alemtuzumab (Campath-1H) has been shown to inhibit or reverse rejection, thus providing clinical evidence supporting an important role for T cells in alloimmunity. In addition to the destructive properties of T cells, subsets of T cells referred to as regulatory T cells have been identified that suppress immune responses (reviewed [2]). The ultimate outcome of transplantation appears to depend on the balance of the destructive and suppressive properties of alloreactive T cells.

Like T cells, B lymphocytes contribute to the destruction of transplanted organs. However, although alloantibodies produced by B cells can mediate rejection, B cells are not necessary for rejection as a variety of tissues are rejected normally by B cell-deficient mice. The role of alloantibodies following transplantation appears to vary depending on the organ transplanted. Following kidney, pancreas or heart transplantation, pre-existing antibodies specific for donor HLA antigens are known to cause significant allograft injury. In contrast, liver allografts appear resistant to the deleterious effects of alloantibodies. The de novo formation of anti-HLA antibodies after transplantation may also mediate acute rejection and has been implicated in the development of chronic allograft injury. Less information is available about the role of alloantibodies in clinical intestinal transplantation although existing data suggest a deleterious role for anti-HLA alloantibodies in the rejection of intestinal allografts [3].

Innate immunity

The innate immune system also contributes to alloimmunity particularly at early time points following transplantation when it acts to amplify adaptive immune responses. Innate immune responses may, themselves, be augmented by graft injury from ischemia/reperfusion (I/R), infection, or trauma. I/R injury is characterized by deposition of complement, up-regulation of vascular adhesion molecules, platelet adherence, release of inflammatory cytokines and graft infiltration by inflammatory cells, including polymorphonuclear leukocytes (PMNs), macrophages, natural killer (NK) cells, and NK T cells. A strategy that targets cells of the innate immune system may blunt this initial destructive response and inhibit rejection. In an experimental model of heart transplantation, the inhibition of PMN migration into the graft by blocking CXCR2, the receptor for two PMN chemokine attractants, synergized with the blockade of costimulatory molecules to prolong allograft survival [4]. Depletion of recipient or donor macrophages has also been shown to improve the survival of intestinal allografts in rats [5]. Although the role of NK and NKT cells in initiating or potentiating alloimmune responses is being increasingly recognized, their role during intestinal allograft rejection is largely unexplored.

Toll-like receptors (TLRs) are highly conserved molecules that contribute to innate immune responses by recognizing specific molecular patterns commonly expressed by pathogenic microorganisms. TLRs are expressed by a variety of cells that may contact infectious agents including epithelial cells, endothelial cells, and dendritic cells (DC). TLR engagement triggers innate immune responses by stimulating selectin expression, chemokine production, DC maturation and the production of antimicrobial peptides. Both experimental and clinical data suggest an important role for TLRs in the alloimmune response. Although the role of TLRs has not been evaluated following intestinal transplantation, these investigations are clearly warranted given the unique relationship of the intestinal graft with enteric flora.

Soluble components of the alloimmune response

Although not capable of independently mediating allograft rejection, soluble components of the immune system such as cytokines, chemokines, and complement play an important role in regulating and amplifying the immune response. Proinflammatory Th1 cytokines such as IFNγ, TNFα, and IL-12 have been associated with allograft rejection while Th2 type cytokines such as IL-4 and IL-10 have been associated with allograft acceptance. TGFβ production by a subset of regulatory T cells has also been associated with long-term allograft acceptance in rodents, nonhuman primates, and humans [6]. Clinically, treatment with an anti-TNFα monoclonal antibody has been reported to reverse intestinal rejection refractory to steroids and OKT3 in a small group of patients [7].

Chemokines also affect the immune response, in large part by regulating the migration of immune responder cells to the graft. Temporal variations in chemokine gene expression and variable expression of chemokine receptors (CCRs) by immune cells of different lineages serve to regulate the migration of cells to transplanted organs. In a murine model of intestinal transplantation several chemokines were found to be upregulated shortly after transplantation, including IP-10, Mig, and MIP1α [8]. Disruption of the interaction of IP-10 with its receptor CXCR3 on T cells significantly impaired T cell migration into the lamina propria and prolonged allograft survival. Components of the complement system also contribute to alloimmunity by mediating chemotaxis and inflammation (C3a and C5a), contributing to formation of the membrane attack complex (C5b) and cell lysis, and by directly affecting T cell activation and function (decay-accelerating factor) [9].

General mechanisms of rejection

Initiation of the immune response

It is widely accepted that antigen presenting cells (APC) of donor origin within a transplanted organ play an important role in a developing alloimmune response. These "passenger leukocytes" migrate from the transplanted organ to the secondary lymphoid organs of the recipient (spleen and lymph nodes) where they prime naïve recipient T cells. This paradigm is supported by the finding that rejection is prevented or significantly delayed in recipient mice that lack all lymph nodes and their spleen [10]. In this model the TCRs of recipient T cells recognize allogeneic MHC molecule/peptide complexes on donor APCs directly (a process referred to as the direct pathway of antigen presentation) resulting in T cell activation. This pathway contrasts with the conventional "indirect pathway" in which recipient APCs take up foreign antigens and process them into peptides that are in turn presented to recipient T cells by MHC molecules on the recipient APCs. It has been estimated that 7% of all T cells are capable of directly recognizing alloantigens [11], whereas fewer than 1 in 100,000 T cells can recognize nominal antigens presented by self MHC molecules. The high precursor frequency of directly alloreactive T cells likely influences the strength of the alloimmune response and may be particularly important in the intestine where a large population of donor APCs are present. Direct antigen recognition predominates in the early posttransplant period while the importance of the indirect pathway of antigen presentation increases at later time points and has been associated with the development of chronic allograft injury [12]. Although the recognition of alloantigens by the TCR is required for T cell activation, this interaction alone is not sufficient to fully activate naïve T cells. Complete T cell activation also requires signals that result from the interactions of costimulatory molecules on the T cell and their ligands expressed by professional APCs. Costimulatory molecules can largely be grouped into two families. The B7 superfamily is best characterized by the interactions of CD28 expressed by T cells with its ligands B7.1 and B7.2 (CD80 and CD86) expressed by activated APCs. Many members of the TNF receptor superfamily, also provide costimulatory signals. The most widely studied of these, CD154, is expressed by T cells and interacts with CD40 that is expressed by activated APCs. Block-

ade of these pathways has been shown to inhibit organ allograft rejection by preventing complete T cell activation [13]. Interestingly, neither of these strategies prevented the rejection of intestinal allografts in mice [14,15] because of the ability of CD8$^+$ T cells to mediate rejection in the absence of the costimulatory signals provided by CD28 and CD154. The demonstration that other costimulatory molecules such as 4–1BB and LTα that belong to the TNF receptor superfamily provide important costimulatory signals to CD8$^+$, alloreactive T cells and inhibit the rejection of intestinal allografts by CD8$^+$ T cells suggests that costimulation blockade may yet be therapeutically important in intestinal transplantation [16,17].

Effector mechanisms

Tissue injury related to brain death, organ procurement, and organ preservation together with contributions from the innate immune response generate an inflammatory environment within a transplanted organ that facilitates the migration of lymphocytes activated in recipient lymphoid organs to the allograft where they mediate damage by direct cytotoxicity or indirectly via the production of cytokines. Generally CD8$^+$ T cells have been associated with cytotoxicity, whereas CD4$^+$ T cells have been associated with cytokine production, although in some settings these roles can be reversed. Mechanisms of direct cytotoxicity include granule exocytosis and engagement of death receptors. Granule exocytosis refers to the targeted release of perforin and granzymes which are stored in preformed cytoplasmic granules in cytotoxic T lymphocytes (CTL). On contact with a target cell, CTLs form a conjugate and release their cytotoxic proteins which are taken up by the target cells. Perforin acts to create pores in the target cell membrane. Granzymes are serine proteases that act to fragment target cell DNA and induce apoptosis. CTLs may also mediate cytolysis via Fas interactions with Fas ligand expressed by target cells. CTLs may also lyse target cells indirectly via the production of cytokines such as TNFα, lymphotoxin α, or IFNγ.

Alloantibodies contribute to hyperacute rejection, acute humoral rejection, and possibly chronic rejection by two main effector mechanisms, including complement activation and antibody-dependent cellular cytotoxicity (ADCC). Complement activation leads to formation of the membrane attack complex, pore formation, and cell lysis. Graft endothelial cells are primary targets for complement deposition detected clinically via immunohistochemical staining for C4d. ADCC refers to the process in which antibody bound to target cells engages Fc receptors on CTL thereby facilitating lysis of the target cell.

Barriers to allograft acceptance posed by preexisting immunity

Like memory B cells and preexisting alloantibodies, memory T cells present a formidable barrier to transplantation. Until recently, T cell memory has not been directly studied in clinical transplantation. T cell memory is often inferred in patients with humoral sensitization detected by cross-matching. However, recent work demonstrates a low correlation between humoral and cellular sensitization and notes significantly worse outcomes in kidney transplant recipients with preexisting antidonor memory T cells [18]. Several unique properties of memory T cells contribute to their propensity to mediate rejection including a reduced threshold for activation, the ability to be primed outside of secondary lymphoid organs, different patterns of migration, and their ability to be primed by nonprofessional APCs. Traditionally memory cells were thought to arise as a result of alloantigen exposure via pregnancy, transfusion, or previous transplantation. More recently heterologous immunity and homeostatic proliferation have been shown to contribute to the pool of potentially alloreactive memory T cells [19,20]. Heterologous immunity refers to the potential of memory T cells generated in response to environmental antigens such as pathologic microorganisms to cross-react with alloantigens. Homeostatic proliferation occurs when a small number of residual T cells expand to repopulate a depleted lymphoid compartment. Strategies to deplete T cells at the time of transplantation have been shown to induce homeostatic proliferation of the remaining T cells, which develop a memory-like phenotype and consequently pose a major barrier to allograft acceptance [21].

Unique aspects of intestinal allograft rejection

The greater immunogenicity of intestinal allografts relative to other types of transplanted organs, observed both experimentally and clinically, suggests that unique aspects of the immune response contribute to the rejection of transplanted intestines. These may include increased susceptibility to immune-mediated injury, alternative mechanisms for generating the immune response, or unique effector mechanisms. Experimental data demonstrate that different organs display a spectrum of injury severity in response to alloantigen-specific CD8$^+$ T cells [22]. Although transplanted intestines were not included in this study, these data support organ-specific differences in the ability of fixed effector mechanisms to mediate alloimmune injury. We have previously shown that unlike the situation in experimental heart transplantation where rejection is dependent on CD4$^+$ T cells, CD8$^+$ T cells are sufficient to mediate rejection of intestinal allografts in mice [1]. These data demonstrate that different mechanisms are, at least in part, responsible for differences in the pattern of rejection of transplanted intestines and hearts in mice.

The large number of passenger leukocytes within the intestine has also been postulated to contribute to the greater immunogenicity of transplanted intestines. In this model, donor leukocytes, specifically professional APCs, migrate from the transplanted intestine to the recipient secondary lymphoid organs where they prime the recipient immune response. A greater number of donor APCs would, in theory, prime a larger recipient alloimmune response. The large number of donor lymphocytes contained within the intestine may also be activated by the inflammatory environment associated with I/R injury, the breakdown of the mucosal barrier, and bacterial translocation. We have shown that activation of donor lymphocytes by non-MHC antigens can exacerbate the recipient immune response to intestinal allografts, as reflected by increased local production of proinflamatory cytokines and an increased incidence of rejection [23].

In addition to donor leukocytes, intestinal grafts also contain large amounts of organized lymphoid tissue (mesenteric lymph nodes and Peyer's patches). We have recently demonstrated that within 24 hours of transplantation large numbers of recipient T cells migrate to the donor lymphoid tissues of the transplanted intestine where they display an activated phenotype, proliferate, and develop effector function as indicated by alloantigen-specific cytokine production [24]. Importantly, the lymphoid organs contained within the transplanted intestine appear to be the primary site of T cell priming in the early period after intestinal

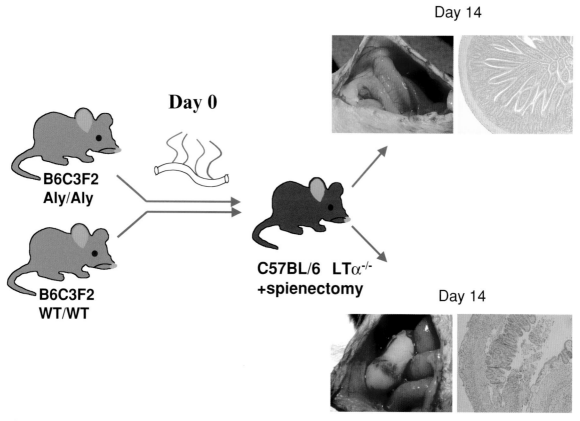

Figure 36.1 Demonstration of the importance of donor lymphoid organs for rejection of transplanted intestines. Splenectomized, lymph node-deficient LTα knockout mice (H2^b) show impaired rejection of intestines from B6C3F2 aly/aly mice (H2K^k) that lack lymphoid organs caused by a mutation in NFκB-inducing kinase (NIK) relative to the rejection of intestines from lymphoid organ-bearing B6C3F2 wild type littermate controls (H2K^k).

transplantation. As shown in Figure 36.1, splenectomized, lymph node-deficient recipients reject wild type intestinal allografts promptly. In contrast, the rejection of intestinal allografts lacking lymphoid organs as a result of a genetic mutation is dramatically impaired confirming the importance of donor origin lymphoid organs to the process of intestinal allograft rejection. These data suggest that strategies aimed at preventing the early migration of recipient T cells to donor lymphoid organs within the transplanted intestine may be useful adjuncts to prevent or delay rejection following intestinal transplantation. Although rejection was significantly delayed in lymphoid organ-deficient donor/recipient pairs, most recipients eventually did reject the transplanted intestines. This observation suggests that unlike other transplanted organs, components of the transplanted intestine may be able to prime the alloimmune response in the complete absence of secondary lymphoid organs. The most likely means by which recipient T cells could be primed in the intestine outside of lymphoid organs would be direct priming by the large number of donor APCs in the relatively inflammatory environment of the intestine or direct priming by epithelial cells as has been reported in vitro [25].

The migration of recipient lymphocytes to epithelial or mucosal surfaces is thought to be regulated by tissue-specific integrins or chemokines. Examples of receptor/ligand pairs shown to preferentially facilitate migration of T cells to the intestine include mucosal addressin cell adhesion molecule-1 (MAdCAM-1) and $\alpha_4\beta_7$, $\alpha_E\beta_7$ (CD103) and E-cadherin, chemokine

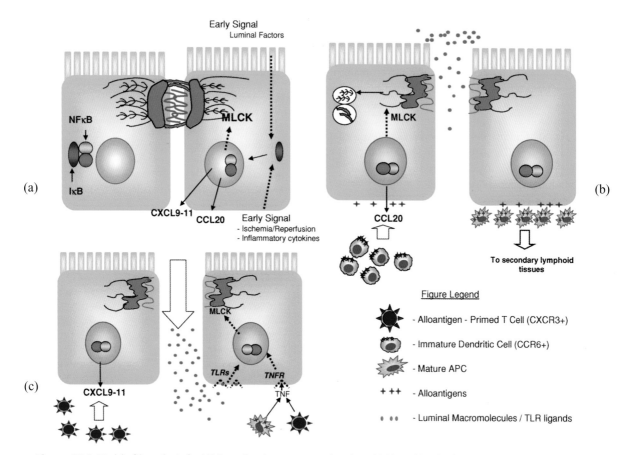

Figure 36.2 Model of hypothesis for NFκB mediated augmentation of small bowel allograft rejection. (a) Early signals trigger NFκB-mediated chemokine induction and (b) myosin light chain kinase (MLCK)-mediated changes in tight junction protein arrangement and function that cause epithelial barrier dysfunction. NFκB dependent chemokines (CCL20) recruit immature (CCR6+) recipient dendritic cells (DCs) that encounter donor alloantigen. Mature DCs facilitate T cell priming in secondary lymphoid tissues or other locations. (c) Chemokines (CXCL9-11) recruit CXCR3+ alloreactive effector T cells to the graft mucosa where they cause rejection. A positive feedback loop of NFκB activation is created by proinflammatory cytokines including TNF, and by epithelial barrier dysfunction which allows passage of luminal microbial products, including toll-like receptor (TLR) ligands, to the basolateral epithelial cell surface where they ligate TLRs that activate NFκB.

receptor 9 (CCR9) and TECK, and CCR6 and CCL20 (MIP-3α). Of these molecules, the pair best studied in the setting of intestinal transplantation is MAdCAM-1, which is expressed by mucosal vessels and the endothelium of gut-associated lymphoid tissue and its ligand $\alpha_4\beta_7$, which is preferentially expressed by T cells displaying gut trophism. It has been demonstrated in a murine model of intestinal transplantation that during rejection allografts are infiltrated by large numbers of $\alpha_4\beta_7^{high}$ T cells and that treatment with a blocking antibody specific for β_7 significantly reduces the cellular infiltrate and inhibits rejection [26]. These findings suggest that agents targeting these unique regulators of lymphocyte trafficking to the intestine may be useful therapeutic adjuncts to prevent rejection of intestinal allografts.

The intimate interaction of intestinal grafts with the external environment may also predispose them toward rejection. The small bowel has the largest epithelial surface of any organ or tissue. Solid organ allografts that have significant potential for interaction between their epithelia and external antigens (i.e. small bowel, lung, and pancreas) have been associated with inferior graft survival. Normally, the density of bacteria in the small bowel is relatively low and increases progressively with proximity to the colon. Accordingly, the normal small bowel epithelium is not specially adapted for defense against micro-organisms or their by-products [27,28], as reflected by the less effective barrier function of the small bowel relative to the colonic epithelium [29]. Animal studies suggest that the SB luminal flora is altered significantly following intestinal transplantation [30,31]. Therefore, in the posttransplant period, products elaborated by the modified luminal flora (i.e. LPS, Zonulin), or generated as a consequence of ischemia/reperfusion or early rejection (TNF), can trigger NFkB-mediated alterations in the junctional proteins. This leads to further compromise in the epithelial barrier function and allows microbial by-products (i.e. LPS, flagellin) to breach the paracellular spaces of the epithelium further enhancing mucosal inflammation and nonspecifically augmenting ongoing alloimmune responses. The net result of this process is to enhance interactions between luminal bacteria and the subepithelial immune system of the transplanted intestine. Given the elaborate immune surveillance system of the small bowel, this scenario may create a volatile environment within the transplanted intestine that is characterized by high levels of proinflammatory cytokines and chemokines as well as increased expression of adhesion molecules and HLA antigens. This hostile environment may lead to the escalation of a mild focal rejection episode to a global "exfoliative" rejection process (Figure 36.2).

Conclusions

It is likely that the immune response to most transplanted organs shares many common features. Consequently, many therapeutic interventions will effectively inhibit rejection of a variety of transplanted organs. However, it is also clear that because of its unique structure and function, the intestinal immune system has developed unique immunologic properties that may contribute to its enhanced immunogenicity. Understanding these unique aspects of the intestinal immune system may provide the opportunity to devise new, relatively intestine-specific approaches to immunosuppression, which have the potential to significantly improve the outcome of intestinal transplantation.

References

1 He G, Hart J, Kim OS, et al. The role of CD8 and CD4 T cells in intestinal allograft rejection: a comparison of monoclonal antibody-treated and knockout mice. *Transplantation* 1999;67:131–137.

2 Wood KJ, Sakaguchi S. Regulatory T cells in transplantation tolerance. *Nat Rev Immunol* 2003;3:199–210.

3 Ruiz P, Garcia M, Pappas P, et al. Mucosal vascular alterations in isolated small-bowel allografts: relationship to humoral sensitization. *Am J Transplant* 2003;3:43–49.

4 El-Sawy T, Belperio JA, Strieter RM, et al. Inhibition of polymorphonuclear leukocyte-mediated graft damage synergizes with short-term costimulatory blockade to prevent cardiac allograft rejection. *Circulation* 2005;112:320–331.

5 Fryer J, Grant D, Jiang J, et al. Influence of macrophage depletion on bacterial translocation and rejection in small bowel transplantation. *Transplantation* 1996;62:553–559.

6 Torrealba JR, Katayama M, Fechner JH, et al. Metastable tolerance to rhesus monkey renal transplants is correlated with allograft TGF-beta 1+CD4+ T regulatory cell infiltrates. *J Immunol* 2004;172:5753–5764.

7 Pascher A, Klupp J, Langrehr JM, Neuhaus P. Anti-TNF-alpha therapy for acute rejection in intestinal transplantation. *Transplant Proc* 2005;37:1635–1636.

8 Zhang Z, Kaptanoglu L, Tang Y, et al. IP-10-induced recruitment of CXCR3 host T cells is required for small bowel allograft rejection. *Gastroenterology* 2004;126:809–818.

9 Heeger PS, Lalli PN, Lin F, et al. Decay-accelerating factor modulates induction of T cell immunity. *J Exp Med* 2005;201:1523–1530.

10 Lakkis FG, Arakelov A, Konieczny BT, Inoue Y. Immunologic "ignorance" of vascularized organ transplants in the absence of secondary lymphoid tissue. *Nat Med* 2000;6:686–688.

11 Suchin EJ, Langmuir PB, Palmer E, et al. Quantifying the frequency of alloreactive T cells in vivo: new answers to an old question. *J Immunol* 2001;166:973–981.

12 Baker RJ, Hernandez-Fuentes MP, Brookes PA, et al. Loss of direct and maintenance of indirect allore-sponses in renal allograft recipients: implications for the pathogenesis of chronic allograft nephropathy. *J Immunol* 2001;167:7199–7206.

13 Larsen CP, Elwood ET, Alexander DZ, et al. Long-term acceptance of skin and cardiac allografts after blocking CD40 and CD28 pathways. *Nature* 1996;381:434–438.

14 Newell KA, He G, Guo Z, et al. Cutting edge: blockade of the CD28/B7 costimulatory pathway inhibits intestinal allograft rejection mediated by CD4+ but not CD8+ T cells. *J Immunol* 1999;163:2358–2362.

15 Guo Z, Meng L, Kim O, et al. CD8 T cell-mediated rejection of intestinal allografts is resistant to inhibition of the CD40/CD154 costimulatory pathway. *Transplantation* 2001;71:1351–1354.

16 Wang J, Guo Z, Dong Y, et al. Role of 4–1BB in allograft rejection mediated by CD8+ T Cells. *Am J Transplant* 2003;3:543–551.

17 Guo Z, Wang J, Meng L, et al. Cutting edge: membrane lymphotoxin regulates cd8(+) t cell-mediated intestinal allograft rejection. *J Immunol* 2001;167:4796–4800.

18 Poggio ED, Clemente M, Hricik DE, Heeger PS. Panel of reactive T cells as a measurement of primed cellular alloimmunity in kidney transplant candidates. *J Am Soc Nephrol* 2006;17:564–572.

19 Adams AB, Pearson TC, Larsen CP. Heterologous immunity: an overlooked barrier to tolerance. *Immunol Rev* 2003;196:147–160.

20 Wu Z, Bensinger SJ, Zhang J, et al. Homeostatic proliferation is a barrier to transplantation tolerance. *Nat Med* 2004;10:87–92.

21 Pearl JP, Parris J, Hale DA, et al. Immunocompetent T-cells with a memory-like phenotype are the dominant cell type following antibody-mediated T-cell depletion. *Am J Transplant* 2005;3:465–474.

22 Jones ND, Turvey SE, Van Maurik A, et al. Differential susceptibility of heart, skin, and islet allografts to T cell-mediated rejection. *J Immunol* 2001;166:2824–2830.

23 Zhang Z, Kaptanoglu L, Haddad W, et al. Donor T cell activation initiates small bowel allograft rejection through an IFN-gamma-inducible protein-10-dependent mechanism. *J Immunol* 2002;168:3205–3212.

24 Wang J, Dong Y, Sun J, et al. Donor lymphoid organs are a major site of alloreactive T cell priming following intestinal transplantation. *Am J Transplant* 2006;6:2563–2571.

25 Li XC, Almawi W, Jevnikar A, et al. Allogeneic lymphocyte proliferation stimulated by small intestine-derived epithelial cells. *Transplantation* 1995;60:82–89.

26 Kellersmann R, Lazarovits A, Grant D, et al. Monoclonal antibody against beta7 integrins, but not beta7 deficiency, attenuates intestinal allograft rejection in mice. *Transplantation* 2002;74:1327–1334.

27 Arvans DL, Vavricka SR, Ren H, et al. Luminal bacterial flora determines physiological expression of intestinal epithelial cytoprotective heat shock proteins 25 and 72. *Am J Physiol Gastrointest Liver Physiol* 2005;288:G696–G704.

28 El Asmar R, Panigrahi P, Bamford P, et al. Host-dependent zonulin secretion causes the impairment of the small intestine barrier function after bacterial exposure. *Gastroenterology* 2002;123:1607–1615.

29 Powell DW, ed. *Intestinal Water and Electrolyte Transport*. New York: Raven Press, 1987.

30 Biffi R, Privitera G, Andreoni B, et al. Luminal bacterial overgrowth and intestinal translocation in pigs given either cyclosporin A or 15-deoxyspergualin after small bowel transplantation. *Eur J Surg* 1995;161:93–96.

31 Browne BJ, Johnson CP, Edmiston CE, et al. Small bowel transplantation promotes bacterial overgrowth and translocation. *J Surg Res* 1991;51:512–517.

37 Histopathology of Intestinal Transplantation

Tong Wu and Anthony J. Demetris

Key points

- Histopathology contributes to almost every aspect of intestinal transplantation, including pretransplant evaluation, posttransplant follow-up, as well as understanding of disease processes and research into new therapeutic approaches.

- Early diagnosis and treatment of intestinal acute cellular rejection (ACR) remains one of the most challenging aspects of postoperative care, which requires close clinicopathologic correlation.

- Histopathologic diagnosis and grading of intestinal ACR is based on assessing the severity of several key histopathologic parameters, including crypt apoptosis, crypt epithelial damage, villous architectural distortion, and mixed inflammatory infiltration.

- Antibody-mediated rejection of human small bowel allografts has not been well documented. Preformed IgG lymphocytotoxic antibodies can be associated with a characteristic clinicopathological syndrome during the early postoperative course.

- The primary histopathologic feature of intestinal allograft chronic rejection is obliterative arteriopathy. Other changes are less specific, including mucosal ulceration, architectural distortion, epithelial regeneration, mucosal fibrosis, and granulation tissue.

Pathology contributes to almost every aspect of intestinal transplantation, including pretransplant eval-

Intestinal Failure: Diagnosis, Management and Transplantation.
Edited by Alan N. Langnas, Olivier Goulet, Eamonn M.M. Quigley and Kelly A. Tappenden. © 2008 Blackwell Publishing.
ISBN 978-1-4051-4637-1.

uation, posttransplant follow-up, as well as understanding of disease processes and research into new therapeutic approaches. This chapter covers several histopathological aspects of intestinal transplantation that have practical implications in the clinical management of patients.

Technical considerations of biopsy monitoring

To monitor for possible development of acute rejection, surveillance endoscopies with multiple guided mucosal biopsies are performed once or twice per week during the early postoperative period. Because the allograft ileum is more susceptible to acute rejection than the jejunum, ileoscopies through a temporary chimney or simple loop ileostomy are the most frequently performed endoscopic examination. Upper endoscopy or enteroscopy are only required for recipients with upper gastrointestinal symptoms, clinical suspicion of rejection with normal ileal biopsy, and other specific indications.

Adequate tissue sampling is necessary for accurate histologic diagnosis. Since the distribution of acute rejection may be patchy, multiple biopsies (usually three to five) are often needed. The obtained tissue should be fixed in 10% neutral buffered formalin for at least 1 hour before processing; multiple sections (usually 10–15) should be examined from each biopsy. In addition to histologic assessment, attention should be paid to the endoscopic findings, because this provides an overall estimation of distribution and magnitude of graft injury. For example, a solitary ulcer near the ileostomy stoma over several weeks with no clinical symptoms is unlikely to represent a moderate or severe acute rejection. Because biopsies obtained close to the ileostomy stoma often have nonspecific inflammatory or regenerative changes, endoscopists should be encouraged to obtain biopsies away from the stoma. Because intestinal allograft rejection is often patchy, biopsies from different regions, including visually involved and noninvolved areas, should be performed to ensure specimen adequacy. In addition, as acute cellular rejection often involves crypts and the graft's donor gut-associated lymphoid tissue, the endoscopic biopsies should be deep enough to include sufficient crypts for evaluation and, ideally, should also include the muscularis mucosae and the upper portion of submucosa.

Preservation/ischemic injury

Preservation injury has been a relatively minor problem in small bowel transplantation. In part, this is likely a result of the intestine's great capacity for epithelial regeneration. Usually, changes of preservation injury are noted during the first few days following transplantation, but resolve within a week posttransplant. Histologically these changes encompass a range of alterations that affect the superficial mucosa, primarily the villi with a variable inflammatory contribution. In pretransplantation specimens, the surface epithelium may be detached from the underlying edematous lamina propria but usually with no active inflammatory infiltration. Shortly after reperfusion, the epithelium often shows pronounced regenerative changes of crypt epithelium characterized by conspicuous mitosis, capillary congestion and shortening of villi with variable degrees of neutrophil-rich inflammatory infiltration. Normal histology is usually present within a week after transplantation. Interestingly, a recent single center retrospective study suggests a protective role of the liver toward intestinal transplantation in pediatric patients, possibly through control of early phase ischemic-reperfusion following transplantation [1].

Because ischemia/preservation injury usually occurs immediately after reperfusion with characteristic histological features that resolve within 2–3 days, in most cases it can be readily differentiated from acute rejection. For patients with delayed recovery from severe ischemia/preservation injury, the diagnosis of early superimposed acute rejection can sometimes be difficult. In this circumstance, the presence of activated lympho-

cytes and eosinophils, ongoing crypt damage, and significant crypt apoptosis points toward acute rejection.

Antibody-mediated rejection of small bowel allografts

Antibodies reactive with donor antigens may have many different effects on small bowel allografts. Animal studies have shown that, although preformed antibodies may cause early small bowel graft failure, they can increase the subsequent duration of graft survival in the long-term [2,3]. These animal studies also suggest that a small bowel graft, similar to a liver graft, may be more resistant to antibody-mediated damage compared to heart and kidney grafts.

Humoral rejection of human small bowel allografts has not been well documented. At our center, we have observed that some patients with preformed IgG lymphocytotoxic antibodies (positive cross-match) developed severe mucosal congestion, darkness, and focal hemorrhage within the small bowel allograft [4]. Mucosal biopsy specimens obtained at this time often show severe congestion, neutrophilic margination and fibrin-platelet thrombi within the lamina propria microvasculature, along with focal hemorrhage (a representative microscopic photograph is shown in Figure 37.1); however, neutrophilic or necrotizing arteritis was not seen and immunofluorescent findings were unremarkable [4]. The long-term significance of these preformed antibodies in human small intestinal transplantation has yet to be determined. Although immunostain for C4d has been used to assist the diagnosis of antibody-mediated rejection in the kidney and heart allografts, we have found that it has limited use in the diagnosis of humoral rejection in the small bowel allograft, largely as a result of the presence of focal capillary staining in normal small bowel mucosa. This impression was also shared by others [5]. However, it remains to be determined whether diffuse capillary C4d staining will have diagnostic value in the small bowel allograft.

Acute cellular rejection of small bowel allografts

The diagnosis and treatment of intestinal acute cellular rejection (ACR) remains one of the most challenging

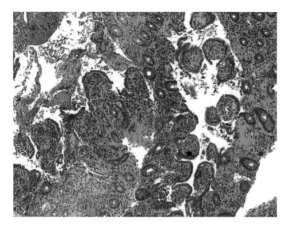

Figure 37.1 Histopathological features of antibody-mediated rejection of the small intestinal allografts. A representative mucosal biopsy obtained within the first 10 days after transplantation. There is prominent intramucosal hemorrhage and congestion with scattered fibrin thrombi in the capillaries, which is not associated with significant inflammation and crypt apoptosis. This is usually accompanied by diffuse C4d positivity.

aspects of postoperative care. Because intestinal acute rejection, if not treated promptly, can rapidly increase in severity and result in graft loss or mortality, early detection and treatment are essential. Several biochemical and functional markers of acute rejection have been proposed in experimental animal models, but they are not practical in the clinical setting. The recognition and diagnosis of intestinal acute rejection rely on the clinical manifestations, endoscopic findings, and histopathological examination of endoscopically guided mucosal biopsy specimens.

The pathogenesis of intestinal acute rejection involves a complex of immunologic events. Following transplantation, the donor intestinal mucosal immune system is replaced gradually by the host's over a period of several weeks to several months after transplantation. Early after transplantation, infiltration of the graft by recipient lymphocytes and the subsequent repopulation of the graft's donor gut-associated lymphoid tissue (GALT) by recipient cells can trigger a mucosal-based mixed lymphocyte response in inadequately-treated recipients. Unless alloreactivity is controlled by adequate immunosuppression, the infiltrated GALT areas become sites of intense immune stimulation and the inflammatory infiltrate begins to extend into the lamina propria and results in epithelial damage and crypt cell apoptosis. As a result of this process, tissue damage, referred to as acute rejection, develops. The normal distribution of GALT likely explains why acute rejection is distributed in a patchy fashion and, most commonly, involves the ileum. The intense host immune reaction to the donor organ rich in lymphoid tissue also explains why heavy immunosuppression is required for intestinal transplant patients.

Recently described histologic criteria represent the current gold standard for the diagnosis and grading of intestinal acute cellular rejection [6], these are based on assessing the severity of several key histopathologic parameters of acute rejection [7,8]: (1) increase in crypt apoptotic bodies; (2) crypt epithelial regeneration (characterized by cytoplasmic basophilia, nuclear enlargement and hyperchromasia, decreased cell height, and mucin depletion) and inflammation; and (3) distortion/atrophy of the villous architecture. Although inflammation can also be seen, it is not a conspicuous finding, nor is it required. The severity of acute rejection is graded as indeterminate, mild, moderate and severe (summarized in Table 37.1). This grading system is practical and has been validated by both retrospective and prospective evaluation of allograft small bowel biopsies from patients receiving different immunosuppressive protocols [6,9].

Indeterminate for acute rejection

Indeterminate for acute rejection is defined, primarily, by increased crypt cell apoptosis that does not reach the threshold needed for mild ACR (<6 apoptotic bodies/10 crypts). The three main features of acute rejection (infiltration by a mixed but primarily mononuclear inflammatory population including blastic or activated lymphocytes; crypt injury and inflammation; and an increase in crypt apoptotic bodies) are variably present, although the inflammatory infiltrate is usually minimal and localized. Indeterminate for acute rejection should not be used as a "wastebasket" diagnosis. Instead, it should be used when the biopsy shows features of rejection, but epithelial injury and apoptosis are less prominent than expected for mild acute rejection. It should not be applied to other non-rejection processes when one is not sure about the diagnosis (Figure 37.2a).

Mild acute rejection

Mild acute rejection is characterized by a generally mild and localized inflammatory infiltrate, which tends to be

Table 37.1 The histopathologic criteria for grading small intestine allograft acute cellular rejection.

Indeterminate for acute cellular rejection
Minimal and localized inflammatory infiltrate; minimal crypt epithelial injury; increased crypt epithelial apoptosis usually with <6 apoptotic bodies/10 crypts; normal to minimal architecture distortion; no mucosa ulceration; changes insufficient for the diagnosis of mild acute rejection.

Mild acute cellular rejection
Mild and localized inflammatory infiltrate with activated lymphocytes; mild crypt epithelium injury, increased crypt epithelial apoptosis usually with >6 apoptotic bodies/10 crypts, mild architectural distortion; no mucosa ulceration.

Moderate acute cellular rejection
Widely dispersed inflammatory infiltrate in lamina propria; diffuse crypt epithelial injury; increased crypt apoptosis with focal confluent apoptosis; more prominent architectural distortion; mild to moderate intimal arteritis may be seen; no mucosa ulceration

Severe acute cellular rejection
Features of moderate acute cellular rejection plus mucosal ulceration. Severe intimal arteritis or transmural arteritis may be seen.

concentrated around small venules in the lamina propria. The mucosa is intact, but the crypt epithelium displays evidence of injury: mucin depletion, cytoplasmic basophilia, decreased cell height, nuclear enlargement and hyperchromasia, and inflammatory infiltration. Apoptosis is increased in crypt epithelial cells, and usually features more than six apoptotic bodies/10 crypts. If sampled by the biopsy specimen, preexisting lymphoid aggregates (Peyer's patches) demonstrate an intense accumulation of activated lymphocytes. The villi are variably shortened and the architecture may be slightly distorted due to expansion of the lamina propria by inflammatory infiltration. A representative microscopic photograph of mild ACR is shown in Figure 37.2b.

Moderate acute rejection

In moderate acute rejection, the inflammatory infiltrate is widely dispersed within the lamina propria. Crypt injury and cryptitis are distributed more diffusely than in mild acute rejection, and the villi tend to have a greater degree of flattening. The number of apoptotic bodies is greater than in mild acute rejection and usually features focal "confluent apoptosis." Mild to moderate intimal arteritis may be seen. However, the mucosa remains intact and without ulceration, although focal superficial erosions can be present. A representative microscopic photograph of moderate ACR is shown in Figure 37.2c.

Severe acute rejection

Severe acute rejection is distinguished by a marked degree of crypt damage and mucosal ulceration, with lymphocytic infiltrates extending deep in the allograft wall and involving nerves and ganglia. As a consequence of the mucosal destruction, luminal contents gain access to the submucosa, prompting a neutrophil-rich infiltrate and an overlying fibropurulent (pseudomembranous) exudate with widespread mucosal sloughing as the final result. The adjacent viable epithelium usually shows rejection-associated changes such as crypt epithelial damage and abundant apoptosis. Severe intimal arteritis or transmural arteritis may be seen. If biopsies are obtained from the necrotic or ulcerated regions or areas with only active inflammation, the deeper rejection-associated changes may not be present in the specimen. Under these circumstances, the overall context and clinical findings then need to be taken into account. A representative microscopic photograph of severe ACR is shown in Figure 37.2d.

"Exfoliative rejection" has been used in some studies to describe a form of severe acute cellular rejection with mucosal exfoliation [10]. This is a descriptive terminology, which is based on the characteristic endoscopic appearance and emphasizes loss of mucosal integrity (diffuse mucosal erosion and/or ulceration). Because the ultimate diagnosis requires histological evaluation and it usually falls into the category of severe ACR

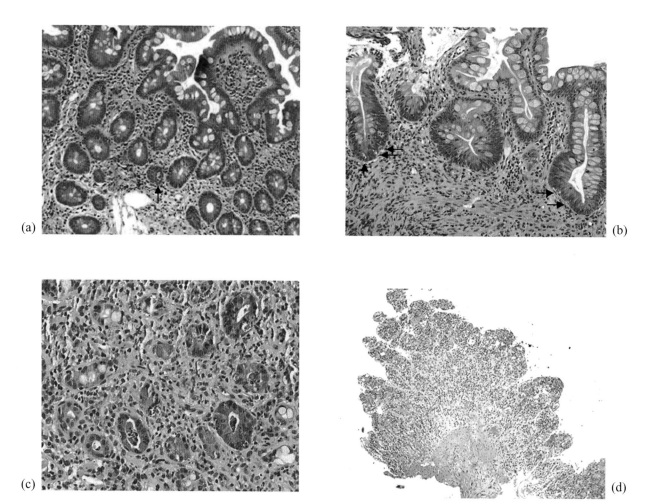

Figure 37.2 Representative microscopic photographs of different severities of small intestine ACR. In contrast to other allografts, infiltration of inflammatory cells above those already present in the lamina propria may or may not be present or conspicuous. Instead, the most important features to monitor are crypt epithelial cell apoptosis epithelial regenerative changes, villous architecture, and evidence of ulceration. (a) Indeterminate for acute rejection is characterized by minimal crypt damage. The apoptotic body count is usually less than 6 apoptotic bodies per 10 crypts. This is usually accompanied by mild regenerative changes but minimal villous atrophy. (b) Mild acute rejection shows crypt epithelial apoptosis involving more than six apoptotic bodies per ten crypts and mild villous shortening and regenerative changes. (c) In moderate acute rejection the number of apoptotic bodies is greater than in mild acute rejection, with focal confluent apoptosis, where apoptotic debris involves at least half of the crypt circumference. The mucosa, however, is not ulcerated. (d) Severe acute rejection is characterized by extensive mucosal destruction, crypt loss, mucosal ulceration, and mixed lymphoplasmacytic, eosinophilic, and neutrophilic infiltration. The residual crypts, if present, often exhibit marked epithelial injury and apoptosis.

based on the established histological grading criteria, in our opinion it probably should not be considered as a separate entity.

As a general rule, early acute rejection episodes (usually within the first 100 days after transplantation) tend to be associated with a greater degree of inflammatory infiltration and less conspicuous apoptosis, while in later rejection episodes, the converse is often seen. The following mechanisms explain the morphological difference between early and later rejection: in early acute rejection the infiltration of donor GALT by recipient's lymphocytes with intense inflammatory reaction is the predominate process; in later rejection episodes the allograft GALT has already been replaced by recipient lymphoid cells and the immune reactivity is directed primarily at the epithelial and stromal cells.

Crypt cell apoptosis is an important process in the physiologic regulation of the intestinal epithelium, and is far more extensive in acute rejection. Apoptotic bodies are characterized by fragmented nuclear debris and cytoplasm contained within a rounded vacuole. The apoptotic bodies should be distinguished from small isolated fragments of nuclear chromatin and intraepithelial neutrophils and eosinophils. We count the apoptotic bodies by scanning the specimen at medium power to identify areas of the greatest concentration and then tallying the total number in ten consecutive crypts.

Although a common feature of rejection, the apoptotic bodies are not specific. Rare apoptotic bodies can be identified in normal mucosa and their number is increased in many inflammatory and immunologic processes including graft-versus-host disease. Nonetheless, normal mucosa generally demonstrates two or fewer apoptotic bodies per ten crypts, whereas counts of more than five per ten crypts are seldom seen except in allograft rejection. It should be remembered, however, that acute rejection is associated with a wide range of apoptotic bodies counts, and, therefore, that the overall findings and context need to be taken into account. It is likely that several mechanisms are responsible for crypt cell apoptosis and the molecules important in this process may include IL-1, TNF-α, Fas, CD40, and cytotoxic T cells. An alternative explanation is that apoptosis may represent merely a nonimmunologic homeostatic process, occurring as a response to increased crypt cell proliferation after epithelial injury.

The quality of the infiltrate (activated lymphocytes admixed with some eosinophils and neutrophils in ACR versus nonactivated lymphocytes in nonspecific enteritis) plays an important role in the differentiation of ACR from other conditions. The intensity of the infiltrate is generally correlated with the severity of ACR (mild infiltrate in mild ACR versus intense infiltrate in severe ACR). In our experience, the area of infiltrate is less reliable, since the infiltrate in low grade ACR can be diffuse despite less intensity. Although eosinophils are frequently seen in the intestinal mucosa, significantly increased eosinophils with coexistent activated lymphocytes and crypt apoptosis point toward acute rejection. Peyer's patches are commonly sampled in mucosal biopsies, especially from the ileum. Although localized Peyer's patches without significant lymphoid activation do not indicate acute rejection, Peyer's patches with lymphoid activation (characterized by lymphoid cells with open chromatin, diffuse infiltration into the surrounding mucosa, or admixed with eosinophils and neutrophils) are frequently associated with acute rejection. The significance of lymphocytic cryptitis (increased lymphocytes in crypt epithelium) is uncertain. Although it is present in some cases of acute rejection, it is also seen in biopsy tissues without ACR (such as nonspecific enteritis, viral infection, or PTLD). Acute cryptitis (increased neutrophils in crypt epithelium) is usually associated with various causes of acute enteritis and is not a diagnostic criterion for acute rejection.

Infections

The heavy immunosuppression required to prevent intestinal allograft rejection places the patients at high risk for the development of infections. The major post transplant infections include cytomegalovirus (CMV), Epstein-Barr Virus (EBV), adenovirus, bacterial and fungal infections. Because these infections can be confused clinically with other causes of intestinal allograft dysfunctions including acute rejection, accurate diagnosis are critical for patient management. CMV infection occurs in approximately one-third of the patients receiving small bowel allografts [11]. Some patients present with multiple episodes of CMV infection in spite of treatment. Histological diagnosis of CMV infection is usually straightforward, because the viral inclusions can be found in endothelial, stromal, and, less often, epithelial cells and can be readily confirmed by immunostaining. However, CMV enteritis can sometimes be associated with increased inflammatory infiltration and increased apoptosis and thus confused with acute cellular rejection; the diagnosis is made by identification of characteristic nuclear/cytoplasmic viral inclusions with confirmatory immunohistochemical staining. EBV infection and PTLD are often associated with significant mononuclear infiltration, and the diagnosis is made by identification of atypical lymphoid cells on H&E sections, immunohistochemical stains for T and B cells, in-situ hybridization for EBER (EBV-early RNA), and clonality analysis. Acute enteritis is often caused by bacterial or viral infection and is characterized by neutrophil-rich infiltration in the lamina propria with acute cryptitis, but, usually, without significantly activated lymphocytes or increased apoptosis.

Posttransplant Lymphoproliferative Disorder (PTLD)

Small bowel transplant recipients are at a relatively high risk of developing PTLD compared to the solid organ transplant population. Approximately 20% of all patients who receive small bowel allografts will develop PTLD. The onset of PTLD varies from 1 to 82 months after transplantation (median onset approximately 8 months) with 2/3 of the cases diagnosed within the first posttransplant year [12]. PTLD is lethal in approximately one-third of all cases. Children are at significantly higher risk than adults. Multivisceral allografts are also at a significantly higher risk to develop PTLD compared to isolated small intestinal grafts. Because the frequency of PTLD can be reduced by modifications of the immunosuppressive regimen and adoption of prophylactic/empirical antiviral therapy, close monitoring for EBV viremia with early diagnosis and treatment of EBV infection is important in reducing the risk of PTLD among intestinal allograft recipients.

The main histological features of PTLD include proliferation of EBV-positive lymphoid cells with malignant potential. EBV infection manifests as a continuum from lymphoid hyperplasia to frankly malignant lymphoid proliferation resembling non-Hodgkin's lymphoma. In the early phase of EBV infection, the tissue is expanded by scattered EBER-positive lymphocytes. With disease progression, the number of positive cells increases, lymphocytes become activated and transformed and, ultimately, tissue architecture is effaced by a malignant lymphoproliferative process. Finn et al. have developed a quantitative method of grading EBV infection in small bowel allograft recipients [13]. Although this method was used in a pediatric population, it can also be readily applied to adult patients. This scheme is based on the number of EBV-positive cells as identified by EBER in-situ hybridization: Grade 1—one to five EBER-positive cells/HPF with most cells being small lymphocytes and scattered mature plasma cells; Grade 2—more than five EBER-positive cells/HPF with atypical features insufficient to warrant categorization as PTLD; Grade 3—more than 15 EBER-positive cells/HPF with features of polymorphous PTLD; Grade 4—more than 15 EBER-positive cells/HPF with features of monomorphic PTLD.

Graft-vs-Host Disease (GVHD)

Because the small intestine is rich in lymphoid tissue, it is not surprising to see that the incidence of GVHD in small bowel transplant patients is higher than in other solid organ transplantation. GVHD occurs in approximately 5% of patients undergoing small bowel transplantation [14,15], which is approximately five to ten times higher than in other solid organ transplantation. Most patients present with a skin rash. Other clinical presentations include ulceration of the oral mucosa, diarrhea, or native liver dysfunction. The onset of clinical symptoms may occur at any time from 8 days to several years postoperatively. The diagnosis is usually established by histopathological criteria, which include keratinocyte necrosis, epithelial apoptosis of the native gastrointestinal tract or oral mucosa. Donor cell infiltration can be demonstrated by several techniques, including immunohistochemistry for mismatched MHC antigens, XY in situ hybridization in sex mismatches, and RFLP analysis. The histological features and diagnostic criteria are similar to those in the classical form of GVHD that occurs after allogenic bone marrow transplantation. The morphological features of intestinal GVHD and acute rejection are very similar. Both conditions manifest, histologically with crypt cell apoptosis and pathogenetically show increased expression of TNF-α and involvement of cytotoxic T lymphocytes. The morphological similarities are most striking with late onset of acute rejection, in which the allograft gut-associated lymphoid tissue has been replaced by recipient lymphoid cells and the immune reactivity is directed primarily at epithelial and stromal cells (this immunologic process is more akin to GVHD). Obviously, because of the morphological similarities between acute rejection and GVHD, histological

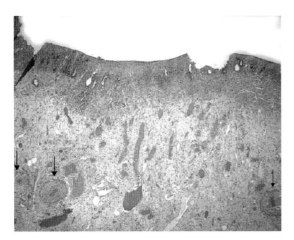

Figure 37.3 Histopathological changes of intestinal chronic rejection. The intestinal allograft was resected as a result of chronic rejection. There is extensive mucosal ulceration and regeneration with fibrosis, mixed inflammation, and crypt loss. Note the presence of severe chronic arteriopathy (arrows).

diagnosis of intestinal GVHD can only be made in the biopsies obtained from the native intestine.

Chronic rejection of small bowel allografts

The primary histologic feature of chronic rejection in the small bowel allograft, as in other solid organ grafts, is obliterative arteriopathy [16], which typically involves the larger arteries within the bowel wall and mesentery. This characteristic arterial pathology is usually observed during evaluation of allograft resection specimens (a representative microscopic photograph is shown in Figure 37.3). Because these vessels are not routinely sampled in the biopsied specimens, a definitive diagnosis of chronic rejection is usually difficult to establish for patients carrying the transplanted intestine grafts. Other features are less specific, but are more apt to be found in mucosal biopsies. These include discrete ulcers accompanied by mucosa showing evidence of prior injury and regeneration (disordered and irregular crypt and villus architecture, epithelial adenomatous changes, mucosal fibrosis, granulation tissue) together with ongoing crypt cell apoptosis. The submucosa can be severely fibrotic, producing a thickened, unyielding bowel wall resembling Crohn's disease. We have observed that some patients develop diffuse mesenteric sclerosis (with or without arterial intimal sclerosis); however, it is unclear whether the mesenteric pathology represents a spectrum of chronic rejection or a separate disease process.

References

1 Jugie M, Canioni D, Le Bihan, et al. Study of the impact of liver transplantation on the outcome of intestinal grafts in children. *Transplantation* 2006;81:992–997.

2 Fujisaki S, Murase N, Demetris AJ, et al. Effects of preformed antibodies induced by whole blood transfusion on small bowel transplantation. *Transplant Proc* 1994;26:1528–1529.

3 Murase N, Fujisaki S, Tanabe M, et al. Small bowel transplantation in sensitized recipients: comparison with heart, kidney, and liver grafts. *Transplant Proc* 1994;26:1517–1518.

4 Wu T, Abu-Elmagd K, Bond G, Demetris AJ. A clinicopathologic study of isolated intestinal allografts with preformed IgG lymphocytotoxic antibodies. *Hum Pathol* 2004;35:1332–1339.

5 Troxell ML, Higgins JP, Kambham N. Evaluation of C4d staining in liver and small intestine allografts. *Arch Pathol Lab Med* 2006;130:1489–1496.

6 Wu T, Abu-Elmagd K, Bond G, et al. A schema for histologic grading of small intestine allograft acute rejection. *Transplantation* 2003;75:1241–1248.

7 Lee RG, Nakamura K, Tsamandas AC, et al. Pathology of human intestinal transplantation. *Gastroenterology* 1996;110:1820–1834.

8 White FV, Reyes J, Jaffe R, Yunis EJ. Pathology of intestinal transplantation in children. *Am J Surg Pathol* 1995;19:687–698.

9 Wu T, Bond G, Dolly M, et al. Histopathologic characteristics of human intestine allograft acute rejection in patients pretreated with thymoglobulin or alemtuzumab. *Am J Gastroenterol* 2006;101:1617–1624.

10 Ishii T, Mazariegos GV, Bueno J, et al. Exfoliative rejection after intestinal transplantation in children. *Pediatr Transplant* 2003;7:185–191.

11 Abu-Elmagd K, Bond G, Reyes J, Fung J. Intestinal transplantation: a coming of age. *Adv Surg* 2002;36:65–101.

12 Nalesnik M, Jaffe R, Reyes J, et al. Posttransplant lymphoproliferative disorders in small bowel allograft recipients. *Transplant Proc* 2000;32:1213.

13 Finn L, Reyes J, Bueno J, Yunis E. Epstein-Barr virus infections in children after transplantation of the small intestine. *Am J Surg Pathol* 1998;22:299–309.

14 Abu-Elmagd K, Reyes J, Todo S, et al. Clinical intestinal transplantation: new perspectives and immunologic considerations. *J Am Coll Surg* 1998;186:512–525; discussion 525–527.

15 Mazariegos GV, Abu-Elmagd K, Jaffe R, et al. Graft versus host disease in intestinal transplantation. *Am J Transplant* 2004;4:1459–1465.

16 Parizhskaya M, Redondo C, Demetris A, et al. Chronic rejection of small bowel grafts: pediatric and adult study of risk factors and morphologic progression. *Pediatr Dev Pathol* 2003;6:240–250.

38 Long-Term Management of Intestinal Transplant Recipients

Frances R. Malone and Simon P. Horslen

Key points

- The improved survival of intestinal transplant recipients has increased the relevance of long-term management. The goal is now to achieve excellent long-term outcomes as well as short-term survival.

- The key to fluid and electrolyte management is close monitoring and compensation for increased intestinal losses.

- Allograft dysfunction has many causes, of particular importance is the differentiation between infection and rejection.

- Careful, detailed discharge from the hospital and, subsequently, to home with the involvement of the entire transplant team and the primary medical provider helps ensure optimal patient and family care.

- Follow-up with an intestinal transplant center is required for the duration of their life as the risk of complications does not appear to decrease over time.

The complexity and challenge of caring for intestinal transplant recipients continues for the duration of graft function. Improved patient survival [1], new immunosuppressive regimens [2] and greater experience have necessitated a shift in our attention to long term management issues. In this chapter, we will present the current approach to the management of the intestinal transplant recipient, the ultimate goal being their resumption of a normal life. Surgical complications, in-

fectious diseases, immunosuppressive medications, rejection, and malignant disorders are distinct and critical issues in patient management, for this reason, they are comprehensively discussed in other chapters of this textbook. Herein, we will address the issues related to immediate posttransplant care, focusing on the transition out of the intensive care unit, we will follow with a discussion on the preparation for discharge, home care issues, routine clinic management, and long-term follow-up and will close with problems and complications specific to recipients of intestinal transplants.

Fluid and electrolyte management

Initially, all patients require intravenous fluid support. As they transition out of the intensive care unit, most patients require parenteral nutrition to meet caloric requirements and additional intravenous fluids to compensate for stomal losses. Parenteral nutrition is continued until the transition to enteral nutrition is complete, commonly by 2–4 weeks following transplantation. All patients will require additional calories posttransplant to facilitate anabolism while promoting wound healing and recovery from major surgery. In some pediatric patients who have had long-term growth failure, a 50–100% increase in calories may be necessary.

Secretory diarrhea is to be expected following resolution of post-op ileus. Stomal fluid losses are replaced to avoid dehydration and electrolyte imbalances [12]. These needs are met with 0.45–0.9% saline ml/ml intravenously for losses in excess of 35 ml/kg/day of ileal effluent. Ostomy output is measured routinely and replacement volume calculated and administered on a 4-hourly basis. As the patient recovers, ostomy output generally diminishes and replacement can be

Intestinal Failure: Diagnosis, Management and Transplantation. Edited by Alan N. Langnas, Olivier Goulet, Eamonn M.M. Quigley and Kelly A. Tappenden. © 2008 Blackwell Publishing. ISBN 978-1-4051-4637-1.

calculated and replaced over 8 and then 12 hours, in preparation for discharge. The aim is to convert the patient to enteral fluid replacements, for stool losses greater than 35–50 ml/kg/day prior to discharge. However, some intestinal transplant patients do require an intravenous fluid replacement plan even after discharge. Bicarbonate wasting is almost universal in the intestinal transplant recipient because of the bicarbonate concentration in various enteric secretions such as pancreatic fluid and bile that are lost in the stomal effluent. This leads to chronic metabolic acidosis, if not supplemented. Potassium requirements tend to be fairly constant in the stable patient and do not usually vary significantly with changes in stomal output volume. For this reason, potassium is avoided in replacement fluids because patients may require very different volumes on different days. Studies have demonstrated that stoma output at 30 days posttransplant averages 37 ml/kg/day [23] and that stoma output volume is a useful guide to monitoring feeding advancement [38]. Stool absorption studies have not been particularly useful in clinical management, although they may have a place in research [15]. If stoma output increases with feeding advancement, the rate of feedings is not advanced until the patient's output returns to their baseline. Occasionally, it is necessary to reduce enteral feeds until stomal output diminishes, after which feeds can be advanced again according to tolerance. Fluid management at times of increased stool output and vomiting, even after enteral feeding has been maximized and parenteral nutrition discontinued, often necessitates short-term administration of replacement fluids intravenously. Periods of high output may suggest a clinical indication for the use of antidiarrheal medications such as loperamide, or somatastatin antagonists. In such cases, a trial of these agents may be worthwhile; however, in most cases, they have not proved to be particularly effective. We would caution against high expectations for these therapies, in this population.

Nutrition

Intestinal transplant recipients require parenteral nutritional support in the early post-op period. Enteral feedings are initiated when graft motility is established by the appearance of gas and effluent from the stoma. This frequently coincides with decreased abdominal distention as the ileal inflammatory response to ischemia-reperfusion injury diminishes (Post-op days 3–7) [12,38]. The route of administration of enteral feeds varies according to unit protocols; some programs routinely administer initial feeds directly into the jejunum, either via a G-J tube or a surgically placed jejunostomy. Delayed gastric emptying often mandates use of transpyloric feeding, even in programs willing to feed directly into the stomach. Low-fat, hypo-osmolar elemental feedings are usually begun although there is little evidence to suggest that fats are any less well tolerated than other nutrients by the newly transplanted bowel [15]. A low-fat diet reduces the risk of chylous ascites, a potential consequence of the lack of lymphatic drainage of the allograft. The feedings start with a dilute formula (usually 15–20 kcal/oz); the rate is slowly increased (in 5–10 ml increments), thereafter. Once the desired optimal rate is obtained, the strength of the formula can be increased along with a transition to oral or gastric feeding in those who had been previously fed directly into the jejunum. Oral intake can be introduced while still advancing tube feeds, particularly in those without oral aversion. Early posttransplantation, the osmolality of feeds does appear to affect stomal output and, for this reason, it is prudent to limit high sugar content foods such as regular sodas, candy, and fruit juices. It is common, in some programs, to avoid dairy products early after transplant because there is thought to be an increased incidence of allergies to food proteins posttransplantation [3] possibly related to altered mucosal permeability and T-cell responses as a result of immunosuppressive medication. The specific food intolerances described after intestinal transplant appear to have IgE mediated symptoms rather than simply being a manifestation of mucosal enzyme inactivity such as lactase deficiency.

Many intestinal transplant recipients and, most notably, but not exclusively, infants, have feeding aversions and may receive worthwhile assistance from occupational, speech, or feeding therapists in reestablishing oral intake. After an intestinal transplant, patients are generally able to achieve linear growth, maintain adequate muscle and fat stores, and transition to an oral diet. Many children are able to achieve positive growth velocity [23]. In long-term survivors of intestinal transplantation, normal growth velocities can be expected; however, catch-up growth sufficient to compensate for pretransplant stunting is rarely seen [10]. Nutritional monitoring of growth and the ability to maintain body weight are essential measures throughout the posttransplant period, as are the periodic evaluation of serum trace elements and vitamins.

Stoma closure

An ileostomy is created in most cases as a means to monitor the allograft. Once it is deemed, on clinical grounds, that elective endoscopic and histologic surveillance of the allograft are no longer necessary, consideration can be given to elective stoma closure. This usually takes place between 6 and 12 months posttransplant but has been achieved earlier in some cases. The stoma site usually heals without difficulty but wound infection and intestinal obstruction may complicate the procedure. Consideration should also be given to the possibility of nosocomial infection; for example, it may not be wise to carry out elective surgery on an immunosuppressed patient at the height of the influenza or respiratory syncitial virus season when the procedure could be safely postponed until the spring or summer.

Allograft function

Intestinal allograft function requires monitoring for the life of the graft. The frequency of clinical assessments decreases over time as the recipient and caregivers gain knowledge and experience with ongoing assessment of stomal appearance and output. Radiologic monitoring may be needed to assess gastric emptying or for evidence of obstruction. The mainstay of graft monitoring is endoscopy with mucosal histology. The intestinal allograft is examined routinely in the early posttransplant weeks by ileoscopy at least once a week. Most centers use routine endoscopic techniques but the Miami group have published their experience with zoom endoscopy [13]. The endoscope is introduced into the transplanted ileum via the stoma (in the case of a double-barreled or loop ileostomy into

both lumens) and advanced as far as is easily accessible, usually 15 to 20 cm. In the case of the distal, or efferent, limb of a loop ileostomy the scope is advanced to the ileo-colonic anastomosis. Mucosal biopsies are obtained from the transplanted intestine with pinch biopsy forceps through the scope. Biopsies (three to four from each site) should, ideally, be at least 5 cm from both the stomal opening and the ileocolonic junction because histology at these sites may be unrepresentative, or misleading. In uncomplicated patients, the frequency of biopsies decreases over time. Following stomal closure, the allograft can only be accessed by standard endoscopic routes. In addition to elective examination, the allograft is examined and biopsied whenever there is an unexplained change in intestinal function, primarily to rule out rejection. Other essential measures of allograft function include: somal/stool output, tolerance of normal feeding regimen, presence of abdominal pain or distention, and the gross appearance of the stomal mucosa. The assessment of the allograft absorption capacity through stool studies may be useful as a research tool, however, it is ungainly, inconvenient, and imprecise in the clinical setting [15].

Graft dysfunction

Determining the cause of gastrointestinal distress in a post intestinal transplant patient may be a difficult endeavor. Common signs of possible graft dysfunction include:
- increased, or decreased, stomal output
- fever
- vomiting, or high gastric residuals
- abdominal pain, or distention
- changes in stomal color, or perfusion
- irritability.

The differential diagnosis to be considered in instances of acute graft dysfunction includes acute cellular rejection, systemic viral or bacterial infection, abdominal sepsis, infective enteritis, and posttransplant lymphoproliferative disorder, as well as surgical complications such as intestinal perforation and obstruction. Blood cultures, viral studies on blood, stool studies, endoscopy and mucosal biopsy, and radiologic studies (ultrasound, contrast studies or CT scanning) may be required to identify the specific diagnosis.

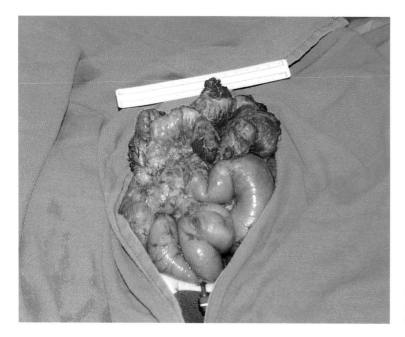

Figure 38.1 Intestinal allograft with chronic rejection requiring allograft enterectomy.

Histopathologic differentiation between viral enteritis, particularly when caused by adenovirus, and acute cellular rejection may be difficult and experienced pathological interpretation is essential. Tissue immunohistochemistry, viral culture and in-situ PCR may assist in diagnosis. Correctly determining the diagnosis is imperative, given that the treatment for rejection involves increasing immunosuppression; an approach that could well prove disastrous in the presence of active infection.

Acute rejection

Allograft function is significantly affected by the occurrence of acute cellular rejection (ACR) [9]. Clinical signs of rejection are nonspecific and may occur late in its progression. After the early posttransplant period of routine endoscopic biopsies the frequency of biopsy is dependent on clinical indicators. The optimal frequency of surveillance biopsies has not been determined and varies between centers. The severity of rejection at the time of diagnosis varies and its scoring is based on standardized histologic criteria [44]. (See Chapter 37).

The treatment of acute rejection starts with intravenous steroid boluses (10–20 mg/kg/day) for 3 days and increased maintenance immunosuppression. Repeated biopsies are performed frequently to document improvement. Antilymphocyte preparations (ATG or OKT3) are reserved for severe or steroid-resistant rejection. Severe exfoliating rejection may necessitate graft enterectomy.

Chronic rejection

Chronic rejection is manifest by a gradual deterioration in allograft function, increased ileal or stool outputs, allograft stricture, or sudden graft loss in the face of an acute dehydrating condition such as rotavirus enteritis. The pathological lesion is one of vascular rejection in the medium sized vessels of the transplant mesentery and in the deeper layers of the bowel wall, and, therefore, mucosal biopsies are rarely diagnostic. Confirmation requires full thickness biopsy, which is usually only undertaken in the context of allograft enterectomy, when graft failure is established. Little is known about the pathophysiology or early changes associated with this condition. There is a suggestion that it may be more common in recipients

Table 38.1 Prophylactic antiviral therapy and duration of use at the 5 intestinal transplant programs surveyed.

Antiviral agent	Omaha	Pittsburgh	Miami	UCLA	Mt Sinai
Cytogam	1 y	2 wk	4 mo		3 mo
Ganciclovir intravenously	2 wk	2 wk (high risk 3 mo)	2–3 wk	100 days	2 wk
Antivirals by mouth	1 y	None (children) 3–6 mo (adults)	6 mo	5 yr	3 mo

(Reproduced from Horslen [8], with permission from the American Gastroenterological Association.)

of isolated intestinal grafts as opposed to those who receive composite liver-intestine or multivisceral grafts [18,35]. The early stages of this lesion are not easily identified and response to modification of immunosuppression is not known, but once chronic rejection is established, increased immunosuppression does not appear to improve graft function and will only predispose to greater risks of infection. Chronic rejection may respond to resection but typically requires complete graft enterectomy (Figure 38.1).

Immunosuppression

Immunosuppression is always a delicate balance after intestinal transplantation. When determining the intensity of immunosuppression, the relative risks of immunosuppression, rejection and infection must be carefully assessed at each stage of the posttransplant recovery process. Underimmunosuppression puts the patient at risk of allograft rejection and potential graft loss, whereas overimmunosuppression increases the potential for local and systemic infections, as well as the incidence of nonimmunologic side effects of the immunosuppressive agents. Currently, the most commonly used immunosuppressive regimens consist of either initial treatment with a IL-2 receptor antagonist followed by tacrolimus and steroids (+/− sirolimus) or a steroid-free protocol with rabbit antithymocyte globulin or alemtuzimab induction followed by tacrolimus monotherapy [21].

Infection prophylaxis and management

Infection is the leading cause of death in intestinal transplant recipients, despite routine bacterial and viral prophylaxis. The intestinal transplant recipient

is susceptible to episodes of bacteremia, fungemia, viremia, and intra-abdominal abscesses as a result of their surgery, immunosuppressed state, and the presence of indwelling intravenous catheters. Bacterial and fungal infections represent the greatest risk in the first 4–6 weeks. Viral pathogens typically cause problems later. Prophylactic regimens vary among transplant centers but, typically, include coverage for pneumocystis jiroveci, cytomegalovirus, and fungal infections in the immediate posttransplant period (Table 38.1) [8]. Co-trimoxazole prophylaxis is prescribed for the first year. Ganciclovir is administered for at least the first 14 days in the low-risk population (cytomegalovirus negative donor to negative recipient) and for 3 months in the high risk recipient (cytomegalovirus positive donor or recipient). Fluconazole is prescribed for the first 14 days. Infections remain the primary reason for readmission at all times following transplantation [1]. Infectious enteritis occurs in 39% of intestinal transplant recipients; two thirds of these cases are attributable to viral agents [45]. Viral pathogens may cause mild gastroenteritis in the general population but can cause severe allograft dysfunction postintestinal transplant [14]. The differentiation of viral infection from rejection is challenging but essential, as an inadvertent misdiagnosis of rejection resulting in an increase in immunosuppression could lead to systemic viral dissemination. Routine viral surveillance is universally performed; however, there is little consistency in its duration (Table 38.2).

Skin care

The skin integrity of the incision, ostomy, intravenous line sites, and pressure points all require close inspection. This population is vulnerable to skin breakdown and infection for a variety of reasons, including general

Table 38.2 Routine viral surveillance on intestinal transplant recipients at the 5 intestinal transplant programs surveyed.

	Omaha	Pittsburgh	Miami	UCLA	Mt Sinai
Cytomegalovirus DNA (blood)		Biweekly for 1 mo then monthly	Weekly for 1 mo, biweekly for 5 mo, then monthly	Biweekly then monthly for 1–2 y	Weekly for 1 mo Monthly for 5 mo
EBV DNA (blood)		Biweekly for 1 mo then monthly	Weekly for 1 mo, biweekly for 5 mo, then monthly	Biweekly then monthly for 1–2 y	Weekly for 1 mo Monthly for 5 mo
Adenovirus DNA (blood)			Monthly for 6 mo		Biweekly
Viral cultures on all allograft biopsy specimens	Yes	No	No	Yes	Yes

(Reproduced from Horslen [8], with permission from the American Gastroenterological Association.)

debilitation, tissue edema and malnutrition, the use of sedative and paralytic agents, and the prolonged recovery time that typifies their postoperative course. The incision is monitored for signs of healing, which may be delayed secondary to both poor nutritional status pretransplant and immunosuppression. Another factor that may complicate wound closure is sheer lack of space for the graft: limited intraperitoneal volume often necessitates delayed abdominal closure in intestinal transplant recipients. Frequently, the fascia is closed but the skin left open because of the risk of wound infection. The ostomy site is monitored for changes in skin integrity or mucosal perfusion, bleeding, prolapse, or breakdown. The use of a two-piece ostomy appliance is useful to permit frequent stomal assessments, bag emptying, the transit of large effluent volumes, and repeated endoscopy. Following stoma takedown, the skin integrity of the recipient's perineum becomes an area of concern. Cholestyramine (in a sugar-free preparation) may help with bile acid-induced diarrhea immediately following stomal takedown, but this settles as the newly recruited colon adapts to the presence of luminal nutrients.

Discharge planning and home care

Planning for discharge begins at evaluation for transplantation but becomes a reality when the patient is transitioned out of the intensive care unit. An ongoing involvement of the care giver in discussions regarding the plan of care and in the daily care of the recipient facilitates the ultimate assumption of their outpatient role. The intestinal transplant recipient is ready to leave the hospital when they can consistently maintain their hydration and nutritional needs. Teaching and preparation for discharge are the combined responsibility of all involved care providers. Specific teaching about the role of posttransplant medications, their administration, and their potential side effects are primarily the domain of the dedicated transplant pharmacy staff. Enteral advancement and nutritional management are presented and reinforced by the transplant dietitian and the nursing staff. Direct patient care is taught and reinforced by the transplant nursing staff and transplant nurse coordinators. Written instructions about each topic discussed with the recipient and family are also provided for their later reference (Table 38.3). Recipients remain in the locale of their transplant center usually for between 3 and 6 months, by which time they are sufficiently stable to consider the transition to home.

Home care issues

Home care services must be available to deliver products to the patient's home and to provide technical support for their feeding and intravenous fluid pumps as well as home nursing support, if needed. The intestinal transplant patient is discharged with a complex fluid and nutrition regimen that will demand a

Table 38.3 Topics for discharge teaching and the discharge handbook. Each of these topics is covered in detail by the Transplant Nurse Coordinator and provided in written form for the families' future reference.

Educational information	• How the digestive system works • Transplant physiology • Immunosuppression/rejection • Medications and side effects
Assessment of the recipient and when/how to call the transplant team	• Inability to tolerate enteral feedings (nausea, vomiting, dehydration) • Difficulty maintaining nutritional status • Sudden increase or decrease in ostomy output • Change in color of stoma, stomal prolapse • Bloody ostomy output • Fever • Enlarged lymph nodes or other "bumps"/localized masses • New onset snoring, drooling, or difficulty swallowing • Persistent headaches • Patient unwell with no obvious cause • Family and primary medical providers are encouraged to contact the transplant team with any questions. These are complex patients in whom serious complications can occur with rather nonspecific signs and symptoms
Nutrition and fluid management	• Home feeding instructions and enteral nutrition taper • Measuring and recording intake and output at home • When to administer supplemental IV fluids • How to administer supplemental IV fluids • How to facilitate oral intake
Wound care	• Wound care • Gastrostomy care and replacement • Ostomy care
Care coordination	• Medication administration and script renewal • Avoidance of nonsteroidal anti-inflammatory agents • Lab work • Lab schedule • Clinic schedule and out patient format for labwork and scripts • Immunizations and exposures • Possibility of readmission is likely in first year

high level of attention from the caregiver. To facilitate their success, the home care providers should have experience in the care of intestinal transplant recipients and be able to offer their staff focused training on the needs of this unique group of patients. The typical patient will be discharged from the hospital with the need for wound and ostomy care supplies, complete enteral nutrition and intravenous fluid supplies, and gastrostomy/jejunostomy appliances.

Transplant clinic follow up

A visit to the intestinal transplant clinic involves the whole transplant team. The patient is seen by their physician and surgeon, transplant coordinator, dietitian, and social worker. Immediately after discharge, the patient is seen in transplant clinic once or twice per week for the first month with laboratory studies being

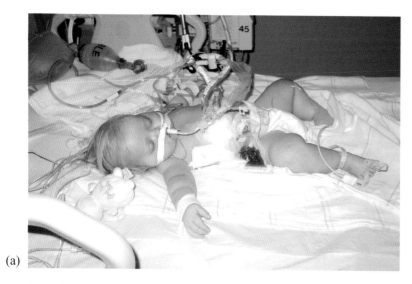

(a)

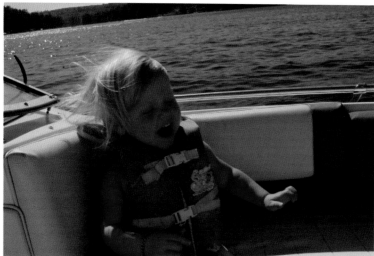

(b)

Figure 38.2 This patient received a liver and intestine transplant in December 2004. This photo (a) is from her pediatric intensive care unit stay immediately posttransplant. Her posttransplant course was complicated by an allograft volvulus that required resection in June of 2005. Here she has recovered and reattained full enteral tolerance (b).

performed immediately before their appointment. Assuming that there are no complications, visits to the transplant center decrease over time. The clinic visit involves an assessment of the patient and of graft function, monitoring of medications, nutrition, hydration, growth; development and social adaptation; as well as making decisions regarding changes in care. Between clinic visits, the patient should communicate with the transplant coordinator regarding any changes in their health. Of particular interest, are any episodes of nausea and/or vomiting outside the patient's norm, fever greater than 38.5°C, changes in stoma appearance or

output, decreased urine output, abdominal pain or distention, rash, or weight loss (see Table 38.3).

Communication with the primary provider

The transplant center should keep the primary medical care provider informed of the patient's progress throughout the transplant process. As the time for transition to home approaches, the primary provider will need detailed information about the patient's health,

Table 38.4 Complications of intestinal transplantation. Complications that may be encountered after intestinal transplant are listed with a selection of available references on the topics.

Surgical complications [6,30,33]	• Vascular thrombosis • Anastomotic leak • Stricture • Wound infections • Fascial dehiscence • Intraabdominal hemorrhage • Stoma prolapse • Obstruction • Perforation
Allograft complications [5,9,11,16,19,26,30]	• Sclerosisng peritonitis • Gastrointestinal bleeding • Persistent chylous ascities with or without pleural effusion • Rejection • Centrolobular necrosis of liver graft in combined transplant
Medication effects [25,36,40,41]	• Renal dysfunction • Hypertension • Posttransplant diabetes • Thrombotic microangiopathy • Thrombocytopenia
Immunologic complications [4,17,22,29,34,39]	• Infection • Posttransplant lymphoproliferative disease and malignancies • Cytopenia • Eosinophilia
Nutrition [23,24,28,42,43]	• Growth • Maintenance of body weight
Other complications [1,3,9,20,27,37,38]	• Rashes • Food sensitivities/allergies • Graft-vs-host disease

and if they feel well supported by the transplant center they are better equipped to support the patient and family. Much of the intestinal transplant recipient's long term care can be performed by their local provider. In addition to the previously listed "Assessment of the recipient and when/how to call the transplant team," (Table 38.3) primary care providers should discuss with the transplant team the occurrence of gastrointestinal illness and the initiation of any new medications in order to ensure there are no interactions with the patient's immunosuppressive regimen.

Problems and complications

There are many potential complications that can occur at any time after intestinal transplant. Recipients are susceptible to the complications inherent to solid organ transplantation and immunosuppression (rejection, infection, and medication toxicity). They may also encounter those specific to the intestinal transplant population (sclerosing peritonitis, stricture, food sensitivities/allergies and malabsorption, gastrointestinal bleeding, persistent ascites, with or without pleural effusion). Severe or prolonged viral enteritis appears to be much more common in intestinal transplant recipients than in other solid organ transplant populations. Infectious complications and acute or chronic rejection are a primary cause of morbidity and mortality in this population. Space limits full discussion of potential complications and their management (summarized in Table 38.4).

Medical issues continue to necessitate readmission to hospital for the intestinal transplant patient even years after successful transplant [1] and they, therefore, require dedicated follow-up and consistent monitoring. Unlike other forms of solid organ transplant, long-term outcomes have not been determined, making it essential that intestinal transplant recipients maintain close contact with a transplant center even years after transplant.

parameters to monitor, and abnormal findings to report to the transplant center. Direct telephone contact with the local physician(s) is highly desirable because few referring physicians will have significant experience with the care of intestinal transplant recipients

References

1 Andersen DA, Horslen S. An analysis of the long-term complications of intestine transplant recipients. 2004;14:277–282.

2 Bond GJ, Mazariegos GV, Sindhi R, et al. Evolutionary experience with immunosuppression in pediatric intestinal transplantation. *J Pediatr Surg* 2005;40:274–279; discussion 279–280.

3 Chehade M, Nowak-Wegrzyn A, Kaufman SS, et al. De novo food allergy after intestinal transplantation: a report of three cases. *J Pediatr Gastroenterol Nutr* 2004;38:545–547.

4 Codeluppi M, Cocchi S, Guaraldi G, et al. Rituximab as treatment of posttransplant lymphoproliferative disorder in patients who underwent small bowel/multivisceral transplantation: report of three cases. *Transplant Proc* 2005;37:2634–2635.

5 D'Errico A, Corti B, Pinna AD, et al. Granzyme B and perforin as predictive markers for acute rejection in human intestinal transplantation. *Transplant Proc* 2003;35:3061–3065.

6 Fishbein TM, Florman S, Gondolesi G, et al. Recurrent portal hypertension after composite liver/small bowel transplantation. *Liver Transpl* 2002;8:639–642.

7 Flynn B, Park BK, Bond G, et al. Immunosuppressant strategies for intestinal transplantation: a review of a tolerogenic regimen. *Prog Transplant* 2005;15:60–64.

8 Horslen SP. Optimal management of the post-intestinal transplant patient. *Gastroenterology* 2006;130:S163–S169.

9 Ishii T, Mazariegos GV, Bueno J, et al. Exfoliative rejection after intestinal transplantation in children. *Pediatr Transplant* 2003;7:185–191.

10 Iyer K, Horslen S, Iverson A, et al. Nutritional outcome and growth of children after intestinal transplantation. *J Pediatr Surg* 2002;37:464–466.

11 Iyer KR, Srinath C, Horslen S, et al. Late graft loss and long-term outcome after isolated intestinal transplantation in children. *J Pediatr Surg* 2002;37:151–154.

12 Jankowski Phillips SK, McGhee B, Reyes J. Pediatric Liver, *Intestine and Multivisceral Transplantation: A Manual of Management and Patient care.* Hudson: Lexi-Comp, Inc., 2003:209.

13 Kato T, Gaynor JJ, Nishida S, et al. Zoom endoscopic monitoring of small bowel allograft rejection. *Surg Endosc* 2006;20:773–782.

14 Kaufman SS, Chatterjee NK, Fuschino ME, et al. Characteristics of human calicivirus enteritis in intestinal transplant recipients. *J Pediatr Gastroenterol Nutr* 2005;40:328–333.

15 Kaufman SS, Lyden ER, Brown CR, et al. Disaccharidase activities and fat assimilation in pediatric patients after intestinal transplantation. *Transplantation* 2000;69:362–365.

16 Lacaille F, Canioni D, Fournet JC, et al. Centrilobular necrosis in children after combined liver and small bowel transplantation. *Transplantation* 2002;73:252–257.

17 Lacaille F, Moes N, Hugot JP, et al. Severe dysimmune cytopenia in children treated with tacrolimus after organ transplantation. *Am J Transplant* 2006;6:1072–1076.

18 Lauro A, Dazzi A, Ercolani G, et al. Results of intestinal and multivisceral transplantation in adult patients: Italian experience. *Transplant Proc* 2006;38:1696–1698.

19 Macedo C, Sindhi R, Mazariegos GV, et al. Sclerosing peritonitis after intestinal transplantation in children. *Pediatr Transplant* 2005;9:187–191.

20 Mazariegos GV, Abu-Elmagd K, Jaffe R, et al. Graft versus host disease in intestinal transplantation. *Am J Transplant* 2004;4:1459–1465.

21 Meier-Kriesche HU, Li S, Gruessner RW, et al. Immunosuppression: evolution in practice and trends, 1994–2004. *Am J Transplant* 2006;6:1111–1131.

22 Nodit L, Murase N, Reyes JD, et al. Transient posttransplant graft-versus-host lymphadenopathy. *Pediatr Dev Pathol* 2004;7:533–537.

23 Nucci AM, Barksdale EM, Jr, Beserock N, et al. Long-term nutritional outcome after pediatric intestinal transplantation. *J Pediatr Surg* 2002;37:460–463.

24 Nucci AM, Reyes J, Yaworski JA, et al. Serum growth factors and growth indices pre- and post-pediatric intestinal transplantation. *J Pediatr Surg* 2003;38:1043–1047.

25 Paramesh AS, Grosskreutz C, Florman SS, et al. Thrombotic microangiopathy associated with combined sirolimus and tacrolimus immunosuppression after intestinal transplantation. *Transplantation* 2004;77:129–131.

26 Parizhskaya M, Redondo C, Demetris A, et al. Chronic rejection of small bowel grafts: pediatric and adult study of risk factors and morphologic progression. *Pediatr Dev Pathol* 2003;6:240–250.

27 Pinna AD, Weppler D, Nery J, et al. Intestinal transplantation at the University of Miami—five years of experience. *Transplant Proc* 2000;32:1226–1227.

28 Porubsky M, Testa G, John E, et al. Pattern of growth after pediatric living-donor small bowel transplantation. *Pediatr Transplant* 2006;10:701–706.

29 Quintini C, Kato T, Gaynor JJ, et al. Analysis of risk factors for the development of posttransplant lymphoproliperative disorder among 119 children who received primary intestinal transplants at a single center. *Transplant Proc* 2006;38:1755–1758.

30 Reyes J, Bueno J, Kocoshis S, et al. Current status of intestinal transplantation in children. *J Pediatr Surg* 1998;33:243–254.

31 Ruiz P, Garcia M, Pappas P, et al. Mucosal vascular alterations in the early posttransplant period of small bowel allograft recipients may reflect humoral-based allograft rejection. *Transplant Proc* 2002;34:869–871.

32 Ruiz P, Perez MT, Garcia M, et al. Semiquantitative measurement of mucosal fibrosis as a means of assessing chronic injury in bowel allografts. *Transplant Proc* 2002;34:874–875.

33 Saggi BH, Farmer DG, Yersiz H, Busuttil RW. Surgical advances in liver and bowel transplantation. *Anesthesiol Clin North Am* 2004;22:713–740.

34 Seda Neto J, Macedo C, Jaffe R, et al. Carcinoma of donor origin after liver-intestine transplantation in a child. *Pediatr Transplant* 2005;9:244–248.

35 Selvaggi G, Kato T, Gaynor JJ, et al. Analysis of rejection episodes in over 100 pediatric intestinal transplant recipients. *Transplant Proc* 2006;38:1711–1712.

36 Selvaggi G, Weppler D, Tzakis A. Liver and gastrointestinal transplantation at the University of Miami. *Clin Transpl* 2003;255–266.

37 Sudan DL, Iverson A, Weseman RA, et al. Assessment of function, growth and development, and long-term quality of life after small bowel transplantation. *Transplant Proc* 2000;32:1211–1212.

38 Sudan DL, Kaufman SS, Shaw BW, et al. Isolated intestinal transplantation for intestinal failure. *Am J Gastroenterol* 2000;95:1506–1515.

39 Talisetti A, Testa G, Holterman M, et al. Successful treatment of posttransplant lymphoproliferative disorder with removal of small bowel graft and subsequent second bowel transplant. *J Pediatr Gastroenterol Nutr* 2005;41:354–356.

40 Tzakis AG, Reyes J, Todo S, et al. Two-year experience with FK 506 in pediatric patients. *Transplant Proc* 1993;25:619–621.

41 Tzakis AG, Todo S, Reyes J, et al. Intestinal transplantation in children under FK 506 immunosuppression. *J Pediatr Surg* 1993;28:1040–1043.

42 Ueno T, Kato T, Revas K, et al. Growth after intestinal transplant in children. *Transplant Proc* 2006;38:1702–1704.

43 Venick RS, Farmer DG, Saikali D, et al. Nutritional outcomes following pediatric intestinal transplantation. *Transplant Proc* 2006;38:1718–1719.

44 Wu T, Abu-Elmagd K, Bond G, et al. A schema for histologic grading of small intestine allograft acute rejection. *Transplantation* 2003;75:1241–1248.

45 Ziring D, Tran R, Edelstein S, et al. Infectious enteritis after intestinal transplantation: incidence, timing, and outcome. *Transplantation* 2005;79:702–709.

39 Management of Posttransplant Lymphoproliferative Disease

Thomas G. Gross

Key points

- Not all Epstein-Barr virus (EBV)-associated disease posttransplant is posttransplant lymphoproliferative disease (PTLD), and not all PTLD is EBV-associated.

- The diagnosis of PTLD is difficult and requires tissue biopsy, demonstration of elevated levels of EBV DNA in peripheral blood is insufficient for diagnosis of PTLD.

- Because of the heterogeneity of PTLD, it has been difficult to consistently identify risk factors, prognostic factors, and uniform treatment approaches to PTLD.

- The role of prophylaxis and preemptive therapy in PTLD has not been proven.

- The treatment of patients with PTLD is challenging as a result of increased risk of rejection, increased susceptibility to infections, and organ toxicity.

General

Following intestinal transplantation, as with all organ transplants, posttransplant lymphoproliferative disease (PTLD) is second only to skin cancer as the most common neoplastic disease posttransplant, and PTLD is the most common cancer in posttransplant children [1]. In this chapter, the spectrum of Epstein-Barr virus (EBV) disease in the posttransplant patient, issues in the diagnosis, prevention, and treatment of PTLD will be

Intestinal Failure: Diagnosis, Management and Transplantation.
Edited by Alan N. Langnas, Olivier Goulet, Eamonn M.M. Quigley and Kelly A. Tappenden. © 2008 Blackwell Publishing. ISBN 978-1-4051-4637-1.

discussed with special attention made to recipients of intestinal transplantation.

Spectrum of EBV-related posttransplant disease

First, not all EBV disease posttransplant is PTLD (Table 39.1). The diagnosis of EBV infection is not trivial in the post-transplant patient. The "monospot" test is not specific for EBV infection and antiviral serology has limited value, as many patients may not have the ability to respond normally or they will have obtained antibodies passively from gammaglobulin or blood products. The detection of EBV DNA in blood by polymerase chain reaction (PCR) provides evidence that the patient has been infected by EBV. Although increased levels of EBV DNA are often seen with EBV-associated disease, the interpretation of EBV "viral loads" results can be problematic in the posttransplant patient since they tend to have higher amounts of EBV DNA than normal healthy individuals presumably due to decreased immunosurveillance of latently EBV infected cells. Serial monitoring of EBV "viral loads" may be helpful in monitoring responses to treatment, though they have not been shown to correlate with response to therapy, especially rituximab [2].

EBV infection or reactivation may be asymptomatic or manifest as a generalized viral syndrome or infectious mononucleosis (Table 39.1). EBV disease post-transplant may manifest as infection in any number of organs. Usually, the designation of PTLD is limited to masses of lymphoproliferation that are often extranodal (frequently in the allograft). Although less common, PTLD may present as a very rapidly progressive, disseminated, disease that clinically resembles septic

Table 39.1 Spectrum of EBV-related posttransplant disease.

EBV infection/reactivation—Evidence of the presence of EBV by serologies, PCR or tissue in-situ (immunohistochemical staining), but no clinical symptoms.

EBV disease—Clinical symptoms associated with EBV infection including: fever, malaise, anorexia, nausea/vomiting, arthralgia, tonsillitis, pharyngitis, hepatitis, lymphoid interstitial pneumonitis, menigno-encephalitis. May include adenopathy with proliferation of interfollicular regions and increased EBV positive B-cells, but absence of nodal effacement or destruction of normal tissue architecture (WHO—Early disease)

PTLD—Lymphoproliferation (nodal or extranodal) with nodal effacement or disruption of normal tissue architecture. Lymphoproliferation may be polyclonal or monoclonal, polymorphic or monomorphic.

shock, which almost always results in death, despite therapy.

The World Health Organization (WHO) classification delineates three subtypes of PTLD: (1) early lesions, (2) polymorphic PTLD, and (3) monomorphic PTLD [3]. Early lesions are not considered PTLD and can be distinguished from PTLD by the lack of disruption of normal tissue architecture or necrosis. Although disruption of normal tissue architecture and/or necrosis is present in polymorphic PTLD, it does not, histologically, resemble non-Hodgkin lymphoma (NHL) as does monomorphic PTLD (Figure 39.1). EBV infection may result in multiple clones of proliferating B cells, and both polymorphic and monomorphic histologies may be present in a single patient or even within the same lesion of PTLD (Figure 39.1). Thus, histology of a single biopsied site may not be representative of the entire disease process.

Not all PTLD is associated with EBV or a B cell phenotype. T cell PTLD is rare and tends to occur many years after transplantation, and, interestingly, 25% of cases of T cell PTLD are EBV-positive. PTLD of Hodgkin's disease (HD) phenotype also tends to occur late, and is generally EBV-positive. Some have suggested that the majority of HD-PTLD is a variant of polymorphic B cell PTLD. EBV-negative B-cell PTLD can also occur and tends also to occur later after transplantation. The wide range of clinical presentations of posttransplant of EBV disease and the heterogeneity of PTLD makes it difficult to evaluate the data on incidence, risk factors, or efficacy of the various treatment approaches for PTLD.

Diagnosis of PTLD

Although many tests have been used to assist in the diagnosis of PTLD, such as C-reactive protein (CRP), total number or subsets of circulating B cells, serum immunoglobulin electrophoresis (assessing clonal

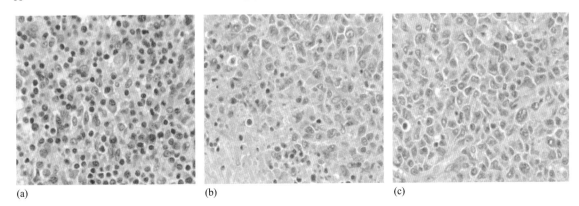

(a) (b) (c)

Figure 39.1 Polymorphic and monomorphic PTLD. (a) Polymorphic PTLD. (b) Areas of polymorphic (left) and monomorphic (right). (c) Monomorphic PTLD.

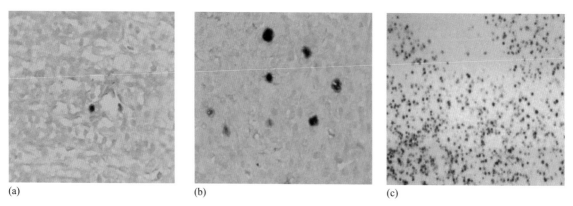

Figure 39.2 EBER staining. (a) Normal—0–1 EBERs (+) cells per high power field (hpf). (b) Posttransplant, but no PTLD—<10 EBER (+) cells per hpf. (c) PTLD—sheets of EBER (+) cells.

spikes), and so on, the diagnosis of PTLD requires a tissue biopsy. These other tests can be supportive of the diagnosis of PTLD but lack specificity and sensitivity as diagnostic tests. Tests for detection of EBV infection, that is, monospots or serology, and even EBV PCR, can be difficult to interpret in an immunocompromised patient. A determination of EBV-associated PTLD is best made by in-situ hybridization with EBV encoded RNA (EBER] probes to identify EBV in tumor cells. Immunohistochemical staining for EBV proteins, for example, latent membrane protein (LMP), does not detect all the EBER positive cases resulting in false negatives in up to 25% of cases. The diagnosis of PTLD requires more than the presence of EBER-positive cells on a tissue biopsy, as posttransplant patients can have increased numbers of EBER-positive cells, making histologic correlation imperative (Figure 39.2). Perhaps the greatest difficulty in making the diagnosis of PTLD occurs in the proliferations that do not produce a mass lesion, but present with disseminated or infiltrative disease in organs and progress very rapidly, resulting in death within hours to days. An examination of the peripheral blood, bone marrow, cerebrospinal fluid (CSF), or other body fluids for the presence of plasmacytoid cells or large B cells can be helpful in these cases, but often this type of PTLD is diagnosed only at autopsy.

Risk factors for PTLD

The strongest risk factor for developing PTLD is EBV seronegativity at the time of transplantatation [4].

Younger recipients have the highest risk of PTLD; therefore a higher incidence of PTLD is observed in children compared to adults [5]. In general, risk is associated with the intensity and T-cell specificity of the immunosuppression [6]. The biggest risk is with the use of ATG or OKT3 serotherapy for treating rejection but not for induction of immunosuppression [6]. PTLD incidence rose with the introduction of calcineurin inhibitors. Early reports suggested more PTLD with tacrolimus but with close attention to the monitoring of levels there appears to be no increased risk compared to cyclosporine [7,8]. Of interest, it does not appear that corticosteroids increase the risk of PTLD; in fact they have activity in treating the EBV disease and PTLD. Although there are less long-term data, it appears that the risk of PTLD is less with the use of mycophenolate mofetil (MMF) or the mTOR inhibitors such as sirolimus [9].

Traditionally, renal, heart, and liver allograft recipients have been considered "lower risk," whereas lung, small bowel, and multiple organ grafts recipients were considered "high risk" for PTLD. The reason is likely multifactorial, that is, median age of the transplant population, amount of immunosuppression required to prevent rejection, and perhaps the amount of donor lymphoid tissue transplanted. In intestinal transplantation, the early experience suggested an incidence of PTLD of as high as 30%; however, the incidence today appears to be about 10%, with children being at the highest risk [10].

Consistent prognostic factors are difficult to ascertain because most studies contain small numbers of patients and uniformity in therapy is rare. Although most studies demonstrate that monomorphic disease and monoclonality confer a worse prognosis, other studies could not confirm this [11,12]. A possible explanation for this is the heterogeneity of disease within a patient or mass, such that a single biopsy may not represent the entire disease process. For example, B cell proliferation may result in a single or multiple clones which does not completely correlate with histology, that is, polymorphic versus monomorphic or polyclonal versus monoclonal disease. In general, monomorphic histology, clonal disease and/or abnormal karyotype predict a poorer prognosis. Classical lymphoma staging has had limited prognostic value in PTLD as a result of the predilection for extranodal involvement, which would render most cases of PTLD high stage (III or IV) disease. The presence of multiple (>2) sites of disease has consistently predicted poorer prognosis, and CNS involvement portends a dismal outcome. PTLD observed greater than 2 years posttransplant, not EBV-associated and/or non-B cell phenotype appear to haves poor prognoses [11]. The exception to this rule is Hodgkin's disease (HD), which is often associated with EBV and responds well to standard therapy for HD.

Prophylaxis for PTLD

Antiviral prophylaxis against EBV, for example, ganciclovir, does not suppress EBV driven B-cell proliferation; however, antivirals may play a role is reducing the incidence of PTLD by reducing the number of infected B-cells in high-risk patients, that is, EBV+ donor into an EBV – recipient. Preemptive treatment, that is, treating patients at times of EBV infection/reactivation (increased levels of EBV in the peripheral blood) may reduce the incidence of PTLD compared to historical controls. The pre-emptive treatment most commonly performed is to reduce immunosuppression with or without antiviral therapy. It has been shown that a low quantity of EBV specific cytotoxic T-cells (EBV-CTL) in the blood is a better predictor of patients who will go on to develop PTLD or develop relapsed disease than is an elevated EBV viral load [13]. Therefore, EBV viral monitoring may serve as a surrogate for overimmunosuppression.

Table 39.2 Treatment for PTLD.

Prophylaxis
1) Ganciclovir may be helpful, especially in EBV(−) recipients and EBV (+) donors

Preemptive therapy
1) Reduction of immunosuppression
2) Ganciclovir
3) ?Rituximab

First line therapy
1) Reduction of immunosuppression
2) Surgery for localized disease
3) ?Rituximab

Second line therapy
1) Rituximab
2) Chemotherapy (standard vs. reduced dose)
3) Combination chemotherapy and rituximab

Treatment of PTLD

The treatment of PTLD presents several therapeutic challenges. These patients are very susceptible to regimen-related toxicity, that is, infections and end-organ toxicity, as well as being at risk of rejecting the transplanted allograft. Therefore, the ideal therapy for PTLD would be minimally toxic, cytotoxic to the B cell proliferation, prevent/treat allograft rejection, and minimize the inhibition of EBV T-cell immune responses.

A reduction or complete withdrawal of immunosuppression remains the cornerstone of PTLD treatment. (Table 39.2) The response to a reduction of immunosuppression varies greatly, from 20 to 80%. This probably reflects differences in the practice of reduction of immunosuppression and the wide spectrum of PTLD, with localized or polymorphic disease more likely to respond. Even for patients that have disease that is responsive to a reduction in immunosuppression, rejection may threaten the viability of the allograft, which may require frequent endoscopy and biopsy, in the case of intestinal transplant recipients. Although an intestinal allograft is not a vital organ, the supply of grafts is limited and, therefore, graft loss is most unfortunate.

Localized disease is one of the strongest favorable prognostic factors. If local control with surgery and/or radiotherapy can be achieved, the outcome is excellent. Even monomorphic, monoclonal, or aggressive histology, that is, Burkitt histology, can be cured by local therapy alone; unfortunately, this represents a small percentage of patients with PTLD. For patients with disease not amenable to local control or that fail reduction of immunosuppression as a result of progressive disease or development of allograft rejection, the outcome has been poor.

Strategies to enhance EBV T-cell immune responses have been attempted. Although remissions have been observed with interferon-α, long-term survival has been poor with many failures because of infection and rejection, as well as recurrent disease. Adoptive T cell therapy is an attractive approach; however, in organ transplantation this strategy is complex. For recipients of cadaveric organs, donor lymphocytes are usually not available. The use of closely matched relatives' lymphocytes runs the risk of both rejection and graft-vs-host disease. HLA-typed, EBV-specific T-cell lines have been established from healthy volunteers and banked for use in the treatment of PTLD patients and have been used with some success. The use of ex vivo generation of EBV-specific cytotoxic T-cells (EBV-CTLs) is being investigated by several groups. The major obstacle for EBV-CTLs when given to solid organ transplant patients, as opposed to when given for PTLD following blood or marrow transplantation, is that the adoptive transferred EBV-CTLs do not persist. Although very exciting, this approach remains prohibitive for most centers because of the high level of technology involved, regulatory issues, and cost.

Early studies employing anti-B-cell monoclonal antibodies (anti-CD21 and anti-CD24) for the treatment of PTLD had a high response rate, but the long-term survival rate was only 50%. There are numerous anecdotal case reports and small series demonstrating efficacy for rituximab in the treatment of PTLD. It appears that as many as two-thirds of patients will achieve remission with rituximab, but relapse occurs in 15–20% of patients. It is unclear how best to use rituximab in the treatment of PTLD. The most common practice is to give 375 mg/m^2 weekly until resolution of disease occurs [14]. The toxicity profile of rituximab has been quite favorable, but prolonged B-cell depletion has been observed and supplementation with IVIG is sometimes required. Additionally, rituximab is very expensive, costing as much as $4000 per infusion for an average-sized adult [15]. More prospective, controlled clinical trials are needed to better define the efficacy, toxicity, and most cost effective strategies for the use of rituximab.

Chemotherapy has traditionally been reserved for the most resistant cases of PTLD because of the high morbidity and mortality associated with such therapy. One benefit of chemotherapy is that the potent level of cytotoxicity directed against the PTLD usually provides sufficient immunosuppression to prevent or treat allograft rejection. The utility of chemotherapy in treating PTLD is difficult to determine, because the published literature contains mainly small, single-center, retrospective experiences with no uniform therapy. Results with standard chemotherapy regimens for NHL, for example, CHOP, ProMACE-CytaBOM, ESHAP, EPOCH, and so on, demonstrate that about 60% of patients will achieve a remission, with relapses and allograft loss being rare events, that is, <5%. However, the 2-year survival remains less than 50%, with the major problem being therapy-related mortality [16]. A particular concern with chemotherapy in intestinal transplant recipients is damage to the gut epithelium. A recently published study reported on 36 children, who had PTLD and who failed to respond to a reduction in immunosuppression and were treated with a low-dose chemotherapy regimen. The 2-year overall survival, relapse-free survival, and failure-free (without PTLD and with functioning original allograft) survival rates were 73%, 69%, and 67%, respectively [17]. For the nine recipients of an intestinal transplant, the 2-year overall survival, relapse-free survival, and failure-free survival rates were 88%, 88%, and 77%, respectively. For the entire 36 patients, the relapse rate was 19%, suggesting that a subset of patients require more intensive therapy. Four patients that presented with disseminated, rapidly progressive disease did very poorly with all dying of progressive disease. Rituximab has been added to this chemotherapy backbone in an attempt to increase efficacy without added toxicity and is currently under investigation in the

Children's Oncology Group (COG), COG ANHL0221. One would expect less therapy-related mortality using this low-dose chemotherapy regimen in adult patients with PTLD, but it remains to be determined if this regimen is effective in controlling PTLD in adult patients. In general, pediatric patients with PTLD have had superior outcomes as compared to adults. PTLD in children tends to occur earlier after transplant, is typically EBV-positive and often associated with primary EBV infection. Therefore, PTLD observed in adults may represent a more malignant disease.

In summary, PTLD continues to be problematic following intestinal transplantation. Because of the heterogeneity of EBV disease and PTLD (Table 39.1), it is difficult to compare data in the literature with regard to incidence, risk and prognostic factors and treatment efficacy. However, it seems clear that EBV seronegative patients are at increased risk for PTLD. Prophylactic antiviral therapy for these patients has not been shown definitively to be of benefit, but probably adds little toxicity or risk. EBV PCR monitoring may play a role in the early posttransplant period, but likely serves as a surrogate marker for overimmunosuppression. Should PTLD be suspected, biopsy is necessary to make the diagnosis, but a single biopsy may not be representative of the entire disease process. The most conservative therapies should still be attempted first, that is, a reduction in immunosuppression and/or surgical resection if possible (Table 39.2). Where this is not feasible or fails, the use of rituximab has become a popular next step, although controlled trials are needed to better define the best way to use rituximab. Finally, for those with the most resistant disease, chemotherapy can cure a percentage of patients; however, approaches to reduce morbidity and mortality associated with chemotherapy, such as lower dosed regimens and the addition of monoclonal antibodies need to be pursued.

References

1 Abu-Elmagd KM, Zak M, Stamos JM, et al. De novo malignancies after intestinal and multivisceral transplantation. *Transplantation* 2004;77:1719–1725.

2 Yang J, Tao Q, Flinn IW, et al. Characterization of Epstein-Barr virus-infected B cells in patients with posttransplantation lymphoproliferative disease: disappearance after rituximab therapy does not predict clinical response. *Blood* 2000;96:4055–4063.

3 Harris NL, Ferry JA, Swerdlow SH. Posttransplant lymphoproliferative disorders: summary of Society for Hematopathology Workshop. *Semin Diagn Pathol* 1997;14:8–14.

4 Ho M, Jaffe R, Miller G, et al. The frequency of Epstein-Barr virus infection and associated lymphoproliferative syndrome after transplantation and its manifestations in children. *Transplantation* 1988;45:719–727.

5 Cox KL, Lawrence-Miyasaki LS, Garcia-Kennedy R, et al. An increased incidence of Epstein-Barr virus infection and lymphoproliferative disorder in young children on FK506 after liver transplantation. *Transplantation* 1995;59:524–529.

6 Opelz G. Dohler BB. Lymphomas after solid organ transplantation: a collaborative transplant study report. *Am J Transplant* 2004;4:222–230.

7 Guthery SL, Heubi JE, Bucuvalas JC, et al. Determination of risk factors for Epstein-Barr virus-associated posttransplant lymphoproliferative disorder in pediatric liver transplant recipients using objective case ascertainment. *Transplantation* 2003;75:987–993.

8 McDiarmid SV, Jordan S, Lee GS, et al. Prevention and preemptive therapy of posttransplant lymphoproliferative disease in pediatric liver recipients. *Transplantation* 1998;66:1604–1611.

9 Buell JF, Gross TG, Woodle ES. Malignancy after transplantation. *Transplantation* 2005;80:S254–S264.

10 Quintini C, Kato T, Gaynor JJ, et al. Analysis of risk factors for the development of posttransplant lymphoproliferative disorder among 119 children who received primary intestinal transplants at a single center. *Transplant Proc* 2006;38:1755–1758.

11 Leblond V, Dhedin N, Mamzer Bruneel MF, et al. Identification of prognostic factors in 61 patients with posttransplantation lymphoproliferative disorders. *J Clin Oncol* 2001;19:772–778.

12 Dror Y, Greenberg M, Taylor G, et al. Lymphoproliferative disorders after organ transplantation in children. *Transplantation* 1999;67:990–998.

13 Smets F, Latinne D, Bazin H, et al. Ratio bewteen Epstein-Barr viral load and anti-Epstein-Barr virus specific T-cell response as a predictive marker of

posttransplant lymphoproliferative disease. *Transplantation* 2002;73:1603–1610.

14 Pescovitz MD. The use of rituximab, anti-CD20 monoclonal antibody, in pediatric transplantation. *Pediatr Transplantation* 2004;8:9–21.

15 Pescovitz MD. Rituximab, an anti-CD20 monoclonal antibody, history and mechanism of action. *Am J Transplant* 2006;6:859–866.

16 Buell JF, Gross TG, Hanaway MJ, et al. Chemotherapy for PTLD: The Israel Penn International Transplant Tumor Registry Experience. *Transplant Proc* 2005;78:956–957.

17 Gross TG, Bucuvalas J, Park J, et al. Low dose chemotherapy for the treatment of refractory posttransplant lymphoproliferative disease in children. *J Clin Oncol* 2005;23:6481–6488.

40 Results of Intestinal Transplantation

David R. Grant and Shimul A. Shah

Key points

- Over the past 20 years, there has been significant improvement in short-term patient survival after intestinal transplantation. These improvements have led to a continued increase in the number of intestinal transplants performed per year.

- Early referral and listing are important in achieving good outcomes after intestinal transplantation.

- Contributing factors that have led to improved survival include center experience, transplantation of a higher ratio of patients who are waiting at home, and the increased use of induction therapy.

- The outcomes of living donor intestinal transplantation are at least comparable to deceased donor transplantation.

- Long-term survival of intestinal transplantation has not improved because of late graft loss, rejection, and patient death for reasons that remain unclear.

Current status of intestinal transplantation

Intestinal transplantation has become the treatment of choice for patients with end-stage gut failure and life-threatening complications on parenteral nutrition. As the results improve, this procedure is poised to become the preferred option for treatment of intestinal failure, much as kidney transplantation is preferred to dialysis for the treatment of end-stage renal disease.

Intestinal Failure: Diagnosis, Management and Transplantation.
Edited by Alan N. Langnas, Olivier Goulet, Eamonn M.M. Quigley and Kelly A. Tappenden. © 2008 Blackwell Publishing. ISBN 978-1-4051-4637-1.

Two factors currently limit deceased donor intestine grafting from more widespread application: (1) a shortage of deceased donor organs, which is associated with a high mortality rate on the waiting list for intestinal transplants; and (2) high rates of late graft and patient loss as a result of rejection and infection [1–3]. The inability to completely control rejection has resulted in heavier immunosuppression; unfortunately, and as a consequence, such attempts to prevent graft loss have led, in some instances, to severe sepsis and eventual death. Newer immunosuppressive regimens and living donor intestinal transplantation may offer theoretical advantages that could help to address these problems.

Patients awaiting intestinal transplants in the United States have the highest mortality of any group on the solid organ waiting list maintained by the UNOS registry (available at http://www.unos.org). Although there are a small number of patients on the waiting list for intestinal transplantation, the waiting time is long, averaging 220 days. The mortality on the waiting list for a deceased donor graft is up to 25% for adult recipients and 60% for pediatric recipients [2,4]. Early referral and living donor intestinal transplantation can reduce waiting time, thus decreasing mortality and preventing progression of the complications caused by TPN [4,5]. UNOS has recently allocated more points to patients waiting for intestinal and liver grafts; whether this change in practice will significantly improve mortality rates remains to be seen.

Currently, the 5-year patient survival rates for all types of intestinal transplants are approximately 50%. In contrast to the dramatic improvement in short-term survival after intestinal grafting, the longer-term survival of grafts in patients who have lived for more than one year after intestinal transplantation has failed to improve (2005 Intestine Registry Report, http://www.Intestinetransplant.org). Graft rejection or infection are still the most common causes of early

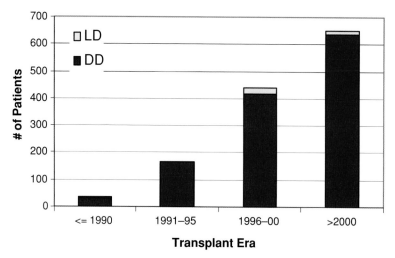

Figure 40.1 Growth of living donor and deceased donor intestine transplantation worldwide by era. LD: living donor; DD: deceased donor.

and late deaths. Potential factors that may reduce the risk of rejection using live donor grafts include: better donor bowel decontamination, improved tissue antigen matching, reduced cold ischemic injury, and optimization of recipient medical status [6].

The surgical techniques for intestinal grafting were first established in dogs [7–9]. Early experiments in rodent, dog, and pig models of intestinal grafting demonstrated a survival advantage with matching of histocompatibility antigens [10,11]. These advantages were subsequently confirmed in mice also [10,12].

Seven attempts were made to transplant the intestine in the 1960s and early 1970s, in the pre-cyclosporine era with limited success. Most failed because of technical complications. It is noteworthy, however, that the longest survivor received an HLA-identical ileal segment from her sister, surviving for 76 days after transplantation [13].

The International Registry report was established to evaluate results of intestinal transplantation and long-term outcomes. There has been a 100% participation rate in the Registry; to the best of our knowledge

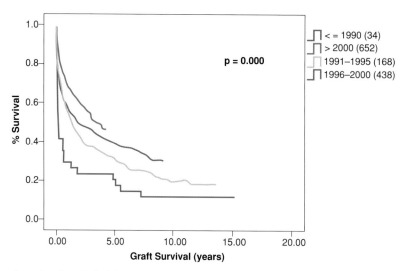

Figure 40.2 Comparison of graft survival of all intestine transplants by era.

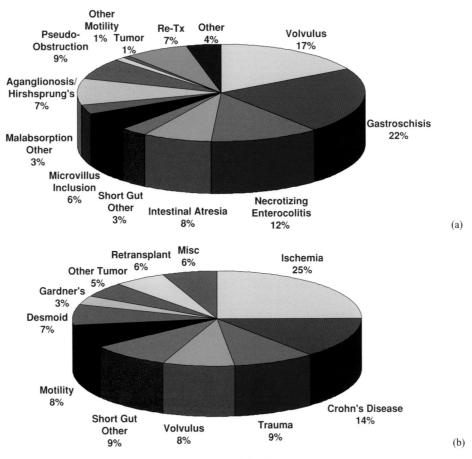

Figure 40.3 Indications for intestinal transplant in children (a) and adults (b).

the Registry captured more than 99% of all intestinal transplants performed worldwide between January 1985 and March 2005.

Current outcomes of intestinal transplantation

Over the last 20 years, there has been a remarkable improvement in short-term graft and patient survival rates after intestinal transplantation and a resulting growth in the application of this procedure (Figures 40.1 and 40.2). Improved outcomes in intestinal transplantation now result in over 170 cases being performed per year worldwide (2006 estimate). Despite this growth, the experience remains skewed; only 25% of all centers have performed more than ten cases.

The Intestinal Transplant Registry contains data on 1292 transplants that have been performed in 1210 patients in 65 centers from twenty countries. Over half of the recipients are still alive today, with the longest patient surviving 16 years with a functioning graft [14]. The types of intestinal transplants performed include small intestine only (44%), liver and small intestine (38%) and multivisceral (18%). There has been an equal sex distribution and 60% of the transplants have been performed in the pediatric population. The most common indication in both children and adults is the short gut syndrome (Figure 40.3). Isolated intestinal transplant is the most common procedure in adults (56%), whereas combined liver and intestine is the most frequent type in children (50%) (Figure 40.4).

Table 40.1 outlines a multivariate analysis of factors potentially relevant to the occurrence of accelerated

Table 40.1 Multivariate analysis of factors affecting survival after intestine transplantation.

	Graft survival		Patient survival	
	p value	AF*	p value	AF*
Grouped transplant year[†]	0.0308	0.58	ns	–
Center size: ≤10 transplants	0.0530	2.11	0.0530	2.14
Pre-transplant status—at home	0.0006	0.43	0.0004	0.40
First transplant	0.0024	0.29	0.0040	0.30
FK506 alone induction	ns	–	0.0098	3.92

*Log normal accelerated failure model.
[†]Groups: <1990; 1990–1995; 1996–2000; 2000–2005.

graft failure. Early referral and listing are important for successful outcomes with intestinal grafting: patients who are called in from home for their intestinal transplant have significantly higher survival rates, irrespective of the type of transplant performed (Figure 40.5a) [1]. Center experience with more than ten intestinal transplants also leads to improved survival rates (Figure 40.5b). As a result of the large lymphoid mass of the graft, the use of antibody induction therapy appears to be particularly important after intestinal transplantation (Figure 40.5c). Either Campath 1-H or anti-IL-2 agents have been shown to improve both graft and patient survival in single center series [1,2,15–17]. Combined liver and intestinal grafts appear to have a slightly higher survival rate (Figure

40.5d), but single center experiences have not had the same results (see later) [2,18,19].

In addition to the Intestinal Transplant Registry, numerous large single center series have added to the advancement of intestinal transplantation. The Pittsburgh group reported their experience of 165 intestinal allografts with patient survival rates of 75%, 54%, and 42% at 1, 5, and 10 years [20]. Improved outcomes were noted in the UCLA experience over 12 years as no patient was lost as a result of cytomegalovirus or Epstein-Barr Virus in their review of 33 patients [21]. In a review of 26 patients who received 28 isolated intestinal allografts, Fishbein reported that high patient survival (3 year—88%) and parenteral nutrition-free survival can be achieved after isolated intestinal

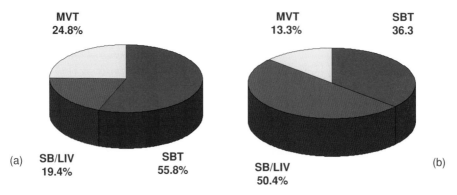

Figure 40.4 Types of intestinal transplants performed for adults (a) and children (b). SBT: small bowel alone; SB/LIV: small bowel liver; MVT: multivisceral.

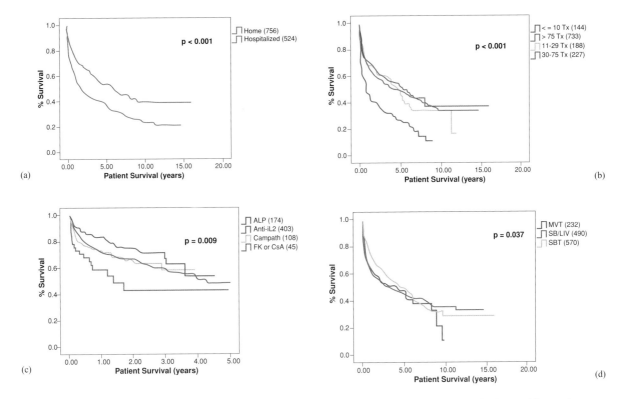

Figure 40.5 Effect of different factors on patient survival. (a) Pretransplant status. (b) Center size. (c) Type of induction. (d) Transplant type.

transplantation [18]. Results from the University of Nebraska confirmed excellent short-term graft survival in 106 patients. Similar to Fishbein's series, they found higher patient survival in isolated intestinal transplants compared to combined intestinal-liver grafts (2 year—82% vs. 60%, respectively) [19].

In the pediatric population, survival has improved steadily over time with 55% (400/721) of recipients alive today. In patients surviving beyond 6 months after transplant, more than 70% enjoy excellent graft function. Improvements in immune suppressive regimens have led to a significant decline in posttransplant lymphoproliferative disease (PTLD) over time. Infants less than 1 year old have similar survival outcomes to those older than 1 year.

Although significant improvements were found in early graft survival, longer-term outcomes have failed to improve over time. No differences were found when conditional survival analyses were performed in 3 month, 6 month, or 1 year survivors grouped according

to era, donor type, or graft type. The most common cause of death in recipients surviving beyond 1 year is sepsis followed by rejection and lymphoma. Severe rejection of the intestine is the final stage of acute rejection. It can be a fatal complication for the recipient or one that, at the very least, necessitates retransplant. This emphasizes the need for prompt diagnosis and control at earlier stages of acute rejection so that severe rejection causing graft failure does not take place [22].

Results of living donor intestinal transplantation

The potential benefits of live donation must be weighed against the potential disadvantages of living donor intestinal transplantation, which include: risk to the donor, inferior graft function because a smaller segment of bowel is transplanted, and a relatively limited

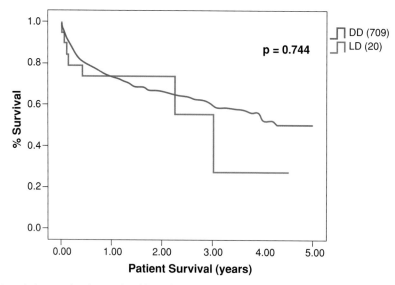

Figure 40.6 Patient survival comparing deceased and living donor intestine transplants.

experience to date, which has been largely confined to adolescents and identical twins [2,23].

Living donor intestinal transplant is not routinely performed and therefore few reports of short- and long-term outcomes exist. The largest series, reported by Benedetti at the University of Illinois at Chicago, included nine patients who underwent transplantation of a 150 to 200 cm segment of terminal ileum proximal to the ileocecal valve. The 1- and 3-year actuarial patient and graft survival rates were 78% and 67%, respectively [4]. No rejection has been documented in six or seven living donor intestinal HLA matched grafts during the first year posttransplant at their institution and all have achieved good long-term graft function (Benedetti, personal communication). Other centers, however, have reported rates with graft rejection comparable to deceased donor organs [6]. Four identical twin intestinal transplants of 150–200 cm small bowel have enjoyed complete recovery with no adverse long-term side affects.

Of 1,292 intestinal transplants performed to date, 41 grafts (3.2%) were obtained from living donors at 16 centers in seven different countries. Volvulus, followed by intestinal ischemia, is the most common indication for live intestinal grafts, which reflects the fact that the procedure is more commonly performed in children. None of the reports of live donor intestinal transplants have described any serious, long-term adverse

effects in the donor and no donor deaths have been reported.

Close to half of the patients who have undergone living donor intestinal transplantation are currently alive today (21/41; 51%). Causes of death included sepsis (29%), liver failure (5%), rejection (5%), and other causes (10%). Only one patient lost their intestinal graft because of vascular thrombosis (2.5%). This suggests that the small vascular pedicle in living donor intestinal transplant is not a significant risk factor for graft loss when compared to deceased donor grafts, as technical results are at least comparable to deceased donors (2.5% vs. 15–20% graft loss, respectively).

Center volume had no effect on graft survival following live donor transplantation, but this may reflect the small number of procedures performed worldwide. There was no difference in graft survival or patient survival (Figure 40.6) when comparing living donor and deceased donor intestinal transplantation.

Thus, living donor intestinal transplantation has become a lifesaving procedure for selected patients with end-stage intestinal failure. The outcomes of living donor intestinal transplant are at least comparable to deceased donor transplantation. More data are needed to: (1) document donor safety; and (2) determine if potential theoretical benefits, such as decreased waiting times and reduced graft rejection rates, can be achieved in clinical practice.

Quality of life after intestinal transplantation

Intestinal transplantation is a life-saving procedure if one avoids the long-term complications from parenteral nutrition such as sepsis, loss of central venous access, thrombosis, and liver failure. In patients with short bowel syndrome and permanent intestinal failure, the survival rate after long-term parenteral nutrition is reported at 87%, 77%, and 44% at 1, 2, and 5 years respectively [24,25].

According to recent reports, more than 80% of infants and children now survive after extensive small bowel resection in the neonatal period [1–3]. Prognosis is related to anatomical factors including age-adjusted intestinal length, preservation of the ileocecal valve and colon and the presence or absence of cholestasis [26–29]. In a long term study, Goulet et al. found that normal long-term growth can be predicted in children with favorable anatomic prognostic factors and a short duration of parenteral nutrition [28]. Children with short bowel syndrome appear to suffer significantly more morbidity in all categories including surgical complications, duration of parenteral nutrition, sepsis, hospital stay, cholestasis, and liver failure [29].

After intestinal transplantation, 1-year patient survival rates of more than 80% are now being achieved. Numerous studies have shown that quality of life in intestinal transplant recipients is excellent and successful intestinal grafting is cost-saving compared with maintenance home parenteral nutrition [20,23,30]. Based on the International Transplant Registry, more than 90% of survivors stop parenteral nutrition, resume oral intake, and return to normal daily activities [1,31].

Few assessments of quality of life have been reported, to date, in children but some have been performed in adults [32–34]. The first study of quality of life in this context was performed by Sudan and colleagues at the University of Nebraska Medical Center. They found that, in pediatric intestinal transplant recipients, their perceived physical and psychosocial functioning was equal to normal children once they had come through the perioperative period. Interestingly, their parents, in contrast, believed that their physical functioning and general health was below that of their peers.

Conclusion

In summary, data remain limited on the experience with intestinal transplantation for end-stage gut failure, worldwide. Improvements in immunosuppresion, early listing and timing of transplant, and center experience have led to dramatic improvements in early outcomes after intestinal transplantation. Unfortunately, long-term survival has not improved. Future research and, especially, studies investigating the causes of late graft loss and severe rejection will be critical in improving long-term outcomes after intestinal transplantation.

References

1 Grant D, Abu-Elmagd K, Reyes J, et al. 2003 report of the intestine transplant registry: a new era has dawned. *Ann Surg* 2005;241:607–613.

2 Fishbein TM. The current state of intestinal transplantation. *Transplantation* 2004;78:175–178.

3 Fishbein TM, Schiano T, LeLeiko N, et al. An integrated approach to intestinal failure: results of a new program with total parenteral nutrition, bowel rehabilitation, and transplantation. *J Gastrointest Surg* 2002;6:554–562.

4 Testa G, Panaro F, Schena S, et al. Living related small bowel transplantation: donor surgical technique. *Ann Surg* 2004;240:779–784.

5 Gruessner RW, Sharp HL. Living-related intestinal transplantation: first report of a standardized surgical technique. *Transplantation* 1997;64:1605–1607.

6 Cicalese L, Rastellini C, Sileri P, et al. Segmental living related small bowel transplantation in adults. *J Gastrointest Surg* 2001;5:168–172.

7 Sarr MG, Duenes JA. Early and long term effects of a model of intestinal autotransplantation on intestinal motor patterns. *Surg Gynecol Obstet* 1990;170:338–346.

8 Libsch KD, Zyromski NJ, Tanaka T, et al. Role of extrinsic innervation in jejunal absorptive adaptation to subtotal small bowel resection: a model of segmental small bowel transplantation. *J Gastrointest Surg* 2002;6:240–247.

9 Tsiotos GG, Kendrick ML, Libsch K, et al. Ileal absorptive adaptation to jejunal resection and extrinsic denervation: implications for living-related small bowel transplantation. *J Gastrointest Surg* 2001;5:517–524.

10 Koltun WA, Madara JL, Smith RJ, Kirkman RL. Metabolic aspects of small bowel transplantation in inbred rats. *J Surg Res* 1987;42:341–347.

11 Murr MM, Miller VM, Sarr MG. Contractile properties of enteric smooth muscle after small bowel transplantation in rats. *Am J Surg* 1996;171:212–217.

12 Kirkman RL, Lear PA, Madara JL, Tilney NL. Small intestine transplantation in the rat—immunology and function. *Surgery* 1984;96:280–287.

13 Fortner JG, Sichuk G, Litwin SD, Beattie EJ, Jr. Immunological responses to an intestinal allograft with HL-A-identical donor-recipient. *Transplantation* 1972;14:531–535.

14 Ruemmele FM, Sauvat F, Colomb V, et al. Seventeen years after successful small bowel transplantation: long term graft acceptance without immune tolerance. *Gut* 2006;55:903–904.

15 Starzl TE, Murase N, Abu-Elmagd K, et al. Tolerogenic immunosuppression for organ transplantation. *Lancet* 2003;361:1502–1510.

16 Reyes J, Mazariegos GV, Abu-Elmagd K, et al. Intestinal transplantation under tacrolimus monotherapy after perioperative lymphoid depletion with rabbit antithymocyte globulin (thymoglobulin). *Am J Transplant* 2005;5:1430–1436.

17 Tzakis AG, Kato T, Nishida S, et al. Preliminary experience with campath 1H (C1H) in intestinal and liver transplantation. *Transplantation* 2003;75:1227–1231.

18 Fishbein TM, Kaufman SS, Florman SS, et al. Isolated intestinal transplantation: proof of clinical efficacy. *Transplantation* 2003;76:636–640.

19 Langnas A, Chinnakotla S, Sudan D, et al. Intestinal transplantation at the University of Nebraska Medical Center: 1990 to 2001. *Transplant Proc* 2002;34:958–960.

20 Abu-Elmagd K, Reyes J, Bond G, et al. Clinical intestinal transplantation: a decade of experience at a single center. *Ann Surg* 2001;234:404–416.

21 Farmer DG, McDiarmid SV, Edelstein S, et al. Improved outcome after intestinal transplantation at a single institution over 12 years. *Transplant Proc* 2004;36:303–304.

22 Tzakis AG, Kato T, Levi DM, et al. 100 multivisceral transplants at a single center. *Ann Surg* 2005;242:480–490.

23 Cicalese L, Sileri P, Gonzales O, et al. Cost-effectiveness of early living related segmental bowel transplantation as therapy for trauma-induced irreversible intestinal failure. *Transplant Proc* 2001;33:3581–3582.

24 Messing B, Crenn P, Beau P, et al. Long-term survival and parenteral nutrition dependence in adult patients with the short bowel syndrome. *Gastroenterology* 1999;117:1043–1050.

25 Cavicchi M, Beau P, Crenn P, Degott C, Messing B. Prevalence of liver disease and contributing factors in patients receiving home parenteral nutrition for permanent intestinal failure. *Ann Intern Med* 2000;132:525–532.

26 Quiros-Tejeira RE, Ament ME, Reyen L, et al. Long-term parenteral nutritional support and intestinal adaptation in children with short bowel syndrome: a 25-year experience. *J Pediatr* 2004;145:157–163.

27 Spencer AU, Neaga A, West B, et al. Pediatric short bowel syndrome: redefining predictors of success. *Ann Surg* 2005;242:403–409.

28 Goulet O, Baglin-Gobet S, Talbotec C, et al. Outcome and long-term growth after extensive small bowel resection in the neonatal period: a survey of 87 children. *Eur J Pediatr Surg* 2005;15:95–101.

29 Wales PW, de Silva N, Kim JH, et al. Neonatal short bowel syndrome: a cohort study. *J Pediatr Surg* 2005;40:755–762.

30 Middleton SJ, Pollard S, Friend PJ, et al. Adult small intestinal transplantation in England and Wales. *Br J Surg* 2003;90:723–727.

31 Grant D. Intestinal transplantation: 1997 report of the international registry. Intestinal Transplant Registry. *Transplantation* 1999;67:1061–1064.

32 Rovera GM, DiMartini A, Schoen RE, et al. Quality of life of patients after intestinal transplantation. *Transplantation* 1998;66:1141–1145.

33 Rovera GM, Sileri P, Rastellini C, et al. Quality of life after living related small bowel transplantation. *Transplant Proc* 2002;34:967–968.

34 Sudan D, Horslen S, Botha J, et al. Quality of life after pediatric intestinal transplantation: the perception of pediatric recipients and their parents. *Am J Transplant* 2004;4:407–413.

Psychosocial Assessment and Management of the Transplant Patient/Family in Intestinal Transplantation

Jodi Gentleman, Leonard W. Penkoski and James H. Sorrell

Key points

- Intestinal transplantation requires a thorough psychosocial assessment to determine psychosocial suitability and supportive needs amenable to intervention.

- Psychosocial management of the patient/family postintestinal transplantation entails facilitation of coping for the patient/caregiver, facilitation of communication with the transplant team, and coordination of resources.

Introduction

Intestinal transplantation has become a viable clinical treatment for patients experiencing intestinal failure. The psychosocial team usually involves Social Work, Psychology, and Psychiatry. The psychosocial assessment utilizes aspects of systems theory. Because of significant psychological challenges and social dynamics involved in intestinal transplantation, it is vital to identify the psychological strengths and weaknesses of each patient and their family early in the process [1,2].

An adequate psychosocial assessment needs to identify several key domains, which are listed in Table 41.1.

Intestinal Failure: Diagnosis, Management and Transplantation.
Edited by Alan N. Langnas, Olivier Goulet, Eamonn M.M. Quigley and Kelly A. Tappenden. © 2008 Blackwell Publishing. ISBN 978-1-4051-4637-1.

Pediatric considerations

The psychosocial assessment of the child differs from that of the adults and in particular carries with it the added dynamic of the patient's parents and other central family members. Considerations for families of pediatric patients that need to be accounted for before transplantation are noted in Table 41.1. Foster placement of an infant or child is a process that may or may not have been instigated before transplant evaluation. If a child is already in a state's custody, assessment of the current family and potential foster parents needs to be completed as well as coordination with the caseworker. Guidance is most often helpful as most caseworkers have not handled a situation of this nature in their previous experience. Coordination with the caseworker may include planning and arranging for temporary foster placement in the patient's local area or in the transplant center area or both. The psychosocial assessment may identify the need for additional support prior to listing for transplant or the need for an alternate caregiver for the infant or child. The psychosocial assessment is an important key in contributing to the transplant team's recommendations to the referring medical team or family.

Adult considerations

As noted in Table 41.1, the majority of adult patients being considered for intestinal transplantation become

Table 41.1 Considerations in the psychosocial assessment of the intestinal transplant candidate.

Medical history
- Chronicity and acuity of illness
- Duration of illness
- Hospitalization history
- Compliance with medical recommendations
- Experience with illness, or health issues
- Nutritional status
- Duration, frequency, and impact of HPN
- Narcotic use for pain management [1,2,5]
- *Geographical distance from medical treatment; visitation/bonding issues

Mental and emotional health [6–7]
- Adaptation to illness by patient and family
- Adaptation to role changes
- Professional services or medication needs
- Perception of stress regarding previous issues and transplantation
- Expectations of transplantation and quality of life
- Previous coping strategies [4,5], and transferability to another location
- Past or current psychiatric issues
- Spiritual/religious strengths
- History of substance abuse
- History of narcotic dependence
- Developing and monitoring a substance abuse compliance program

Family support system
- Immediate family support
- Married, single, divorced, widowed
- Supportive or conflicted relationship(s)
- Custody issues of children
- Care-partners
- Extended family support; supportive or conflicted
- *Additional pregnancies of mother/caregiver
- *Level of concern or lack of support requiring temporary or permanent foster placement

Social support system
- Church/community of faith network
- Peer group
- Community support
- Employer support and flexibility for patient/caregiver

Financial resources
- Maintenance of insurance benefits
- Healthcare issues for care-partner's/family support away from health network
- Transportation [3–5]
- Loss of income
- Maintaining existing rent/mortgage, vehicle [1], and other household expenses
- Fund-raising

*Denotes specific to pediatrics

addicted to narcotics [1,2,5]. This can be the result of multiple surgeries, the chronicity of the illness, functional impairments, that is, losses in activities of daily living, independence, and mobility, and chronic pain. A complete substance abuse history is necessary to determine the presence of substance/polysubstance dependence in the patient or care-partner. Recommendations may be made by the multidisciplinary team that the patient be "weaned off" all narcotics before transplantation, when feasible. Patients with chronic pain can be referred to a pain management clinic to assist in this. Random drug screens may be required to determine patient compliance with the medical team's requirements. Patients or care-partners with underlying co-morbid substance abuse/dependency will need to be referred to a treatment program. This may include referral to an inpatient treatment program, intensive outpatient program, outpatient treatment, aftercare or relapse prevention program, Alcoholics Anonymous, or Narcotics Anonymous.

Other considerations

Particular attention needs to be paid to the family's support plan. The lengthy time required to recover post transplantation, as both an inpatient and outpatient requires a comprehensive plan that includes the availability of a care-partner. Given the varying individual strengths and constellations of support available to each patient, a variety of plans are appropriate [4]. Financial resources are a significant challenge for most patients and families facing intestinal transplantation. Most likely, their financial capacity has been diminished by the extensive medical care they have received before transplantation. Many families are not financially stable in their lives before the onset of the medical illness. The challenges this creates include having sufficient funds for copays, deductibles, out-of-pocket expenses, medications or services that may not be covered by their particular insurance plan. Other significant financial challenges are listed in Table 41.1. It is important to assist families in identifying financial needs and possible community resources for assistance [6–7].

The final key element before transplantation that must be assessed and arranged is transportation. Transportation is dependent on the type of insurance coverage the potential recipient has at the time of transplantation. This cost can be up to $18,000, or more, depending on the distance from the transplant center and can be prohibitive. However, the patient may elect to relocate to the transplant center before transplantation. Relocating to the vicinity of the transplant center can add additional stress related to the move itself, as well as issues such as loss of existing social support, job loss, potential loss of insurance, obtaining affordable housing, and establishing new medical support.

Finally, the goal of assessment is to establish a positive rapport, allowing for a continuum of support to the patient and family throughout the entire transplant process [6,7].

Psychosocial management of the patient/family posttransplantation

Intestinal transplantation often necessitates a lengthy stay at the transplant center of six months or longer, depending on the individual transplant course. This period of time could include multiple setbacks related to infection, perforation, or rejection episodes. The hospital and outpatient stay are continually uncomfortable and frustrating [1]. Stenn et al (1992) noted that small bowel transplantation placed more stress on the family or caregiver in comparison to the stress experienced by families for other organ transplants such as kidney, liver, and heart. Although little research, in this area, has focused on small intestinal transplantation, research in liver transplantation has demonstrated the emergence of adverse psychological and psychiatric sequelae not present before transplantation [3,8,9].

Facilitation of coping for patient/caregiver

In the immediate time following transplantation, patient and care-partners often experience a myriad of emotions ranging from elation to exhaustion. Patients and families may experience anxiety as they anticipate being discharged to an outpatient setting. There are a multitude of responsibilities being placed on the patient/caregiver in terms of medical care. They will have to manage clinic appointments, daily lab draws, scheduled or nonscheduled biopsies, feeding and medication pumps, daily or weekly medication and feeding adjustments, physical and occupational therapy visits, daily or weekly feeding appointments, and school and homework updates and assignments for families of pediatric patients. The patient/caregiver is also responsible for updating friends and relatives on their progress or setbacks. Brief home nursing visits, nurse coordinators, and other multidisciplinary staff continue to provide emotional and practical support, along with friends and other family acquaintances in the area.

The transplant team can anticipate significant role changes in family systems because of the disruptive force of being ill and separation from other members of the family. Single parent families with families in which there are other children to care for are particularly vulnerable. Families experiencing strain on their everyday relationships as a result of the distance from friends/family are prone to a sense of emotional fatigue and isolation. There are major stresses that are experienced by the patient, spouse, and other children because of the changing roles that are assumed when the patient becomes ill. Once transplantation occurs, role reversal and reluctance on the part of family members to relinquish assumed roles can, and often do, create conflict within the patient and family unit.

In families of children receiving a transplant, there are emotional struggles that they face in meeting the needs of both or all of their children. Patient and family members are constantly pulled in different directions with competing needs from all different areas in their life. Staff can assist the family through these issues by listening to what they are experiencing, acknowledging their associated emotions, providing accurate medical and resource information, clarifying their understanding of the patient's condition, and assisting them problem solve or set attainable goals [4]. Managing the exhaustion and the adjustments often experienced by the patients and their families involves a multidisciplinary team approach. Pastoral Care may coordinate with volunteers for practical daily needs through community churches, spiritual support, and counseling, if desired. Psychologists provide clinical recommendations and opportunities for therapeutic sessions to meet already existing or maladaptive coping mechanisms in the patients/families [4]. Volunteer Services can provide transportation, emotional, and social support.

Social Work provides brief, supportive counseling, coordination of services, and referrals to community, medical, and psychiatric resources when indicated [1].

An essential element of any transplant program is the establishment of a support group. The support group facilitates communication, reduces stress/anxiety, and helps the patient/family members to establish equilibrium. This can be facilitated by transplant recipients, social work, nurse coordinators, or pastoral care. The provision of a biweekly educational/informational group for pediatric families enhances communication among the patients, their families, and team members.

Often overlooked in the optimism and enthusiasm for transplantation is the real possibility of death [4]. While in the transplant center families interact, establish relationships with each other, and assist other families if a patient dies. Families are then clearly reminded that their child, spouse/significant other, or sibling is at similar risk and may become terrified that their child also might die, despite everything they've endured so far.

When a patient is critically ill and the medical team has done all that is possible, it becomes the responsibility of the transplant team to support the family through their loved one's death. At this time, the team redirects treatment to comfort care and emotional support for the patient and family. It is important for staff to recognize each family's individual needs throughout the dying process. Social Work or other support staff can assist them through the end-of-life decisions. End-of-life decisions may include: when a ventilator can be removed, when they can hold the patient as they die (primarily if the patient is their infant or child), who can be present at the time of death, and what is the involvement of siblings, extended family and friends. Once the patient has died, assisting families with basic issues such as the grief process, funeral arrangements, and making plans for the family's return home is a vital role for the transplant team.

Communication

As in liver transplantation, a small bowel transplant patient's condition can change rapidly, it is necessary for the patient and family to be updated with new information as soon as possible. It is important to answer questions posed by the family as quickly as possible to decrease anxiety [4]. The transplant team works on communicating with the patient and family by encouraging participation in daily medical rounds. It is important for staff to acknowledge any concerns or needs of the patient and family shortly following transplant. Information from the pretransplant evaluation should be reviewed and updated, new information from the family and from staff should be included in a plan of care [4].

For adult intestinal and pediatric transplant patients, family care conferences are established on an as needed basis. For example, the pediatric social worker may schedule a 2-week, posttransplant care conference for staff and parents to discuss the child's medical condition, progress, issues causing concern, and address any questions. Short- and long-term goals for emotional support, developmental, and physical growth are established with the parents' contributions. Parents or staff can gather for additional care conferences at other times, as needed. If there are specific concerns identified by family or staff regarding the level of understanding of the patient's medical condition, Social Work and the transplant nurse coordinator often meet with the parents to provide clarification and support. Additionally, a useful tool to facilitate communication and coordination of the patient's care among the multidisciplinary team is to hold a weekly meet with nursing staff, transplant nurse coordinators, Educational Support, Social Work, Psychology, Pastoral Care, Child Life, Physical Therapy, and Occupational Therapy.

Coordination of resources

Social Work can assist families in meeting these financial responsibilities with many different resources. Families with or without insurance benefits for nonmedical expenses are encouraged to seek assistance from their extended family members, friends, community, workplaces, or church organizations in fundraising efforts. When families do not have any of these options available to them, internal emergency funds can be used and outside transplant organizations are accessed if appropriate.

The transplant team encourages visits from immediate and extended family members as often as possible. The caregiver is also encouraged to return to their home area at times to promote healthy coping. Social Work can assist in organizing these plans and provide access to resources for travel/finances through various transplant organizations or discounted or complimentary travel programs.

Social Work also assists patients in maintaining their current insurance, Medicaid, and disability programs despite the many challenges, paperwork, phone calls, and confusion as a result of circumstances being beyond what is within normal policy.

Summary

Intestinal transplantation is a psychosocial challenge for all families who experience it. Managing patients and families before, and following, transplantation takes an entire multidisciplinary team effort and great dedication to maintaining care provider health. It is only with a steady and proactive approach by multiple disciplines within the hospital, community, and family that an intestinal transplant will be successful. Further research into both the assessment and management of the psychosocial issues associated with small intestinal transplantation is clearly indicated.

References

1 Stenn PG, Lammens P, Grant D. Psychiatric psychosocial and ethical aspects of small bowel transplantation. *Transplant Proc* 1992;24:1251–1252.
2 DiMartini A, Fitzgerald M, et al. Psychiatric evaluations of small intestine transplantation patients. *Gen Hosp Psychiatry* 1996;18:25S–29S.
3 Kennard J. Nurse education. A helping hand? *Nurs Times* 1991;87:39–40.
4 Benning CR, Smith A. Psychosocial needs of family members of liver transplant patients *Clin Nurse Spe* 1994;8:280–288.
5 Stowe J, Kotz, M. Addiction medicine in organ transplantation. *Prog Transplant* 2001;11:50–57.
6 Andersen D, Devoll-Zabrocki A, Brown C, et al. Intestinal Transplantation in Pediatric Patients: A Nursing Challenge: Part One: Evaluation for Intestinal Transplantation. *Gastroenterol Nurs* 2000;23:3–9.

7 Andersen D, Devoll-Zabrocki A, Brown C. Intestinal Transplantation in Pediatric Patients: A Nursing Challenge Part 2: Intestinal Transplantation and the Immediate Postoperative Period. *Gastroenterol Nurs* 2000;23:203–209.

8 House RM, Thompson TL. Psychiatric aspects of organ transplantation. *JAMA* 1988;360:535–539.

9 Frierson RL, Lippman SB. Heart transplant candidates rejected on psychiatric indications. *Psychosomatics* 1987;28:347–355.

42 Financial, Economic and Insurance Issues Pertaining to Intestinal Transplantation: When Is Too Much Not Enough?

Roger W. Evans

Key points

- Clinical innovation offers many hospitals a marketing advantage, but it increasingly comes at a price hospitals are unable to afford.

- For specific indications, and for patients who are transplanted at selected centers, intestinal transplantation is considered therapeutic.

- Over 225,000 persons in the United States require some form of maintenance nutritional support, few of whom would qualify for intestinal transplantation.

- Sales of clinical nutrition products in the United States are expected to exceed $13.6 billion in 2008, with parenteral nutrition products estimated at $2.0 billion.

- The annual per-patient expense of maintenance nutritional support is between $75,000 and $250,000, with some estimates exceeding $300,000.

- The aggregate expenditures associated with intestinal transplantation will remain low due to an intractable shortage of donor organs.

- The total first-year per-patient billed charges for intestinal transplantation in the United States are estimated by actuaries to exceed $800,000.

- Because of insufficient experience and incomplete data, no definitive study has established the cost-effectiveness of intestinal transplantation.

- Intestinal transplantation does not assure immortality; therefore, it cannot be justified on grounds that it is less expensive than the cost of dying.

- The expense of intestinal transplantation must be considered relative to what is often called the "payback period."

- The significance of the distinction between insurance *coverage* and *reimbursement* cannot be underestimated.

- Relative to their actual accounting costs, many hospitals in the United States perform life-saving organ transplants at a substantial financial loss.

- Medicare reimbursement for intestinal transplantation in the United States is abysmal, with many hospitals incapable of covering their costs.

- Hospitals in the United States use a variety of pricing strategies, all of which are intended to maximize reimbursement relative to accounting costs.

- With the expectation of sustained financial losses, many hospitals in the United States may be unable and unwilling to offer intestinal transplantation.

- Consumer-directed health care, with increased cost-sharing by patients, may make transplantation unaffordable and death the preferred option.

- Academic health centers are no longer in a financial position enabling them to be everything to everyone, making it necessary to prioritize services.

Intestinal Failure: Diagnosis, Management and Transplantation.
Edited by Alan N. Langnas, Olivier Goulet, Eamonn M.M. Quigley and Kelly A. Tappenden. © 2008 Blackwell Publishing.
ISBN 978-1-4051-4637-1.

Introduction

Intestinal and multivisceral transplantation can be life-saving procedures for carefully selected patients with irreversible or multivisceral organ failure who can no longer be maintained on total parenteral nutrition (TPN) [1–6]. In the United States, this has prompted third-party payers, including Medicare, to make favorable, although restrictive, coverage determinations [7].

Unfortunately, regardless of the combination of organs involved, intestinal transplantation is an exceedingly expensive procedure, raising difficult questions for patients, providers, insurers, and health care policy makers [8,9]. The primary treatment alternative—TPN—is also costly, making cost-effectiveness an issue, but one that has only been superficially addressed [9,10].

The number of persons with intestinal failure is increasing, as is the demand for intestinal transplantation [11,12]. Donor organs remain in short supply, constraining the aggregate health care expenditures associated with the procedure.

Despite favorable coverage determinations, transplant hospitals are now facing some serious challenges—reimbursement is often insufficient to cover their accounting costs. In other words, intestinal transplant centers typically provide life-saving procedures at a financial loss.

Hospitals cannot sustain significant losses for extended periods of time. Although clinical innovation provides hospitals with a marketing advantage, the management mantra—"no money, no mission"—is an obvious truism. Consequently, many transplant hospitals are being forced to set priorities, which, in some cases, may mean suspending clinical programs that are no longer financially viable.

Despite limited experience, and scant evidence, this chapter will directly confront the economic and financial reality surrounding intestinal transplantation in the United States. Multiple perspectives will be considered, as thorny issues are conveyed. There are no straightforward answers when life hangs in the balance. A significant conclusion will become readily apparent: technology at the edge can become an ethical protuberance.

Table 42.1 Prevalence of home parenteral nutrition patients in selected countries and locations.

Country/Location	Patients per Million Population	Year of Data
United Kingdom	9.0	2001
Scotland	14.0	2001
North West England	14.0	2001
West Midlands	4.0	2002
Wales	6.0	2003
Denmark	12.7	1999
United States	156.0	1992

Source: Reference [13], page 3, except the U.S. figure, which is based on reference [11].

Prevalence of parenteral and enteral nutrition

In 1992, there were approximately 40,000 parenteral and 152,000 home enteral nutrition patients in the United States [11]. The usage of home parenteral and enteral nutrition doubled between 1989 and 1992, suggesting that the prevalence of maintenance nutritional support in the United States was 4 to 10 times higher than in other Western countries [11].

In a recent position paper, the British Association for Parenteral & Enteral Nutrition estimated that 500 persons in England were receiving home TPN at any one time [13]. However, the report noted that there were major differences in the incidence and prevalence of home TPN in different regions. This is apparent from Table 42.1, and led the authors to conclude that there is currently "inequity of access" to home parenteral nutrition in the United Kingdom.

Although registry data are no longer available, today it is estimated that more than 225,000 persons in the United States require maintenance total parenteral or enteral nutrition.

The economics of parenteral and enteral nutrition

Numerous efforts have been made to assess the aggregate, as well as the per patient expenditures, or "costs," of parenteral and enteral nutrition. In 1992, the aggregate expenditures associated with home parenteral nutrition were estimated to be $780 million, compared with $357 million for home enteral therapy [11,14].

More recently, two consultancy analyses have been published concerning the "market" for clinical nutrition products in the United States [15,16]. The market was estimated to be $10.3 billion in 2003, $12.0 billion in 2005, with revenues expected to rise to $13.6 billion by 2008. In 2003, sales of parenteral nutrition products reached $1.8 billion, with sales in 2008 projected to exceed $2.0 billion.

Published estimates of per patient per year "costs" of parenteral and enteral nutrition are highly variable. Parenteral nutrition is expensive, ranging from $75,000 to $250,000 per year [9,10]. Some estimates within the foregoing range exclude the expenses associated with home nursing support, equipment, and materials [9]. Elsewhere, it is reported that home health agencies "charge" the patient's insurance or Medicare from $3,000 to $6,000 per week for TPN (i.e., $156,000 to $312,000 per year]. [12].

There is some debate concerning the comparative cost advantages of enteral over parenteral nutritional therapy. To address this issue, Reddy and Malone derived estimates for parenteral and enteral nutrition *solutions* over the period 1991 to 1996 [17]. Based on Medicare charges, they concluded that the average (mean) annual cost per patient for parenteral *solutions* was $55,193 (±$30,596), compared with $9,605 (±$9,327) for enteral tube feedings.

However, a review of the economics of enteral nutrition and oral nutrition supplements conducted for the National Institute for Health and Clinical Excellence (NICE) in the United Kingdom concluded that although "there is some evidence to indicate economic advantages of enteral over parenteral nutrition, there is a lack of well-designed studies taking a broad view of relevant comparators, costs, and outcomes" [18].

Home parenteral nutrition on a per diem basis is somewhat less expensive than in-hospital care. For one group of patients in a Canadian study, home care costs averaged $405 (±$129) per day, compared with $660 (±$144) for inpatient care. In a second group of patients, all with underlying malignancy, the mean inpatient per diem costs were $660 (±$169), compared

with $463 (±$146) for outpatients [19]. (All cost figures are in Canadian dollars for 2002).

In a second Canadian study, based on data from 1996 to 2001, the estimated monthly savings per patient maintained on home parenteral nutrition, compared with hospital-based parental nutrition, were $4,860, thus leading the authors to conclude that home parenteral nutrition is cost-saving compared to hospital-based parenteral nutrition [20]. The cost-effectiveness of home parenteral nutrition was systematically reviewed, and a report published in 1997 by the Health Technology Assessment Programme in the United Kingdom [21]. Two, now dated, cost-utility analyses included in the review showed a favorable cost per quality-adjusted life year (QALY) for home parenteral nutrition. Moreover, the studies included in the review concluded that home parenteral nutrition was 65–80% less expensive than the alternative of hospital treatment.

The need and the demand for intestinal transplantation

It is within the preceding context that the various financial issues associated with intestinal transplantation must be considered. Both aggregate and per procedure perspectives are relevant to this analysis.

Aggregate expenditures are largely a function of the number of intestinal transplants performed per year, multiplied by per procedure costs, with donor organ availability serving as the major constraint on overall transplant activity.

Based on the indications for total parenteral, as well as enteral, nutrition, the *need* for intestinal transplantation, as suggested earlier, is considerable, although it is unlikely that all patients with intestinal failure requiring maintenance nutritional support would qualify for intestinal transplantation.

Currently in the United States, 224 patients are awaiting an intestinal transplant, up from 69 patients in 1995 [22]. Meanwhile, the number of intestinal transplants performed per year has increased from 46 in 1995, to 152 in 2004 [23].

In contrast to the *need* for intestinal transplantation, the *demand* for intestinal transplantation is functionally equivalent to the number of persons who are

Table 42.2 Summary of the average cost of the initial hospitalization for intestinal transplantation.

Type of allograft	Published cost of intestinal transplant procedures at the University of Pittsburgh, 1994–1998	Cost of intestinal transplantation at the University of Nebraska Medical Center, 2002–2003
Isolated intestine	$132,285	$135,000
Liver/small bowel	$214,716	$207,000
Multivisceral	$219,098	N/A

(Reprinted from Sudan [9] page S159, with permission from the American Gastroenterological Association.)

eventually placed on the transplant waiting list [24]. At this time, the *demand*, let alone the *need* for intestinal transplantation, cannot be met because donor organs are simply unavailable. Therefore, the aggregate health care expenditures associated with intestinal transplantation are necessarily constrained. This, in turn, is reflected by the very low per member per month costs actuaries project that health plans will experience in relation to intestinal transplantation (i.e., about 3 cents per person per month in the United States) [25].

Intestinal Transplantation Procedure Charges

Sudan has recently published the results of a cost-outcome analysis of intestinal transplantation [9]. In her report, she reviews previous attempts to estimate procedure "costs," and then presents the experience of the University of Nebraska Medical Center.

Sudan's estimates for the initial transplant hospitalization are summarized in Table 42.2 [9]. As shown, there is considerable variation by procedure type, with an isolated intestine transplant being the least expensive option.

Sudan's report underscores the myriad problems that are associated with the analysis of financial data. The same terminology is often used to describe similar concepts. In this regard, Table 42.3 summarizes the definitions of the key concepts used in accounting, actuarial, and economic analyses [26,27]. It goes without saying that accountants, actuaries, and economists of-

Table 42.3 Financial concepts in health care.

Concept	Definition
Cost	The economic value of both the labor and resource inputs required to provide a service or perform a procedure, excluding markup (i.e., production cost).
Charge	The amount a patient or third-party payer is actually billed by a health care organization or provider of health care services (i.e., list price).
Reimbursement	The amount a patient or third-party payer actually pays based on billed charges determined retrospectively or prospectively. There is often a substantial difference between what is charged and what is reimbursed.
Price	The amount a third-party payer, usually a managed care plan, has determined in advance (i.e., prospectively) that it will pay for a service or procedure individually or in the aggregate (i.e., capitation).
Margin	The difference between the amount it actually costs to provide a service or procedure and the amount ultimately reimbursed or paid. Margin is sometimes referred to as profit, or net operating income.
Discount	The difference between what is charged for a service or a procedure and what is paid, expressed as a percent.

See references [26] and [27].

ten use similar financial data in very different ways, frequently arriving at inconsistent conclusions.

As Sudan notes, further problems are encountered when attempting to estimate all relevant charges for purposes of cost estimation [9]. Costs associated with hospital readmissions, maintenance immunosuppressive drugs, and other drugs required for the management of co-morbid conditions may be excluded from the analyses.

There are ways to overcome many of the foregoing problems through the application of what is commonly referred to as resource use modeling [28,29].

Table 42.4 Estimates of the charges associated with those services that may comprise a negotiated case rate for various types of intestinal transplantation.

| Transplant procedure | Services that may comprise a negotiated case rate | | | |
	Organ procurement ($)	Hospital ($)	Physician ($)	Total ($)
Intestine only	74,600	549,400	70,700	694,700
Liver-intestine	132,000	492,000	70,700	694,700
Liver-pancreas-intestine	199,200	476,000	70,700	745,900
Pancreas-intestine	141,800	490,600	70,700	703,100

See reference [25], page 5.

Unfortunately, although resource use modeling can be considered the "gold standard" for cost analyses, it is infrequently used in the United States. Instead, charge data are accumulated for the most relevant items and services, with relatively crude cost-to-charge ratios used to estimate accounting costs (as defined in Table 42.3) [30,31].

Since 1993, the actuarial firm Milliman (formerly Milliman & Robertson) has published numerous reports on what it refers to as "cost estimates" for organ and tissue transplantation. In their most recent report, they have included intestinal transplantation [25].

Actuaries are persons who assess risks and then establish rates and premiums for insurance companies and managed care organizations. Like most analysts, actuaries primarily rely on billed charge data. Not surprisingly, all of the Milliman reports are based on billed charges derived from administrative, or claims, databases. Most of their data are considered proprietary, or are licensed through various vendors.

Today, most transplant centers are contracted to provide transplant services based on "case rates" through what are often referred to as "centers of excellence" networks [25–27]. Although intriguing, this terminology is largely a misnomer, because there is persuasive evidence that many networks are willing to sacrifice some level of quality for a more favorable price. This has prompted some critics to refer to centers of excellence networks as "discount centers."

The sheer prevalence of contracting based on case rates has prompted Milliman to revise the format of the estimates included in its most recent report [25]. First, Milliman estimates average first-year billed charges per transplant based on a case rate—a rate that is ultimately much less than billed charges. A second estimate is provided for services not usually part of a negotiated case rate.

Milliman defines their "charge estimates" as follows: [25].
• Typical (Negotiated) Case Rate Services: Hospitals typically charge one negotiated case rate that combines hospital and physician charges. Although organ procurement charges may be included in the negotiated case rate, they typically reflect slight, if any, discounts from billed levels.
• Services Not Usually Part of a (Negotiated) Case Rate: Rarely do case rates cover transplant evaluation, follow-up, or maintenance outpatient immunosuppression. A majority of follow-up charges occur within the first 90 days post-hospital discharge. Outpatient immunosuppression is a lifelong proposition. A transplant recipient may continue to receive care at their transplant center, or they may go to other local providers. Table 42.4 summarizes the charges subject to case rate negotiation for four types of intestinal transplantation—intestine only, liver-intestine, liver-pancreas-intestine, and pancreas-intestine [25].

As shown, there is wide variation in organ procurement, as well as hospital charges. Physician fees are assumed to be constant.

The total billed charges for the initial intestinal transplant hospital stay range from $694,700 to $745,900. These billed charges are then negotiated with the payor. One major center of excellence network claims that its negotiated case rates are 40–45 percent below billed "industry standard" charges (the foregoing range once discounted at 40% would then be $416,820 to $447,540) [32].

Table 42.5 Estimates of the charges not usually part of a negotiated case rate for various types of intestinal transplantation.

| Transplant procedure | Services not usually part of a negotiated case rate | | | |
	Evaluation ($)	Follow-up ($)	Maintenance therapy: outpatient immunosuppressive drugs ($)	Total ($)
Intestine only	34,300	64,600	20,000	118,900
Liver-intestine	34,300	74,800	26,400	135,500
Liver-pancreas-intestine	34,300	74,800	30,600	139,700
Pancreas-intestine	34,300	64,600	30,100	129,000

See reference [25], page 5.

Table 42.5 provides a second set of estimates for first-year services not usually included in the case rate [25]. The three major components are: transplant evaluation, follow-up care post-transplant hospital discharge, and maintenance immunosuppression. As shown, with a range between $118,900 and $139,700, there is little variability.

An estimate of the total first-year charges associated with intestinal transplantation can be derived by adding the figures included in Tables 42.4 and 42.5. The final figures, or grand totals, are as follows: intestine only transplantation, $813,600; liver-intestine transplantation, $830,200; liver-pancreas-intestine transplantation, $885,600; and pancreas-intestine transplantation, $832,100.

It is noteworthy that the foregoing figures exclude estimated charges for what is commonly referred to as the transplant "candidacy period" [26,27,33]. Few patients are immediately transplanted once they are placed on the waiting list. Instead, while they await donor organs, they are cared for medically and surgically using conventional means. For an intestinal transplant candidate, this would include nutritional support, the charges for which are excluded from all of the Milliman estimates.

The cost of living...and dying

Organ transplantation is often justified on the basis that it "...costs more to die than to perform a transplant."

This observation is unequivocally false [26,27,33]. It would be true only if an organ transplant assured immortality. Unfortunately, all transplant recipients will eventually die and, given inflation and technology, it is often less expensive to die today than tomorrow.

However, when it comes to dying, there are some nuances associated with organ transplantation which deserve special consideration [33]. For a heart, liver, or a lung transplant candidate, there is no highly efficacious long-term treatment option. In contrast, kidney dialysis is an acceptable treatment modality for patients with end-stage renal disease. Likewise, it can be argued that nutritional support is a worthy option for patients in need of an intestinal transplant.

Because there are multiple treatment options for intestinal failure, cost-effectiveness analyses have merit, and can eventually be performed as relevant data are accumulated. Unfortunately, at this time, sufficient data do not exist and, therefore, simple cost-outcome analyses are an instructive, although an inferior alternative [8,9]. In such studies, treatment "costs" are reported alongside patient survival and quality of life data, often with the implication that intestinal transplantation is "cost-effective."

As described here, maintenance nutritional support therapy is an expensive treatment option, with serious complications. This means that, eventually, intestinal transplantation will need to be examined from the perspective of the expected "payback period." The underlying issue can be posed as a question: given the long-term expenses associated with nutritional support therapy, and the relatively high expenditures that accompany intestinal transplantation, how long does a patient need to survive to "payback" the costs of an intestinal transplant?

It is noteworthy that the payback period for kidney transplantation has been favorably analyzed relative to maintenance kidney dialysis. Eggers initially reported the payback period to be 3.9 years for living donor, and 4.9 years for deceased donor kidney transplantation [34].

The perverse implications of coverage and reimbursement policy

Third party payors distinguish between the concepts of *coverage* and *reimbursement* [35,36]. Coverage refers to what an insurer is contractually obligated to pay for under an insurance policy. Reimbursement is the amount an insurer pays for a covered procedure, service, or item, often reflecting a discount on billed charges.

When it comes to transplantation, there are many anomalies associated with coverage and reimbursement policy. For example, it is not unusual for insurers to cover a procedure, but establish a reimbursement rate that is so abysmal no hospital can afford to offer the procedure without incurring a substantial loss. In this regard, public payers, namely, Medicare and Medicaid, are amongst the worst offenders.

Medicare coverage for intestinal transplantation is an excellent example of the perversity that often surrounds coverage and reimbursement policy.

On April 1, 2001, the Health Care Financing Administration (now the Centers for Medicare and Medicaid Services) announced that Medicare was going to cover intestinal transplants "...for beneficiaries with irreversible intestinal failure" at three Medicare-approved centers [7]. In announcing the decision, Department of Health and Human Services Secretary Tommy G. Thompson said, "Although only a few people may benefit from this coverage, it reflects our commitment to providing all of the nearly 40 million Medicare beneficiaries with access to proven new treatments and technologies." In his press release, Thompson pointed out that fewer than 1,000 intestinal transplants had been performed in the United States, with approximately two-thirds of the patients being children [7].

Table 42.6 Medicare payment policy for intestinal and multivisceral transplantation inpatient services: a summary.

- If an intestinal transplantation alone is performed on a patient with an intestinal principal diagnosis, the case would be assigned to either DRG 148 (Major Small & Large Bowel Procedures With Complications or Comorbidities) or DRG 149 (Major Small & Large Bowel Procedures Without Complications or Comorbidities).
- If intestinal transplantation and liver transplantation are performed simultaneously, or if a multivisceral transplantation includes a liver, the case would be assigned to DRG 480 (Liver Transplant). If a multivisceral transplantation that does not include a liver is performed, the case would be assigned to either DRG 148 or DRG 149.
- Presently, the Medicare regulations do not authorize payment of organ acquisition costs on a reasonable cost basis for organs other than heart, liver, lung, kidney, or pancreas. Hospitals should report any acquisition charges they incur for intestine, stomach, or colon on the bill for the transplant procedure. However, no interim pass-through acquisition payment will be made for these costs, and hospitals should not include the costs in the preparation of the Schedule D-6 of their cost report. Acquisition costs for liver and pancreas may be paid on a reasonable cost basis and reported on the cost report.

See reference [38], page 4.

This situation gives rise to the first anomaly: very few children qualify for Medicare and, when they do, it is usually because their parents are Medicare beneficiaries. Moreover, parents with young children who qualify for Medicare are usually disabled (they are not elderly). Thus, as Secretary Thompson noted, Medicare can be expected to pay for very few intestinal transplants.

A second anomaly associated with Medicare coverage concerns the broader intent of a favorable coverage determination. Typically, private insurers modify their coverage policies to reflect those of Medicare. Thus, Secretary Thompson had an unstated objective in mind—to positively influence private health insurer policies with respect to coverage of intestinal transplantation. This is precisely what happened on February 9, 1984, when Medicare coverage was extended to children with biliary atresia who required a liver transplant [37].

The last anomaly underscores the financial perversity often associated with Medicare coverage and

Table 42.7 Intestinal transplant centers in the United States, 2006.

Transplant center/hospital/medical center	Number of intestine transplants performed in 2004	Medicare approval date
University of Pittsburgh Medical Center—Presbyterian	33	04/01/01
University of Miami—Jackson Memorial Hospital	16	04/01/01
Mount Sinai Medical Center, New York	8	04/01/01
Nebraska Health System	21	05/01/01
UCLA Medical Center	8	05/23/03
Georgetown University Hospital	11	06/24/04
Clarian Health Methodist—Indiana University—Riley	4	06/07/05
Northwestern Memorial Hospital	0	01/05/06
Children's Hospital of Pittsburgh	20	01/05/06
Children's Hospital of Los Angeles	1	Not Approved
Stanford University Medical Center	11	Not Approved
Children's Memorial Hospital, Chicago	2	Not Approved
University of Illinois Medical Center, Chicago	5	Not Approved
Children's Hospital, Boston	1	Not Approved
New York Presbyterian Hospital/Weill Cornell Medical Center	1	Not Approved
Children's Hospital Medical Center, Cincinnati	4	Not Approved
University of Wisconsin	5	Not Approved
University of Minnesota Medical Center	0	Not Approved
Medical University of South Carolina	0	Not Approved
Baylor University Medical Center, Dallas, TX	0	Not Approved

reimbursement policy. Unlike kidney, heart, liver, pancreas, and lung transplantation, the Centers for Medicare and Medicaid Services (CMS) has never established a separate diagnosis-related group (DRG) for intestinal transplantation. In the United States, hospitals are reimbursed for Medicare inpatient services (often referred to as Part A) based on a DRG.

CMS decided to use existing DRGs for reimbursement purposes. In a reissued and revised Program Memorandum dated March 27, 2002, CMS outlined its policy, which is summarized in Table 42.6 [38]. To state what will soon become obvious, there are some profound issues associated with Medicare's reimbursement policy for intestinal transplantation.

Medicare reimbursement for intestinal transplantation

Unfortunately, many transplant centers in the United States experience significant losses in relation to the provision of transplant services. The problem is often acute for both small and large centers, with an adverse patient case-mix and an unfavorable payer-mix both factoring into the losses.

Based on Medicare reimbursement policies for intestinal transplantation, the losses could be staggering for any center that performs an intestinal transplant on a Medicare beneficiary or one's dependent. Moreover, to the extent that other public and private payors attempt to mimic Medicare policies, the losses hospitals experience could be substantial for patients in all payor categories.

Nine centers/hospitals now qualify as Medicare-approved intestinal transplant centers (as of June 30, 2006) [39]. However, in 2004, 16 transplant centers in the United States performed one or more intestinal transplants [40]. The centers are listed in Table 42.7. For purposes of this analysis, it is instructive to examine each hospital's Medicare experience with respect to DRGs 148, 149, and 480, using two data resources maintained by CMS. They are: the 2004 Medicare

Table 42.8 Financials for DRG 148—major small and large bowel procedures with complications or co-morbidities.

Transplant center/ hospital/medical center	Number of medicare inpatients	Average length of stay (days)	Average charges ($)	Average reimbursed ($)	Average cost ($)	Net operating income or loss per case ($)
1	211	12.06	131,110	24,141	22,640	1,501
2	50	16.46	99,549	34,468	36,216	(1,748)
3	231	18.60	71,122	30,636	32,209	(1,573)
4	113	13.54	70,387	22,101	25,243	(3,142)
5	79	13.51	90,876	30,394	30,216	178
6	57	20.67	130,236	38,073	46,563	(8,490)
7	192	15.47	59,190	26,261	29,645	(3,384)
8	121	10.93	57,817	23,182	24,532	(1,350)
11	91	12.75	122,345	32,909	35,438	(2,529)
13	40	13.43	76,872	34,534	36,645	(2,111)
15	278	12.65	70,308	31,390	29,625	1,765
17	79	12.34	46,158	21,821	24,748	(2,927)
Averages	129	14.37	85,498	29,159	31,143	(1,984)

Note: This table excludes any hospitals that had ten or fewer Medicare inpatient admissions for DRG 148 in 2004. Numbers in parentheses indicate a loss.

Provider Review and Analysis (MEDPAR) database, and the Healthcare Cost Reporting Information System (HCRIS) [41,42]. The relevant financials are summarized in Tables 42.8, 42.9, and 42.10. If a hospital had ten or fewer Medicare admissions for a DRG, it is omitted from the table. For example, five hospitals had ten or fewer Medicare patient admissions for DRG 148 (i.e., hospitals 9,10,12,14, and 16).

As shown in Table 42.8, for the 12 hospitals with more than ten Medicare admissions for DRG 148— major small and large bowel procedures with complications or co-morbidities—the range for patient

Table 42.9 Financials for DRG 149—major small and large bowel procedures without complications or co-morbidities.

Transplant center/ hospital/medical center	Number of medicare inpatients	Average length of stay (days)	Average charges ($)	Average reimbursed ($)	Average cost ($)	Net operating income or loss per case ($)
1	18	4.83	57,308	7,158	8,517	(1,359)
3	42	6.14	29,481	12,897	13,689	(792)
4	19	6.37	30,976	7,658	10,982	(3,324)
5	12	4.58	27,165	8,952	9,353	(401)
7	20	6.00	22,943	8,611	11,339	(2,728)
8	32	5.56	27,381	8,846	13,509	(4,663)
11	11	6.27	52,187	10,774	14,447	(3,673)
13	20	6.10	27,998	13,160	14,165	(1,005)
15	62	5.16	28,771	12,576	11,026	1,550
17	18	6.22	19,728	9,145	10,628	(1,483)
Averages	25	5.72	32,394	9,978	11,766	(1,788)

Note: This table excludes any hospitals that had ten or fewer Medicare inpatient admissions for DRG 149 in 2004. Numbers in parentheses indicate a loss.

Table 42.10 Financials for DRG 480—liver transplant.

Transplant center/ hospital/medical center	Number of medicare inpatients	Average length of stay (days)	Average charges ($)	Average reimbursed ($)	Average cost ($)	Net operating income or loss per case ($)
1	40	15.72	385,589	62,492	102,740	(40,248)
3	12	13.83	154,974	80,669	102,565	(21,896)
4	14	11.86	164,298	64,540	84,501	(19,961)
7	30	18.23	185,837	79,177	114,619	(35,442)
8	21	13.43	260,829	73,075	143,313	(70,238)
17	23	29.87	239,208	75,035	145,591	(70,556)
Averages	23	17.16	231,789	72,498	115,555	(43,057)

Note: This table excludes any hospitals that had ten or fewer Medicare inpatient admissions for DRG 480 in 2004. Numbers in parentheses indicate a loss.

admissions was 40 to 278. The average length of hospital stay was 10.93 to 20.67 days. The ranges for the four financial indicators are as follows: average billed charges, $46,158 to $131,110; average reimbursement, $21,821 to $38,073; average cost, $22,640 to $46,563; net operating income or loss per case, −$8,490 to +$1,765.

Table 42.9 summarizes the same data for DRG 149—major small and large bowel procedures without complications or co-morbidities—for the ten hospitals with

more than ten Medicare patient admissions in 2004. The relevant ranges are as follows: admissions, 11 to 62; length of hospital stay, 4.58 to 6.37 days; charges, $19,728 to $57,308; reimbursement, $7,158 to $13,160; cost, $8,517 to $14,447; net operating income or loss per case, −$4,663 to +$1,550.

Only five hospitals included in this analysis performed more than ten liver transplants (DRG 480) on Medicare beneficiaries in 2004. The data are summarized in Table 42.10. The pertinent ranges are as

Table 42.11 Intestinal transplant center financials—cost and markup.

Transplant center/ hospital/medical center	Cost (as a percentage of charges)			Mark-up (charges as a percentage over cost)		
	DRG 148	DRG 149	DRG 480	DRG 148	DRG 149	DRG 480
1	17.3%	14.9%	26.6%	579.1%	672.9%	375.3%
2	36.4%			274.9%		
3	45.3%	46.4%	66.2%	220.8%	215.4%	151.1%
4	35.9%	35.5%	51.4%	278.8%	282.1%	194.4%
5	33.2%	34.4%		300.8%	290.4%	
6	35.8%			279.7%		
7	50.1%	49.4%	61.7%	199.7%	202.3%	162.1%
8	42.4%	49.3%	54.9%	235.7%	202.7%	182.0%
11	29.0%	27.7%		345.2%	361.2%	
13	47.7%	50.6%		209.8%	197.7%	
15	42.1%	38.3%		237.3%	260.9%	
17	53.6%	53.9%	60.9%	186.5%	185.6%	164.3%
Averages	39.1%	40.0%	53.6%	279.0%	287.1%	204.9%

Note: This table excludes any hospitals that had ten or fewer Medicare inpatient admissions for DRGs 148, 149, and 480 in 2004. Also, if no value is shown, it indicates that the hospital had ten or fewer Medicare admissions for the DRGs included in the table.

Table 42.12 Intestinal transplant center financials—reimbursement and margin.

Transplant center/ hospital/medical center	Reimbursement (percentage of charges paid)			Margin (reimbursement over cost)		
	DRG 148	DRG 149	DRG 480	DRG 148	DRG 149	DRG 480
1	18.4%	12.5%	16.2%	1.1%	−2.4%	−10.4%
2	34.6%			−1.8%		
3	43.1%	43.7%	52.1%	−2.2%	−2.7%	−14.1%
4	31.4%	24.7%	39.3%	−4.5%	−10.7%	−12.1%
5	33.4%	33.0%		0.2%	−1.5%	
6	29.2%			−6.5%		
7	44.4%	37.5%	42.6%	−5.7%	−11.9%	−19.1%
8	40.1%	32.3%	28.0%	−2.3%	−17.0%	−26.9%
11	26.9%	20.6%		−2.1%	−7.0%	
13	44.9%	47.0%		−2.7%	−3.6%	
15	44.6%	43.7%		2.5%	5.4%	
17	47.3%	46.4%	31.4%	−6.3%	−7.5%	−29.5%
Averages	36.5%	34.1%	34.9%	−2.5%	−5.9%	−18.7%

Note: This table excludes any hospitals that had ten or fewer Medicare inpatient admissions for DRGs 148, 149, and 480 in 2004. Also, if no value is shown, it indicates that the hospital had ten or fewer Medicare admissions for the DRGs included in the table.

follows: admissions, 12 to 40; length of hospital stay; 11.86 to 29.87 days; charges, $154,974 to $385,589; reimbursement, $62,492 to $80,669; cost, $84,501 to $145,591; net operating income or loss per case, −$19,961 to −$70,556. Clearly, based on the foregoing data, Medicare reimbursement for intestinal transplantation is an issue—an issue that can be further underscored based on hospital resource utilization, of which hospital length of stay is one indicator. The mean hospital length of stay for intestinal transplantation is as follows: isolated intestine, 60 days; intestinal and liver transplant, 77 days; and multivisceral, 80 days [43]. The average hospital lengths of stay for DRGs 148, 149, and 480 are as follows: 14, 6, and 17 days, respectively. Obviously, there is a problem in including intestinal transplantation within the three existing DRGs.

Hospital pricing strategies and related financials

Hospitals use a variety of strategies to price their services. For example, some hospitals have much higher mark-ups than others [26,27]. This allows for substantial discounting, which has become a managed care

expectation. Other hospitals are more traditional in their approach—offering modest discounts relative to low markups.

Consistent with the data presented earlier in this chapter, Tables 42.11 and 42.12 put hospital costs, markups, reimbursement, and margin into a simplified context for DRGs 148, 149, and 480. Hospitals with ten or fewer Medicare admissions for all three DRGs are omitted from the tables. For the remaining hospitals, the absence of a value indicates that there were ten or fewer Medicare admissions for a particular DRG.

As shown in Table 42.11, the relationship between costs and charges is highly variable, although the averages for DRG 148 and 149 are similar.

Markups—charges as a percentage over cost—are even more variable. Compared with Center 17, Center 1 has a remarkably high markup for all three DRGs. Meanwhile, the range for DRG 148 is from 186.5 to 579.1 percent.

The reimbursement experience is noteworthy. Hospitals with higher billed charges often collect a smaller percentage of their charges. For example, Center 1 consistently collects a lower percentage of its charges. The opposite is true for Center 17, a center with lower markups.

Table 42.13 Estimated hospital charges, cost, reimbursement, and loss per case for intestinal transplantation: initial transplant procedure stay only.

Transplant center/ hospital/medical center	Estimates ($)		Estimated reimbursement per case ($)		Estimated loss per case ($)	
	Charges	Cost	Low	High	Low	High
1	502,000	133,758	7,158	62,492	(71,266)	(126,600)
3	201,761	133,530	12,897	80,669	(52,861)	(120,633)
4	213,900	110,012	7,658	64,540	(45,472)	(102,354)
7	241,942	149,223	8,611	79,177	(70,046)	(140,612)
8	339,574	186,580	8,846	73,075	(113,505)	(177,734)
17	311,426	189,546	9,145	75,035	(114,511)	(180,401)
Averages	301,767	150,441	9,053	72,498	(77,943)	(141,389)

Note: This table excludes any hospitals that had ten or fewer Medicare inpatient admissions for DRG 480 in 2004. Numbers in parentheses indicate a loss.

The margins shown in Table 42.12 poignantly emphasize what is well recognized—many hospitals, medical centers, and transplant centers consistently lose money on Medicare patients. For liver transplantation, the losses can be substantial, from 10.4 to 29.5 percent per case, with an average loss of 18.7 percent per case.

Can U.S. hospitals afford to offer intestinal transplantation?

The data presented here collectively underscore one of the most critical points of this analysis. If Medicare reimbursement for intestinal transplantation is based on DRGs 148, 149, and 480, hospitals and transplant centers in the United States will experience unsustainable losses.

The reimbursement figures for DRGs 148, 149, and 480 must be compared and contrasted with the Milliman actuarial estimates presented in Table 42.4 [25]. According to Milliman, undiscounted average billed hospital charges for an intestinal transplant range between $476,000 and $549,400 (see Table 42.4). Meanwhile, for the hospitals included in this analysis, the average Medicare reimbursement amounts for DRGs 148, 149, and 480 are as follows: $29,159, $9,978, and $72,498, respectively (see Tables 42.8, 42.9, and 42.10).

It also can be assumed that only a portion of the organ procurement charges associated with intestinal

transplantation will be subject to the Medicare pass-through and, therefore, reimbursed on a reasonable cost basis (see Table 42.6). This means hospitals are subject to even greater losses during the patient's initial transplant hospitalization.

It is impossible to definitively state the size of any losses hospitals might experience relative to Medicare reimbursement. However, assuming the average billed charge for an intestinal transplant is $502,000 at Center 1, it is possible to derive estimated financials for all intestinal transplant centers that performed liver transplants on more than ten Medicare beneficiaries in 2004. The relevant data are presented in Table 42.13.

As shown in Table 42.13, the expected losses are considerable for all centers, with Centers 8 and 17 having the worst financial forecasts. Center 4 has the most favorable outlook, with estimated losses for the initial hospital stay between $45,472 and $102,354 per case. On average, hospitals can expect to lose between $77,943 and $141,389 per intestinal transplant.

Conclusions

Intestinal transplantation is an important, but expensive clinical innovation. It is clearly a decisive alternative to total parenteral nutrition for the treatment of intestinal failure, yet its true cost-effectiveness remains to be established. The results of simple cost-outcome analyses have been persuasive to the extent they have served as the basis for favorable coverage determinations on behalf of third-party payers.

Because of the donor organ shortage, aggregate expenditures for intestinal transplantation are unlikely to be an issue, although procedure-specific costs will be a concern for patients, insurers, providers, and health care policy makers. In an era of consumer-directed health care, with ever-increasing patient out-of-pocket costs, patients and their families are certain to face wrenching decisions about the value of life [44,45]. Some may choose to forego treatment because the expense is simply beyond their financial means. In an effort to contain their costs, insurers will adhere to relatively rigid coverage criteria. Their goal will be to limit their risk exposure, while maximizing patient outcomes, and minimizing costs. In other words, payors will do everything they can to positively influence the overall cost-effectiveness of intestinal transplantation. In part, this will be accomplished through conservative patient selection and the designation of transplant centers which meet criteria that are philosophically aligned with payor objectives. Transplant hospitals are by no means passive participants in this process. They face at least one serious dilemma that could limit their interest. In many cases, the level of reimbursement available for intestinal transplantation is insufficient to cover their accounting costs. Thus, with each transplant the hospital performs, a substantial loss accrues to the bottom line. Today, hospitals are in a vulnerable position whenever financially nonviable clinical programs are promoted as misleading marketing misadventures. Intestinal transplantation could fall into this category, as clinical enthusiasm turns to administrative disgust.

The future of expensive clinical innovation has never been in more doubt than it is today. Academic health centers are finding it difficult, if not impossible, to generate the level of net operating income (profit) necessary to subsidize cutting-edge clinical programs, particularly those programs with long-term potential, yet excessively high short-term costs. For many hospitals, an intestinal transplantation program could fall into the category of "nice, but more than we can afford," an important realization for those academic health centers which have come to appreciate the fact that they can no longer be everything to everyone [46]. In a perverse way, this may actually facilitate progress in the field, as greater experience is concentrated in fewer centers.

References

1 Sudan D, DiBaise J, Torres C, et al. A multidisciplinary approach to the treatment of intestinal failure. *J Gastrointest Surg* 2005;9:165–176.

2 Sudan DL, Kaufmann SS, Shaw BW, Jr., et al. Isoloated intestinal transplantation for intestinal failure. *Am J Gastroenterol* 2000;95:1506–1515.

3 Fryer JP. Intestinal transplantation: an update. *Curr Opin Gastroenterol* 2005;21:162–168.

4 Fishbein TM, Matsumoto CS. Intestinal replacement therapy: timing and indications for referral of patients to an intestinal rehabilitation and transplant program. *Gastroenterology* 2006;130:S147–S151.

5 Reyes J, Mazariegos GV, Bond GM, et al. Pediatric intestinal transplantation: historical notes, principles and controversies. *Pediatr Transplant* 2002;6:193–207.

6 Abu-Elmagd K, Reyes J, Fung JJ. Clinical intestinal transplantation: recent advances and future considerations. In: Norman DJ, Turka LA, eds. *Primer on Transplantation*. 2nd Edition. Mt. Laurel, NY: American Society of Transplantation, 2001:610–625.

7 Medicare begins coverage of intestinal transplants. Accessed May 30, 2006. Available at: http://www.cms.hhs.gov/apps/media/press/release.asp?Counter=280.

8 Abu-Elmagd KM, Reyes J, Fung JJ, et al. Evolution of clinical intestinal transplantation: improved outcome and cost-effectiveness. *Transplant Proc* 1999;31:582–584.

9 Sudan D. Cost and quality of life after intestinal transplantation. *Gastroenterology* 2006;130:S158–S162.

10 Puntis JW. The economics of home parenteral nutrition. *Nutrition* 1998;14:809–812.

11 Howard L, Ament M, Fleming CR, et al. Current use and clinical outcome of home parenteral and enteral nutrition therapies in the United States. *Gastroenterology* 1995;109:355–365.

12 Lovvorn D. Total parenteral nutrition. Accessed June 2, 2006. Available at: http://www.scleroderma.org/medical/gastro_articles/lovvorn_1998summer.htm.

13 British Association for Parenteral & Enteral Nutrition. Home Parenteral Nutrition in the United Kingdom: A Position Paper. Accessed May 31, 2006. Available at: http://www.bapen.org.uk/documents/home-parenteral-nutrition.doc.

14 Oley publishes research on the cost-benefit of HPEN therapy. Accessed May 31, 2006. Available at: http://www.oley.org/lifeline/95–038.htm.

15 Crandall MA. GA-112R The U.S. Market for Ethical Nutrition in Health Care. Accessed May 30, 2006. Available at: http://www.bccresearch.com/food/GA112R.html.

16 Ingredients Used in the Clinical & Medical Nutrition Market, 2006. Accessed May 30, 2006. Available at: http://www.ubic-consulting.com/brochures/Clinical%20nutrition.pdf.

17 Reddy P, Malone M. Cost and outcome analysis of home parenteral and enteral nutrition. *JPEN J Parenter Enteral Nutr* 1998;22:302–310.

18 Pritchard C, Duffy S, Edington J, Pang F. Enteral nutrition and oral nutrition supplements: a review of the economics literature. *JPEN J Parenter Enteral Nutr* 2006;30:52–59.

19 Marshall JK, Gadowsky SL, Childs A, Armstrong D. Economic analysis of home vs. hospital-based parenteral nutrition in Ontario, Canada. *JPEN J Parenter Enteral Nutr* 2005;29:266–269.

20 Gadowsky S, Armstrong D, Childs A, Marshall JK. Home parenteral nutrition is cost-saving regardless of age or malignancy. Accessed May 30, 2006. Available at: http://www.cag-acg.org/cddw/cddw2003/ abs/abs082.htm.

21 Richards DM, Deeks JJ, Sheldon TA, Shaffer JL. Home Parenteral Nutrition: A Systematic Review. Health Technol Assess 1997;1(1).:i–iii, 1–59. Accessed May 30, 2006. Available at: http://www.ncchta.org.

22 Intestinal transplant waiting list, the United Network for Organ Sharing, Richmond, VA. Accessed June 7, 2006. Available at: http://www.optn.org/data/default.asp?displayType=usData.

23 Shiffman ML, Saab S, Feng S, et al. Liver and intestine transplantation in the United States, 1995–2004. *Am J Transplant* 2006;6:1170–1187.

24 Evans RW. Coming to terms with reality: why xenotransplantation is a necessity. In: Platt JL, ed. *Xenotransplantation*. Washington, D.C.: ASM Press, Inc., 2001:29–51.

25 Ortner NJ. 2005 US Organ and Tissue Transplant Cost Estimates and Discussion. Brookfield, WI: Milliman, 2005. Accessed May 30, 2000. Available at: http://www.milliman.com/pubs/Healthcare/content/research_reports/US-Organ-Tissue-Transplant-2005-RR.pdf.

26 Evans RW, Kitzmann DJ. Contracting for services: liver transplantation in the era of mismanaged care. *Clin Liver Dis* 1997;1:287–303.

27 Evans RW. Economic, actuarial, and contracting perspectives on liver transplantation. In: Maddrey WC, Schiff ER, Sorrell MF, eds. *Transplantation of the Liver*. Philadelphia, PA: Lippincott Williams & Wilkins, 2000:479–489.

28 Drummond MF, McGuire A, eds. *Economic Evaluation in Health Care: Merging Theory with Practice*. New York: Oxford University Press, 2001.

29 Gold MR, Siegel JE, Russell LB, Weinstein MC. *Cost-Effectiveness in Health and Medicine*. New York: Oxford University Press, 1996.

30 Finkler SA, ed. *Issues in Cost Accounting for Health Care Organizations*. Gaithersburg, MD: Aspen Publishers, Inc., 1994.

31 Finkler SA. *Essentials of Cost Accounting for Health Care Organizations*. Gaithersburg, MD: Aspen Publishers, Inc., 1994.

32 Centers of Excellence Networks, United Resource Networks. Accessed June 7, 2006. Available at: http://www.urnweb.com/gateway/public/employers/centersOfExcellenceNetworks.jsp.

33 Evans RW. Cost-effectiveness analysis of transplantation. *Surg Clin North Am* 1986;66:603–616.

34 Eggers PW. Comparison of treatment costs between dialysis and transplantation. *Semin Nephrol* 1992;12:284–289.

35 Towery OB, Perry S. The scientific basis for coverage decisions by third party payers. *JAMA* 1981;245:59–61.

36 Tunis SR. Why Medicare has not established criteria for coverage decisions. *N Engl J Med* 2004;350:2196–2198.

37 Medicare Coverage Issues Manual, Transmittal 142, July 17, 2001. Accessed June 7, 2006. Available at: http://www.cms.hhs.gov/transmittals/downloads/R142CIM.pdf.

38 Program Memorandum Intermediaries/Carriers. Transmittal AB-02-040, Intestinal and Multi-Visceral Transplantation. Baltimore, MD: Centers for Medicare and Medicaid Services, March 27, 2002. Accessed May 30, 2006. Available at: http://www.cms.hhs.gov/Transmittals/Downloads/AB02040.pdf.

39 Medicare Approved Intestinal Transplant Centers. Accessed June 7, 2006. Available at: http://www.cms.hhs.gov/ApprovedTransplantCenters/downloads/intestinal_list.pdf.

40 Intestinal transplants by transplant center. Accessed June 7, 2006. Available at: http://www. optn.org/AR2005/1015_IN.htm.

41 Medicare Provider Analysis and Review (MEDPAR) File. Accessed June 7, 2006. Available at: http://www.cms.hhs.gov/IdentifiableDataFiles/05_MedicareProviderAnalysisandReviewFile.asp.

42 Healthcare Provider Cost Reporting Information System (HCRIS). Accessed June 7, 2006. Available at: http://

www.cms.hhs.gov/CostReports/Downloads/CRGeneral
Info.pdf.

43 International Intestinal Transplant Registry. Intestinal
transplant registry report. Updated 2003 December. Accessed June 4, 2006. Available at: http://www.
intestinaltransplant.org/ITR_Reports/Report_2003/ITR%
202003%20FINAL%20Summary%20slides.htm.

44 Robinson JC. Managed consumerism in health care.
Health Affairs 2005;24:1478–1489.

45 Wilensky GR. Consumer-driven health plans: early evidence and potential impact on hospitals. *Health Affairs*
2006;25:174–185.

46 Envisioning the Future of Academic Health Centers:
Final Report of the Commonwealth Fund Task Force
on Academic Health Centers. New York: The Commonwealth Fund, 2003. Accessed June 7, 2006. Available at:
http://www.cmwf.org/usr_doc/ahc_envisioningfuture_
600.pdf.

Index

Entries followed by *f* refer to material found in figures; entries followed by *t* refer to material found in tables.

Index

Index

GI Epidemiology

Edited by

Nicholas J Talley, MD MMedSc (ClinEpid) PhD, *Chair, Department of Internal Medicine, Mayo Clinic College of Medicine, Jacksonville, Florida, USA*

G Richard Locke III, MD, *Division of Gastroenterology and Hepatology, Mayo Clinic College of Medicine, Rochester, Minnesota, USA*

Yuri A Saito, MD MPH, *Division of Gastroenterology and Hepatology, Mayo Clinic College of Medicine, Rochester, Minnesota, USA*

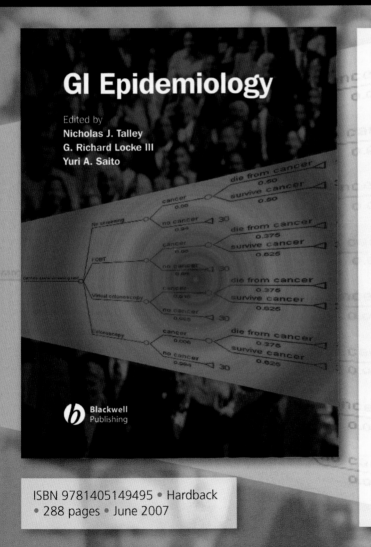

GI Epidemiology

Edited by
Nicholas J. Talley
G. Richard Locke III
Yuri A. Saito

Blackwell Publishing

ISBN 9781405149495 • Hardback
• 288 pages • June 2007

Provides an authoritative evidence-based text on epidemiology of gastrointestinal diseases inspired by the course run by the Mayo Clinic

- Focuses on population-based information and studies looking at principles and approaches to diagnosis and treatment of diseases

- Serves as both a useful refresher and a reliable reference on the methods and techniques used in epidemiological studies for consultants and researchers in gastroenterology

- Appeals to fellows/trainees in gastroenterology and candidates for recertification in the combined disciplines of gastroenterology, pediatric gastroenterology and colorectal surgery

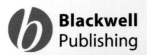

Blackwell Publishing

To order or view a sample chapter visit
www.BlackwellGastroenterology.com

TEXTBOOK OF
HEPATOLOGY

From Basic Science to Clinical Practice

THIRD EDITION

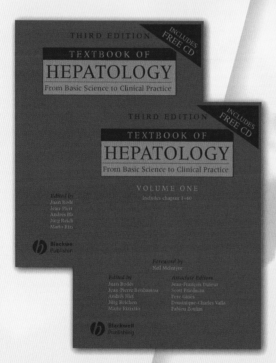

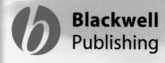